Chemotherapy of Parasitic Diseases

Chemotherapy of Parasitic Diseases

Edited by
WILLIAM C. CAMPBELL
Merck Institute for Therapeutic Research
Rahway, New Jersey
and
ROBERT S. REW
Merck Sharp & Dohme Research Laboratories
Rahway, New Jersey

PLENUM PRESS • NEW YORK AND LONDON

Library of Congress Cataloging in Publication Data

Main entry under title:

Chemotherapy of parasitic diseases.

Includes bibliographies and index.
1. Parasitic diseases—Chemotherapy. 2. Anthelmintics. I. Campbell, William C.
(William Cecil), 1930–   . II. Rew, Robert S. [DNLM: 1. Anthelmintics. 2. Anti-
protozoal Agents. 3. Insecticides. 4. Parasitic Diseases—drug therapy. WC 695
C5175]
RC119.C393   1985   616.9′6061   85-19377
ISBN-13:978-1-4684-1235-2   e-ISBN-13:978-1-4684-1233-8
DOI: 10.1007/978-1-4684-1233-8

© 1986 Plenum Press, New York
Softcover reprint of the hardcover 1st edition 1986

A Division of Plenum Publishing Corporation
233 Spring Street, New York, N.Y. 10013

Contributors

PETER ANDREWS • Institut für Chemotherapie, Bayer AG, Pharma-Forschungs-zentrum, D-5600 Wuppertal 1, West Germany

JAMES ARMOUR • Department of Veterinary Parasitology, University of Glasgow Veterinary School, Glasgow G61 1QH, Scotland

J. H. ARUNDEL • Veterinary Clinical Centre, University of Melbourne, Werribee, Victoria, Australia 3030

WILLIAM N. BEESLEY • Department of Veterinary Parasitology, Liverpool School of Tropical Medicine, Liverpool L3 5QA, England

JAMES L. BENNETT • Department of Pharmacology and Toxicology, Michigan State University, East Lansing, Michigan 48824

LYNDIA SLAYTON BLAIR • Merck Institute for Therapeutic Research, Rahway, New Jersey 07065

GERHARD BONSE • Chemische Forschung, Pflanzenschutzzentrum Monheim, D-5090 Leverkusen-Bayerwerk, West Germany

J. C. BORAY • Department of Agriculture, New South Wales, Central Veterinary Laboratory, Glenfield, New South Wales 2167, Australia

DAVID BOTERO • Section of Parasitology, School of Medicine, University of Antioquia, Medellin, Colombia

WILLIAM C. CAMPBELL • Merck Institute for Therapeutic Research, Rahway, New Jersey 07065

JOHN C. CHABALA • Merck Sharp & Dohme Research Laboratories, Rahway, New Jersey 07065

DAVID A. DENHAM • London School of Hygiene & Tropical Medicine, London WC1E 7HT, England

ROGER O. DRUMMOND • U.S. Livestock Insects Laboratory, U.S. Department of Agriculture, Agricultural Research Service, Kerrville, Texas 78028

S. ALLEN EDGAR • Department of Poultry Science, Auburn University, Auburn, Alabama 36849

RAYMOND H. FETTERER • Animal Parasitology Institute, Agricultural Research Service, U.S. Department of Agriculture, Beltsville, Maryland 20705

MICHAEL H. FISHER • Merck Sharp & Dohme Research Laboratories, Rahway, New Jersey 07065

EDITO G. GARCIA • Department of Parasitology, Institute of Public Health, University of The Philippines, Ermita, Manila 2801, Philippines

TIMOTHY G. GEARY • Department of Microbiology and Public Health, Michigan State University, East Lansing, Michigan 48824

JOHN E. GEORGE • U.S. Department of Agriculture, Agricultural Research Service, Southern Plains Area, U.S. Livestock Insects Laboratory, Kerrville, Texas 78029

RICHARD JOHN HART • Wellcome Research Laboratories, Berkhamsted Hill, Berkhamsted HP4 2DY, United Kingdom

G. WAYNE IVIE • Veterinary Toxicology and Entomology Research Laboratory, Agricultural Research Service, U.S. Department of Agriculture, College Station, Texas 77841

JAMES B. JENSEN • Department of Microbiology and Public Health, Michigan State University, East Lansing, Michigan 48824

THOMAS R. KLEI • Department of Veterinary Science, Louisiana Agricultural Experimental Station, Louisiana State University and Agricultural and Mechanical College, Baton Rouge, Louisiana 70803

JOSEPH A. KOVACS • Critical Care Medicine Department, Clinical Center National Institutes of Health, Bethesda, Maryland 20205

JULIUS P. KREIER • Department of Microbiology, Ohio State University, Columbus, Ohio 43210

KENNETH L. KUTTLER • U.S. Department of Agriculture, Agricultural Research Service, Hemoparasitic Diseases Research Unit, Washington State University, Pullman, Washington 99164

DOUGLAS L. LOOKER • Division of Infectious Disease, University of Colorado, Health Sciences Center, Denver, Colorado 80262

J. JOSEPH MARR • Division of Infectious Disease, University of Colorado, Health Sciences Center, Denver, Colorado 80262

SUSAN MARRINER • Department of Veterinary Pharmacology, University of Glasgow Veterinary School, Glasgow G61 1QH, Scotland

PHILIP D. MARSDEN • Nucleo de Medicina e Nutricao, Faculdade de Ciencias de Saude, Universidade de Brasilia, Brasilia DF 70,000, Brazil

HENRY MASUR • Critical Care Medicine Department, Clinical Center, National Institutes of Health, Bethesda, Maryland 20205

LARRY R. McDOUGALD • Department of Poultry Science, University of Georgia, Athens, Georgia 30602

PATRICK B. McGREEVY • Department of Parasitology, Division of Experimental Therapeutics, Walter Reed Army Institute of Research, Walter Reed Army Medical Center, Washington, D.C. 20307

MAX W. MILLER • School of Pharmacy, The University of Connecticut, Storrs, Connecticut 06268

HELMUT MROZIK • Merck Sharp & Dohme Research Laboratories, Rahway, New Jersey 07065

JAMES NOLAN • CSIRO, Division of Tropical Animal Science, Long Pocket Laboratories, Indooroopilly, Queensland 4068, Australia

ROGER K. PRICHARD • Institute of Parasitology, McGill University, Macdonald College, Ste. Anne-de-Bellevue, Quebec H9X 1CO, Canada

ROBERT S. REW • Merck Sharp & Dohme Research Laboratories, Rahway, New Jersey 07065

LOYD D. ROWE • Veterinary Toxicology and Entomology Research Laboratory, Agricultural Research Service, U.S. Department of Agriculture, College Station, Texas 77841

HERBERT J. SCHNITZERLING • CSIRO, Division of Tropical Animal Science, Long Pocket Laboratories, Indooroopilly, Queensland 4068, Australia

RONALD L. STOTISH • Merck Institute for Therapeutic Research, Rahway, New Jersey 07065. *Present address*: Department of Chemotherapy and Immunology, American Cyanamid, Princeton, New Jersey 08540

DAVID P. THOMPSON • Department of Pharmacology and Toxicology, Michigan State University, East Lansing, Michigan 48824

HUGO VANDEN BOSSCHE • Laboratory of Comparative Biochemistry, Department of Life Sciences, Janssen Pharmaceutica Research Laboratories, B-2340 Beerse, Belgium

PETER J. WALLER • McMaster Laboratory, CSIRO, Division of Animal Health, Glebe, New South Wales 2037, Australia

GERALD WEBBE • Department of Medical Helminthology, London School of Hygiene & Tropical Medicine, Winches Farm Field Station, St. Albans, Hertfordshire AL4 OXQ, England

Preface

"Have a chew of dulse," said Crubog . . .
"What is it?" asked Potter, half-suspiciously.
"Seaweed."
"Is it good for the virility? . . ."
"And what is the virility?" asked the old man.
"Does it make you more attractive to women?" Potter
shouted in his ear.
"No."
"What is it good for then?"
"Worms."
"Worms?"
"Intestinal worms. You'll never again pass a worm if you
eat a fistful of dulse first thing in the morning and last thing at
night."
"If it's an anthelmintic, I'll try a spot of it," said Potter.
— From *Bogmail*, a novel by
Patrick McGinley (1981)

With modern techniques of chemical isolation and structure determination, the old distinction between herbal and chemical remedies has largely been broken down. By *chemotherapy* we now mean simply the treatment of disease by drugs (the word *medicines* has unhappily been eclipsed). The distinction made between chemotherapy and non-chemical therapy (e.g., radiation, physiotherapy, surgical intervention, immunomodulation) remains useful despite some minor overlapping. The present work thus deals with drugs and their use in parasitic disease. (Since we are dealing with the treatment of incipient as well as established infection, *chemotherapy* subsumes chemoprophylaxis as well as chemotherapeusis *per se*.)

Definition of parasitism as a biological *modus vivendi*, although important in itself, need not concern us here. We need simply delimit the scope of the book, and that is easily done. Included are the organisms that are, by almost universal convention, called *parasites*—the traditional subjects of parasitology. These organisms fall within the following groups: protozoa (single-cell organisms), nematodes (roundworms), trematodes (flukes), cestodes (tapeworms), acarines (ticks and mites), and insects. Excluded are the bacteria and viruses, which, their parasitic lifestyle notwithstanding, do not fall within the generally accepted boundaries of parasitology. Information on drug effects on those organisms is widely available in microbiological source books.

Information on the chemotherapy of parasitic infections is not so readily available. A vast literature on the subject has been built up, but a comprehensive source book is lacking. Specialized reviews have appeared (an outstanding example being Peters's volume on the chemotherapy of malaria), but, for the most part, reviews have been scattered both in time and in place. *Experimental Chemotherapy* (R. J. Schnitzer and F. Hawking, eds., 1963) covered a vast amount of territory but was devoted to investigational aspects rather than to clinical or field usage and is now a couple of decades old. Other volumes, such as *Chemotherapy of Helminthiasis* (R. Cavier and F. Hawking, eds., 1973), dealt with some of the major parasitic infections, but by no means all of them, and they too have inevitably become outdated with the rapid advance of knowledge in this field. The book entitled *Parasitic Diseases*, Vol. 2: *The Chemotherapy* (J. M. Mansfield, ed., 1984) is indeed modern but was not intended to be comprehensive. It deals only with malaria, the trypanosomiases, leishmaniasis, and schistosomiasis, and addresses, almost exclusively, these diseases in man. Furthermore, reviews of chemotherapy have not always stuck to their subject. *Antiparasitic Chemotherapy* (H. Schonfeld, ed., 1981) would seem to have been inappropriately titled. In several chapters more than one-half the text is devoted to information on the history, biology, and pathology of the infections, and one chapter devotes 21 of 23 pages to such nonchemotherapeutic matters. A working knowledge of the diseases being treated is a prequisite for successful experimental or clinical therapy, but it is not our present intention to provide such background information. Source books of zoological, medical, and veterinary parasitology are abundantly available; in the present volume we have tried to make sure that every penny a purchaser puts down for chemotherapeutic information will actually be spent for such information.

The advance of knowledge in the field of chemotherapy has been very rapid, and the reasons are not hard to find. We depend on drugs. Whether we should do so is another issue; the fact remains that we rely on medication to promote and preserve the welfare of our livestock, our pets, and ourselves. Nowhere is this dependence more evident than in the case of infectious diseases, including those caused by parasites. In the control of infectious disease in general, vaccination, livestock management, and human hygiene have played roles that cannot be emphasized too much, but in the case of parasitic disease, most of the starring roles have been played by drugs. It is to be hoped that those other factors will achieve greater success in the future, but it is safe to say that the medicinal approach will continue to be of critical importance in the foreseeable future.

This volume is directed toward members of the many technical disciplines associated with parasites and the drugs that are active against them. Most obvious, perhaps, are the members of the medical, paramedical, and veterinary professions, who use drugs daily in the prevention and treatment of disease. In the preparation of this book, attention has therefore been paid to the practical aspects of drug use. Its scope, however, goes beyond the human or veterinary clinic. The experimental chemotherapist will find information on experimental methods as well as on drugs new and old. For the medicinal chemist, there is information on chemical properties and structure–activity relationships. For the biochemist, there is information on the mode of action of drugs.

The book is, indeed, intended to serve as a comprehensive source book for all who deal with parasites and drugs, be they clinical, academic, or industrial workers.

A source book, to be truly useful, should be orderly. We have developed a format that does not seem to have been tried before. In so doing, we have tried to keep in mind the needs of those who may consult the book. A glance at the table of contents will reveal a common pattern within each major parasitological category. First, there is a chapter on the chemistry of the drugs used against parasites of that category. There follows a series of chapters on the particular parasitic infections and the drugs used to treat them. Finally, there is a chapter on the biochemical action of the drugs in question and, where appropriate, a chapter on drug resistance. The individual chapters differ in their internal organization because of the difference in subject matter and because we considered it desirable to give the authors as much latitude as was compatible with the overall objectives of the book.

Drugs are referred to by their generic or nonproprietary names. In many cases trade names are provided in the text as additional information; their use does not imply endorsement of a product and does not necessarily mean that there are not other names for a given medication. The book does not presume to prescribe—for every patient is unique, and one paddock is not the same as another.

W. C. C.
R. S. R.

ACKNOWLEDGMENTS. The senior editor would particularly like to express his gratitude to Dr. Dickson D. Despommier for proposing the preparation of this volume. During the early stages of planning, Dr. D. A. Denham and Ms. L. S. Blair contributed, as always, criticism and advice of the most constructive kind. The editors also wish to thank Mrs. June Wood for her expert typing of portions of the manuscript, as well as Mr. Kirk Jensen, Mr. Alan Winick, Mr. John Hirschfeld, and Ms. Eve Greenwood of Plenum Press for their expert handling of the publication of the book.

Contents

I. INTRODUCTION

II. PROTOZOA

Chapter 3

Protozoan Infections of Man: Malaria

TIMOTHY G. GEARY and JAMES B. JENSEN

Chapter 4

Protozoan Infections of Man: American Trypanosomiasis and Leishmaniasis

PATRICK B. MCGREEVY and PHILIP D. MARSDEN

Chapter 5

Protozoan Infections of Man: African Trypanosomiasis

ROBERT S. REW

Chapter 6

Protozoan Infections of Man: Other Infections

JOSEPH A. KOVACS and HENRY MASUR

Chapter 7

Protozoan Infections of Domestic Animals: Coccidian and Related Infections

L. R. McDougald

Chapter 8

Hemoprotozoan Infections of Domestic Animals: Trypanosomiasis, Babesiosis, and Anaplasmosis

KENNETH L. KUTTLER and JULIUS P. KREIER

III. NEMATODES

Chapter 12

Nematode Infections of Man: Intestinal Infections

DAVID BOTERO

Chapter 13

Nematode Infections of Man: Extraintestinal Infections

DAVID A. DENHAM

Chapter 14

Nematode Infections of Domestic Animals: Gastrointestinal Infections

SUSAN MARRINER and JAMES ARMOUR

Chapter 15

Nematode Infections of Domestic Animals: Extraintestinal Infections

LYNDIA SLAYTON BLAIR and THOMAS R. KLEI

Chapter 16

Mode of Action of Antinematodal Drugs

ROBERT S. REW and RAYMOND H. FETTERER

Chapter 17

Drug Resistance in Nematodes

PETER J. WALLER and ROGER K. PRICHARD

IV. TREMATODES

Chapter 18

Chemistry of Antitrematodal Agents

HELMUT MROZIK

Chapter 19

Trematode Infections of Man

WILLIAM C. CAMPBELL and EDITO G. GARCIA

Chapter 20

Trematode Infections of Domestic Animals

J. C. BORAY

Chapter 21

Mode of Action of Antitrematodal Agents

JAMES L. BENNETT and DAVID P. THOMPSON

V. CESTODES

Chapter 25

Mode of Action of Anticestodal Agents

HUGO VANDEN BOSSCHE

VI. ARTHROPODS

Chapter 26

Chemistry of Drugs Used against Arthropod Parasites

G. WAYNE IVIE and LOYD D. ROWE

Chapter 27

Insect Infestations of Man

    WILLIAM C. CAMPBELL

Chapter 28

Acarine Infestations of Man

    JOHN E. GEORGE

Chapter 29

Insect Infestations of Domestic Animals

WILLIAM N. BEESLEY

Chapter 30

Acarine Infestation of Domestic Animals

ROGER O. DRUMMOND

Chapter 31

Mode of Action of Agents Used against Arthropod Parasites

RICHARD JOHN HART

Chapter 32

Drug Resistance in Arthropod Parasites

JAMES NOLAN and HERBERT J. SCHNITZERLING

I

Introduction

1

Historical Introduction

WILLIAM C. CAMPBELL

Speak to me no more of these fine things; I am not a
man for drugs.
Napoleon Bonaparte

1. THE MISSION

The treatment of parasitic diseases has undoubtedly been going on for as long as such diseases have been known—literally for thousands of years. Some parasites, especially the larger intestinal worms, were known in ancient times. The microscopic parasites (and many macroscopic ones, too) were not known, but the diseases that they cause were known. Then, as now, diseases of known or unknown etiology evoked an attempt to treat them.

For most of recorded history, medicines were primarily herbal, working (when they worked) by virtue of their unknown chemical content or their placebo effect. Animals and minerals were not totally excluded as drug sources, and old records testify to the medicinal use of such items as exotic feces, oil of swallows, wine of vipers, raspings of a hanged man's skull, and metals of every form and hue. Centuries ago, as Turner (1958) aptly put it "remedies were esteemed according to whether they were rare, complex or unpleasant. A drug which combined all three qualities was irresistible." It is easy to disparage such therapy as unscientific, but we would do well to bear in mind that medicinal science is like any other science in that many of its achievements have been transmuted by time from the reasonable to the ridiculous. At any moment in history, those who ministered to the sick included many who were at the forefront of the science of their day. Even in our own day, that is the best we can hope for.

In this brief chapter, it will be necessary to exclude from systematic consideration

WILLIAM C. CAMPBELL • Merck Institute for Therapeutic Research, Rahway, New Jersey 07065.

the vast accumulation of animal, vegetable, and mineral nostrums of unknown or unproven principle. Information on such materials may be found in the innumerable herbals and pharmacopeias of the past. A valuable survey of ancient antiparasitic lore has been provided by Hoeppli (1959), and the history of antiparasitic therapy up to the middle of the present century was reviewed in considerable detail by Hawking (1963*a*). Here a brief note will be made on the general evolution of antiparasitic chemotherapy and on the methods it employs; within each major category of parasite (protozoa, helminths, arthropods) a miscellany of events will be recorded, chosen rather arbitrarily and eschewing any claims of completeness. Recent developments, no matter how "historic" they might seem, are left for consideration in other chapters.

2. GENERAL EVOLUTION

Chemotherapy, as distinct from herbal medicine, is often said to have begun with Ehrlich, and to a degree that is true. Ehrlich defined chemotherapy as the treatment of a systemic parasitic disease with a chemical of known constitution, his intention being to exclude the treatment of wounds with topical antiseptics and the use of immune serum (Marshall, 1964). It is true that in pre-twentieth-century medicine, the chemical composition of drugs was usually unknown. However, the stranglehold exercised by Galen's dogmatic herbalism from about 200 AD through the Middle Ages began to be broken during the Renaissance when Paracelsus introduced chemistry of a sort by attempting to cure specific diseases with laboratory-produced mineral drugs (Ackerknecht, 1970). Of perhaps greater significance, Paracelsus also taught that experience was more valuable than tradition. The seventeenth century was a period of therapeutic confusion but saw the introduction of two outstanding remedies. They were among the very first of the successful specifics and were introduced for the treatment of what subsequently turned out to be parasitic diseases—cinchona bark for intermittent fevers (which we would call malaria) and ipecac for dysentery (often representing amebiasis). The eighteenth century too was a period of therapeutic confusion and conflict in which folk remedies such as digitalis and belladonna were incorporated into medical practice but in which bleeding, purging, and the use of emetics was continued. Vaccination was introduced, and poisons such as the heavy metals were widely abused.

In looking at nineteenth century chemotherapy, one is struck by the sheer vastness of the "knowledge" that was accumulated—knowledge that was mostly to die with the century itself. Much of what seemed useful was rather abruptly shown to be useless with the advent of the controlled laboratory and clinical trial and the new learning in chemistry, microbiology, and physiology. A small volume on the homeopathic treatment of malaria (Douglas, 1853) contained page after page of prescriptions in which hundreds of drugs were correlated with hundreds of symptoms. Other texts were more reputable, but they too would soon be reduced to absurdity. Heavy dispensatories and pharmacopeias abounded, their pages replete with the findings of innumerable pharmacists and physicians, and it is a salutary experience to browse through those pages in the realization that they were, for the most part, the work of *bona fide* experts. Some of the information, to be sure, was to survive into our own age, but it is the rubbish that is truly awesome in retrospect. Yet order began to be established out of therapeutic chaos in the middle of the nineteenth century as experimental physiology and pharmacology began to provide a scientific basis for therapeutics. Indeed the nineteenth century was a crucial transition period in the evolution of chemotherapy, and it is worth mentioning two of the factors that were important in bridging the gap between the previous centuries of botanical and apothecarial dogmata and the abrupt flowering of chemotherapy in the twentieth century. One was the expanding knowledge of chemistry, which made it possible to isolate and identify the chemicals in many of the old remedies. Classic examples relating to parasitic disease were the isolation of the active ingredients of the two great antiprotozoal agents introduced in the seventeenth century: in 1820, Caventou and Pelletier isolated quinine from cinchona bark; and in 1822, Pelletier and Magendie isolated emetin from ipecac. Such advances made it possible for an investigator to reach the conclusion (now so very self-evident that we find it hard to appreciate) that "there can be no reasonable doubt that a relation exists between the physiological action of a substance and its chemical composition" (Crellin, 1981; see also Ackerknecht, 1970). Another factor in bridging the gap was the advance in microbiology, not merely in the establishment of a secure "germ theory" but in the production of infections for research purposes—leading by the end of the nineteenth century to the availability of laboratory animals experimentally infected with tubercle bacilli (mice), pneumococci (mice), trypanosomes (mice and rats), and *Treponema* (rabbits) (Marshall, 1964; and see following sections). The use of immune antisera at the end of the nineteenth century also brought a new awareness of the possibilities of therapeutic specificity.

The stage was thus set for the entrance of the star performer. The story of Paul Ehrlich is now an old one, featured prominently in any history of chemotherapy. His contribution to our particular branch of the subject, the treatment of parasitic infections, was essentially confined to studies on malaria (methylene blue) and trypanosomiasis (arsenicals). Ehrlich himself acknowledged that "from the very origin of the art of healing, chemotherapy has been in existence, since almost all of the medicaments that we employ are chemical." Herken, however, has pointed out that Ehrlich's term "chemotherapy" is incomplete without Ehrlich's adjective "specifica" (Parascandola, 1981). Chemotherapy meant the use of chemical substances, especially those produced synthetically, to destroy pathogenic microorganisms within the body (Parascandola, 1981). Since Ehrlich's day, many drugs have been products of the soil and the fermentation vat rather than the chemist's flask, but the skills of the chemist have provided identification and molecular modification as well as methods of production and even synthesis of such drugs. Thus has the distinction between natural and synthetic drugs happily been blurred.

3. EXPERIMENTAL METHODS

3.1. Concept and Control

The evolution of modern chemotherapy has inevitably been linked to, and indeed determined by, the evolution of methods of drug discovery and assessment. For many centuries new drugs for use in man were discovered and tested by administering them to patients, although some were selected because they fitted a particular theory of disease and their efficacy was simply presumed. Even those physicians who claimed to be empiricists, relying on clinical experience, were probably influenced most of all by tradition and by the opinion of the medical profession (Ackerknecht, 1970). As far back as the third century BC, attempts were made to draw conclusions from repeated clinical experiences, and throughout the intervening years periodic advances were made toward controlled experimentation. In evaluating a treatment for burns in 1537, Pare compared healing in treated and untreated parts of the body, and in treated and untreated patients (Sigerist, 1944). In 1747 Lind conducted a controlled trial on the prevention of scurvy. These were exceptional events, however, and Withering's book of 1785 on digitalis showed that a mere compilation of case histories, if carried out by an astute observer, could be of the utmost value. Controlled drug trials in human medicine, being fraught with ethical and practical difficulties and the constraints of tradition, did not become common until modern times.

Several eighteenth century investigators used laboratory animals to study drugs, but apparently not to demonstrate efficacy against parasitic or other infectious disease. Substantial methodological progress, however, came in the early nineteenth century when advances in chemistry made it possible for experimental pharmacologists to work with chemically identifiable and reproducible substances such as urea, the alkaloids, and the halogens. As already indicated, this progress was accelerated by pharmacological and parasitological developments later in the century.

3.2. Some Specific Assay Applications

A trypanosome assay played a crucial role in the most famous of the early breakthroughs in experimental chemotherapy—the discovery of a "magic bullet" for syphilis. In 1902 it was reported by Laveran and Mesnil that trypanosomes from horses could be maintained in rats by inoculation of blood from rat to rat and that compounds could be tested in mice similarly infected (Hawking, 1963a; Marshall, 1964). Ehrlich and his assistant Shiga used trypanosome-infected mice first for testing dyes. They discovered the efficacy of Trypan Red, which thus became the first synthetic drug to cure an infection in any animal (Marshall, 1964). Unfortunately it was not active *in vitro* or in the natural horse host, thereby raising a methodological problem that continues to perplex the experimental chemotherapist. Later Ehrlich and Hata used the mouse system to test trypanocidal arsenical compounds. The progress made in improving the therapeutic index of these compounds was exploited in experimental *Treponema* infections in mice (*Treponema* then being considered a relative of *Trypanosoma*) and led to the discovery of arsphenamine, or Salvarsan 606, in 1910.

The search for synthetic antimalarials before and during World War II (*vide infra*) depended on extensive "molecule manipulation" and *in vivo* testing. This had become feasible in 1926 with the development of an assay using canaries infected with *Plasmodium relictum*. During the war, testing was directed against avian species of the parasite in chickens, ducks, and turkeys; after the war emphasis was switched to the newly discovered mammalian species *P. berghei,* which could easily be passaged in laboratory mice. In the German studies of the 1930s and 1940s about 12,000 compounds were tested, while the number tested in the United States during the early 1940s was more than 17,000 (Black *et al.,* 1981). An intensive program was also conducted in the United Kingdom both during and after the war. Early studies on the testing of compounds against *Plasmodium knowlesi, P. falciparum,* and *P. gallinaceum* in tissue culture were reported in 1945–1946 by Ball, Berliner, and Tonkin, respectively (Findlay, 1951). After the war, the utility of conducting advanced testing against simian species of *Plasmodium* in monkeys was established, and in the late 1960s such testing was even further refined with the use of *Aotus* monkeys infected with human species of *Plasmodium.* The importance of this development was accentuated by the cessation, on ethical grounds, of conducting tests in prison volunteers or other experimentally infected human volunteers. During the period 1963–1975, coincident with the emergence of drug resistance and renewed warfare in southeast Asia, a mouse–malaria model was used in the United States to screen more than 250,000 compounds.

It is hardly surprising that macroscopic parasites were subjected intentionally to drug exposure earlier than their microscopic counterparts. *In vitro* experiments for the detection of anthelmintics were carried out as long ago as the seventeenth century. In 1684, after describing 39 *in vitro* experiments using earthworms and leeches and 12 experiments using parasitic helminths, the Italian Savant Redi concluded that some substances were active against both earthworms and parasitic worms (de Carneri and Vita, 1973). This finding anticipates the legendary incident in which a teacher immerses an earthworm in alcohol and asks what lesson is to be learned from its early demise. A pupil replies "that if you drink alcohol you won't have worms." This response is a bit more sensible than the expected one; yet, while alcohol has been reported to have at least some anthelmintic effect *in vivo,* the limited value of earthworm tests soon became evident. It has been said that Redi was "the originator of experimental studies on the therapy of helminthic infections" and was "in all probability also the first worker to adopt the experimental approach to chemotherapy in the broad sense of the term" (de Carneri and Vita, 1973).

According to Kuchenmeister (1857), several investigators looked for *in vitro* effects on worms between the time of Redi's experiments and the reporting of his own forays into this field. Rejecting both nonparasitic worms and expelled effete human roundworms as test organisms, Kuchenmeister advocated the use of ascarids freshly taken from dogs or cats and incubated at body temperature in a suitable medium, especially egg albumen. He also conducted anticestode assays by rotating tapeworms in egg albumin and determining the time taken for them to die when test substances were added to the medium. Using his ascarid assay, he tested more than 50 substances, paying attention not only to the mortality of the worms, but also to the time taken for the worms to die and to the solubility of the test material. Later developments in assaying anthelmintic efficacy *in vitro* included the discovery of the activity of hexylresorcinol in an *Ascaris* immersion test and the use of graphic records of nematode muscle contractions or whole-worm contractions (Cavier, 1973). During the 1950s, Yokagawa tested drugs against excysted metacercariae of *Paragonimus in vitro* and discovered the efficacy of bithionol, which was subsequently found effective and safe for dogs and humans.

During the mid-nineteenth century, Kuchenmeister used *in vivo* experiments to test substances that were especially active *in vitro* or that were of alleged clinical value (Kuchenmeister, 1857). He used dogs or cats with naturally acquired ascarid infections. The use of natural helminth infections was also suggested in several doctoral dissertations of the latter half of the nineteenth century, and in the early decades of the present century workers in the Far East tested drugs against natural infections of *Opisthorchis* in cats and *Paragonimus* in dogs. It was not until the middle of the twentieth century, however, that emphasis began to be placed on natural small-animal infections as models for assay purposes. The use of natural *Passalurus*–rabbit infection for anthelmintic assay was reported by Erhard and Gieser in 1941, *Ascaridia*–pigeon infection by Guilhon in 1947, *Syphacia*–mouse infection by Deschiens in 1944, and *Aspiculurus*–mouse infection by Reinertson and Thompson in 1951 (Cavier, 1973). Similarly, a century was to elapse after Kuchenmeister's trials (actually begun in 1851) before advantage began to be taken of the convenience and reproducibility of experimentally induced infections in chemotherapeutic studies. Experimental infection was used in a *Nippostrongylus*–rat model reported by Whitlock and Bliss in 1943, an *Aspiculurus*–mouse model by Wells in 1951, a *Syphacia*–mouse model by Chan in 1952, a *Nematospiroides*–mouse model by Hewitt and Gumble in 1957, and a *Heterakis*–rat model by Steward in 1955 (Cavier, 1973). In modern times, various other assays have been introduced.

4. ANTIPROTOZOAL AGENTS

Accounts of the origins of malaria chemotherapy invariably include an apocryphal story about the countess of Cinchon, wife of a Spanish viceroy in Lima, Peru, in the seventeenth century. It is said that she recovered dramatically from a severe attack of malaria when she took a remedy proffered by a local Spanish official. The celebrity status and charitable nature of this patient, it is alleged, were responsible for the widespread use of the remedy in question—a remedy prepared from the bark of a native tree. The role of the countess in introducing "Peruvian bark" into western medicine is discounted by modern historians (Guerra, 1977; Black *et al.*, 1981). What is accepted, however, is that the use of Peruvian bark was introduced to Europe in the mid-seventeenth century, probably by missionary priests returning from Peru to Spain. Peruvian bark was included in the *London Pharmacopeia* by 1677. Its reputation benefited from successful use against the fevers of the king of England, the dauphin of France (1682), and the emperor of China (1692). In deference to the legend of the countess, Linnaeus in 1749 gave the name *Cinchona* to the tree from which the bark was obtained. Reference has already been made to the importance of the isolation of quinine from the bark of *Cinchona* in the mid-nineteenth century. After two centuries of more or less continuous use of crude powders and infusions, a chemically defined preparation was now available (quinine being the most useful of the several alkaloids isolated) and soon became the standard remedy for intermittent fevers.

During the 1920s and 1930s, workers in the German pharmaceutical industry attempted to develop a synthetic alternative to quinine (for test methods, see above). By marketing quinacrine in 1932, they were able to challenge the virtual monopoly on quinine production enjoyed by the Dutch (by virtue of their *Cinchona* plantations in the East Indies). In World War II, Japanese military actions in the Pacific jeopardized (and subsequently cut off) the East Indian quinine supply, and this called for urgent countermeasures by the Allies. Quinacrine was evaluated by American, British, and Australian research teams and was introduced, under the name Atebrine or Mepacrine, as the standard malarial suppressive drug for military personnel. It was better than quinine for this purpose but was not exactly popular. An American marine later recalled that "Everyone was ordered to swallow Atabrine tablets daily. Many mutinied at this; the drug left its takers sicklied o'er with a pale yellow cast and scuttlebutt had it that it made men impotent. In the end the pills were doled out in chow lines. A corpsman popped a tablet on your tongue, then peered down your throat to be sure you had swallowed it. Still, there were those who managed to avoid it, and those who gulped it down and then worried about it. Personally I wasn't troubled by the pills. Being potent hadn't done me much good" (Manchester, 1979). The skin discoloration was responsible for a secret wartime project—an attempt to develop a face powder to offset this side effect in female military personnel (G. F. Otto, personal communication). The drug was used effectively by Allied forces in southeast Asia and the southwest Pacific, and it has been stated that "there is no exaggeration in saying that this probably changed the course of modern history" (Black *et al.*, 1981).

During the mid-1930s, the 4-aminoquinoline compound chloroquine was synthesized by the same industrial group and tested in birds and humans. Because of reservations about its safety, it was set aside in favor of its methyl derivative, sontaquine (which was widely investigated before and during World War II and eventually discarded). Chloroquine was again synthesized, in 1944, as part of the wartime antimalarial program in the United States (the action being based on chemical insight, knowledge of German patents on 4-aminoquinolines, a prewar link between German and American pharmaceutical companies, and fragmentary data in a Russian journal). The superiority of this compound soon became apparent, and a vast testing program was initiated—a program that led to the acceptance, at the end of World War II, of chloroquine as the drug of choice for the prevention and treatment of malaria. Chloroquine was to become a drug of monumental importance.

The recent flurry of interest in febrifugine and artemisinin as antimalarial agents is the latest development in the evolution of very old treatments (Klayman, 1985). The plants from which they are extracted have been used to treat intermittent fevers for centuries. For further information on the history of antimalarial drugs (including pamoquin, proquanil, and pyrimethamine), see Black *et al.* (1981), Peters (1970, 1980), Hawking (1963*a*), Coatney (1963), and Findlay (1951). For information on *Cinchona* and the various national attempts to cultivate it, see Duran-Reynals (1946), Taylor (1965), and Warshaw (1949).

Eimeria is phylogenetically related to *Plasmodium,* and there is some chemotherapeutic correlation between them, but the drugs used for the control of poultry coccidiosis and human malaria are in practice quite different. The efficacy of sulfanilamide in poultry coccidiosis was demonstrated almost as soon as the drug was introduced into human medicine. Levine (1939) found it prophylactically effective when administered in the feed, but the safety margin was not adequate, especially at the dietary concentrations needed to control *Eimeria tenella* and *E. necatrix*. Other sulfa drugs were tested during World War II, several of which proved superior (Delaplane *et al.*, 1947). One of them, sulfaquinoxaline, was studied intensively under the guidance of Dr. D. F. Green and Dr. A. C. Cuckler and was introduced commercially for the dietary prevention of coccidiosis in 1948. On the basis of studies by Dr. E. Waletzky, nitrophenide was introduced in 1951. Soon the control of coccidiosis, and indeed the efficiency of poultry production, was transformed by the widespread use of medicated feed.

Arsenic, which has been important in treating trypanosomiasis in humans, was first tried against the corresponding disease (nagana) in horses. The investigator was the redoubtable missionary-explorer David Livingstone, the year was 1847 or 1848, and the investigator did not know the etiology of the disease he was treating (Kean *et al.*, 1978). Inorganic arsenic had been used orally for centuries for the treatment of malaria (and many other ailments), and it would have made sense to try it against any "new" disease. At the turn of the century, Laveran and Mesnil found arsenious acid active but lethal in trypanosome-infected mice, and soon Thomas found that the organic derivative atoxyl could cure mice without killing them (Marshall, 1964). Arsenicals later became the focus of Ehrlich's program of chemical synthesis and indeed became the mainstay of treatment of several varieties of trypanosomiasis in humans and domestic animals. Their use in strategic treatment campaigns in Africa has been reviewed by Duggan (1970). One arsenical, named atoxyl for its alleged safety, had caused blindness in 800 trypanosomiasis patients in Cameroun in 1932. Although these patients would have been doomed to die of sleeping sickness in the absence of treatment and their blindness was attributable to misuse (overdose) of the drug, the tragedy stimulated Dr. E. A. H. Friedheim, to synthesize a series of arsenicals in a quest for increasing safety (Chesterman, 1979). By the end of World War II, he had developed melarsoprol, which not only remains in clinical use after heavy metals have generally been abandoned but is an indispensable tool for saving the lives of patients with trypanosomal invasion of the central nervous system.

In 1912 a young Brazilian physician, Dr. G. Vianna, reported the successful use of tartar emetic (potassium antimony tartrate) in cutaneous leishmaniasis. His clinical trial had been prompted by the successful use of the drug in trypanosomiasis (Vianna, 1912). A few years later, Di Cristina and Caronia used it intravenously against visceral leishmaniasis in Italy; the value of this treatment was soon made apparent in Asia (Beveridge, 1963). The inconvenience and toxicity of the treatment, however, were also apparent, leading to the development of the improved antimonial drugs that subsequently revolutionized the control of leishmaniasis.

Successful treatment of *Babesia* infection dates from 1909, when the efficacy of Trypan Blue (sodium ditolyldiazo-bis-8-amino-1-naphthol-3,6-disulfonate) was demonstrated by Nuttal (Joyner *et al.*, 1963).

5. ANTHELMINTIC AGENTS

5.1. Roundworms (Nematoda)

Alexander of Tralles, who lived from 525 to 605 AD., was something of a specialist on intestinal worms and listed the following as anthelmintics: celery, leek, parsley, garlic, mint, pomegranate pips, cress, castor oil, walnuts, cabbage seeds in olive oil with rue and portulaca, fern root, wormwood, chenopodium, and santonin. The last four-mentioned plant substances became established anthelmintics in the 19th Century and remained in use even until modern times (Leake, 1975). This is not so impressive as might at first appear, because herbal remedies were prescribed for "worms" with such lack of discrimination that it would be difficult to avoid the fortuitous inclusion of a few real anthelmintics.

In our grandfathers' day, pharmacists concocted and collected their favorite treatment recipes, as cooks collected and concocted recipes of favorite dishes—with the remedies usually containing one widely accepted ingredient aided and abetted (or perhaps merely obscured) with a dash of this, that, and the other. The mixture often included a laxative and perhaps a "tonic" to improve the condition of the intestine or the blood, as in the following example taken from Powell (1854): lime water, oil of wormwood, spirits of turpentine, tincture of myrrh, essence of anise, molasses, oil of Tansy, castor oil, and croton oil.

The treatment of parasitic disease, like other branches of medicine, has had a commercial component since antiquity. Patent protection and advertising have been employed widely, and the ethical standards associated with these endeavors have ranged over the spectrum characteristic of a given time and place. In 1796 a patent was granted in England to John Ching for an anthelmintic medication consisting of calomel (mercurous chloride), sugar, and saffron and prepared in the form of lozenges (Jackson, 1972). Ching' worm lozenges were used for many decades and were apparently responsible for the death of at least one child from mercury poisoning.

Two herbal anthelmintics have been particularly prominent in the treatment of intestinal roundworms, namely wormwood (Artemisia) and wormseed or epazote (Chenopodium). The historical persistence and wide geographic distribution of these remedies strongly suggest that they are efficacious, yet evidence of their usefulness under folk-medicine conditions has been difficult to obtain.

Medicinal wormwood in its crude form consists of the dried unexpanded flower heads of Artemisia (= Santonica). It is sometimes called Levant wormseed, though it does not consist of seeds. (Absinthe, too, is obtained from Artemisia sp. and is sometimes called wormwood.) The flowers of Artemisia cina have been prescribed under homeopathic medicine, with the "proof" of the remedy being attributed to Hahnemann, the founder of that cult. The symptoms of worm infection were given as "sickly, pale face, with rings around the eyes; gritting of the teeth at night; canine hunger, or variable appetite; the child picks its nose and cries out in its sleep; jerking of hands and feet; urine milky." The "mental" symptoms attributed to the drug, which were presumably held to resemble the effects of the infection, were given as "children awake in a fright, scream, tremble and cannot be quieted; they are proof against all caresses; are cross, irritable, nervous and peevish; they want to be rocked" (Dewey, 1908). *Artemisia* is the source of santonin, a sesquiterpene lactone believed to be the active principle and an essential oil that may also have some anthelmintic activity. As recently as 1964, it was reported that *Artemisia kurramensis* was cultivated in the Kurram Valley, resulting in the production of more than 1000 tons of santonin annually by a Lahore Factory (Kreig, 1964). Santonin was described in the 25th edition of the United States Dispensatory (1955) but has not been listed in a U.S. medical compendium since the 11th edition of the *National Formulary* (1960).

American wormseed, the leaves, seeds, flowers, and sometimes roots of *Chenopodium ambrosioides* var. *anthelminticum,* has been used for centuries in Latin America as *epazote* or *paico* (Kliks, 1985). Early in the eighteenth century its use by native and colonial Americans was reported in Europe, where it soon became an established remedy. It had become established in China by the nineteenth century. In the nineteenth and early twentieth centuries, the drug was chiefly used in the form of a volatile oil distilled from the plant. Oil of chenopodium, listed in the *National Formulary* up to 1960 contains an active principle, ascaridole, which has been identified as 1-methyl-4-(1-methylethyl)-2,3-dioxabicyclo[2.2.2]-oct-5-ene. Ascaridole has been used in both synthetic and natural form, and its efficacy and toxicity have been documented. Attempts have been made to define the efficacy of the various decoctions of *C. ambrosioides* used in folk remedies, but these have generally failed to demonstrate anything more than a modest suppression of worm egg production. This enigma was analyzed in depth by Kliks, who pointed out that the crude plant preparations increase intestinal peristalsis and are mildly laxative and that the transient effect on worm egg production suggests an adverse, though not lethal, effect on the worms. He further pointed out that "in areas of hyperendemic transmission the dramatic passage of large numbers of ascarids in the feces is a common occurrence" and went on to suggest "that the chance association of therapeusis and spontaneous self-cure events (aided perhaps by mechanical stimulation of the bowel), even if infrequent, repeated over millennia has resulted in the belief that decoctions of *epazote* have a direct and immediate anthelmintic action, particularly in children." Kliks concluded that "this general line of reasoning may well explain the plethora of reputed anthelmintics, particularly those designated as being specific for *Ascaris.*"

An *Ascaris* specific containing baked earthworm and baked toad was among the prescriptions compiled by Chinese imperial officials in the year 1111 (Chao, 1940). The prescriptions also included a rectal suppository for *Enterobius* treatment; it consisted of mercury and steamed dates, and was connected to the outside world with a strip of silk for the purpose of terminating treatment. In traditional Chinese medicine, the proper use of anthelmintics often required quiet (so as not to alarm the worms) and the preparation of aromatic food to induce the worms to point toward the patient's mouth (especially in the second half of the month when such reorientation was held to be especially needed).

The discovery of the "germ of laziness," the alleged cause of the physical and economic woes of the American "poor white trash," was announced, to a mixed chorus of cheers and jeers, at the dawn of the present century. The germ was the hookworm, *Necator americanus;* it was indeed responsible for much anemia and debilitation, hence at least the demeanor of laziness, in the United States and Puerto Rico. The hookworm control campaign that soon followed and was the earliest medical crusade of Rockefeller philanthropy, has been described in detail (Sullivan, 1930; Williams, 1969; Ettling, 1981). It constitutes a major historical event in the chemotherapy of worm diseases. At first, thymol was the drug used against hookworm, with a purge given both before and after. The efficacy of this drug (and male fern extract) had been discovered by Italian physicians grappling with the hookworm epidemic that had struck the workers building the St. Gotthard Tunnel in the Alps in 1879–1880 (Chandler, 1929). Thymol, 5-methyl-2-(methylethyl)phenol, isolated in 1719 from the plant *Thymus vulgaris,* was neither very effective nor very well tolerated. During the period 1917–1922, it was largely replaced by oil of chenopodium, which had been used elsewhere for some time. It, too, left much to be desired, especially in terms of safety, and was in turn replaced during the period 1922–1929 by carbon tetrachloride. This drug was the contribution of M. C. Hall, who had noticed the expulsion of worms from animals anesthetized with chloroform and had pursued the notion of hydrocarbon treatment to the point of demonstrating the powerful efficacy of carbon tetrachloride against hookworm in dogs and conducting small but daring safety experiments on primates such as monkeys and Dr. Hall himself. [According to reports cited by Cavier (1973), chloroform itself had been used against hookworm in miners as early as 1885.] Hundreds of thousands of patients were treated with this cheap cleaning fluid and fire extinguisher, accompanied by a purgative dose of salts, intended to speed the intestinal passage of the drug and thereby reduce liver damage from absorbed drug. In 1925, Hall reported that tetrachlorethylene was better than carbon tetrachloride and that it required no purging. By this time, the physicians involved in the hookworm campaign were just learning how to use carbon tetrachloride with a minimum of toxic mishaps, but gradually they switched to the new drug, which eventually became the drug of choice, not only in the Rockefeller-sponsored programs but in medical practice in general (Williams, 1969). Tetrachlorethylene remained in use until recent years and is probably still used where cheapness of drug is the prime consideration in treatment. Among the numerous unproven anthelmintics scattered throughout the medical literature is "powdered rust of iron" (Chase, 1876), raising the possibility that this usage may have stemmed from clinical observation of the benefits of treating anemia in severe hookworm disease.

With one exception, i.e., phenothiazine, the modern medium-spectrum and broad-spectrum anthelmintics (Table I) were discovered and developed by scientists employed by pharmaceutical companies. Developed for use in domestic animals, many of these agents were subsequently introduced into human medicine. Such technology transfer is by no means confined to the new or the good. For example, during the mid-sixteenth century, shepherds used mercury to deworm their flocks, inspiring Fallopius to tout its use as an anthelmintic in man (Mathison, 1958). An example of transfer in the opposite direction is provided by piperazine; the story of the discovery and development of this drug as an anthelmintic has been told by Goodwin (1980). Phenothiazine,

Table 1. Increasing Potency in the Evolution of Medium- and
Broad-Spectrum Anthelmintics[a,b]

Time of major market introduction	Compound class	Dosage (mg/kg)
Early 1940s	phenothiazine	600
Late 1950s	organophosphates	50–100
Early 1960s	thiabendazole	45
Mid-1960s	pyrantel	25
Late 1960s	tetramisole	15
Early 1970s	morantel	10
Early 1970s	levamisole	7.5
Mid-1970s	new benzimidazoles[c]	5–10
Early 1980s	ivermectin	0.2

[a]A simplification based on the approximate dosage required to give optimum efficacy (for that drug) when given to sheep as a single oral dose.
[b]Reprinted by permission from Campbell (1983).
[c]Includes albendazole, fenbendazole, mebendazole, oxfendazole, oxibendazole and benzimidazole pro-drugs. Benzimidazoles of intermediate potency (cambendazole, parbendazole) were introduced between the introduction of thiabendazole and the new benzimidazoles.

a veterinary anthelmintic that did not find use in man, was being evaluated as an insecticide by scientists of the U.S. Department of Agriculture when its anthelmintic properties were observed.

The antinematodal drugs mentioned thus far have been directed primarily against intestinal worms. The extraintestinal roundworms have presented exceptional difficulty. Small-animal models for filarial infections have been notoriously unsatisfactory, and the drugs in use have been grossly deficient, if not downright dangerous. The efficacy of two antifilarial compounds was first discovered in human trials. Potassium antimony tartrate was reported active against *Wuchereria* by Rogers in 1920 (Hawking, 1963b). Other antimonials were examined later, but the class was eventually discarded as unsuitable for antifilarial treatment in man or beast. Suramin was found active against *Onchocerca* by Van Hoof during the course of treating trypanosomiasis patients in 1945 (Hawking, 1963b) and remains an important antifilarial drug. The antifilarial activity of diethylcarbamazine was discovered just after World War II as a result of screening compounds in cotton rats infected with *Litomosoides carinii*.

Reports of the efficacy of arsenic in filarial infections go back at least as far as 1905. That year it was reported that clinical improvement had been seen in heartworm-infected dogs after administration of sodium arsenite (Blair, 1905), but supporting parasitological evidence was not provided. Arsenicals were found to be microfilaricidal by Hawking in 1940 (Hawking, 1963b), but their significance in filarial infections resides in an effect discovered by Otto and Maren a few years later, namely their efficacy against adult *Dirofilaria* in dogs (Otto and Maren, 1947).

Over the past century, the clinical severity of some *Trichinella* infections in man resulted in the testing of almost every conceivable, and some barely conceivable, medications in man or mouse (Campbell and Blair, 1974). The results were monotonously unfavorable until some of the modern broad-spectrum anthelmintics proved to have sufficient systemic absorption and sufficient activity against the muscle stage of the parasite to permit successful therapy of human trichinosis.

5.2. Flukes (Trematoda)

Trematodes, like hookworms (vide supra) were sometimes "cleaned out" with carbon tetrachloride. The drug was used against adult Fasciola in cattle, and the American medical missionary Barlow used it against Fasciolopsis in man. Indeed both the infection and the treatment were in the form of experiments that Barlow conducted on himself in China in 1923 (Barlow, 1925). The infection caused much pain and discomfort; the treatment did likewise, but it worked. β-Naphtol worked too, but was even more toxic.

Schistosomiasis, the most important of the fluke diseases of man, has been the subject of much chemotherapeutic investigation. The first specific remedy, at least in western medicine, was organic antimony, which was introduced by a British physician working in the Sudan during World War I (Christopherson, 1918). This was the beginning of an association between schistosomiasis and antimony that was to last until very recent times. One derivative was named fuadin in honor of the royal family of Egypt, but eventually the compound, like the royal family, was unceremoniously deposed.

Some modern drugs are active against liver fluke and hookworm (perhaps because they both are blood feeders), and this unexpected correlation goes back to one of the very first observations on the treatment of those two very different worms. It has been noted above that male fern extract (aspidium) has been found active against hookworm by Perroncito and colleagues during the construction of the St. Gotthard Tunnel in 1879–1880. I am indebted to Dr. J. C. Boray for pointing out that the same workers found the same drug active in fascioliasis (Perroncito, 1913). Dr. Boray adds that this observation served as the basis for the development of the first commercial liver fluke remedy, which was produced in Hungary in 1917 and which consisted of an extract of aspidium in gelatin capsules. It was sold initially under the name Distol and subsequently sold in England under the name Danistol.

5.3. Tapeworms (Cestoda)

Tapeworms have always been a delight to physicians and quacks. They are big, and after certain treatments they are readily, if incompletely, evacuated from the gut for all to see (or at least for the interested parties to see). They are relatively benign, yet are known to and abhorred by the layman. Thus they have long provided satisfaction to patient and physician, who like to obtain palpable results, as well as to those on the fringes of medicine who like to exploit the commercial opportunities offered by feared, though not truly fearsome, diseases. Traveling quacks who touted tapeworm cures in days gone by were said to give capsules containing fake tapeworms to members of their audiences, with instructions that they should examine their stool the next morning. Since the victims of this trick were not accomplices of the salesman, their subsequent reports of the passage of a tapeworm in the stool had an excellent effect on business (Mathison, 1958). It was undoubtedly scientific naivety rather than knavery that lay behind the patent application submitted by one Alpheus Myers, M.D. for the invention of a tapeworm trap. Novelty is what counts in these matters, and the patent was issued in 1854 as United States patent No. 11,942. The trap was to be baited with food, swallowed by the patient and retrieved with a string—and was thus an alternative to chemotherapy rather than an example of it.

Kuchenmeister (1857) recorded a case of human tapeworm infection that was subjected to a bizarre, if not fraudulent, treatment. He cited the following from an Arabian narrative:

> Then God tried him with a disagreeable disorder . . . which consists in a worm (fixing itself) at the issue of his anus, which gnawed the intestine and neighboring parts. Then large rams' tails were brought in order that he might insert them into him, so that the worm (or worms) might gnaw these instead of him, and he might thus obtain a little rest. When these were again drawn out, they were all gnawed to pieces by the worm, and new ones were then applied to the anus. The worms, however, did not cease to gnaw until his genitals fell off, and he in consequence died."

The case was thought to be one of rectal cancer with incidental tapeworm infection.

In his classic treatise on the parasites of man, Kuchenmeister (1857) devoted 30 pages to the treatment of tapeworm infections. He pulled no punches and roundly condemned medical practices that he considered unhelpful, dishonorable or cruel. He insisted that a good tapeworm remedy should result in removal of the scolex. He quickly dismissed more than 40 reported remedies, mostly herbal. He gave some consideration to a handful of other remedies, including turpentine, tin compounds (derivatives of which were used against tapeworm in poultry in modern times) and kousso (*vide infra*) but devoted most of his attention to the merits and faults of various preparations of male fern and pomegranate bark. Both remedies have had a remarkably enduring acceptance, being mentioned by Dioscorides during the first century and continuing in use virtually to the present.

Pomegranate bark was largely ignored in Europe until the beginning of the nineteenth century, when the English physician Buchanan reintroduced it from the East Indies, where it had long been popular. Kuchenmeister rejected reports that when a decoction of the bark was poured over tapeworms they "curled themselves up . . . appeared to experience pain, and died within five minutes in convulsions." Should such reports of pain be revived in our time, the whole subject matter of this volume may become considerably complicated. Kuchenmeister endorsed the use of pomegranate bark for tapeworm infection, and soon after the publication of his book the active principle was isolated. This alkaloid, 1-(2-piperidinyl)-2-propanone, was named pelletierine, and its tannate became a standard remedy in both human and veterinary medicine.

The other great classic of tapeworm therapy, male fern (*Dryopteris filix-mas*) has had a more continuous history of usage, at least in Western medicine. It was used through the centuries, however, not because it was so good but because the alternatives were so bad. It was the object of a minor *faux pas* in eighteenth century France. In 1775, Madame Nouffer inherited from her husband a remedy that she subsequently popularized as Madame Nouffer's Tapeworm Cure. King Louis XVI paid a large sum of money to learn her secret, only to find that the active ingredient was male fern and that the method of use—buttered toast followed by enemas followed by male fern, calomel, and the herbal purgatives scammony and gamboge, washed down with hot tea—went back to the time of Dioscorides. It must be one of the earliest examples of taxpayers' money being spent on a well-intentioned, well-conceived, yet unproductive search for a new drug.

Male fern is one of three unrelated plants that produce phloroglucinol compounds and which, apparently by virtue of these compounds, have been used as folk remedies for tapeworms, the others being *Mallotus phillipinesis,* used as kamala, and *Hagenia abbyssinica* (= *Brayera anthelmintica*) used as kousso (de Carneri and Vita, 1973). Male fern has been commonly used as oleoresin of aspidium, an ether extract of the rhizome, and the active ingredients (e.g., filicic acid) were isolated by Boehm at the end of the last century. Aspidium was included in the 16th revision of the U.S. Pharmacopeia in 1960. Its clinical use was described in full in the U.S. Dispensatory as recently as 1973 (27th edition), at which time the drug was no longer included in the U.S. Pharmacopeia or the National Formulary. It was listed as an alternative drug for tapeworms in *The Medical Letter on Drugs and Therapeutics* in 1969 but not in 1978.

6. ECTOPARASITES

For the most part, drugs used against ectoparasites constitute a subset of insecticides. They have traditionally been applied topically (i.e., to the skin of the infested host), and there is no clear generic distinction between these agents and the chemicals used to control agricultural or household pests. In recent years, systemic treatment has also been used, with the drugs being given orally, injected parenterally, or even applied topically in skin-penetrating formulations.

As in the case of endoparasites, the development of insecticides is rooted in antiquity and was for many centuries characterized by folk remedies of little or no demonstrable efficacy. The period from the mid-nineteenth to the mid-twentieth century was characterized by the use of nonspecific toxins. These consisted mostly of arsenical and mercury compounds, plant products such as nicotine and derris, and coal tar and petroleum derivatives. The nonspecific toxins had some specific triumphs. For example, the large-scale dipping of cattle in arsenical solutions resulted in the eradication of the *Boophilus* tick, and thus the eradication of bovine babesiosis (Texas fever) from the United States. The blunderbus biocides did not have the field entirely to themselves, and this period saw the introduction of the specific plant insecticide pyrethrum and the chemical identification of the active principles of both pyrethrum and derris (Busvine, 1980).

The modern era of insecticides could be said to have begun in 1939 with the discovery of the activity of DDT and might be said to consist of three component parts, not sequential periods but coexisting or overlapping branches: (1) the widespread use of insecticidal synthetic chemicals, consisting first of chlorinated hydrocarbons such as DDT, but subsequently including organophosphates, carbamates, pyrethroids (chemical analogues of pyrethrum), and formamidines; (2) the development of insect growth regulators i.e., agents that are responsible in nature for controlling growth, moulting, and other developmental processes, or synthetic mimics of such agents; and (3) microbial products (avermectins, milbemycins) of known chemical structure, but produced by microbial fermentation. These modern insecticides and ectoparasiticides are discussed elsewhere in this volume (Chapters 26–32), as are modern methods of application such as cattle eartags or dog collars consisting of insecticide-impregnated plastic. Beyond the scope of either this chapter or this book lie the nonchemotherapeutic approaches to arthropod control, including the use of pathogens (e.g., *Bacillus thuringiensis*), release of sterile male insects, and the use of pheromone-baited traps.

One way to put the modern ectoparasiticides (Chapters 25–31) into historical perspective is to record some of the recommendations of expert advisors at the turn of the century. A report issued by the U.S. Department of Agriculture (1896) gives the following advice for psoroptic and chorioptic mange in cattle:

> It is of the utmost importance to cleanse the skin, removing crusts, etc., before the parasites can be effectually eradicated . . . to kill the mites apply thoroughly, with a brush, the following mixture: creolin, 1 ounce; oil of tar, 1 ounce; soft soap, ½ pint; sulphur, ½ pound; alcohol, 1 pint. Wash it off in 2 days with soap and water. Three or 4 days later a second application should be made to destroy all remaining acari. It is essential that the stable or stalls where affected cattle have been should be cleansed and white-washed, or saturated with sulphuric acid 1 pint to 3 gallons of water.

For lice on cattle, the recommendation was as follows:

> Take a half pound . . . of *Cocculus Indicus*—fish berries . . . for each animal, pound fine, then add 2 quarts of vinegar, and set it on the stove to simmer for an hour. Apply this thoroughly by rubbing it well into the hair over the infested region. This will not injure the skin or sicken the animal, and it remains effective long enough to kill all the young lice as they are hatched from the nits. Professor Riley's kerosene emulsion is also very effective, and is made as follows: Kerosene, 2 gallons; common or whale oil soap, ¼ pound; water 1 gallon. Heat the solution of soap and add it boiling hot to the kerosene; churn the mixture for 5 to 10 minutes. Dilute the emulsion with 8 parts of water, and apply it to the animal by a thorough rubbing.

Referring to Buffalo gnats (*Simulium*), the report states:

> When an animal has been weakened by an attack of these gnats, give from 1 to 2 drams of carbonate of ammonia in 4 ounces of whisky every 4 hours. Keep the animal in a cool, dark place. Occasional immersion in cold water has been beneficial.

The rapid advance of therapeutics in the twentieth century, relative to the slow and unsteady progress of earlier times, may also be seen in comparing the advice given for the treatment of bots (*Gastrophilus*) in the seventeenth, eighteenth, and nineteenth centuries. In a treatise on horses, de Gray (1639) recommended for bots (and worms) a mixture that included fern root, savin (juniper), brimstone and soot, but pointed out that bots in the rectum of horses could best be removed manually. Gibson (1754) wrote (the letter "f" being used to approximate the antiquated typography of the original):

> If a Horfe is troubled with Bots, he may be relieved without much expense or trouble, only by giving him a fpoonful of Savin, cut very small, once or twice every day, in oats or bran moiftened, and if three or four cloves of chopped Garlick be mixed with the Savin, it will do better, for Garlick is alfo a great deterfive, attenuates vifcid matter, and keeps the Body open, which is of great fervice in all thefe complaints.

Little progress, if any, is reflected in a report issued 149 years later (U.S. Department of Agriculture, 1903), stating that horse bots "do not require special treatment unless they lodge in the rectum, in which case they may be dislodged by injecting tobacco water" into the rectum.

The oral use of drugs to remove stomach bots from horses represents an early example of systemic treatment of arthropod parasites; but stomach bots, being endoparasitic, hardly qualify as typical arthropod parasites. Successful systemic treatment directed against a skin-piercing insect was reported by Lindquist et al., (1944), who demonstrated the lethal effect of DDT and pyrethrum on bedbugs fed on rabbits that had been treated orally. Soon thereafter, systemic efficacy against an acarine ectoparasite was reported by DeMeillon (1946), who gave lindane orally to tick-infected rabbits.

7. THE PAST AS PROLOGUE

The history of antiparasitic chemotherapy has been sketched; the present state of the field is the subject of the rest of this book. As always, the accomplishments of yesterday and today tell us little about tomorrow. Since the current emphasis on prevention will undoubtedly continue, there is the hope that vaccination will replace chemotherapy. Nevertheless it seems likely that drugs will remain the cornerstone of prevention of parasitic diseases until the end of the present century.

By the beginning of the twenty-first century vaccines will probably be playing a significant role in the control of certain diseases—especially in the prevention of poultry coccidiosis and human malaria. The technological problems will probably be solved well before then, but the economic and political ones will be more intractable. And what of the longer term? The question will probably become moot, because the physicochemical basis of the immune response should eventually become so thoroughly understood that chemical manipulation of, or even simulation of, the immune response would become practicable.

Perhaps mankind will one day become completely successful in preventing parasitic diseases through immunochemical ingenuity and through political and social progress—including the provision of clean water and the other elements of hygiene. Then books such as this one will be obsolete. " 'Tis a consummation devoutly to be wished."

ACKNOWLEDGMENTS. The author thanks Dr. Gilbert F. Otto for reviewing the manuscript. He is also indebted to Dr. Otto and Dr. Mary H. Pritchard for information about the tapeworm trap, and to Dr. Michael M. Kliks for a prepublication copy of his paper on *Chenopodium*.

REFERENCES

Ackerknecht, E. H., 1970, Historical aspects of medicinal drug control, in: *Safeguarding the Public* (J. B. Blake, ed.), pp. 51–58, Johns Hopkins Press, Baltimore.

Barlow, C. H., 1925, The life cycle of the human intestinal fluke *Fasciolopsis buski* (Lankester), *Am. J. Hygiene Monogr. Series*, No. 4, pp. 93.

Beveridge, E., 1963, Chemotherapy of leishmaniasis, in: *Experimental Chemotherapy* (R. J. Schnitzer and F. Hawking, eds.), pp. 257–287, Academic Press, New York.

Black, R. H., Canfield, C. J., Clyde, D. F., Peters, W., and Wernsdorfer, W. H., 1981, *in: Chemotherapy of Malaria* (L. J. Bruce-Chwatt, ed.), pp. 9–19, World Health Organization, Geneva.

Blair, W. R., 1905, Filariae, *Am. Vet. Rev.* 18:1147–1151.

Busvine, J. R., 1980, *Insects and Hygiene*, Chapman and Hall, London.

Campbell, W. C., 1983, Progress and prospects in the chemotherapy of nematode infections of man and other animals, *J. Nematol.* 15:608–615.

Campbell, W. C., and Blair, L. S., 1974, Chemotherapy of *Trichinella spiralis* infections (a review), *Exp. Parasitol.* 35:304–334.

Cavier, R., 1973, Chemotherapy of intestinal nematodes, in: *Chemotherapy of Helminthiases* (R. Cavier and F. Hawking, eds.), pp. 215–436, Pergamon Press, Oxford.

Chandler, A. C., 1929, *Hookworm Disease*, Macmillan, New York, 494 pp.

Chao, C. S., 1940, Chinese anthelmintic prescriptions: Examples from the Han period to the present time, *Chinese Med. J.* 57:251–289.

Chase, A. W., 1876, *Dr. Chase's Recipes*, R. A. Beal, Ann Arbor, Michigan.

Chesterman, C., 1979, Dr. Ernst A. H. Friedheim: A tribute on his eightieth birthday, *Trans. R. Soc. Trop. Med. Hyg.* 73:597–598.

Christopherson, J. B., 1918, The successful use of antimony in bilharziosis, *Lancet* 325–327.

Coatney, G. R., 1963, Pitfalls in a discovery: The chronicle of chloroquine. *Am. J. Trop. Med. Hyg.* 12:121–128.

Crellin, J. K., 1981, Internal antisepsis or the dawn of chemotherapy, *J. Hist. Med. Allied Sci.* 36:9–18.

de Carneri, I., and Vita, G., 1973, Drugs used in cestode diseases, in: *Chemotherapy of Helminthiasis* (R. Cavier and F. Hawking, eds.), pp. 145–213, Pergamon Press, Oxford.

de Gray, T. 1639. *The Compleat Horseman and Expert Ferrier*, Vol. 2, pp. 97–100, Harper, London.

Delaplane, J. F., Batchelder, R. M., and Higgins, T. C., 1947, Sulfaquinoxaline in the prevention of *Eimeria tenella* infections in chickens, *North Am. Vet.* 28:19–24.

DeMeillon, B., 1946, Effect on some bloodsucking arthropods of Gammexane when fed to a rabbit, *Nature (Lond.)* 158:839.

Dewey, W. A., 1908, *Essentials of Homoepathic Materia Medica and Homoepathic Pharmacy*, Boericke and Fatel, Philadelphia, 372 pp.

Douglas, J. S., 1853, *Homoeopathic Treatment of Intermittent Fevers*, William Radde, New York, 108 pp.

Duggan, A. J., 1970, An historical perspective, in: *The African Trypanosomiases* (H. W. Mulligan, Ed.), pp. xli–lxxxviii, Wiley, New York.

Duran-Reynals, M. L., 1946, *The Fever Bark Tree*, Doubleday, Garden City, New York, 275 pp.

Ettling, J., 1981, *The Germ of Laziness, Rockefeller Philanthropy and Public Health in the New South*, Harvard University Press, Cambridge, Massachusetts, 263 pp.

Findlay, G. M., 1951, *Recent Advances in Chemotherapy*, Vol. 2, Blakiston, Philadelphia.

Gibson, W., 1754, *A New Treatise on the Diseases of Horses*, A. Millar, London, Vol. 2, 428 pp.

Goodwin, L. G., 1980, New drugs for old diseases, *Trans. Roy. Soc. Trop. Med. Hyg.* 74:1–7.

Guerra, F., 1977, The introduction of cinchona in the treatment of malaria, *J. Trop. Med. Hyg.* 80:112–118, 135–139.

Hawking, F., 1963a, History of chemotherapy, in: *Experimental Chemotherapy* (R. J. Schnitzer and F. Hawking, eds.), pp. 1–24, Academic Press, New York.

Hawking, F., 1963b, Chemotherapy of filariasis, in: *Experimental Chemotherapy* (R. J. Schnitzer and F. Hawking, eds.), pp. 893–912, Academic Press, New York.

Hoeppli, R., 1959, *Parasites and Parasitic Infections in Early Medicine and Science*, University of Malaya Press, Singapore, 526 pp.

Jackson, W. A., 1972, Ching's worm lozenges, *Pharm. J.* 209:614.

Joyner, L. P., Davies, S. F. M., and Kendall, S. B., 1963, Chemotherapy of babesiasis, in: *Experimental Chemotherapy* (R. J. Schnitzer and F. Hawking, eds.), pp. 603–624, Academic Press, New York.

Kean, B. H., Mott, K. E., and Russell, A. J., 1978, *Tropical Medicine and Parasitology*, Cornell University Press, Ithaca, New York, 2 vols., 677 pp.

Klayman, D. L., 1985, Qinghaosu (artemesinin): an antimalarial drug from China, *Science* 228:1049–1055.

Kliks, M. M., 1985, Studies on the traditional herbal anthelmintic *Chenopodium ambrosoides*, *Soc. Sci. Med. in press*.

Kreig, M. B., 1964, *Green Medicine*, Rand McNally, Chicago, 462 pp.

Kuchenmeister, F., 1857, *Animal and Vegetable Parasites of the Human Body*, translated by E. Lankester, The Sydenham Society, London, Vol. 1, 452 pp.

Leake, C. D., 1975, *An Historical Account of Pharmacology to the 20th Century*, Charles C Thomas, Springfield, Illinois, 210 pp.

Levine, P. P., 1939, The effect of sulfanilamide on the course of experimental avian coccidiosis, *Cornell Vet.* 29:309–320.

Lindquist, A. W., Knipling, E. F., Jones, H. A., and Madden, A. H., 1944, Mortality of bedbugs in rabbits given oral doses of DDT and pyrethrum, *J. Econ. Entomol.* 237:128.

Manchester, W., 1979, *Goodbye, Darkness—A Memoir of the Pacific War*, Little, Brown, Boston, p. 182.

Marshall, E. K., 1964, Historical perspectives in chemotherapy, in: *Advances in Chemotherapy* (A. Goldin and F. Hawking, eds.), pp. 1–8, Academic Press, New York.

Mathison, R. R., 1958, *The Eternal Search*, G. P. Putnam's Sons, New York.

Otto, G. F., and Maren, T. H., 1947, Filaricidal activity of substituted phenyl arsenoxides, *Science* 106:105–107.

Parascandola, J., 1981, The theoretical basis of Paul Ehrlich's chemotherapy, *J. Hist. Med. Allied Sci.* 36:19–43.

Perroncito, E., 1913, Sulla cura della distomatosis epatica, *Ann. Acad. Agric. Torino* 56:212–217.

Peters, W., 1970, *Chemotherapy and Drug Resistance in Malaria*, Academic Press, London.

Peters, W., 1980, Chemotherapy of malaria, in: *Malaria* (J. P. Kreier, ed.), Vol. 1, pp. 145–283, Academic Press, New York.

Powell, W. B., 1854, *The Eclectic Practice of Medicine*, H. W. Derby, Cincinnati, 1084 pp.

Sigerist, H. E., 1944, Ambroise Pare's onion treatment of burns, *Bull. Hist. Med.* 15:143–149

Sullivan, M., 1930, *Our Times, The United States 1900–1925*, Vol. 3, 586 pp. Charles Scribner's Sons, New York.

Taylor, N., 1965, *Plant Drugs that Changed the World*, Dodd, Mead, New York, 275 pp.

Turner, E. S., 1958, *Call the Doctor: A Social History of Medical Men*, p. 320, Michael Joseph, London.

United States Department of Agriculture, 1896, *Special Report on Diseases of Cattle*, pp. 325–348, U.S. Government Printing Office, Washington, D.C.

United States Department of Agriculture, 1903, *Special Report on Diseases of the Horse*, pp. 34–74, U.S. Government Printing Office, Washington, D.C.

Vianna, G., 1912, Tratamento da leishmaniose tegumenter por injeccoes intravenosas de tartaro emetico, *Ann. VII Congr. Brasileiro Med. Cirurgia* 4:426–428 (Translation in Kean *et al.* 1978).

Warshaw, L. J., 1949, *Malaria, The Biography of a Killer*, Rinehart, New York, 348 pp.

Williams, G., 1969, *The Plague Killers*, Charles Scribner's sons, New York, 345 pp.

II

Protozoa

II

Protozoa

2

Chemistry of Antiprotozoal Agents

JOHN C. CHABALA and MAX W. MILLER

1. INTRODUCTION

The search for agents useful for the prevention or cure of the protozoal diseases malaria and sleeping sickness was closely linked to the early development of medicinal chemistry (see Chapter 1). Unlike antibacterial agents, for which a few chemical structural classes exhibit a wide spectrum of biological activity, antiprotozoal activity exists in a wide variety of chemical classes, each of which possesses only a narrow chemotherapeutic spectrum. Antiprotozoal agents may be usefully subdivided into three broad categories: organometallics, carbocyclics, and heterocyclics. Each category may in turn be further subdivided on the basis of structural similarities among its members. The members of each group and subgroup as well as the protozoal genera against which each is currently used are outlined in the following section. Detailed descriptions of each compound (by number) are given in Section 3.

The descriptions in Section 3 include the name (and synonyms), *Chemical Abstracts* registry number (CARN), chemical formula, molecular weight, a structural representation, and physical and biological properties of each compound. Among the latter are data, or reference thereto, covering preparation, solubility, toxicity, metabolism, and mechanism of action, as well as references to published reviews.

2. STRUCTURAL CATEGORIES

2.1. Organometallic Compounds

The earliest described and most toxic of antiprotozoal agents are the organic compounds of the group V metals: arsenic, antimony, and bismuth. The arsenicals

---

JOHN C. CHABALA • Merck Sharp & Dohme Research Laboratories, Rahway, New Jersey 07065.
MAX W. MILLER • School of Pharmacy, The University of Connecticut, Storrs, Connecticut 06268.

currently in use are all substituted benzene arsonic acid salts or esters and include tryparsamide (1), Melarsen (2) and its cyclic reduced dithioester melarsoprol (3)—all used in the treatment of *Trypanosoma*—as well as roxarsone (4, *Eimeria*), nitarsone (5, *Histomonas*), and carbarsone (6, *Histomonas, Balantidia, Eimeria,* and *Entamoeba*). Even the simplest member of this series, arsanilic acid (7) still finds use in the treatment of *Eimeria* infections in poultry. Glycobiarsol (8, *Entamoeba, Trichomona*) is a bismuth ester of a benzene arsonic acid. In contrast to the arsenicals, only one antiprotozoal anti-monial (Neostibosan, 9) contains a carbon–metal bond, while all others are antimonate esters (10–14). Antimonials are used exclusively for the treatment of *Leishmania*. Only one organometallic compound that does not contain a group V metal (butynorate, 15, *Eimeria*) is currently used.

2.2. Substituted Carbocyclic Compounds

The second broad class of antiprotozoal agents to be exploited are substituted aromatic compounds. These structures vary from moderately simple monocyclic aro-matics to the highly complex tetracyclines. Other members of this class may be cate-gorized according to the nature and position of their aromatic substituents. Although there are no broad-spectrum aromatic antiprotozoals, members of this structural class have been discovered that exhibit activity against most protozoal infections. In contrast, only one purely acyclic nonorganometallic antiprotozoal, gloxazone (16, *Anaplasma*), is currently used.

2.2.1. Sulfonic Acids and Ureas

The highly complex aromatic sulfonic acids, suramin (17, *Trypanosoma*) and trypan blue (18, *Babesia*), were among the first antiprotozoals. These structures have been progressively simplified to provide imidocarb (19, *Babesia*), the drug of choice in the treatment of babesiosis, and the still simpler nicarbazin (20, *Eimeria*). Although not strictly a simple aromatic urea, the bisquinoline quinuronium sulfate (21, *Babesia*) is structurally similar to both nicarbazin and imidocarb.

2.2.2. Bisamidines

Compounds bearing two amidine functionalities separated by an aromatic spacer have been a fruitful source of antiprotozoal agents. Amicarbalide (22, *Babesia*) bridges the structural gap between this group and the ureas mentioned above, with particular structural similarity to imidocarb (19). All other bisamidines are *p*-substituted, but a variety of bridging groups have been employed to expand the spectrum of this series. The simplest members are phenamidine (23, *Babesia*) and stilbamidine (24, *Leishmania*), which are bridged by an oxygen and an ethylene, respectively. Diminazene (25, *Trypanosoma, Babesia*) possesses a triazene bridge; pentamidine (26, *Leishmania, Pneumocytis, Trypanosoma, Babesia*) has the longest bridge and also the widest spectrum within this group.

2.2.3. Other Symmetrical Diphenyls

The symmetrical arrangement of two substituted phenyl rings as seen in the aforementioned ureas and amidines is a common feature of several otherwise structurally disparate antiprotozoals. In the case of robenidine (27, *Eimeria*), the phenyl rings each bear a *p*-chlorine in lieu of an amidine and are bridged by a bisbenzylideneamino-guanidine. A sulfone moiety joins the two phenyl rings in dapsone (28, *Plasmodium*) and in its acetylated relative acedapsone (29, *Plasmodium*).

2.2.4. Monocyclic Aromatics

Although compounds possessing two phenyl rings predominate in the aromatic carbocyclic series, several useful compounds have been discovered that contain only one phenyl ring. These may be subdivided into the arylbiguanides and the arylamides. The biguanides, used solely in the treatment of malaria, include chlorguanide (30, *Plasmodium*) and the more highly chlorinated chlorproguanil (31, *Plasmodium*). The discovery that 30 is cyclized oxidatively *in vivo* to an active metabolite led to the introduction of cycloguanil (32, *Plasmodium*). The arylamides are a heterogeneous class that include the coccidiostats dinitolmide (33, *Eimeria*) and ethopabate (34, *Eimeria*), as well as the antiamebic diloxanide (35, *Entamoeba*).

2.2.5. Polycyclic Aromatics

Recently the bicyclic naphthoquinone menoctone (36, *Theileria*, *Plasmodium*) has demonstrated useful potency against East Coast Fever and malaria. The last class of carbocyclic antiprotozoals are the tetracyclines, better known for their antibacterial properties. The members of this group exhibit the broadest spectrum of any antiprotozoal agents and include tetracycline (37, *Plasmodium*, *Entamoeba*, *Anaplasma*), oxytetracycline (38, *Balantidia*, *Theileria*, *Entamoeba*), chlortetracycline (39, *Theileria*, *Anaplasma*), and doxycycline (40, *Plasmodium*).

2.3. Heterocyclic Compounds

Heterocyclic structures form the majority of antiprotozoal agents. This monolithic class, like the carbocycles, may be subdivided into several smaller groups: compounds elaborated from pyridine and pyrimidine nuclei, several azaonium species, nitro-substituted pentacycles, sulfas, polyether ionophores, and a mixed group of structures incorporating a glycoside moiety.

2.3.1. Monocyclic and Fused Pyridines

A substantial number of structures possessing antiprotozoal properties incorporate a pyridine ring as a structural element. Although monocyclic pyridines are represented only by clopidol (41, *Eimeria*), the bicyclic fused quinolines and isoquinolines form the basis of several active structures. The discovery and structural elucidation of quinine (42, *Plasmodium*, *Babesia*) led to the preparation of a long series of quinoline antiprotozoals, including chloroquin (43, *Plasmodium, Babesia, Entamoeba*) and hydroxychloroquin (44, *Plasmodium*), primaquin (45, *Plasmodium*), amodiaquin (46, *Plasmodium*), and most recently mefloquin (47, *Plasmodium*). Two quinolones are currently used as coccidiostats: decoquinate (48, *Eimeria*) and buquinolate (49, *Eimeria*). Even highly simplified structures such as oxyquinoline (50, *Balantidia*) and its diiodinated homologue iodoquinol (51, *Entamoeba*) retain useful activity. In contrast to their well-represented isomers, only two isoquinolines are currently employed in antiprotozoal chemotherapy: emetine (52, *Entamoeba*) and dehydroemetine (53, *Entamoeba*). The fusion of an additional phenyl ring onto the quinoline ring system provides the acridines quinacrine (54, *Plasmodium, Giardia*) and acranil (55, *Giardia*) and their simpler relative acriflavin (56, *Babesia*).

2.3.2. Pyrimidines and Fused Pyrimidines

The monocyclic pyrimidines are represented by the folate antagonists pyrimethamine (57, *Plasmodium, Pneumocystis, Toxoplasma, Isospora*) and trimethoprim (58, *Pneumocystis, Toxoplasma, Isospora*) and by the thiamine antagonist amprolium (59, *Eimeria*). Active structures have also been described wherein the pyrimidine ring is fused to a phenyl ring to form the quinazoline halofuginone (60, *Eimeria*), or to an imidazole to form the purines arprinocid (61, *Eimeria*) and sinefungin (62, *Trypanosoma*).

2.3.3. Azaonium Species

In several cases, active azaheterocycles are known in which ring nitrogen atoms are alkylated to form permanently positively charged species. Such compounds are used exclusively in the treatment of trypanosomiasis and include the phenanthridiniums metamidium (63), homidium (64), and prothidium (65), as well as the doubly alkylated quinapyramine (66).

2.3.4. Nitroheterocycles

The incorporation of a nitro substituent onto a furan or imidazole ring has provided a number of antiprotozoal compounds. These structures exhibit particularly potent activity against trichomonal and histomonal infections and are the drugs of choice for these diseases in spite of their reported mutagenicity. Among the 5-nitroimidazoles, metronidazole (67, *Trichomonas, Giardia*, and *Entamoeba*) is perhaps the best known, but tinidazole (68, *Trichomonas* and *Giardia*) and nimorazole (69, *Trichomonas, Giardia*) have found their place for the treatment of trichomonal and giardial infections. Ipronidazole (70,), ronidazole (71), and dimetridazole (72) are used in the treatment of *Histomonas* infections in turkeys. In contrast, the 2-nitroimidazole benzenidazole (73, *Trypanosoma cruzi*) is useful in the treatment of Chagas' disease. Although not nitrated, clotrimazole (74, *Naegleria*), known largely for its antifungal properties, has been used as one of the very few treatments for *Naegleria* infections.

Among the nitrofurans, nitrofurazone (75, *Trypanosoma, Eimeria*) and furazolidinone (76, *Trichomonas, Giardia, Histomonas*) have the longest history of use, whereas more recently nifursol (77, *Histomonas*) has been used to treat turkey blackhead disease, and nifurtimox (78, *Trypanosoma cruzi*) has been introduced as one of the few treatments for Chagas' disease.

2.3.5. Sulfas

Although used primarily as antibacterial agents, a few sulfonamide folate antagonists have been applied to the treatment of protozoal infections, often as components of combination therapies. Five sulfas are currently in use: sulfalene (79, *Plasmodium*), sulfaquinoxaline (80, *Eimeria*), sulfadimethoxine (81, *Eimeria*), sulfamethoxazole (82, *Pneumocystis, Toxoplasma, Isospora*), and sulfadiazene (83, *Pneumocystis, Toxoplasma, Isospora*).

2.3.6. Polyether Ionophores

After the spectacular success of monensin (84, *Eimeria*) in the treatment of poultry coccidial infections, a total of four additional ionophores have been introduced, all for the prevention of coccidiosis. Of these, monensin (84), salinomycin (85), narasin (86), and maduramicin (87) are monovalent and cation specific, whereas lasalocid (88) binds both mono- and divalent cations.

2.3.7. Glycosides

A heterogeneous group of glycoside-containing structures form the last group of antiprotozoal agents. These compounds, better known for, and more widely applied to, the treatment of fungal or bacterial infections, include the macrolides spiramycin (89, *Cryptosporidia, Toxoplasma*) and amphotericin B (90, *Naegleria, Leishmania*) and the aminoglycosides paromomycin (91, *Entamoeba, Giardia, Balantidia, Leishmania*) and clindamycin (92, *Plasmodium, Babesia, Toxoplasma*).

3. PROPERTIES OF ANTIPROTOZOAL AGENTS

1. TRYPARSAMIDE

CARN: 554-72-3

$C_8H_{10}AsN_2NaO_4$ mol. wt. 296.08

(4-[(2-Amino-2-oxoethyl)amino]phenylarsonic acid monosodium salt

Synonyms: Glyphenarsine; Tryparsone; Tryponarsyl; Trypothane.

Hemihydrate (mol. wt. 323.10), platelets, air stable, light sensitive.
Solubility: approx. 0.5 g/ml H_2O (pH of a 1 : 20 aq. soln. = 6.5); sl. sol. C_2H_5OH; insol. $(C_2H_5)_2O$, $CHCl_3$.
Keep in tight containers at preferably <20°C, protected from light.
Preparation: Jacobs and Heidelberger (1919).

2. MELARSEN

CARN: 3599-28-8
$C_9H_9AsN_6Na_2O_3$ mol. wt. 370.11
N-(4,6-Diamino-*s*-triazin-2-yl)arsanilic acid disodium salt
Synonyms: 4-melaminylphenylarsonic acid disodium salt.

Acid:
$C_9H_{11}AsN_6O_3$ mol. wt. 326.15
Amorphous powder, stable at 300°C, chars without melting at 300–350°C.
Preparation: Friedheim (1944).

3. MELARSOPROL

CARN: 494-79-1
$C_{12}H_{15}AsN_6OS_2$ mol. wt. 398.34
2-(4-[(4,6-Diamino-1,3,5-triazin-2-yl)amino]phenyl)-1,3,2-dithiarsolane-4-methanol
Synonyms: Mel B; Arsobal.

Solubility: practically insol. H_2O, CH_3OH, cold C_2H_5OH; sol. in propylene glycol.
Preparation: Friedheim (1953, 1956).

4. ROXARSONE

CARN: 121-19-7
$C_6H_6AsNO_6$ mol. wt. 263.03
4-Hydroxy-3-nitrobenzenearsonic acid

Synonyms: NSC-2101; Ren-O-sal; Ristat

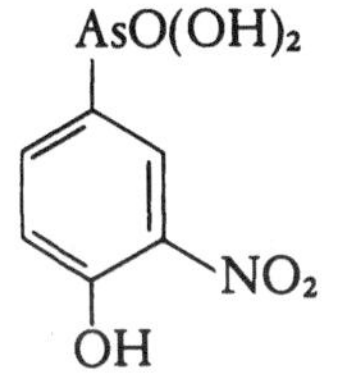

$$AsO(OH)_2$$

[structure: benzene ring with AsO(OH)₂ at top, NO₂ at right, OH at bottom]

NO_2

OH

Tufts of pale yellow needles or rhombohedral plates from H_2O; puffs up and deflagrates upon heating.

Solubility: sl. sol. cold H_2O, sol. in about 30 parts boiling H_2O; freely soluble in CH_3OH, C_2H_5OH, CH_3COOH, $(CH_3)_2CO$, alkalies; sparingly sol. in dil. mineral acids; insol. in $(C_2H_5)_2O$, $CH_3CO_2C_2H_5$.

Forms mono-, di-, and trisodium salts.

Toxicity: LD_{50} rats 155 mg/kg po, 66 mg/kg ip; LD_{50} chickens: 110–123 mg/kg po, 34 mg/kg ip. (Kerr *et al.*, 1963).

Preparation: Benda and Bertheim (1911).

5. NITARSONE

CARN: 98-72-6

$C_6H_6AsNO_5$ mol. wt. 247.04

4-Nitrophenylarsonic acid

Synonyms: *p*-nitrophenylarsonic acid.

$$\begin{array}{c} O \\ \| \\ HO-As-OH \end{array}$$

[structure: benzene ring with arsonic acid group at top and NO₂ at bottom]

NO_2

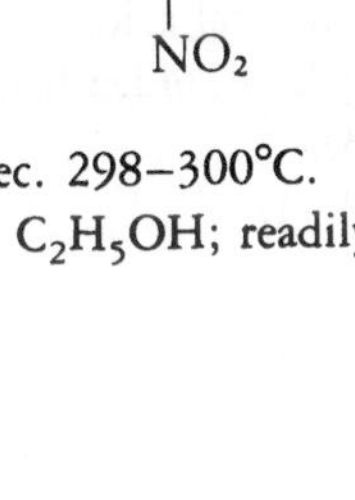

Pale yellow leaflets from H_2O, dec. 298–300°C.

Solubility: very sl. sol. cold H_2O, C_2H_5OH; readily sol. warm H_2O, C_2H_5OH.

Preparation: Jacobs *et al.* (1918).

6. CARBARSONE

CARN: 121-59-5

$C_7H_9AsN_2O_4$ mol. wt. 260.07

(4-[(Aminocarbonyl)amino]phenyl)arsonic acid

Synonyms: N-carbamoylarsanilic acid; Amebevan; Ameban; Amibiarson; Arsambide; Carb-O-Sep; Histocarb; Fenarsone; Leucarsone; Aminarsone; Amebarsone.

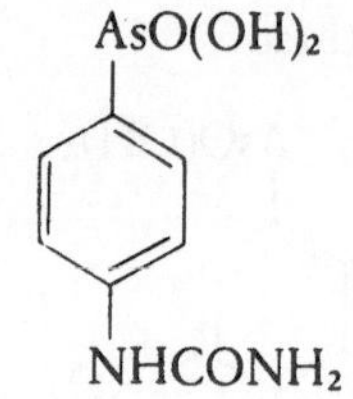

$$AsO(OH)_2$$

$$NHCONH_2$$

White powder, m.p. 174°C.

Solubility: sl. sol. H_2O, C_2H_5OH (sat. aq. solns. are acid to litmus); sol. in solns. of alkali hydroxides and carbonates; nearly insol. in $(C_2H_5)_2O$ and $CHCl_3$.

Toxicity: LD_{50} rats 510 mg/kg po (Windholz *et al.*, 1983).

Preparation: Stickings (1928); Nakatsu and Kawase (1956).

7. ARSANILIC ACID

CARN: 98-50-0

$C_6H_8AsNO_3$ mol. wt. 217.04

(4-Aminophenyl)arsonic acid

Synonyms: *p*-aminophenylarsonic acid; atoxylic acid; AS 101.

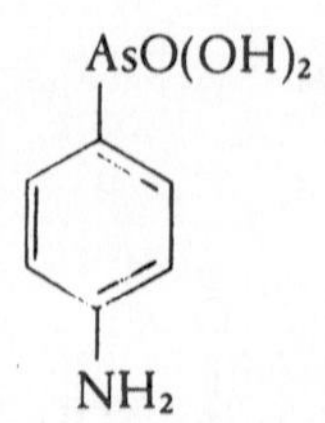

$$AsO(OH)_2$$

$$NH_2$$

Needles from H_2O or C_2H_5OH.

Solubility: sl. sol. cold H_2O, C_2H_5OH, CH_3COOH; sol. hot H_2O, amyl alcohol, solns. of alkali carbonates; mod. sol. in conc. mineral acids; insol. $(CH_3)_2CO$, C_6H_6, $CHCl_3$, $(C_2H_5)_2O$, mod. dil. mineral acids.

Toxicity: LD_{50} male rats >1000 mg/kg (Goldenthal, 1971).

Toxicology: swine (Ledet *et al.*, 1973).

Preparation: Lewis and Cheetham (1941).

8. GLYCOBIARSOL

CARN: 116-49-4

$C_8H_9AsBiNO_6$ mol. wt 499.07

([4-([Hydroxyacetyl]amino)phenyl]arsonato(1^-)-O^{As}) oxobismuth

Synonyms: bismuth glycoloylarsanilate; Broxolin; Dysentulin; Milibis; Viasept; Wintodon.

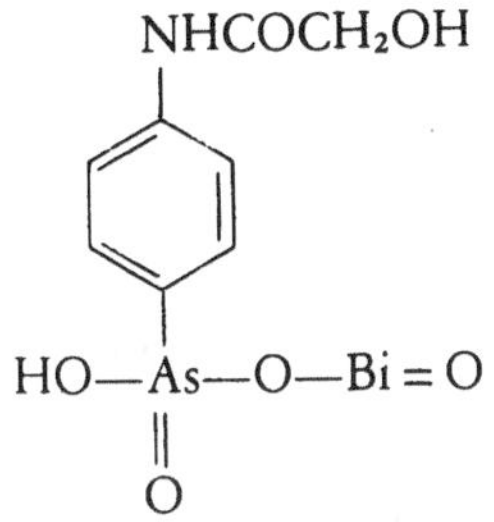

NHCOCH₂OH

$$\text{HO—As—O—Bi} = \text{O}$$

Yellowish to pink powder, dec. on heating.
Solubility: very sl. sol. H_2O, C_2H_5OH; practically insol. $(C_2H_5)_2O$, $CHCl_3$, C_6H_6.
Toxicity: LD_{50} male rats >10 g/kg/day po (McChesney and Hoppe, 1950).
Preparation: Auterhoff *et al.* (1958).
Note: A derivative containing additional bismuth is marketed as Garbisil.

9. NEOSTIBOSAN

CARN: 554-76-7
No definite formula   mol. wt. undefined
Ethylstibamine
Synonyms: Stibosamine; Astaril; 693 B.

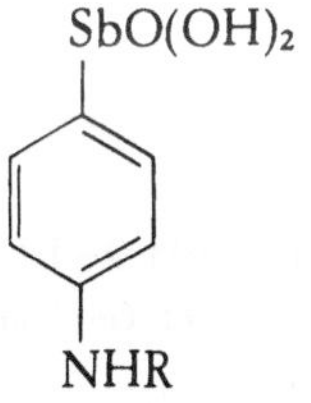

SbO(OH)₂

9a.   R = H

9b.   R = COCH₃

NHR

An approx. $1:2:1:3$ complex of *p*-aminobenzenestibonic acid (9a, largely as
   tetramer), *p*-acetylaminobenzenestibonic acid (9b, largely as dimer), antimonic
   acid, and diethylamine. Contains 41–44% organic pentavalent antimony.
Light yellow to yellowish-brown powder.
Solubility: freely sol. in H_2O forming neutral colloids (pH of 5% aq. soln. $= 6.5–7.6$);
   a 25% solution is isotonic.
Unstable on heating or standing.
Solutions must be prepared immediately before use.
Toxicity: varies greatly with slight differences in preparation (Schmidt, 1930).

10. TARTAR EMETIC

CARN: 28300-74-5
$C_4H_4KO_7Sb$ mol. wt. 324.92
Antimony potassium tartrate
Synonyms: tartrated antimony; tartarized antimony.

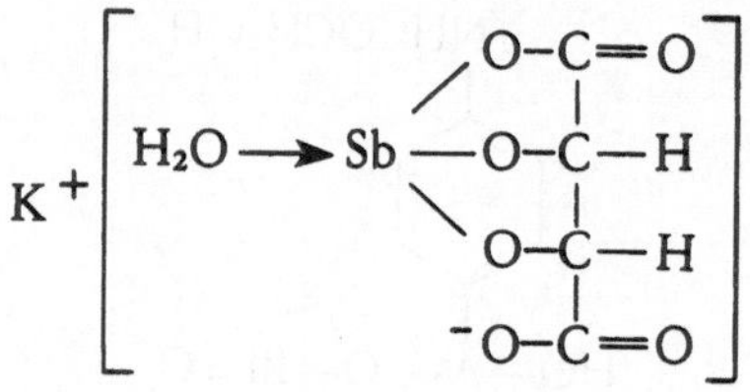

$$K^+ \left[H_2O \longrightarrow Sb \begin{matrix} O-C=O \\ O-C-H \\ O-C-H \\ ^-O-C=O \end{matrix} \right]$$

Hemihydrate (mol. wt. 351.94), transparent crystals, effluoresces on exposure to air, loses 0.5 mol H_2O at 100°C, loses 1 mol H_2O at 210°C (Pfeiffer and Schmitz, 1949).

Optical rotation: $[\alpha]_D^{20}$ +140.69° (c = 2 [H_2O]), +139.25° (c = 2 [glycerol]).

Solubility: 1 g/12 ml H_2O (to form a sl. acid soln.), 1 g/3 ml boiling H_2O, 1 g/15 ml glycerol; insol. in C_2H_5OH.

Toxicity: LD_{50} mice 55 mg/kg sc, 65 mg/kg iv (Ercoli, 1968).

Incompatabilities: Tannic acid, alkalies, alkali carbonates, lead salts, astringent infusions (e.g., cinchona, rhubarb), acacia, antipyrine, mercury bichloride.

Preparation: Davies (1943, 1945).

11. ANTIMONY SODIUM GLUCONATE

CARN: 16037-91-5

Trivalent antimonyl sodium gluconate

$C_6H_8NaO_7Sb$ mol. wt. 336.88

Synonyms: Triostam; T.S.A.G.

Amorphous powder.

Solubility: sol. H_2O (pH of 2% aq. soln. = 9–10); at pH 9–10 aq. solns. are unstable and should be adjusted with gluconic acid to pH 6–7 and used immediately.

Preparation: Das Gupta (1953), Chyan *et al.* (1956).

Pentavalent sodium antimonyl gluconate

Synonyms: Pentostam; Myostibin; Solustibosan; Solyusurmin; Stibanate; Stibanose; Stibatin; Stibinol.

Contains 28–29.5% Sb.

Crystals.

Solubility: freely sol. H_2O (pH 10% aq. soln. = 5.4–5.6); ampuled solutions should be stored at room temperature.

Preparation: Bose and Ghosh (1949).

12. UREA STIBAMINE

CARN: 1340-35-8

No definite formula   mol. wt. undefined

Synonym: Carbostibamine.

No definitely known and agreed-upon structure; antimony content of commercial samples varies between 39 and 42%.

White powder.
Solubility: sol. H_2O; partly sol. C_2H_5OH, $(C_2H_5)_2O$.
Preparation: Datta *et al.* (1946).

13. STIBOPHEN

CARN: 15489-16-4
$C_{12}H_{18}Na_5O_{23}S_4Sb$ mol. wt. 895.21
Bis[4,5-dihydroxy-1,3-benzenedisulfonato(4^-)-O^4,O^5]antimonate(5^-)   pentasodium
   heptahydrate
Synonyms: sodium antimony bis(pyrocatechol-2,4-disulfonate); Sdt 91; Fuadin; Fouadin;
   Pyrostib; Corystibin; Trimon; Fantorin; Repodral; Neoantimosan; Sodium
   Antimosan.

Fine crystals.
Solubility: readily sol. cold H_2O (if a neutral aq. soln. is not acidified, it soon acquires a
   yellowish tint, ultimately turning lemon yellow); almost insol. in abs. C_2H_5OH,
   $(C_2H_5)_2O$, $CHCl_3$, $(CH_3)_2CO$, petroleum ether.
Toxicity: MLD rabbits 80 mg/kg iv (Windholz *et al.*, 1983)
Incompatabilities: Iron and iron compounds.
Preparation: Schmidt (1930).

Potassium salt
$C_{12}H_{18}K_5O_{23}S_4Sb$ mol. wt. 975.75
Synonyms: Antimosan; Heyden 611.

14. GLUCANTIME

CARN: 133-51-7
$C_7H_{18}NO_8Sb$ mol. wt. 365.97
N-Methylglucamine antimonate
Synonyms: Protostib; RP 2168.
Powder.
Solubility: about 35% (*w/w*) in H_2O (pH of aq. solns. = 6.7); practically insol.
   C_2H_5OH, $(C_2H_5)_2O$, $CHCl_3$.
Toxicity: human mild irritant (Windholz *et al.*, 1983).
Preparation: Carcassi (1948).

15. BUTYNORATE

CARN: 77-58-7
$C_{32}H_{64}O_4Sn$ mol. wt. 631.55

Dibutylbis[(1-oxododecyl)oxy]stannane
Synonyms: dibutylbis(lauroyloxy)tin; Davainex; Tinostat.

$$(CH_3 (CH_2)_{10} \overset{\overset{\text{O}}{\|}}{C}O)_2 - Sn - (CH_2CH_2CH_2CH_3)_2$$

Soft crystals, m.p. 22–24°C, or yellow liquid n_D^{20} 1.4683.
Solubility: practically insol. H_2O, CH_3OH; sol. petroleum ether, C_6H_6, $(CH_3)_2CO$, CCl_4, $(C_2H_5)_2O$, organic esters.
Preparation: Sheverdina *et al.* (1962).

16. GLOXAZONE

CARN: 2507-91-7
$C_8H_{16}N_6OS_2$ mol. wt. 276.38
2,2′-[1-(1-Ethoxyethyl)-1,2-ethanediylidene]bishydrazinecarbothioamide
Synonyms: Contrapar; BW 356-C-61; NSC 82116, KTS.

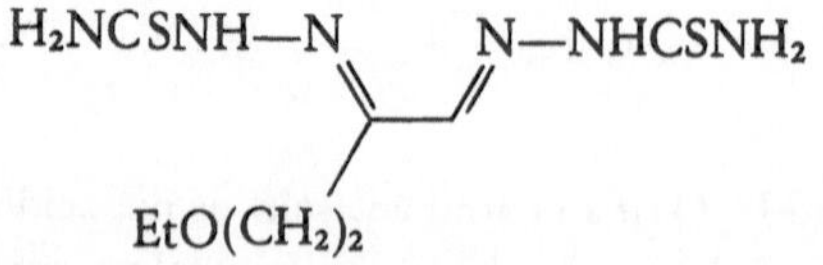

H₂NCSNH—N   N—NHCSNH₂

EtO(CH₂)₂

Crystals from CH_3OH, m.p. 202–204°C; uv max: 232, 270, 340, 347 nm (ε 9000,
    7500, 47850, 49150).
Toxicology: LD_{50} mice 2.62 g/kg ip one dose (Petering *et al.*, 1964).
Preparation: Petering *et al.* (1964).

17. SURAMIN

CARN: 129-46-4
$C_{51}H_{34}N_6Na_6O_{23}S_6$ mol. wt. 1429.21
8,8′-(Carbonylbis[imino-3,1-phenylenecarbonylimino(4-methyl-3,1-phenylene)car-
    bonylimino])bis-1,3,5-naphthalenetrisulfonic acid hexasodium salt
Synonyms: Bayer 205; 309F; Antrypol; Germanin; Moranyl; Naganol; Naganin;
    Naphuride Sodium.

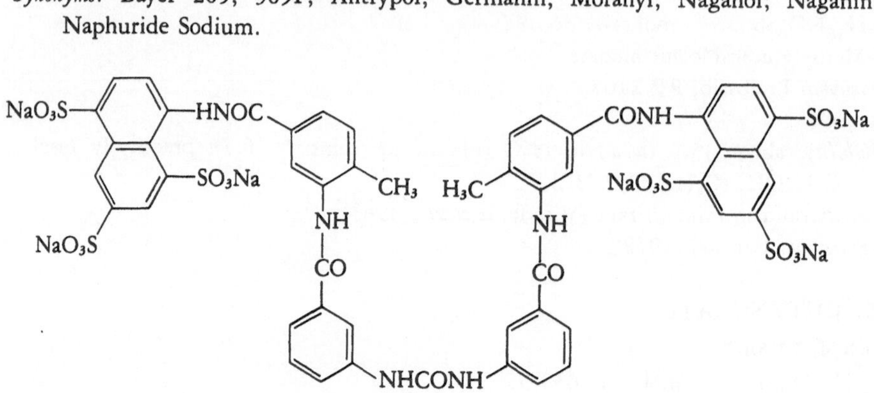

White or slightly pink or cream-colored powder; sl. bitter taste; hygroscopic.
Solubility: freely sol. H_2O (solns. neutral to litmus), physiological salt soln.; sparingly
   sol. 95% C_2H_5OH; insol. C_6H_6, $(C_2H_5)_2O$, $CHCl_3$, pet. ether.
Toxicity: LD_{50} mice 40 mg/kg iv (Windholz *et al.*, 1983).
Preparation: Fourneau *et al.* (1924).
Review: Olenick (1975*a*).

18. TRYPAN BLUE

CARN: 72-57-1
$C_{34}H_{24}N_6Na_4O_{14}S_4$ mol. wt. 960.83
3,3'-([3,3'-Dimethyl(1,1'-biphenyl)-4,4'-diyl]bis[azo])bis(5-amino-4-hydroxy-2,7-
   naphthalenedisulfonic acid) tetrasodium salt
Synonyms: sodium ditolyl-diazobis-8-amino-1-naphthol-3,6-disulfonate; Benzamine
   Blue; Diamine Blue; Benzo Blue; Congo Blue; Dianil Blue; Naphthylamine Blue;
   Niagara Blue.

Bluish-gray powder.
Solubility: sol. in H_2O forming a deep blue soln. with a violet tinge; almost insol. in
   C_2H_5OH.
Toxicity: LD_{50} rats 300 mg/kg iv (Anderson *et al.*, 1934).
Teratogenicity: Cahen (1964).
Preparation: Lewers and Lowry (1925).

19. IMIDOCARB

CARN: 27885-92-3
$C_{19}H_{20}N_6O$ mol. wt. 348.41
N,N'-Bis[3-(4,5-dihydro-*1H*-imidazol-2-yl)phenyl]urea

Preparation: Fischer and Hirt (1965).

Dihydrochloride
$C_{19}H_{22}Cl_2N_6O$ mol. wt. 421.33
Synonyms: imizocarb; 4A65.

Solid, m.p. 350°C (dec).

Toxicity: LD_{50} mice 107 mg/kg sc; LD_{50} rats 150 mg/kg sc (Beveridge, 1969).

Dipropionate

$C_{25}H_{32}N_6O_7$ mol. wt. 528.57

Synonyms: imizol; Imizad Equine Injection.

20. NICARBAZIN

CARN: 330-95-0

$C_{19}H_{18}N_6O_6$ mol. wt. 426.38

N,N'-Bis(4-nitrophenyl)urea, compound with 4,6-dimethyl-2(*1H*)-pyrimidone

Synonyms: 4,4'-dinitrocarbanilide compound with 4,6-dimethyl-2-pyrimidinol; Nicarb; Nicoxin; Nicrazin.

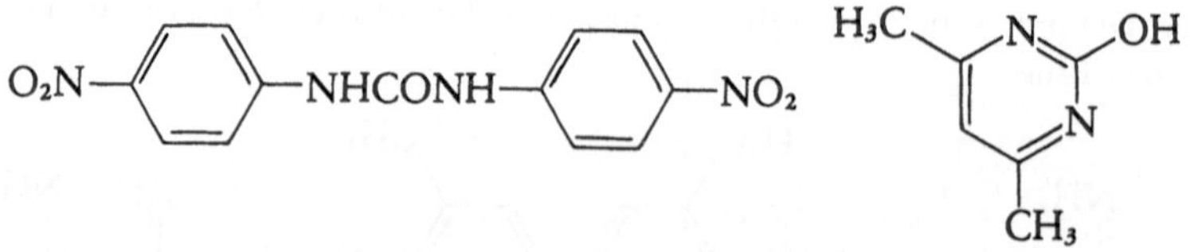

Crystals, dec. 265–275°C; uv max (conc. H_2SO_4) 298 nm ($A_{1cm}^{1\%}$ 670); complex slowly dec. by trituration with H_2O, or more rapidly with dil. aq. acids; dry crystals are strongly electrostatic and present some dry mixing problems.

Solubility: practically insol. H_2O.

Preparation: Cuckler *et al.* (1955).

21. QUINURONIUM SULFATE

$C_{23}H_{26}N_4O_9S_2$ mol. wt. 566.61

1,3-Di-6-quinolylurea bismethosulfate

Synonyms: SN 5870; Acaprin; Zothelone; Baburan; Pirevan; Pyroplasmin; Atral.

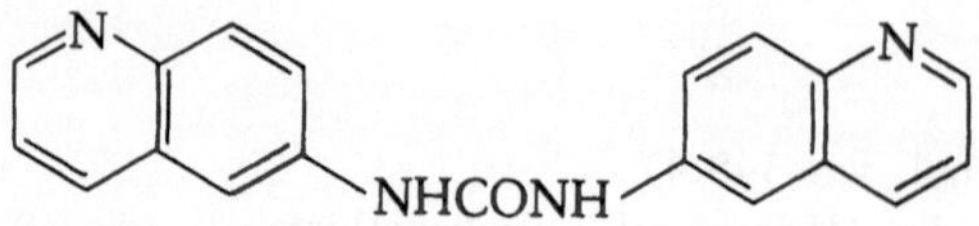

Yellow crystals from methanol, dec. 237°C.

Solubility: freely soluble in H_2O.

Free base

CARN: 532-05-8

$C_{19}H_{14}N_4O$ mol. wt. 314.33

1,3-Di-6-quinolylurea

Synonym: Babesan.

Crystals from pyridine, m.p. 262°C.

Solubility: sol. in dil. acid.

Preparation: Schönhöfer and Henecka (1933); Haskelberg (1947).

22. AMICARBALIDE

CARN: 3459-96-9
$C_{15}H_{16}N_6O$ mol. wt. 296.34
3,3'-(Carbonyldiimino)bisbenzenecarboximidamide
Synonyms: N,N'-di(m-amidinophenyl)urea.

Diisethionate
$C_{19}H_{28}N_6O_9S_2$ mol. wt. 548.56
Synonyms: M & B 5062A; Diampron.
Crystals, m.p. 209°C, dec. 256°C.
Solubility: approx. 1 g/ml H_2O.
Toxicity: LD_{50} mice 120 mg/kg sc (Windholz *et al.*, 1983)
Preparation: Ashley *et al.* (1960).

23. PHENAMIDINE

CARN: 620-90-6
$C_{18}H_{26}N_4O_9S_2$ mol. wt. 506.57
4,4'-Oxydibenzamidine diisethionate
Synonyms: phenamidine isethionate.

Crystals, m.p. 225°C (with dec.).
Solubility: 1 part in 1.4 parts H_2O; 1 part in 300 parts C_2H_5OH; practically insol.
   $(C_2H_5)_2O$, $CHCl_3$.

Free base
CARN: 101-62-2
$C_{14}H_{14}N_4O$ mol. wt. 254.29
m.p. 201–202°C.
Preparation: Newberry and Easson (1946a); Slack *et al.* (1946).

24. STILBAMIDINE

CARN: 3784-99-4
$C_{20}H_{28}N_4O_8S_2$ mol. wt. 516.59
2-Hydroxyethanesulfonic acid compound with 4,4-(1,2-ethenediyl)bis(benzenecarb-
   oximidamide) (2 : 1)

Synonyms: stilbamidine isethionate; stilbamidine diisethionate; 4,4'-stilbenedicarbox-
amidine; M & B 744; stilbemidine isethionate.

$$H_2N \diagdown C - \diag<\diagright> - CH = CH - \diagleft\diagright> - C \diagup NH_2 \bullet 2HOCH_2CH_2SO_3H$$

Crystals, dec. 290°C, discolored by light; uv max: 330 nm ($E_{1cm}^{1\%}$ 750); neutral or
alkaline solutions are unstable, thermal stability of aq. solns. depends on pH;
solutions can be sterilized by brief autoclaving if pH is not too high.
Solubility: approx. 1 g in 2.5–3 ml H_2O (pH of 0.5% aq. soln. = 5.5–6.5); 1.5 g/100
ml CH_3OH.
Preparation: Ashley *et al.* (1942).
Review: Festy (1979).

25. DIMINAZENE

CARN: 908-54-3
$C_{22}H_{29}N_9O_6$ mol. wt. 515.54
N-Acetylglycine compound with 4,4'-(diazoamino)dibenzamidine
Synonyms: diminazene aceturate; diminazene diaceturate; Azidin; Ganasag; Berenil.

$$H_2N - C - \diagup\diagdown - NHN = NH - \diagup\diagdown - C - NH_2 \bullet 2(HOOCCH_2NHC - CH_3)$$

Yellow solid, dec. 217°C.
Solubility: sol. in 14 parts H_2O (20°C); sl. sol. C_2H_5OH; very sl. sol. $(C_2H_5)_2O$,
$CHCl_3$.

Dilactate
$C_{20}H_{27}N_7O_6$ mol. wt. 461.48
Synonym: Babesin.
Preparation: Brodersen *et al.* (1958).
Review: Newton (1975).

26. PENTAMIDINE

CARN: 140-64-7
$C_{23}H_{36}N_4O_{10}S_2$ mol. wt. 592.68
4,4'-(Pentamethylenedioxy)dibenzamidine bis(2-hydroxyethanesulfonate)
Synonyms: pentamidine isethionate; 4,4'-diamidinodiphenoxypentane; M & B 800; RP
2512; Lomidine.

$$\underset{NH_2}{\overset{NH}{C}} - \diagup\diagdown - OCH_2(CH_2)_3CH_2O - \diagup\diagdown - \underset{NH_2}{\overset{NH}{C}} \bullet 2 \underset{CH_2SO_3H}{\overset{CH_2OH}{|}}$$

Hygroscopic, very bitter crystals, m.p. about 180°C; slight butyric odor.

Solubility: sol. in about 10 parts H_2O (25°C), in about 4 parts H_2O (100°C) (pH of a 5% w/v aq. soln. = 4.5–6.5); sol. in glycerol, more readily on warming; sl. sol. C_2H_5OH; insol. $(C_2H_5)_2O$, $(CH_3)_2CO$, $CHCl_3$, liq. petroleum.

Preparation: Newberry and Easson (1946*b*)

27. ROBENIDINE

CARN: 25875-51-8
$C_{15}H_{13}Cl_2N_5$ mol. wt. 334.21
1,3-Bis[(4-chlorobenzylidene)amino]guanidine

Hydrochloride

$C_{15}H_{14}Cl_3N_5$ mol. wt. 370.67
Synonyms: robenzidene; Cycostat; Robenz.
Crystals from C_2H_5OH, m.p. 289–290°C.
Preparation: Tomcufcik (1970).
Metabolism: Zulalian *et al.* (1972*a,b*).

28. DAPSONE

CARN: 80-08-0
$C_{12}H_{12}N_2O_2S$ mol. wt. 248.30
4,4'-Sulfonylbisbenzeneamine
Synonyms: 4,4'-sulfonyldianiline; bis(4-aminophenyl)sulfone; DDS, diaphenylsulfone; DADPS; 1358F; Dumitone; Avlosulphone; Sulfona-Mae; Croysulfone; Croysulphone; Sulphadione; Avlosulfon; Eporal; Diphone; Novophone; Diphenasone; Udolac.

Crystals from 95% C_2H_5OH, m.p. 175–176°C (also a higher melting form, m.p. 180.5°C); pK_b 13.0.
Solubility: Sol. CH_3OH, C_2H_5OH, $(CH_3)_2CO$, dil. hydrochloric acid; practically insol. H_2O.
Mechanism of toxic action: Wu and DuBois (1970).
Preparation: Ferry *et al.* (1955).
Review: Orzech *et al.* (1976).

29. ACEDAPSONE

CARN: 77-46-3
$C_{16}H_{16}N_2O_4S$ mol. wt. 332.37

4,4'-Sulfonylbis(acetanilide)

Synonyms: bis(4-acetamidophenyl)sulfone; DADDS; diacetyldapsone; sulfadiamine; 1399F; CI 556; Hansolar; Rodilone.

$$CH_3CONH-\!\!\!\bigcirc\!\!\!-SO_2-\!\!\!\bigcirc\!\!\!-NHCOCH_3$$

Crystalline solid, m.p. 289–292°C; uv max (CH_3OH) 256, 284 nm (ϵ 25500, 36200).
Solubility: 0.003 mg/ml H_2O; 0.026 mg/ml in benzyl benzoate–castor oil (2 : 3).
Preparation: Fromm and Wittmann (1908); Raiziss *et al.* (1939).

30. CHLORGUANIDE

CARN: 500-92-5
$C_{11}H_{16}ClN_5$ mol. wt. 253.75
N-(4-Chlorophenyl)-*N'*-(1-methylethyl)imidodicarbonimidic diamide
Synonyms: 1-(*p*-chlorophenyl)-5-isopropylbiguanide; chloroguanide; M 4888; RP 3359; SN 12837; Diguanyl; Drinupal; Guanatol; Palusil; Proguanil; Tirian.

$$Cl-\!\!\!\bigcirc\!\!\!-\overset{\overset{NH}{\|}}{NHCNHCNHCH(CH_3)_2}$$

Rectangular plates from toluene, m.p. 129°C.
Metabolism: converted to cycloguanil (Carrington *et al.*, 1951).
Preparation: Curd and Rose (1946).

Acetate
$C_{13}H_{20}ClN_5O_2$ mol. wt. 313.79
Crystals from $(CH_3)_2CO$, m.p. 189–190°C.
Preparation: Gailliot (1952)

Hydrochloride
$C_{11}H_{17}Cl_2H_5$ mol. wt. 290.20
Synonym: Paludrin.
Crystals from H_2O or C_2H_5OH, m.p. 243–244°C; uv max (C_2H_5OH): 259 nm.
Solubility: sol. C_2H_5OH; sl. sol. H_2O (pH of satd. soln. = 5.8–6.3); practically insol. $CHCl_3$ and $(C_2H_5)_2O$.
Toxicity: LD_{50} rats 200 mg/kg po (Schmidt *et al.*, 1947).

31. CHLORPROGUANIL

CARN: 537-21-3
$C_{11}H_{15}Cl_2N_5$ mol. wt. 288.18
N-(3,4-Dichlorophenyl)-*N'*-(1-methylethyl)imidocarbonimidic diamide
Synonyms: 1-(3,4-dichlorophenyl)-5-isopropylbiguanide; M5943.

Preparation: Crowther *et al.* (1951).

Hydrochloride
$C_{11}H_{16}Cl_3N_5$ mol. wt. 324.64
Synonym: Lapudrine.
Crystals, m.p. 246–247°C.
Solubility: 1 g/100 ml H_2O; solutions may be boiled without dec.

32. CYCLOGUANIL

CARN: 516-21-2
$C_{11}H_{14}ClN_5$ mol. wt. 251.73
1-(4-Chlorophenyl)-1,6-dihydro-6,6-dimethyl-1,3,5-triazine-2,4-diamine
Synonyms: 4,6-diamino-1-(*p*-chlorophenyl)-1,2-dihydro-2,2-dimethyl-*s*-triazine; chlorazine; chlorguanide triazine; TCl; 10,580; M 10580; D-20.

Prisms from $CHCl_3$ + $(C_2H_5)_2O$, m.p. 146°C; uv max (H_2O): 241 nm (ϵ 12900).
Preparation: Modest *et al.* (1952); Modest (1956).

Hydrochloride
$C_{11}H_{15}Cl_2N_5$ mol. wt. 288.18
Prisms from H_2O, m.p. 210–215°C; uv max (H_2O): 241 nm (ϵ 13200).

Dihydrochloride
$C_{11}H_{16}Cl_3N_5$ mol. wt. 324.64
Crystals from $(CH_3)_2CO$, m.p. 190–196°C.

Pamoate
$C_{45}H_{44}Cl_2N_{10}O_6$ mol. wt. 891.82
Synonyms: cycloguanil embonate; CI-501; Camolar.
Yellow crystals, m.p. 231–234°C.
Solubility: sol. H_2O 0.003%.

33. DINITOLMIDE

CARN: 148-01-6

$C_8H_7N_3O_5$ mol. wt. 225.16

2-Methyl-3,5-dinitrobenzamide

Synonyms: 3,5-dinitro-*o*-toluamide; Zoalene; Zoamix.

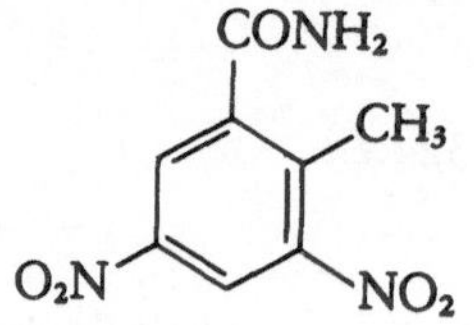

Crystals from dil. C_2H_5OH, m.p. 181°C.

Metabolism: Smith *et al.* (1963); Smith (1964).

Preparation: McGookin *et al.* (1940).

34. ETHOPABATE

CARN: 59-06-3

$C_{12}H_{15}NO_4$ mol. wt. 237.25

4-Acetamido-2-ethoxybenzoic acid methyl ester

Synonyms: methyl 4-acetamido-2-ethoxybenzoate; ethyl pabate; Amprol Plus (when mixed with amprolium, *q.v.*).

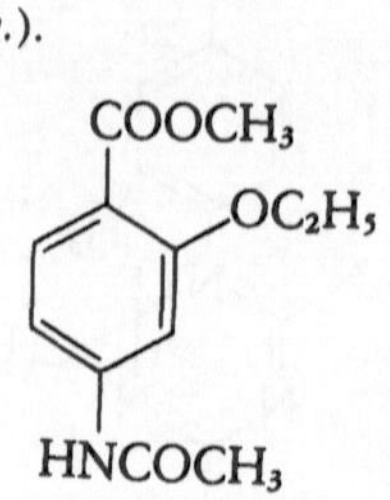

White to pinkish-white, practically odorless crystals from CH_3OH and H_2O, m.p. 148–149°C; uv max (CH_3OH): 298, 267 nm ($A_{1\ cm}^{1\%}$ 805, 365).

Solubility: sol. CH_3OH, C_2H_5OH, $(CH_3)_2CO$, CH_3CN; sparingly sol. isopropanol, *p*-dioxane, $CH_3CO_2C_2H_5$, CH_2Cl_2; very sl. sol. H_2O and isooctane.

Metabolism: in chickens (Buhs *et al.*, 1966).

Preparation: Grimme and Schmitz (1954).

35. DILOXANIDE

CARN: 579-3804

$C_9H_9Cl_2NO_2$ mol. wt. 234.09

2,2-Dichloro-*N*-(4-hydroxyphenyl)-*N*-methylacetamide

Synonyms: 2,2-dichloro-4'-hydroxy-*N*-methylacetanilide; Entamide; Ame-Boots.

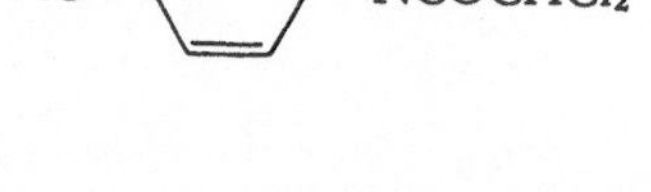

Crystals from $CH_3CO_2C_2H_5$, m.p. 175°C.
Preparation: Oxley *et al.* (1959).

Furoate
$C_{14}H_{11}Cl_2NO_5$ mol. wt. 344.15
Synonyms: diloxanide 2-furoic acid ester; Furamide (*do not confuse with the amide of furoic acid*); Histomibal; Miforon.

36. MENOCTONE

CARN: 14561-42-3
$C_{24}H_{32}O_3$ mol. wt. 368.52
2-(8-Cyclohexyloctyl)-3-hydroxy-1,4-naphthoquinone
Synonyms: Win 11,530; WR 49808; Menocton.

Crystals from CH_3OH, m.p. 79–80°C.
Preparation: Fieser *et al.* (1967).
Review: Hudson (1984).

37. TETRACYCLINE

CARN: 60-54-8
$C_{22}H_{24}N_2O_8$ mol. wt. 444.43
4-(Dimethylamino)-1,4,4a,5,5a,6,11,12a-octahydro-3,6,10,12,12a-pentahydroxy-6-methyl-1,11-dioxo-2-naphthacenecarboxamide
Synonyms: deschlorobiomycin; tsiklomitsin; Abricycline; Achromycin; Agromicina; Ambramicina; Ambramycin; Bio-Tetra; Bristaciclina; Cefracycline suspension; Criseociclina; Cyclomycin; Democracin; Hostacyclin; Omegamycin; Panmycin; Polycycline; Purocyclina; Sanclomycine; Steclin; Tetrabon; Tetracyn; Tetradecin.

Trihydrate (mol. wt. 498.49), crystals, dec. 170–175°C (swells at 165°C), becomes anhydrous by drying *in vacuo* at 60°C for 8 hr; $[\alpha]_D^{25}$ −257.9° (0.1 N HCl), $[\alpha]_D^{25}$ −239° (CH_3OH); uv max (0.1 N HCl): 220, 268, 355 nm (ϵ 13000, 18040, 13320); pK$_a$ (50% aq. DMF): 8.3, 10.2; stable in neutral and alkaline soln.

Solubility: at about 28°C, 1.7 mg/ml H_2O and >20 mg/ml CH_3OH; for solubility
   studies, see Weiss *et al.* (1957).
Toxicity: LD_{50} rats 807 mg/kg po; LD_{50} mice 808 mg/kg po (Goldenthal, 1971).
Mechanism of action: Kaji and Ryoji (1979).
Preparation: Boothe *et al.* (1953).
Total synthesis: Boothe *et al.* (1959); Conover *et al.* (1962).
Review: Evans (1968).

Hydrochloride

$C_{22}H_{25}ClN_2O_8$ mol. wt. 480.91

Synonyms: Achro; Achromycin V; Ala Tet; Ambracyn; Artomycin; Cefracycline tablets;
   Cyclopar; Diacycline; Dumocyclin; Mephacyclin; Partex; Quadracycline; Quatrex;
   Remicyclin; Ricycline; Stilciclina; Subamycin; Supramycin; Sustamycin; Tefilin;
   Teline; Telotrex; Tetrabakat; Tetrabid; Tetrablet; Tetrachel; Tetracompren;
   Tetra-D; Tetrakap; Tetralution; Tetramavan; Tetramycin; Tetrasol; Tetra-Wedel;
   Topicycline; Totomycin; Triphacyclin; Unicin; Unimycin; Vetquamycin-324.
Crystals from butanol + HCl, dec. 214°C; $[\alpha]_D^{25}$ −257.9° (c = 0.5 in 0.1 N HCl).
Solubility: freely sol. H_2O (pH 2% aq. soln. = 2.1–2.3); sol. CH_3OH, C_2H_5OH;
   insol. $(C_2H_5)_2O_9$ hydrocarbons.
Toxicity: LD_{50} rats 6443 mg/kg po (Goldenthal, 1971).

38. OXYTETRACYCLINE

CARN: 79-57-2
$C_{22}H_{24}N_2O_9$ mol. wt. 460.44
4-(Dimethylamino)-1,4,4a,5,5a,6,11,12a-octahydro-3,5,6,10,12,12a-hexahy-
   droxy-6-methyl-1,11-dioxo-2-naphthacenecarboxamide
Synonyms: glomycin; terrafungine; riomitsin; hydroxytetracycline; Berkmycin; Biostat;
   Imperacin (tablets); Oxacyclin; Oxatets; Oxydon; Oxy-Dumocyclin; Oxymycin;
   Oxypan; Oxytetracid; Ryomycin; Stevacin; Terraject; Terramycin; Tetramel;
   Tetran; Vendarcin; Vendracin.

Oxytetracycline crystals shows no potency loss on heating for 4 days at 100°C.
Isolation: Regna and Solomons (1950); Regna *et al.* (1951).
Total synthesis: Muxfeldt *et al.* (1979).

Dihydrate

Synonyms: Abbocin; Clinimycin.
Needles from H_2O or CH_3OH, dec. 181–182°C; $[\alpha]_D^{25}$ −196.6° (0.1 N HCl), $[\alpha]_D^{25}$

$-2.1°$ (0.1 N NaOH), $[\alpha]_D^{25}$ $+26.5°$ (CH_3OH); uv max (pH 4.5 phosphate buffer 0.1 M): 249, 276, 353 nm ($E_{1cm}^{1\%}$ 240, 322, 301).

Solubility: in H_2O varies with pH; abs. C_2H_5OH 12 mg/ml, 95% C_2H_5OH 0.2 mg/ml; for additional solubility data, see Weiss *et al.* (1957).

Hydrochloride

$C_{22}H_{25}ClN_2O_9$ mol. wt. 496.91

Synonyms: Aquacycline; Arcospectron; Bio-Mycin; Duphacycline; Geomycin; Gynamousse; Imperacin (capsuls); Macocyn; Macodyn; Occrycetin; Oxlopar; Oxybiocyclin; Oxybiotic; Oxycycline; Oxyject; Stecsolin; Tetra-Tablinen; Toxinal.

Yellow platelets from H_2O.

Solubility: very sol. H_2O (1 g/ml), conc. aq. solns. at neutral pH hydrolyze on standing and deposit crystals of oxytetracycline; sol. abs. C_2H_5OH 12 mg/ml, 95% C_2H_5OH 33 mg/ml; for additional solubility data, see Weiss *et al.* (1957).

Disodium salt dihydrate

$C_{22}H_{26}N_2Na_2O_{11}$ mol. wt. 540.44

Yellow crystals, darkens on standing; aq. solns. soon lose potency.

Solubility: CH_3OH 1.5 mg/ml; abs. C_2H_5OH 8 mg/ml.

39. CHLORTETRACYCLINE

CARN: 57-62-5

$C_{22}H_{23}ClN_2O_8$ mol. wt. 478.88

7-Chloro-4-dimethylamino-1,4,4a,5,5a,6,11,12a-octahydro-3,6,10,12,12a-pentahydroxy-6-methyl-1,11-dioxo-2-naphthacenecarboxamide

Synonyms: 7-chlorotetracycline; Acronize; Aureocina; Aureomycin; Biomitsin; Biomycin; Chrysomykine.

Golden-yellow crystals, m.p. 168–169°C; $[\alpha]_D^{25}$ $-275.0°$ (CH_3OH); uv max (0.1 N HCl): 230, 262.5, 367.5 nm; uv max (0.1 N NaOH): 255, 285, 345 nm.

Solubility: 0.5–0.6 g/ml H_2O, very sol. in aq. solns. above pH 8.5; freely sol. Cellosolves, dioxane, Carbitol; sl. sol. CH_3OH, C_2H_5OH, butanol, $(CH_3)_2CO$, $CH_3CO_2C_2H_5$, C_6H_6; practically insol. $(C_2H_5)_2O$, petroleum ether.

Isolation: Duggar (1948).

Review: Schwartzman *et al.* (1979).

Hydrochloride

$C_{22}H_{24}Cl_2N_2O_8$ mol. wt. 515.35

Synonyms: Aureociclina; Isphamycin.

Bitter, yellow rhomboid crystals, dec above 210°C; $[\alpha]_D^{23}$ −240°.

Solubility: 8.6 mg/ml H_2O (pH sat. aq. soln. = 2.8–2.9); 17.4 mg/ml CH_3OH; 1.7 mg/ml C_2H_5OH; sol. in solns. of alkali hydroxides and carbonates; practically insol. $(CH_3)_2CO$, $(C_2H_5)_2O$, $CHCl_3$, dioxane.

Toxicity: LD_{50} rats 10.3 g/kg po (Goldenthal, 1971).

40. DOXYCYCLINE

CARN: 564-25-0

$C_{22}H_{24}N_2O_8 \cdot H_2O$ mol. wt. 462.46

4-(Dimethylamino)-1,4,4*a*,5,5*a*,6,9,11,12*a*-octahydro-3,5,10,12,12*a*-pentahydroxy-6-methyl-1,11-dioxo-2-naphthacenecarboxamide monohydrate

Synonyms: α-6-deoxy-5-hydroxytetracycline monohydrate; GS-3065; Doxitard; Liviatin; Vibramycin; Vibravenös.

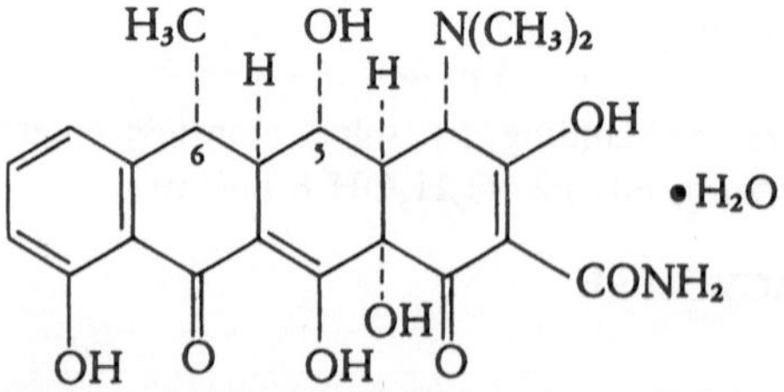

Pharmacology: Fabre *et al.* (1966); Gibaldi (1967).

Preparation: von Wittenau *et al.* (1962).

Review: Edwards (1979).

Hydrochloride

$C_{22}H_{25}ClN_2O_8$ mol. wt. 480.91

Synonyms: doxycycline hyclate; Vibramycin Hyclate; Doxy-II (caps); Doxy-Tablinen; Vibra-Tabs; Retens; Liomycin; Ecodox; Novadox; Midoxin; Samecin; Vibradox; Nivocilin; Tanamicin; Tetradox; Hydramycin; Dixigalumicina; Tecacin; Mespafin; Roximycin.

Light yellow powder that crystallizes from C_2H_5OH + HCl as the hemihydrate hemialcoholate, chars without melting at about 201°C, the C_2H_5OH and H_2O of crystallization are lost by drying at 100°C under reduced pressure; $[\alpha]_D^{25}$ − 110° (*c* = 1 [0.01 N methanolic HCl]); uv max (0.01 N methanolic HCl): 267, 351 nm (ε 17400, 13200).

Toxicity: LD_{50} rats 262 mg/kg ip (Goldenthal, 1971).

41. CLOPIDOL

CARN: 2971-90-6

C_7H_7NO mol. wt. 192.06

3,5-Dichloro-2,6-dimethyl-4-pyridinol

Synonyms: meticlorpindol; clopidol; Coyden.

Solid, m.p. >320°C.
Solubility: practically insol. H_2O.
Toxicity: LD_{50} rats 18 g/kg po (Plisek *et al.*, 1971).
Metabolism: in chickens (Smith, 1969); in rats (Smith and Watson, 1969).
Preparation: Stevenson (1965).

42. QUININE

CARN: 130-95-0
$C_{20}H_{24}N_2O_2$ mol. wt. 324.41
6'-Methoxycinchonan-9-ol
Synonyms: 6-methoxy-α-(5-vinyl-2-quinuclidinyl)-4-quinolinemethanol.

Triboluminescent, orthorhombic needles from abs. C_2H_5OH, m.p. 177°C (some dec.); sublimes in high vacuum at 170–180°C; $[\alpha]_D^{15} -169°$ (c = 2 [97% C_2H_5OH]), $[\alpha]_D^{17} -117°$ (c = 1.5 [$CHCl_3$]), $[\alpha]_D^{15} -285°$ (c = 0.4 M [0.1 N H_2SO_4]); pK_1 = 5.07 (at 18°C), pK_2 = 9.7; the blue fluorescence is particularly strong in dil. H_2SO_4 (Rabe and Marschall, 1911).
Solubility: 1 g dissolves in 1900 ml H_2O (pH of a sat. aq. soln. = 8.8), 760 ml boiling H_2O, 0.8 ml C_2H_5OH, 80 ml C_6H_6 (18 ml C_6H_6 at 50°C), 250 ml dry $(C_2H_5)_2O$, 1.2 ml $CHCl_3$, 20 ml glycerol, 1900 ml of 10% ammonia water; almost insol. in petroleum ether.
Total synthesis: Woodward and Doering (1944).
Review: Hahn (1979).

Trihydrate
Microcrystalline powder, m.p. 57°C; effluorescent; loses 1 H_2O in air, 2 H_2O over H_2SO_4, anhydr. at 125°C.

43. CHLOROQUINE

CARN: 54-05-7

$C_{18}H_{26}ClN_3$ mol. wt. 319.89

N^4-(7-Chloro-4-quinolinyl)-N,N'-diethyl-1,4-pentanediamine

Synonyms: 7-chloro-4-(4-diethylamino-1-methylbutylamino)quinoline; SN7618; RP 3377; Aralen; Nivaquine B; Sanoquin; Artrichin; Bipiquin; Reumachlor; Bemaphate; Résoquine.

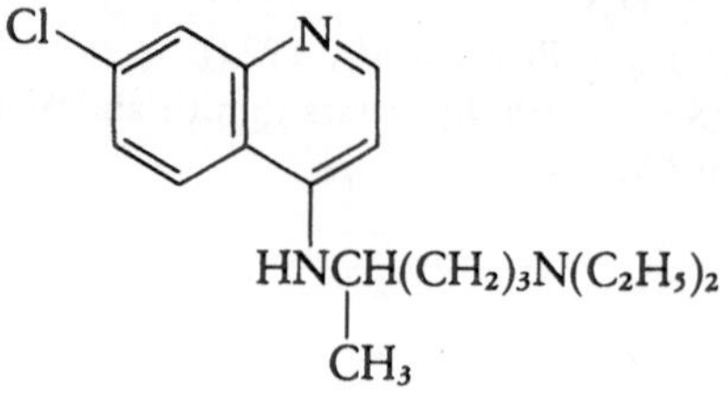

$$Cl—\underset{\underset{CH_3}{|}}{HNCH}(CH_2)_3N(C_2H_5)_2$$

m.p. 87°C.

Preparation: Surrey and Hammer (1946).

Review: Hahn (1975); Hong (1976).

Diphosphate

$C_{18}H_{32}ClN_3O_8P_2$ mol. wt. 515.87

Synonyms: Arechin; Avloclor; Imagon; Malaquin; Resochin; Silbesan; Tresochin.

Bitter, colorless crystals, dimorphic m.p. 193–195°C and 215–218°C; stable to heat in solns. of pH 4.0–6.5.

Solubility: freely soluble in H_2O (pH of 1% aq. soln. = about 4.5); less sol. at neutral and alkaline pH; practically insol. C_2H_5OH, C_6H_6, $CHCl_3$, $(C_2H_5)_2O$.

Sulfate

$C_{18}H_{28}ClN_3O_4S$ mol. wt. 417.96

Synonym: Nivaquine.

44. HYDROXYCHLOROQUIN

CARN: 118-42-3

$C_{18}H_{26}ClN_3O$ mol. wt. 335.87

2-[(4-[(7-Chloro-4-quinolinyl)amino]pentyl)ethylamino]ethanol

Synonyms: 7-chloro-4-(4-[ethyl(2-hydroxyethyl)amino]-1-methylbutylamino)quinoline; oxychloroquin; oxichlorochine.

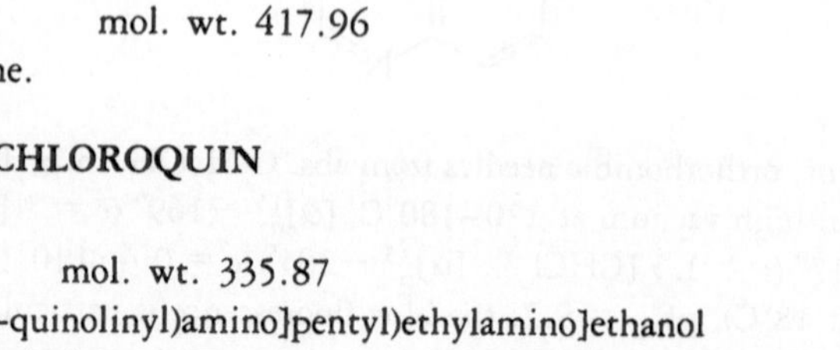

$$Cl—\underset{\underset{CH_3}{|}}{HNCH}CH_2CH_2CH_2N\overset{\displaystyle CH_2CH_2OH}{\underset{\displaystyle CH_2CH_3}{}}$$

Crystals from ethylene dichloride and Skellysolve B, m.p. 89–91°C.

Preparation: Surrey and Hammer (1950).

Sulfate

$C_{18}H_{28}ClN_3O_5S$ mol. wt. 433.96

Synonyms: Ercoquin; Plaquenil Sulfate; Quensyl.

Odorless, bitter, white crystalline powder, exists in two forms: m.p. about 240°C and m.p. about 198°C.

Solubility: freely soluble in H_2O (pH of aq. solns. = about 4.5); practically insol. C_2H_5OH, $CHCl_3$, $(C_2H_5O)_2O$.

45. PRIMAQUINE

CARN: 90-34-6

$C_{15}H_{21}N_3O$ mol. wt. 259.34

N^4-(6-methoxy-8-quinolinyl)-1,4-pentanediamine

Synonyms: 8-(4-amino-1-methylbutylamino)-6-methoxyquinoline; SN 13272

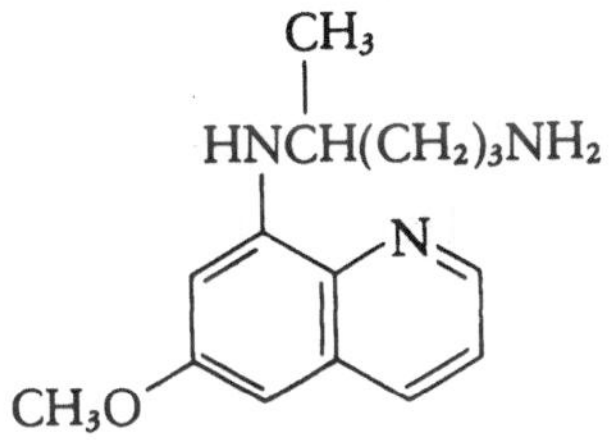

Viscous liquid, b.p.$_{0.2}$ 175–179°C.

Solubility: sol. in $(C_2H_5)_2O$.

Preparation: Elderfield *et al.* (1946).

Review: Olenick (1975*b*).

Diphosphate

$C_{15}H_{27}N_3O_9P_2$ mol. wt. 455.34

Yellow crystals from 90% C_2H_5OH, m.p. 197–198°C.

Solubility: mod. sol. H_2O.

46. AMODIAQUIN

CARN: 86-42-0

$C_{20}H_{22}ClN_3O$ mol. wt. 355.86

4-[(7-Chloro-4-quinolinyl)amino]-2-[(diethylamino)methyl]phenol

Synonyms: 4-[(7-chloro-4-quinolinyl)amino]-α-(diethylamino)-*o*-cresol; SN 10751.

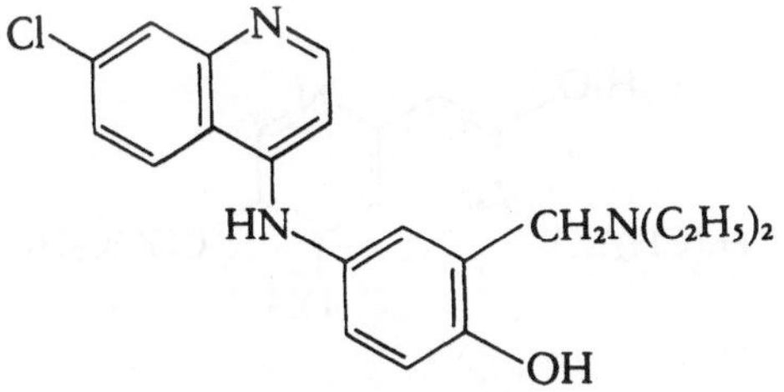

Crystals from Cellosolve, m.p. 208°C.
Preparation: Burckhalter *et al.* (1948).

Dihydrochloride dihydrate
$C_{20}H_{28}Cl_3N_3O_3$ mol. wt. 464.82
Synonyms: CAM-AQl; Camoquin; Flavoquin; Miaquin.
Yellow, bitter crystals, dec. 150–160°C; uv max: 224, 342 nm ($E_{1\ cm}^{1\%}$ 394–410).
Solubility: sol. in H_2O (pH of a 1% aq. soln. = 4.0–4.8); sparingly sol. C_2H_5OH; very
    sl. sol. C_6H_6, $CHCl_3$, $(C_2H_5)_2O$.

47. MEFLOQUIN

CARN: 49752-90-1
$C_{17}H_{16}F_6N_2O$ mol. wt. 378.32
α-(2-Piperidinyl)-2,8-bis(trifluoromethyl)-4-quinolinemethanol
Synonym: Ro 21-5998.

Hydrochloride
$C_{17}H_{17}ClF_6N_2O$ mol. wt. 414.78
Crystals from CH_3CN, m.p. 259–260°C (dec.); uv max (CH_3OH): 283, 304, 318 nm.
Metabolism: rat (Jauch *et al.*, 1980).
Preparation: Ohnmacht *et al.* (1971).

48. DECOQUINATE

CARN: 18507-89-6
$C_{24}H_{35}NO_5$ mol. wt. 417.53
6-Decyloxy-7-ethoxy-4-hydroxy-3-quinolinecarboxylic acid ethyl ester
Synonyms: ethyl 6-(*n*-decyloxy)-7-ethoxy-4-hydroxyquinoline-3-carboxylate; M & B
    15497; Deccox.

Metabolism: Craine *et al.* (1971); Kouba *et al.* (1971).

Description: Ball *et al.* (1968).

49. BUQUINOLATE

CARN: 5486-03-3

$C_{20}H_{27}NO_5$ mol. wt. 361.42

4-Hydroxy-6,7-bis(methylpropoxy)-3-quinolinecarboxylic acid ethyl ester

Synonyms: 4-hydroxy-6,7-diisobutoxy-3-quinolinecarboxylic acid ethyl ester; ethyl 6,7-diisobutoxy-4-hydroxyquinoline-3-carboxylate; Bonaid.

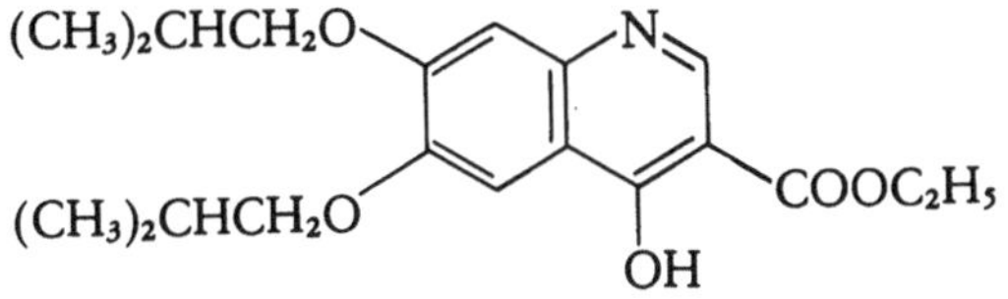

Crystals, m.p. 288–291°C.

Preparation: Watson (1965).

50. OXYQUINOLINE

CARN: 148-24-3

C_9H_7NO mol. wt. 145.15

8-Hydroxyquinoline.

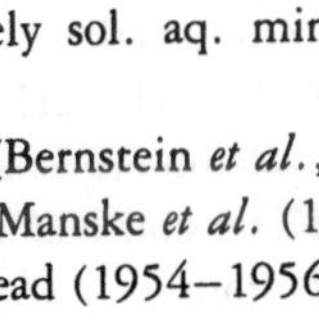

White crystals or crystalline powder, m.p. 76°C, b.p. approx. 267°C.

Solubility: almost insol. H_2O; freely sol. aq. mineral acids, C_2H_5OH, $(CH_3)_2CO$, $CHCl_3$, C_6H_6.

Toxicity: LD_{50} mice 48 mg/kg ip (Bernstein *et al.*, 1963).

Preparation: Skraup (1880, 1882); Manske *et al.* (1949).

Review: Phillips (1956); Hollingshead (1954–1956).

51. IODOQUINOL

CARN: 83-73-8

$C_9H_5I_2NO$ mol. wt. 396.98

5,7-Diiodo-9-quinolinol

Synonyms: 5,7-diiodo-8-hydroxyquinoline; SS 578; Diodoquin; Di-Quinol; Disoquin; Floraquin; Dyodin; Dinoleine; Searlequin; Diodoxylin; Moebiquin; Rafembin; Ioquin; Direxiode; Stanquinate; Quinadome; Yodoxin; Zoaquin; Enterosept; Embequin.

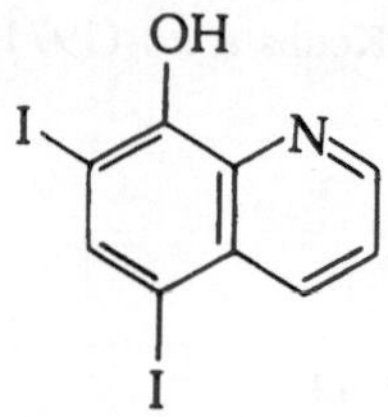

Crystals from xylene, medicinal grade is a yellowish-brown powder, m.p. 200–215°C (extensive dec.).

Solubility: almost insol. H_2O; sparingly sol. C_2H_5OH, $(C_2H_5)_2O$, $(CH_3)_2CO$; sol. hot pyridine, hot dioxane.

Preparation: Papesch and Burtner (1936).

52. EMETINE

CARN: 483-18-1

$C_{29}H_{40}N_2O_4$ mol. wt. 480.63

$6',7',10,11$-Tetramethoxyemetan

Synonym: cephaeline methyl ether.

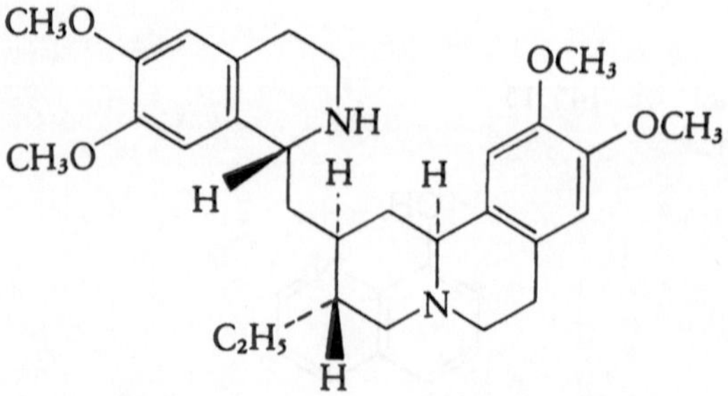

White, amorphous powder, m.p. 74°C; turns yellow on exposure to light and heat; $[\alpha]_D^{20}$ −50° (c = 2 [$CHCl_3$]); strong alkaline reaction, pK_1 5.77, pK_2 6.64.

Solubility: freely soluble in CH_3OH, C_2H_5OH, $(CH_3)_2CO$, $CH_3CO_2C_2H_5$, $(C_2H_5)_2O$, $CHCl_3$; sparingly sol. H_2O, petroleum ether; mod. sol. dil. ammonium hydroxide; sparingly sol. in solns. of KOH and NaOH.

Toxicity: LD_{50} rats 12.1 mg/kg ip (Radomski *et al.*, 1952).

Total synthesis: Evstigneeva *et al.* (1950); Van Tamelen *et al.* (1969).

Review: Grollman and Jarkovsky (1975).

Hydrochloride

CARN: 316-42-7

$C_{29}H_{42}Cl_2N_2O_4$ mol. wt. 553.56

Emetine dihydrochloride.

Contains 3–8 H_2O of crystallization; clusters of needles after drying at 105°C have m.p. 235–255°C (dec.); $[\alpha]_D$ +11° (c = 1) to $[\alpha]_D$ +21° (c = 8) calculated for anhydrous salt; solid and solns. turn yellow on exposure to light or heat.

Solubility: 1 g hydrated salt in about 7 ml H_2O (pH aq. soln. [1 g/50 ml] = 5.6); sol. C_2H_5OH.

Toxicity: LD_{50} mice 32 mg/kg sc, 30 mg/kg po (calculated as base) (Child *et al.*, 1964).

Review: Feyns and Grady (1981).

53. DEHYDROEMETINE

CARN: 4914-30-1
$C_{29}H_{38}N_2O_4$　　　mol. wt. 478.61
2,3-Dehydro-6',7',10,11-tetramethoxyemetan
Synonyms: 2,3-dehydroemetine; 2-dehydroemetine; Mebadin.

Synthesis: Brossi *et al.* (1959); Clark *et al.* (1962).

(±)-2,3-Dehydroemetine hydrochloride
$C_{29}H_{39}ClN_2O_4$　　　mol. wt. 515.10
Crystals from C_2H_5OH + $(C_2H_5)_2O$, m.p. 235°C.
Toxicity: LD_{50} mice 70 mg/kg sc (Windholz *et al.*, 1983).

(−)-2,3-Dehydroemetine
$C_{29}H_{38}N_2O_4$　　　mol. wt. 478.61
Crystals from isopropyl ether, m.p. 94–96°C; $[\alpha]_D$ −183°.

(−)-2,3-Dehydroemetine dihydrobromide
$C_{29}H_{40}Br_2N_2O_4$　　　mol. wt. 643.381
Crystals, m.p. 243–245°C; $[\alpha]_D$ −97° (CH_3OH); uv max (C_2H_5OH): 282 ·nm (ε 7300).
Toxicity: LD_{50} mice 50 mg/kg sc (Windholz *et al.*, 1983).

(+)-2,3-Dehydroemetine dihydrobromide
$C_{29}H_{40}Br_2N_2O_4$　　　mol. wt. 643.381
Crystals, m.p. 241–243°C; $[\alpha]_D$ +95° (CH_3OH); uv max (C_2H_5OH): 282 nm (ε 7350).

(±)-2,3-Dehydroisoemetine hydrochloride
$C_{29}H_{39}ClN_2O_4$　　　mol. wt. 515.10
Crystals from C_2H_5OH + $(C_2H_5)_2O$, m.p. 220–225°C.

(−)-2,3-Dehydroisoemetine dihydrobromide
$C_{29}H_{40}Br_2N_2O_4$　　　mol. wt. 643.381

Crystals, m.p. 257–260°C; $[\alpha]_D$ −107° (CH_3OH); uv max (C_2H_5OH): 285 nm (ϵ 7400).

Toxicity: LD_{50} mice 700 mg/kg sc (Windholz *et al.*, 1983).

(+)-2,3-Dehydroisoemetine Dihydrobromide

$C_{29}H_{40}Br_2N_2O_4$ mol. wt. 643.381

Crystals, m.p. 257–258°C; $[\alpha]_D$ +109° (CH_3OH); uv max (C_2H_5OH): 285 nm (ϵ 7450).

54. QUINACRINE HYDROCHLORIDE

CARN: 69-05-6

$C_{23}H_{32}Cl_3N_3O$ mol. wt. 472.88

N^4-(6-Chloro-2-methoxy-9-acridinyl)-N^1,N^1-diethyl-1,4-pentanediamine dihydrochloride

Synonyms: 6-chloro-9-([4-(diethylamino)-1-methylbutyl]amino)-2-methoxyacridine dihydrochloride; mepacrine hydrochloride; RP 866; SN 390; Atabrine dihydrochloride; Atebrin hydrochloride; Chinacrin hydrochloride; Erion; Acriquine; Acrichine; Palacrin; Metoquin; Italchin.

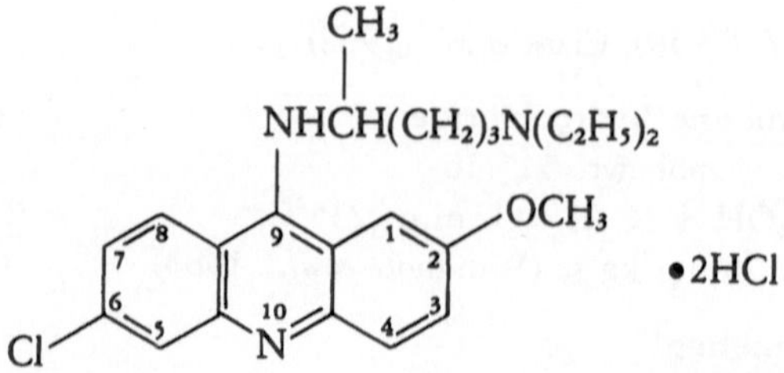

Bitter, bright yellow crystals, dec. 248–250°C (m.p. poorly discernible); under uv light the yellow aq. solns. exhibit vivid fluorescence detectable at 1 : 5,000,000 dilution.

Solubility: 1 g in about 35 ml H_2O, much more sol. in hot H_2O (pH of a 1% aq. soln. = about 4.5); sl. sol. C_2H_5OH; somewhat more sol. CH_3OH; insol. $(C_2H_5)_2O$, C_6H_6, $(CH_3)_2CO$.

Toxicity: LD_{50} mice 7000 mg/kg po (Yamamoto *et al.*, (1973).

Preparation: Stenbuck and Hood (1962); Roth *et al.* (1980*a,b*).

Review: Burchall (1975); Manius (1978).

55. ACRANIL®

CARN: 260-94-6

$C_{21}H_{28}Cl_3N_3O_2$ mol. wt. 460.82

1-[(6-Chloro-2-methoxy-9-acridyl)amino]-3-(diethylamino)-2-propanol dihydrochloride

Synonyms: SKF 16214-A2; SN 186.

$$\text{OH}$$
$$\text{CH}_2\text{CHCH}_2\text{N}(\text{C}_2\text{H}_5)_2$$

(structure of acridine derivative with HN, OCH$_3$, Cl substituents)   • 2HCl

Bitter, yellow crystals, m.p. 237–239°C (dec).
Solubility: sol. H_2O.
Preparation: Mietzsch and Mauss (1934).

Free base
$C_{21}H_{26}ClN_3O_2$ mol. wt. 387.91
Yellow crystals, m.p. 105–107°C.
Solubility: sparingly sol. $(C_2H_5)_2O$.

56. ACRIFLAVINE

CARN: 8048-52-0
mol. formula varies   mol. wt. indefinite
3,6-Diamino-10-methylacridinium chloride mixture with 3,6-acridinediamine
Synonyms: neutral acriflavine; euflavine; trypaflavine; neutroflavine; gonacrine.

(chemical structures: 3,6-diamino-10-methylacridinium cation with Cl⁻, and 3,6-acridinediamine)

Contains 30–40% unmethylated compound; deep orange, granular powder; aq. solns.
   are reddish-orange and fluoresce on dilution.
Solubility: 1 g in about 3 ml H_2O (pH 1% aq. soln. = approx. 3.5); incompletely sol.
   C_2H_5OH; nearly insol. in $(C_2H_5)_2O$, $CHCl_3$, fixed oils.
Preparation: Benda (1912); Gaillot (1934).
Toxicology: Ungar and Robinson (1944).
Review: Adrien (1966); Acheson (1973).

Dihydrochloride
mol. formula varies   mol. wt. indefinite
Synonyms: acid acriflavine; acid trypaflavine; acriflavine hydrochloride; Panflavin.
Deep reddish-brown, crystalline powder; pH 1% aq. soln. = approx. 1.5.

57. PYRIMETHAMINE

CARN: 289-95-2

$C_{12}H_{13}ClN_4$ mol. wt. 248.71

5-(4-Chlorophenyl)-6-ethyl-2,4-pyridinediamine

Synonyms: RP 4753; Daraprim; Chloridin; Darapram; Malocide; Tindurin.

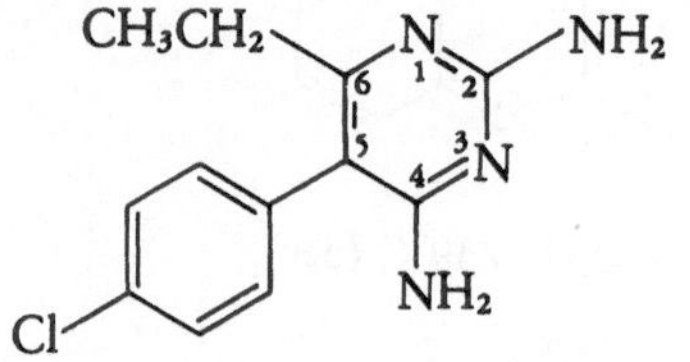

Crystals, m.p. 233–234°C (capillary), m.p. 240–242°C (copper block).

Solubility: practically insol. H_2O; about 9 g/liter C_2H_5OH, about 25 g/liter boiling C_2H_5OH; about 5 g/liter dil. HCl; very sparingly sol. propylene glycol, dimethylacetamide at 70°C.

Preparation: Russell and Hitchings (1951).

Review: Burchall (1975).

58. TRIMETHOPRIM

CARN: 738-70-5

$C_{14}H_{18}N_4O_3$ mol. wt. 290.32

5-[(3,4,5-Trimethoxyphenyl)methyl]-2,4-pyrimidinediamine

Synonyms: 2,4-diamino-5-(3,4,5-trimethoxybenzyl)pyrimidine; Monotrim; Proloprim; Syraprim; Tiempe; Trimanyl; Trimopan; Trimpex; Wellcoprim.

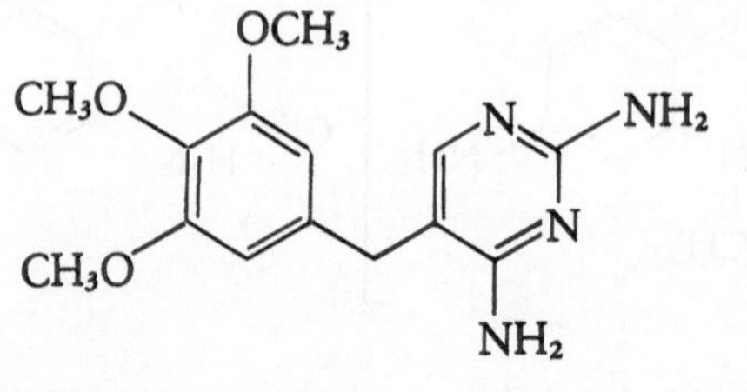

White to cream, bitter crystalline powder, m.p. 199–203°C; pK_a 6.6.

Solubility: (g/100 ml at 25°C): 13.86 DMAC; 7.29 benzyl alcohol; 2.57 propylene glycol; 1.82 $CHCl_3$; 1.21 CH_3OH; 0.04 H_2O; 0.003 $(C_2H_5)_2O$; 0.002 C_6H_6.

Toxicity: LD_{50} mice 7000 mg/kg po (Yamamoto *et al.*, 1973).

Preparation: Stenbuck and Hood (1962); Roth *et al.* (1980*a,b*).

Review: Burchall (1975); Manius (1978).

59. AMPROLIUM

CARN: 121-25-5

$C_{14}H_{19}ClN_4$ mol. wt. 278.78

1-[(4-Amino-2-propyl-5-pyrimidinyl)methyl]-2-methylpyridinium chloride
Synonyms: 1-[(4-amino-2-propyl-5-pyrimidinyl)methyl]-2-picolinium chloride; Corid.

Hydrochloride

$C_{14}H_{20}Cl_2N_4$ mol. wt. 315.25

Synonym: Amprol.

Crystals from CH_3OH + C_2H_5OH, dec. 248–249°C.

Solubility: freely sol. H_2O (pH 10% aq. soln. = 2.5–3.0), CH_3OH, 95% C_2H_5OH, dimethylformamide; sparingly sol. abs. C_2H_5OH; practically insol. isopropanol, butanol, dioxane, $(CH_3)_2CO$, $CH_3CO_2C_2H_5$, CH_3CN, isooctane.

Preparation: Rogers *et al.* (1960).

60. HALOFUGINONE

CARN: 55837-20-2

$C_{16}H_{17}BrClN_3O_3$ mol. wt. 414.70

7-Bromo-6-chloro-3-[3-(3-hydroxy-2-piperidinyl)-2-oxopropyl]-4(3H)-quinazolinone

Synonym: 7-bromo-6-chlorofebrifugine.

Toxicity: to freshwater organisms (Canton and Van Esch, 1976).

Preparation: Waletzky *et al.* (1967).

Hydrobromide

$C_{16}H_{18}Br_2ClN_3O_3$ mol. wt. 495.61

Synonyms: RU-19110; Stenorol.

Crystals, m.p. 247°C (dec.).

61. ARPRINOCID

CARN: 55779-18-5

$C_{12}H_9ClFN_5$ mol. wt. 277.69

9-[(2-Chloro-6-fluorophenyl)methyl]-9H-purin-6-amine

Synonyms: 9-(2-chloro-6-fluorobenzyl)adenine; MK-302; Arpocox.

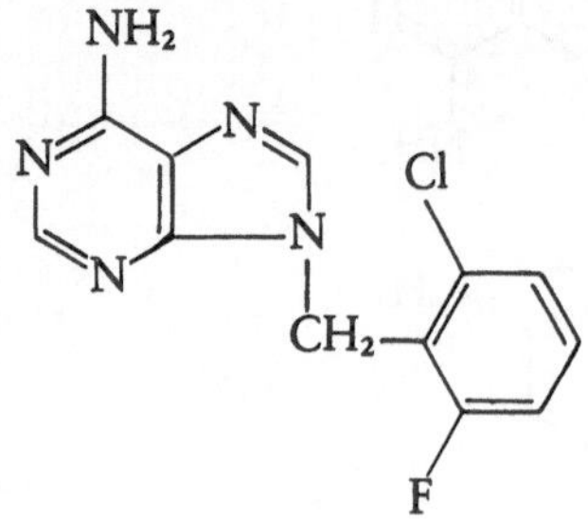

Crystals from CH_3OH/H_2O, m.p. 245–246°C.

Preparation: Lira *et al.* (1972); Hartman *et al.* (1978).

62. SINEFUNGIN

CARN: 58944-73-3

$C_{15}H_{23}N_7O_5$ mol. wt. 381.39

6,9-Diamino-1-(6-amino-9H-purin-9-yl)-1,5,6,7,8,9-hexadeoxydecofuranuronic acid

Synonyms: RP 32232; A 9145.

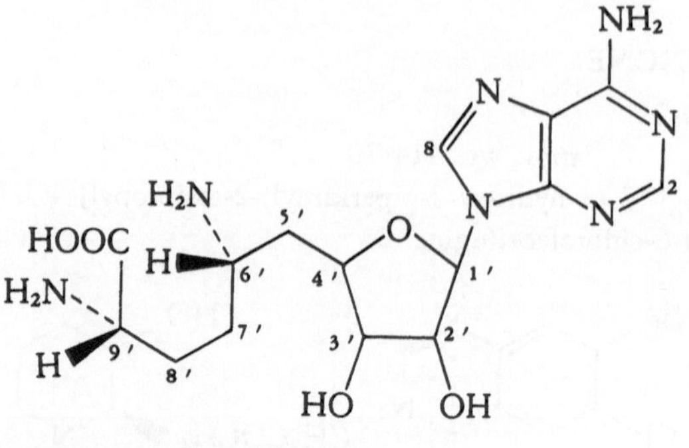

Isolation: Hamill and Hoehn (1971).

Total synthesis: Mock and Moffat (1982); Geze *et al.* (1983).

63. ISOMETAMIDIUM CHLORIDE

CARN: 34301-55-8

$C_{28}H_{26}ClN_7$ mol. wt. 496.04

3-Amino-8-(3-[3-(aminoiminomethyl)phenyl]-1-triazenyl)-5-ethyl-6-phenanthridi-
nium chloride

Synonyms: metamidium; M & B 4180 A; Samorin.

Red crystals from aq. CH_3OH, m.p. 244–245°C.
Preparation: Wragg *et al.* (1958).

64. HOMIDIUM

CARN: 3546-21-2
$C_{21}H_{20}N_3^+$ mol. wt. 314.41
3,8-Diamino-5-ethyl-6-phenanthridinium
Synonyms: ethidium; RD 1572; Novidium; Babidium.

Bromide
$C_{21}H_{20}BrN_3$ mol. wt. 394.32
Synonym: Dromilac.
Bitter-tasting, dark red crystals from C_2H_5OH, m.p. 238–240°C.
Solubility: sol. in 20 parts H_2O (20°C); 750 parts $CHCl_3$ (20°C).

Chloride
$C_{21}H_{20}ClN_3$ mol. wt. 349.87
Dark red crystalline powder; crystallizes with 1 mole C_2H_5OH.
Solubility: sol. in 5 parts H_2O at room temperature.
Preparation: Watkins (1952).
Review: LePecq (1971); Waring (1975).

65. PROTHIDIUM BROMIDE

CARN: 14222-46-9
$C_{26}H_{26}Br_2N_6$ mol. wt. 582.36
3-Amino-8-[(2-amino-1,6-dimethyl-4(1H)-pyrimidinylidene)amino]-6-(4-ami-
    nophenyl)-5-methylphenanthridinium bromide hydrobromide
Synonyms: pyrithidium; pyritidium bromide.

Elongated red plates from CH_3OH-ethylene dichloride, m.p. 299°C.
Preparation: Watkins (1958).

66. QUINAPYRAMINE

CARN: 20493-41-8
4-Amino-6-[(2-amino-1,6-dimethylpyrimidinium-4-yl)amino]quinolinium
Synonyms: M7555; Antrycide.

Preparation: Curd and Davey (1950).

Dimethosulfate
$C_{19}H_{28}N_6O_8S_2$ mol. wt. 532.60
Creamy white crystals from CH_3OH, m.p. 265–266°C.
Solubility: Freely sol. H_2O.
Toxicity: LD_{50} mice 10–15 mg/kg iv (Curd and Davey, 1950).

Dichloride
$C_{17}H_{22}Cl_2N_6$ mol. wt. 381.31
Crystals from H_2O, m.p. 316–317°C.
Solubility: Sparingly sol. H_2O.
Toxicity: LD_{50} mice 10–15 mg/kg iv (Curd and Davey, 1950).

67. METRONIDAZOLE

CARN: 443-48-1
$C_6H_9N_3O_3$ mol. wt. 171.16
2-Methyl-5-nitroimidazole-1-ethanol

Synonyms: 1-(2-hydroxyethyl)-2-methyl-5-nitroimidazole; Bayer 5630; RP 8823; Arilin; Clont; Cont; Danizol; Deflamon; Flagyl; Fossysol; Gineflavir; Klion; Orvagil; Sanatrichom; Trichazol; Trivazol; Vagilen; Vagimid.

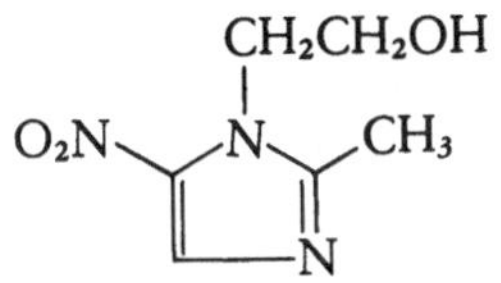

$$CH_2CH_2OH$$

$$O_2N-N-CH_3$$

Cream-colored crystals, m.p. 158–160°C.

Solubility: 1.0 H_2O g/100 ml (20°C) (pH sat. aq. soln. = 5.8); 0.5 g/100 ml (20°C) C_2H_5OH; <0.05 g/100 ml (20°C) $(C_2H_5)_2O$, $CHCl_3$; sparingly sol. dimethylformamide; sol. dil. acids.

Preparation: Jacob *et al.* (1960).

Metabolism: Ings *et al.* (1966).

Review: Wearly and Anthony (1976); Brogden *et al.* (1978).

Hydrochloride

$C_6H_{10}ClN_3O_3$ mol. wt. 207.62

Synonyms: SC-32642; Flagyl I.V.

68. TINIDAZOLE

CARN: 19387-91-8

$C_8H_{13}N_3O_4S$ mol. wt. 247.26

1-[2-(Ethylsulfonyl)ethyl]-2-methyl-5-nitroimidazole

Synonyms: CP 12574; Fasigin; Fasigyn; Pletil; Simplotan; Sorquetan; Tricolam.

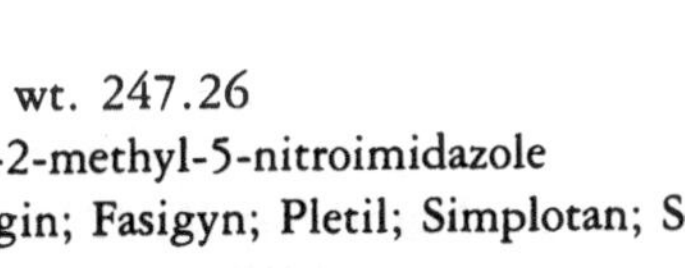

$$CH_2CH_2SO_2CH_2CH_3$$

$$O_2N-N-CH_3$$

Colorless crystals from C_6H_6, m.p. 127–128°C.

Toxicity: LD_{50} mice >3600 mg/kg po, >2300 mg/kg ip (Miller *et al.*, 1970).

Pharmacokinetics: human and murine (Taylor *et al.*, 1970).

Preparation: Butler (1968); Miller *et al.* (1970).

Review: Nord and Phillips (1982).

69. NIMORAZOLE

CARN: 6506-37-2

$C_9H_{14}N_4O_3$ mol. wt. 226.23

4-[2-(5-Nitroimidazol-1-yl)ethyl]morpholine

Synonyms: N-2-morpholinoethyl-5-nitroimidazole; nitrimidazine; K 1900; Acterol; Esclama; Naxofem; Naxogin; Nulogyl; Sirledi.

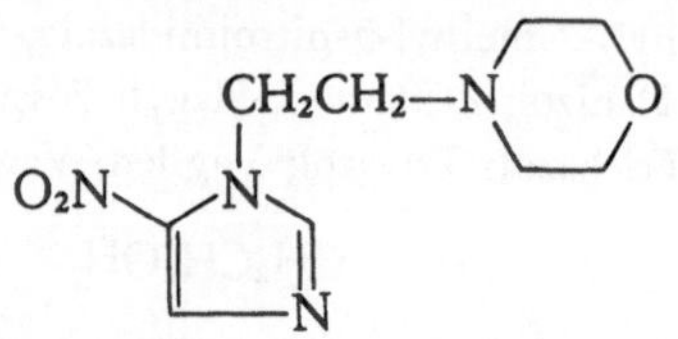

CH$_2$CH$_2$—N O

O$_2$N N

N

Crystals from H$_2$O, m.p. 110–111°C.
Solubility: Slightly sol. H$_2$O at room temperature; sol. alcohols, (CH$_3$)$_2$CO, CHCl$_3$.
Toxicity: LD$_{50}$ Wistar rats 3180 mg/kg po (Windholz *et al.*, 1983).
Preparation: Giraldi and Mariotti (1968).
Pharmacology and toxicology: Barbieri *et al.* (1972).
Metabolism: Giraldi *et al.* (1971).

70. IPRONIDAZOLE

CARN: 14885-29-1
C$_7$H$_{11}$N$_3$O$_2$ mol. wt. 169.18
1-Methyl-2-(1-methylethyl)-5-nitro-*1H*-imidazole
Synonyms: 2-isopropyl-1-methyl-5-nitroimidazole; Ro 7-15554; Ipropran.

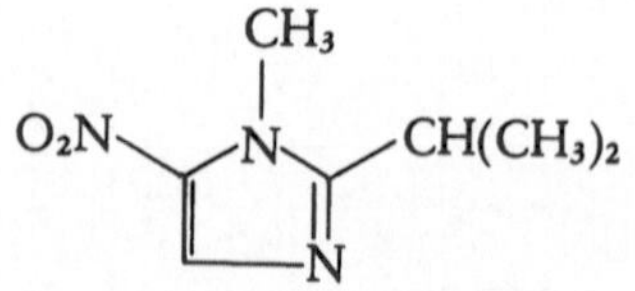

CH$_3$

O$_2$N N CH(CH$_3$)$_2$

N

White plates, m.p. 60°C
Toxicity: LD$_{50}$ poults 640 ± 25 po (Marusich *et al.*, 1970).
Structure–activity relationships: Butler *et al.* (1967).
Preparation: Hoffer and Mitrovic (1968).

Hydrochloride
C$_7$H$_{12}$ClN$_3$O$_2$ mol. wt. 201.66
m.p. 177–182°C.
Solubility: H$_2$O sol.

71. RONIDAZOLE

CARN: 7681-76-7
C$_6$H$_8$N$_4$O$_4$ mol. wt. 200.16
1-Methyl-5-nitroimidazole-2-methanol carbamate (ester)
Synonyms: 1-methyl-2-[(carbamoyloxy)methyl]-5-nitroimidazole;   MCMN;   Dugro;
Ridzol.

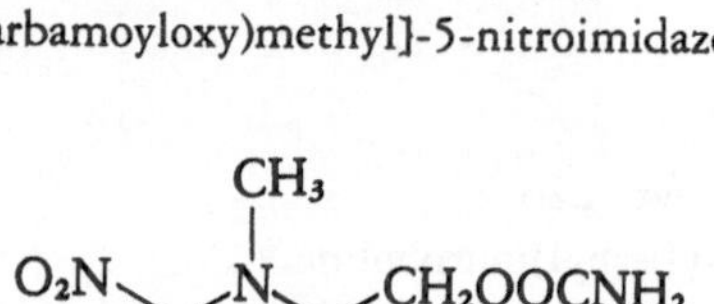

CH$_3$

O$_2$N N CH$_2$OOCNH$_2$

N

Pale yellow crystals, m.p. 167–169°C; unstable in alkaline solns; pK_a 1.2.
Solubility: about 2.9 mg/ml H_2O at pH 6.5 at room temperature, more sol. in acid
solns.; freely sol. $(CH_3)_2CO$; sol. CH_3OH, C_2H_5OH, $CHCl_3$, $CH_3CO_2C_2H_5$.
Preparation: Hoff *et al.* (1967).

72. DIMETRIDAZOLE

CARN: 551-92-8
$C_5H_7N_3O_2$ mol. wt. 141.13
1,2-Dimethyl-5-nitro-*1H*-imidazole
Synonyms: RP 8595; Emtrylvet; Unizole.

Needles from H_2O, m.p. 138–139°C.
Solubility: Freely sol. C_2H_5OH; sparingly sol. cold H_2O, $(C_2H_5)_2O$.
Preparation: Bhagwat and Pyman (1925).

Hydrochloride
$C_5H_8ClN_3O_2$ mol. wt. 177.59
Prisms from dil. HCl, m.p. 195°C.
Solubility: freely sol. H_2O, C_2H_5OH; sparingly sol. $(CH_3)_2CO$.

73. BENZNIDAZOLE

CARN: 22994-85-0
$C_{12}H_{12}N_4O_3$ mol. wt. 260.26
2-Nitro-*N*-(phenylmethyl)-*1H*-imidazole-1-acetamide
Synonyms: Ro 7-1051; Radanil; Rochagan.

Crystals from C_2H_5OH, m.p. 188.5–190°C; uv max (C_2H_5OH): 313 nm (ϵ 7600).
Solubility: 40 mg/ml H_2O at 37°C (Raaflaub and Ziegler, 1979).
Toxicity: mammalian cells *in vitro* (Adams *et al.*, 1980).
Mutagenicity: Voogd *et al.* (1979).
Pharmacokinetics: Raaflaub and Ziegler (1979).
Preparation: Beaman *et al.* (1969).

74. CLOTRIMAZOLE

CARN: 23593-75-1

$C_{22}H_{17}ClN_2$ mol. wt. 344.84

1-[(2-Chlorophenyl)diphenylmethyl]-$1H$-imidazole

Synonyms: FB 5097; BAY b 5097; Canesten; Empecid; Gyne-Lotrimin; Lotrimin; My-
celax; Mycosporin; Trimysten.

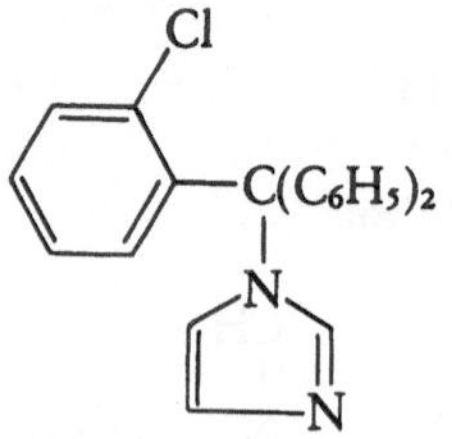

Crystals, m.p. 147–149°C; a weak base; rapidly hydrolyzes upon heating in aq. acids.
Solubility: sl. sol. H_2O, C_6H_6, toluene; sol. $(CH_3)_2CO$, $CHCl_3$, $CH_3CO_2C_2H_5$, DMF.
Toxicity: LD_{50} mice 923 mg/kg po; LD_{50} rats 708 mg/kg po (Tettenborn, 1972).
Pharmacology: Plempel *et al.* (1970), von Duhm *et al.* (1972).
Preparation: Buechel *et al.* (1969), von Büchel *et al.* (1972).
Review: Hoogerheide and Wyka (1982).

75. NITROFURAZONE

CARN: 59-87-0

$C_6H_6N_4O_4$ mol. wt. 198.14

2-[(5-Nitro-2-furanyl)methylene]hydrazinecarboxamide

Synonyms: 5-nitro-2-furaldehyde semicarbazone; Amifur; Furacin; Chemofuran; Furesol;
Nifuzon; Nitrofural; Nitrozone; Furacinetten; Furacoccid; Furazol W; Mammex;
Furaplast; Coxistat; Aldomycin; Nefco; Vabrocid.

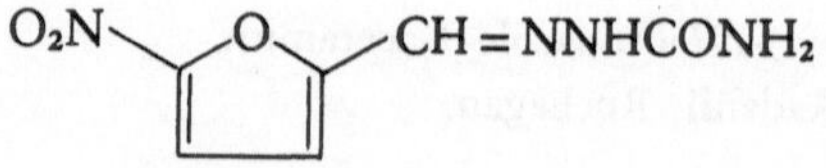

Pale yellow needles, m.p. 236–240°C; bitter aftertaste; darkens on prolonged exposure
to light; uv max: 260, 375 nm.
Solubility: very sl. sol. H_2O (1 : 4200), pH of a sat. aq. soln. = 6.0–6.5; sol. in alkaline
solns. with a dark orange color; sl. sol. C_2H_5OH (1 : 590), propylene glycol
(1 : 350); insol. $(C_2H_5)_2O$
Toxicity: LD_{50} rats 0.59 g/kg po, 3.0 g/kg sc (Godwin *et al.*, 1947).
Tumorigenic activity: Morris *et al.* (1969); Ertürk *et al.* (1970).
Preparation: Stillman and Scott (1947).

76. FURAZOLIDONE

CARN: 67-45-8

$C_8H_7N_3O_5$ mol. wt. 225.16

3-([(5-Nitro-2-furanyl)methylene]amino)-2-oxazolidinone
Synonyms: 3-(5-nitrofurfurylideneamino)-2-oxazolidinone; NF 180; Furovag; Furoxane; Furoxone; Giarlam; Giardil; Medaron; Neftin; Nicolen; Nifulidone; Ortazol; Roptazol; Tikofuran; Topazone.

Yellow crystals, dec. 275°C; dec. by alkali; darkens under strong light.
Solubility: approx. 40 mg/liter H_2O (pH 6).
Toxicity: Yurchenko *et al.* (1953); Rogers *et al.* (1956).
Pharmacology and toxicology: Ali (1983).
Preparation: Drake and Hayes (1956).

77. NIFURSOL

CARN: 16915-70-1
$C_{12}H_7N_5O_9$ mol. wt. 365.22
2-Hydroxy-3,5-dinitrobenzoic acid ([5-nitro-2-furanyl]methylene)hydrazide
Synonyms: 3,5-dinitrosalicylic acid (5-nitrofurfurylidene)hydrazide; Histomon; Salfuride.

Preparation: Berndt *et al.* (1969).

78. NIFURTIMOX

CARN: 23256-30-6
$C_{10}H_{13}N_3O_5S$ mol. wt. 287.29
4-([5-Nitrofurfurylidene]amino)-3-methylthiomorpholine-1,1-dioxide
Synonyms: BAY 2502; Lampit

Orange-red crystals from dil. CH_3COOH, m.p. 180–182°C.
Toxicity: LD_{50} mice 3720 mg/kg po; LD_{50} rats 4050 mg/kg po (Hoffman, 1972).

Review: Gönnert (1972).
Preparation: Herlinger *et al.* (1964).

79. SULFALENE

CARN: 152-47-6

$C_{11}H_{11}N_4O_3S$ mol. wt. 280.32

4-Amino-*N*-(3-methoxypyrazinyl)benzenesulfonamide

Synonyms: sulfamethopyrazine; 2-sulfanilamido-3-methoxypyrazine; sulfamethoxy-
pyrazine; sulfapyrazinemethoxyine; Farmitalia 204/122; Kelfizina; Longum;
Dalysep; Polycidal.

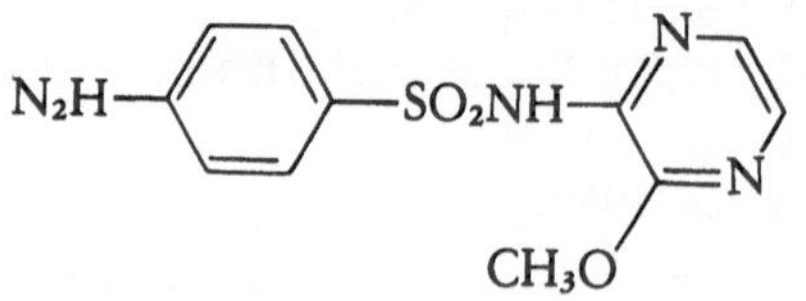

Crystals from C_2H_5OH, m.p. 176°C.
Toxicity: LD_{50} mice 2.164 g/kg po, 1.41 g/kg iv (Windholz *et al.*, 1983).
Preparation: Camerino and Palamidessi (1960).
Review: Gasparini (1971).

80. SULFAQUINOXALINE

CARN: 59-40-5

$C_{14}H_{12}N_4O_2S$ mol. wt. 300.33

4-Amino-*N*-2-quinoxalinylbenzenesulfonamide

Synonyms: 2-sulfanilamidoquinoxaline; sulfabenzpyrazine; Compound 3-120; Sulfa-Q
20; Sulquin.

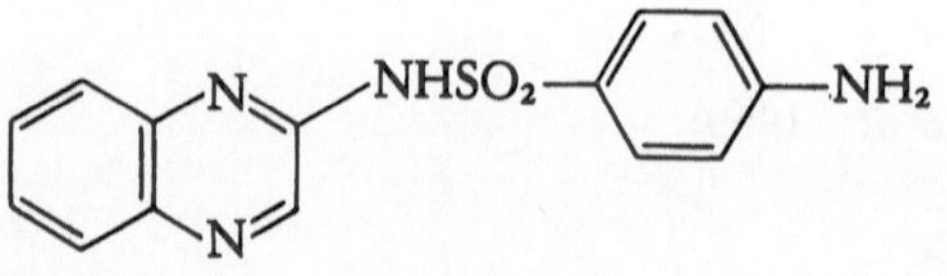

Minute crystals, m.p. 247–248°C; uv max (pH 6.6 H_2O): 252, 360 nm ($E_{1cm}^{1\%}$ 1110,
275).
Solubility: 0.75 mg/100 ml H_2O pH 7; 73 mg/100 ml 95% C_2H_5OH; 430 mg/100 ml
$(CH_3)_2CO$; sol. aq. Na_2CO_3 and NaOH solns.

Sodium salt
$C_{14}H_{11}N_4NaO_2S$ mol. wt. 322.32
Synonyms: Aviochina; Embazin.
The pH of a 1% aq. soln. = about 10; the amorphous salt is deliquescent and absorbs
CO_2, which liberates the practically insol. sulfaquinoxaline.
Solubility: Very sol. in H_2O.
Preparation: Weijlard *et al.* (1944).

81. SULFADIMETHOXINE

CARN: 122-11-2

$C_{12}H_{14}N_4O_4S$ mol. wt. 310.33

4-Amino-N-(2,6-dimethoxy-4-pyrimidinyl)benzenesulfonamide

Synonyms: 2,6-dimethoxy-4-sulfanilamidopyrimidine; Agribon; Albon; Madribon; Sulxin; Bactrovet; Dinosol; Sudine; Radonin; Dimetazina; Memcozine; Metoxidon; Neostreptal; Sulfasol; Theracanzan; Symbio; Suldixine; Diasulfa; Arnosulfan; Maxulvet; Diasulfyl; Roscosulf.

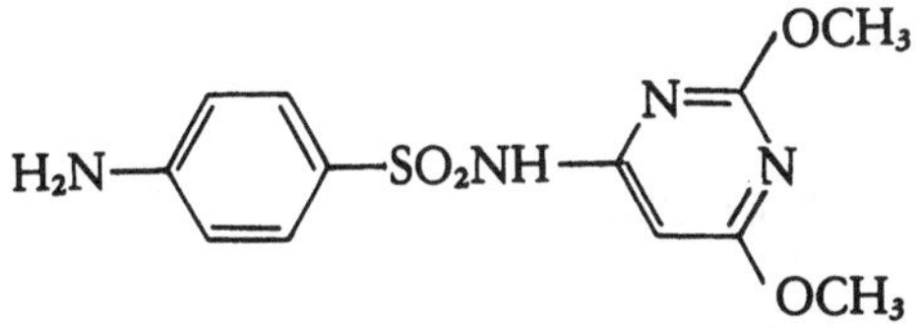

Crystals from dil. C_2H_5OH, m.p. 201–203°C.

Solubility: Sol. dil. HCl and aq. solns. of Na_2CO_3; sol. H_2O (mg/dl) at 37°C: 4.6 at pH 4.10, 29.5 at pH 6.7, 58.0 at pH 7.06, 5170 at pH 8.71.

Toxicity: LD_{50} mice >10 g/kg po (Seki *et al.*, 1965).

Toxicology and pharmacokinetics: Böhni *et al.* (1969).

Preparation: Bretschneider and Klötzer (1955).

Sodium salt

$C_{12}H_{13}N_4NaO_4S$ mol. wt. 332.56

Crystals from CH_3OH + $(C_2H_5)_2O$; pH of a 5% aq. soln. = 8.1; pH of a 10% aq. soln. = 8.6.

Solubility: freely sol. H_2O.

82. SULFAMETHOXAZOLE

CARN: 723-46-6

$C_{10}H_{11}N_3O_3S$ mol. wt. 253.31

4-Amino-N-(5-methyl-3-isoxazolyl)benzenesulfonamide

Synonyms: 5-methyl-3-sulfanilamidoisoxazole; sulfisomezole; sulfamethylisoxazole; sulfamthoxizole; Gantanol; Sinomin.

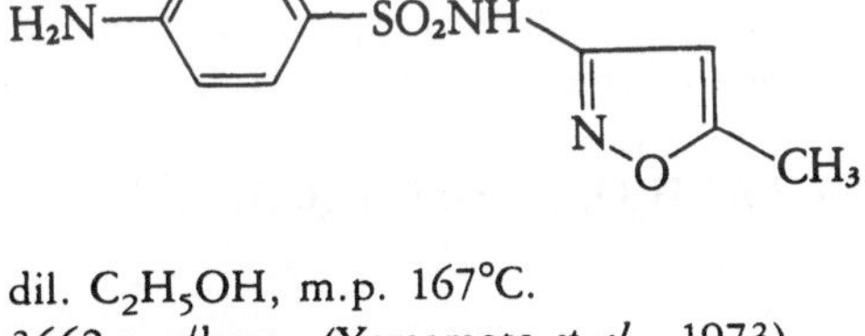

Bitter crystals from dil. C_2H_5OH, m.p. 167°C.

Toxicity: LD_{50} mice 3662 mg/kg po (Yamamoto *et al.*, 1973).

Preparation: Kano *et al.* (1959).

Review: Rudy and Senkowski (1973).

Mixture with trimethoprim

Usually 5 : 1.

Synonyms: co-trimoxazole, Abacin; Bactramin; Bactrim; Baktar; Bactromin; Drylin; Eusaprim; Gantaprim; Gantrim; Kepinol; Momentol; Nopil; Omsat; Septra; Septrim; Sigaprim; Sulfotrim; Sulfotrimin; Sulprim; Sumetrolim; Suprim; Tacumil; Teleprim; TMS 480; Trigonyl; Linaris; Eltrianyl; Microtrim; Trimesulf; Apo-Sulfatrim; Fectrim; Trimforte; Uro-Septra.

Toxicity: LD_{50} mice 5513 mg/kg (Yamamoto *et al.*, 1973).

83. SULFADIAZINE

CARN: 68-35-9

$C_{10}H_{10}N_4O_2S$ mol. wt. 250.28

4-Amino-*N*-2-pyrimidinylbenzenesulfonamide

Synonyms: 2-sulfanilamidopyrimidine; sulfapyrimidine; Pyrimal; Debenal; Diazyl; Sterazine; Sulfolex; Adiazine; Ultradiazin; Eskadiazine.

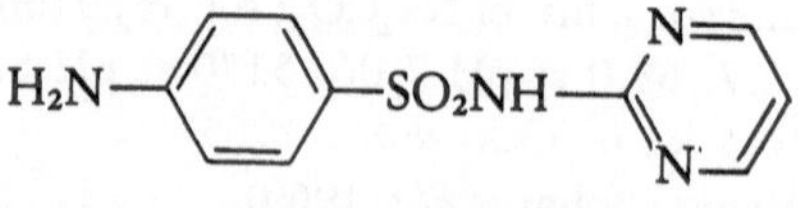

White or slightly yellow powder, m.p. 252–256°C.

Solubility: sparingly sol. H_2O at 37°C: 13 mg/dl at pH 5.5, 200 mg/dl at pH 7.5; sparingly sol. C_2H_5OH, $(CH_3)_2CO$; freely sol. in dil. acids and solns. of NaOH and KOH and in ammonia water.

Toxicology and pharmacokinetics: Böhni *et al.* (1969).

Preparation: Roblin *et al.* (1940).

Review: Stober and DeWitte (1982).

Mixture with trimethoprim

Usually 5 : 1.

Synonyms: co-trimazine; Triglobe; Coptin.

Sodium salt

CARN: 547-32-0

$C_{10}H_9N_4NaO_2S$ mol. wt. 272.28

4-Amino-*N*-2-pyrimidinylbenzenesulfonamide sodium salt

Synonym: soluble sulfadiazine.

White powder; absorbs CO_2 on prolonged exposure to humid air with liberation of sulfadiazine, becoming completely insol. on H_2O; aq. solutions are alkaline to phenolphthalein (pH 9–11).

Solubility: 1 g in about 2 ml H_2O; sl. sol. C_2H_5OH.

84. MONENSIN

CARN: 17090-79-8

$C_{36}H_{62}O_{11}$ mol. wt. 670.90

2-[5-Ethyltetrahydro-5-(tetrahydro-3-methyl-5-[tetrahydro-6-hydroxy-6-(hydroxymethyl)-3,5-dimethyl-2H-pyran-2-yl]-2-furyl]-2-furyl]-9-hydroxy-β-meth-
oxy-α,γ,2,8-tetramethyl-1,6-dioxaspiro[4.5]decane-7-butyric acid

Synonym: A 3823A.

Monohydrate: crystals, m.p. 103–105°C; [α]$_D$ +47.7°; pK$_a$ 6.6 (in 66% DMF); very
stable under alkaline conditions.
Solubility: slightly sol. H$_2$O; more sol. hydrocarbons; very sol. other organic solvents.
Toxicity: LD$_{50}$ mice 43.8 ± 5.2 mg/kg po, LD$_{50}$ chicks 284 ± 47 mg/kg po (Haney
and Hoehn, 1967).
Isolation: Haney and Hoehn (1967).
Total synthesis: Fukayama *et al.* (1979).
Review: Stark (1969).

Sodium salt
C$_{36}$H$_{61}$NaO$_{11}$ mol. wt. 649.00
Synonyms: Coban; Romensin; Rumensin.
m.p. 267–269°C; [α]$_D$ +57.3 (CH$_3$OH).
Solubility: slightly sol. H$_2$O; more sol. hydrocarbons; very sol. other organic solvents.

85. SALINOMYCIN

CARN: 53003-10-4
C$_{42}$H$_{70}$O$_{11}$ mol. wt. 751.02
Synonym: Coxistac.

Solid, m.p. 112.5–113.5°C; [α]$_D^{25}$ −63°(c = 1 [C$_2$H$_5$OH]); pK$_a$' 6.4 (DMF); uv max
(2:1 C$_2$H$_5$OH:H$_2$O): 284 nm (ε 126).
Toxicity: LD$_{50}$ mice 18 mg/kg ip, 50 mg/kg po (Miyazaki *et al.*, 1974).
Production: Miyazaki *et al.* (1972).
Total synthesis: Kishi *et al.* (1982).

86. NARASIN

CARN: 55134-13-9

$C_{43}H_{72}O_{11}$ mol. wt. 765.05

4-Methylsalinomycin

Synonyms: narasin A; Compound 79891; Antibiotic A-28086; factor A; C-7819B; Monteban.

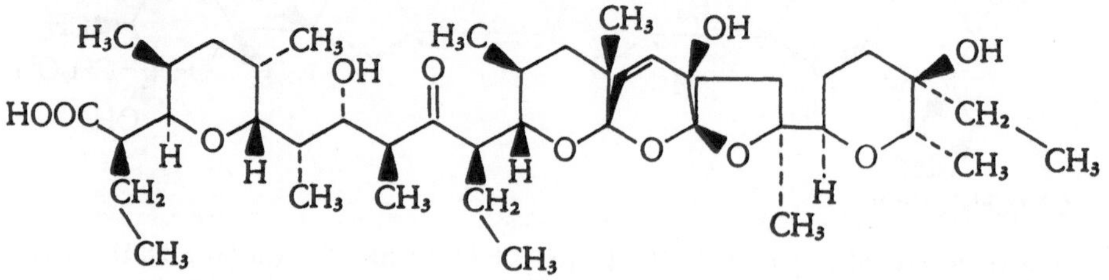

Crystals from $(CH_3)_2CO-H_2O$, m.p. 98–100°C, resoldifies and remelts 198–200°C; uv max (C_2H_5OH): 285 nm (ϵ 58); $[\alpha]_D^{25}$ −54° (c = 2 [CH_3OH]); pK$_a$ 7.9 (80% aq. DMF).

Solubility: sol. in alcohols, $(CH_3)_2CO$, DMF, DMSO,C_6H_6, $CHCl_3$, $CH_3CO_2C_2H_5$; insol. H_2O.

Toxicity: LD$_{50}$ mice 7.15 mg/kg ip (Berg *et al.*, 1975).

Production: Berg *et al.* (1975).

Total synthesis: Kishi *et al.* (1982).

87. MADURAMICIN

CARN: 79356-08-4

$C_{47}H_{79}NaO_{17}$ mol. wt. 939.13

Synonyms: X-14868A; CL 259,971; Cygro; Prinocin.

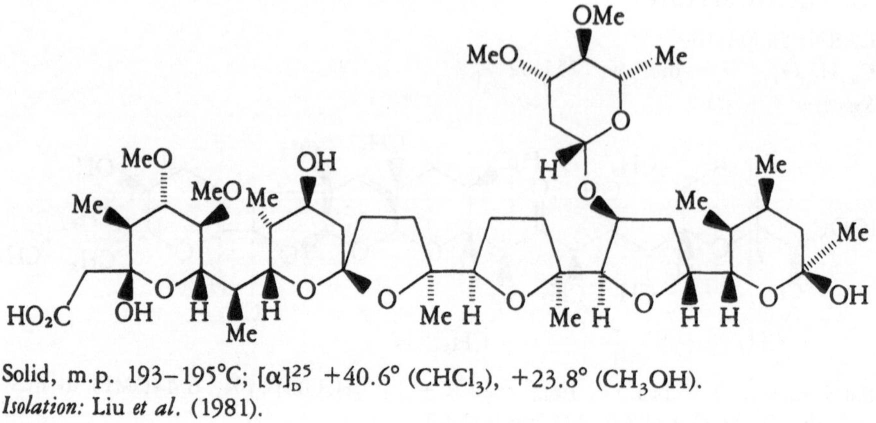

Solid, m.p. 193–195°C; $[\alpha]_D^{25}$ +40.6° ($CHCl_3$), +23.8° (CH_3OH).

Isolation: Liu *et al.* (1981).

88. LASALOCID A

CARN: 25999-31-9

$C_{34}H_{54}O_8$ mol. wt. 590.80

6-(7R-[5S-Ethyl-5-(5R-ethyltetrahydro-5-hydroxy-6S-methyl-2H-pyran-2R-yl)tetra-
hydro-3S-methyl-2S-furanyl]-4S-hydroxy-3R,5S-dimethyl-6-oxononyl)-2-hy-
droxy-3-methylbenzoic acid
Synonyms: antibiotic X-537A; ionophore X-4537A; Ro 2-2985; Bovatec.

Crystals, m.p. 110–114°C; $[\alpha]_D^{25}$ −7.55° (CH_3OH); uv max (50% aq. isopropanol):
248, 318 nm (ϵ 6750, 4300).
Solubility: sol. organic solvents; insol. H_2O.
Toxicity: LD_{50} mice 40 mg/kg ip (Berger *et al.*, 1951); 64 mg/kg ip, 146 mg/kg po
(Westley, 1978).
Mode of action: Lin and Kun (1973).
Preparation: Stempel and Westley (1971).
Total synthesis: Nakata *et al.* (1978).

Sodium salt
$C_{34}H_{53}NaO_8$ mol. wt. 612.79
Synonym: Avatec.
Crystals from C_6H_6-ligroine, m.p. 191–192°C (dec.), also reported as 168–171°C;
$[\alpha]_D^{25}$ −30° (c = 1 [CH_3OH]); uv max (50% aq. isopropanol): 308 nm (ϵ 4100).

89. SPIRAMYCIN

CARN: 8025-81-8
Synonyms: RP 5337; Sequamycin; Selectomycin; Foromacidin; Rovamicina; Rovamycin;
Provamycin.

Amorphous base; $[\alpha]_D^{20}$ $-80°$ (CH_3OH); uv max (C_2H_5OH): 231 nm; separable into 3 components.

Solubility: Slightly sol. H_2O; sol. in most organic solvents.

Toxicity: LD_{50} rats 9400 mg/kg po, 1000 mg/kg sc, 170 mg/kg iv (Sous *et al.*, 1958).

Production: Cosar *et al.* (1952).

Structure: Freiberg *et al.* (1974).

Hexanedioate

Synonyms: spiramycin adipate; Suanovil; Suanozil; Calactin vet.

Spiramycin I (R = H)
$C_{43}H_{74}N_2O_{14}$ mol. wt. 843.07
Synonym: Foromacidin A.
Crystals, m.p. 134–137°C; $[\alpha]_D^{20}$ $-96°$.

Spiramycin II (R = $COCH_3$)
$C_{45}H_{76}N_2O_{15}$ mol. wt. 885.11
Synonym: Foromacidin B.
Crystals, m.p. 130–133°C; $[\alpha]_D^{20}$ $-86°$.

Spiramycin III (R = $COCH_2CH_3$)
Synonym: Foromacidin C.
Crystals, m.p. 128–131°C; $[\alpha]_D^{20}$ $-83°$.

90. AMPHOTERICIN B

CARN: 1397–89-3
$C_{47}H_{73}NO_{17}$ mol. wt. 924.11
Synonyms: Amphozone; Fungizone; Fungilin; Ampho-Moronal.

Deep yellow prisms or needles from DMF; dec. gradually above 170°C; uv max (CH_3OH): 406, 382, 363, 345 nm; $[\alpha]_D^{24}$ $+333°$ (acidic DMF), $-33.6°$ (0.1 N methanolic HCl); solids and solutions appear stable for long periods at pH 4–10 when stored at moderate temp. out of contact with light and air.

Solubility: insol. H_2O at pH 6–7, sol. approx. 0.1 mg/ml in H_2O at pH 2 or 11; sol. in H_2O increased by sodium desoxycholate; sol. 2–4 mg/ml in DMF; 60–80 mg/ml in DMF + HCl; 30–40 mg/ml in DMSO.

Toxicity: LD_{50} mice 40 mg/kg ip (Berger, 1951), 65 mg/kg ip (Westley, 1978).

Mechanism of action: Holz (1979).

Production: Gold *et al.* (1955–1956).

Structure: Mechlinski *et al.* (1970); Borowski *et al.* (1970).

Review: Asher (1977).

91. PAROMOMYCIN

CARN: 7542-37-2

$C_{23}H_{45}N_5O_{14}$ mol. wt. 615.65

O-2-Amino-2-deoxy-α-D-glucopyranosyl-(1→4)-O-[O-2,6-diamino-2,6-dideoxy-β-L-idopyranosyl-(1→3)-β-D-ribofuranosyl-(1→5)]-2-deoxy-D-streptamine

Synonyms: paromomycin I; aminosidine; amminosidin; catenulin; crestomycin; estomycin; hydroxymycin; monomycin A; neomycin E; paucimycin; R 400.

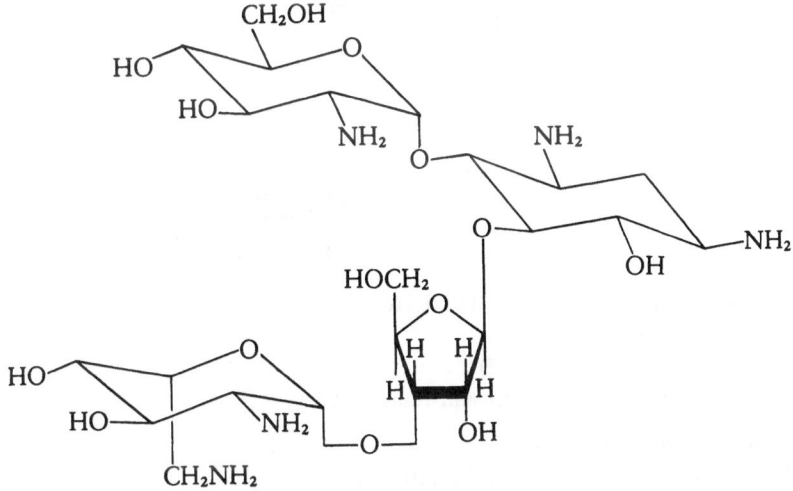

Amorphous white powder; $[\alpha]_D^{25}$ +65° ±3°.

Solubility: sol. H_2O; mod. sol. CH_3OH; sparingly sol. abs. C_2H_5OH.

Toxicity: LD_{50} rats >1625 mg/kg po, >659 mg/kg sc, 156 mg/kg iv; LD_{50} mice >2275 mg/kg po, 423 mg/kg sc, 90 mg/kg iv (Coffey *et al.*, 1959).

Pharmacology: Gasparini and Pignatelli (1972).

Isolation: Frohardt *et al.* (1959); Davisson and Finlay (1959); Canevazzi and Scotti (1959).

Structure: Haskell *et al.* (1959*a,b*).

Sulfate

CARN: 7205-49-4

$C_{23}H_{47}N_5O_{18}S$ mol. wt. 713.72

Synonyms: 1600 Antibiotic; Farmiglucin; Farminosidin; Fi 5858; Gabbromicina; Gab-
   bromycin; Gabbroral; Humatin; Pargonyl; Paramicina; Paricina.

$[\alpha]_D^{25}$ +50.5° (c = 1.5 [H_2O pH 6]).

Toxicity: LD_{50} mice approx. 15,000 mg/kg po, 700 mg/kg sc, 110 mg/kg iv (Di
   Marco and Bertazzoli, 1963).

92. CLINDAMYCIN

CARN: 18323-44-9

$C_{18}H_{33}ClN_2O_5S$ mol. wt. 424.98

Methyl   7-chloro-6,7,8-trideoxy-6-({1-methyl-4-propyl-2-pyrrolidinyl)carbonyl]ami-
   no)- 1-thio-L-*threo*-α-D-*galacto*-octopyranoside

Synonyms: 7(S)-chloro-7-deoxylincomycin; U-21251; Cleocin; Dalacin C; Sobelin.

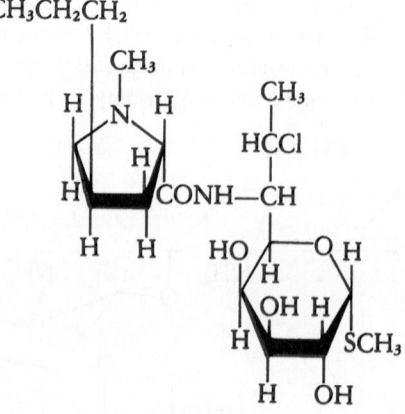

Yellow, amorphous solid; $[\alpha]_D$ +214° ($CHCl_3$).

Toxicology: Gray *et al.* (1972).

Preparation: Magerlein *et al.* (1967).

Synthesis and structure: Birkenmeyer and Kagan (1970).

Hydrochloride monohydrate

$C_{18}H_{36}Cl_2N_2O_6S$ mol. wt. 447.40

Synonym: Dalactine.

White crystals from C_2H_5OH–$CH_3CO_2C_2H_5$, m.p. 141–143°C; $[\alpha]_D$ +144° (H_2O);
   pK_a 7.6.

Solubility: sol. H_2O, pyridine, C_2H_5OH, DMF.

Toxicity: LD_{50} mice 245 mg/kg iv, 361 mg/kg ip, 2618 mg/kg po (Gray *et al.*, 1972).

REFERENCES

Acheson, R. M., 1973, *Acridines,* Wiley–Interscience, New York.

Adams, G. E., Stratford, I. J., Wallace, R. G., Wardman, P. and Watts, M. E., 1980, Toxicity of nitro
   compounds towards hypoxic mammalian cells in vitro: Dependence on reduction potential, *J. Natl.
   Cancer Inst.* 64:555–560.

Adrien, A., 1966, *The Acridines*, St. Martin's Press, New York.

Ali, B. H., 1983, Some pharmacological and toxicological properties of furazolidone, *Vet. Res. Commun.* 6:1–11.

Anderson, H. A., Emerson, G. A., and Fisher, B. H., 1934, Acute toxicity of trypan blue, gentian violet and brilliant green, *Proc. Soc. Exp. Biol. Med.* 31:825–828.

Asher, I. M., 1977, Amphotericin B, in: *Analytical Profiles of Drug Substances* (K. Florey, ed.), Vol. 6, pp. 1–42, Academic Press, New York.

Ashley, J. N., Barber, H. J., Ewins, A. J., Newberry, G., and Self, A. D. H., 1942, A chemotherapeutic comparison of the trypanocidal action of some aromatic diamidines, *J. Chem. Soc.* 103–116.

Ashley, J. N., Berg, S. S., and Lucas, J. M. S., 1960, 3,3′-Diamidinocarbanilide: A new drug active against babesial infections, *Nature (Lond.)* 185:461.

Auterhoff, H., Neuwald, F., and Schmid, W. (eds.), 1958, Glycobiarsol, *Pharm. Prax.* I (Suppl. 2), 1:759.

Ball, S. J., Davis, M., Hodgson, J. N., Lucas, J. M. S., Parnell, E. W., Sharp, B. W., and Warburton, D., 1968, *Chem. Ind. (Lond.)* 56–57.

Barbieri, P., Beltrame, D., Bloch, K., Guidi, P., Passerini, N., and Tamassia, V., 1972, Characteristics of the action of nitrimidazine (nimorazole), a new systemic trichomonacide. II. Pharmacology and toxicology, *Boll. Chim. Pharm.* 111: 541–554; *Chem. Abstr.* 78:52828f.

Beaman, A. G., Duschinsky, R., and Tautz, W. P., 1969, *Br. Patent* 1,138,529.

Benda, L., 1912, On 3,6-diamino-acridine, *Ber.* 45:1787–1799.

Benda, L., and Bertheim, A., 1911, On nitro-oxy-aryl-arsinic acids, *Ber.* 44:3446.

Berg, D. H., Hamill, R. L., Hoehn, M. M., and Nakatsukasa, W. M., 1975, Antibiotic A-28086, *Ger. Patent* 2,525,095.

Berger, J., Rachlin, A. I., Scott, W. E., Sternbach, L. H., and Goldberg, M. W., 1951, The isolation of a new crystalline antibiotic from streptomyces, *J. Am. Chem. Soc.* 73:5295–5298.

Berndt, E. W., Van Essen, H., Held, B. G., and Vatne, R. D., 1969, 3,5-Dinitrosalicylic acid (5-nitrofurfurylidene)hydrazide, a potent preventative of histomoniasis in turkeys, *J. Med. Chem.* 12:371–374.

Bernstein, E. H., Pienta, P. W., and Gershon, H., 1963, Acute toxicity studies on 8-quinolinol and some derivatives, *Toxicol. Appl. Pharmacol.* 5:599–604.

Beveridge, E., 1969, Babesicidal effect of basically substituted carbanilides. II. Imidocarb in rats and mice: Toxicity and activity against *Babesia rodhaini*, *Res. Vet. Sci.* 10:534–539.

Bhagwat, V. K., and Pyman, F. L., 1925, The 4- and 5-nitro-1:2-dimethylglyoxalines, *J. Chem. Soc.* 127:1832–1836.

Birkenmeyer, R. D., and Kagan, F., 1970, Lincomycin. XI. Synthesis and structure of clindamycin a potent antibacterial agent, *J. Med. Chem.* 13:616–619.

Böhni, E., Fust, B., Rieder, J., Schaerer, K., and Havas, L., 1969, Comparative toxicological, chemotherapeutic and pharmacokinetic studies with sulphormethoxine and other sulfonamides in animals and man, *Chemotherapy* 14:195–226.

Boothe, J. H., Morton, J. II, Petisi, J. P., Wilkinson, R. G., and Williams, J. H., 1953, Tetracycline, *J. Am. Chem. Soc.* 75:4621.

Boothe, J. H., Kende, A. S., Fields, T. L., and Wilkinson, R. G., 1959, Total synthesis of tetracycline. I. (±)-Dedimethylamino-12a-deoxy-6-demethylanhydrochlorotetracycline, *J. Am. Chem. Soc.* 81:1006–1007.

Borowski, E., Zielinski, J., Ziminski, T., Falkowski, L., Kolodziejczyk, P., Golik, J., and Jereczek, E., 1970, Chemical studies with amphotericin B. III. The complete structure of the antibiotic, *Tetrahedron Lett.* 3909–3914.

Bose, A. N., and Ghosh, T. N., 1949, A note on the pharmacopeial characteristics of injection of sodium antimony (V) gluconate (concentrated), *Indian J. Pharm.* 11:155–157.

Bretschneider, H., and Klötzer, W., 1955, Benzenesulfonamides with therapeutic activity, U.S. Patent 2,703,800.

Broderson, R., Loewe, H., and Ott, H., 1958, Soluble, stable salts of 1,3-bis(4-amidinophenyl)triazene and a process of preparing them, U.S. Patent 2,838,485.

Brogden, R. N., Heel, R. C., Speight, T. M., and Avery, G. S., 1978, Metronidazole in anaerobic infections: A review of its activity, pharmacokinetics and therapeutic use, *Drugs* 16:387–417.

Brossi, A., Baumann, M., Chopard-dit-Jean, L. H., Würsch, J., Schneider, F. and Schnider, O., 1959, Racemic 2-dehydro-emetine, *Helv. Chim. Acta* 42:772–788.

Buechel, K. H., Regel, E., and Plempel, M., 1969, N-Tritylimidazoles as antimycotics, South Afr. Patent 68 05,392.

Buhs, R. P., Polin, D., Beattie, J. O., Beck, J. L., Smith, J. L., Speth, O. C., and Trenner, N. R., 1966, The metabolism of ethopabate in chickens, *J. Pharmacol. Exp. Ther.* 154:357–363.

Burchall, J. J., 1975, Trimethoprim and pyrimethimine, in: *Antibiotics* (J. W. Corcoran, and F. E. Hahn, eds.), Vol. 3, pp. 312–320, Springer-Verlag, New York.

Burckhalter, J. H., Tendick, F. H., Jones, E. M., Jones, P. A., Holcomb, W. F., and Rawlins, A. L., 1948, Aminoalkylphenols as antimalarials. II. (Heterocyclic-amino)-α-amino-*o*-cresols. The synthesis of camoquin, *J. Am. Chem. Soc.* 70:1363.

Butler, K., 1968, 1-(Lower alkyl)sulfonylalkyl-2-(lower alkyl)-5-nitroimidazoles, U.S. Patent 3,376,311.

Butler, K., Howes, H. L., Lynch, J. E., and Pirie, D. K., 1967, Nitroimidazole derivatives. Relationship between structure and antitrichomonal activity, *J. Med. Chem.* 10:891–897.

Cahen, R. L., 1964, Evaluation of the teratogenicity of drugs, *Clin. Pharmacol. Ther.* 5:480–514.

Camerino, B., and Palamidessi, G., 1960, Pyrazine derivatives—Note II. Sulfonamidopyrazines, *Gazz. Chim. Ital.* 90:1815–1820.

Canevazzi, G., and Scotti, T., 1959, Description of a new species of streptomycetes (*Streptomyces chrestomyrceticus*) producing a new antibiotic, amminosidin, *Giorn. Microbiol.* 7:242–250.

Canton, J. H., and Van Esch, G. J., 1976, The short-term toxicity of some feed additives to different freshwater organisms, *Bull. Environ. Contam. Toxicol.* 15:720–725.

Carcassi, U., 1948, Treatment of visceral leishmaniasis. First observations on employment in Italy of N-methylglucamine antimonate (glucantime, 2168 RP), *Progr. Med.* 5:426–428; 1949, *Abstr. World. Med.* 5:511; *Chem. Abstr.* 46:5208h.

Carrington, H. C., Crowther, A. F., Davy, D. G., Levi, A. A., and Rose, F. L., 1951, A metabolite of "Paludrine" with high antimalarial activity, *Nature (Lond.)* 168:1080.

Child, K. J., Davis, B., Dodds, M. G., and Tomich, E. G., 1964, Toxicity and tissue distribution studies on the hydrochloride, bismuth iodide complex and a resinate of emetine, *J. Pharm. Pharmacol.* 16:65–71.

Chyan, W.-H., Lu, X.-T., Soong, H.-T., and Chang, C.-C., 1956, Studies on the antimonials for schistosomiasis. I. Water-soluble organic trivalent antimony compounds, *Yao Hsueh Hsueh Pao* 4:295–299; 1958, *Chem. Abstr.* 52:9963d.

Clark, D. E., Holton, P. G., Meredith, R. F. K., Ritchie, A. C., Walker, T., and Whiting, K. D. E., 1962, Emetine and related compounds. Part II. The stereospecific synthesis of (±)-2,3-dehydroisoemetine, *J. Chem. Soc.* 2479–2490.

Coffey, G. L., Anderson, L. E., Fisher, M. W., Galbraith, M. M., Hillegas, A. B., Kohberger, D. L., Thompson, P. E., Weston, K. S., and Ehrlich, J., 1959, Biological studies of paromomycin, *Antibiot. Chemother.* 9:730–738.

Conover, L. H., Butler, K., Johnston, J. D., Korst, J. J., and Woodward, R. B., 1962, The total synthesis of 6-demethyl-6-deoxytetracycline, *J. Am. Chem. Soc.* 84:3222–3224.

Cosar, C., Ninet, L., Pinnert-Sindico, S., and Preud'homme, J., 1952, Trypanocidal activity of an antibiotic produced by a streptomyces, *C. R. Soc. Biol.* 234:1498–1499.

Craine, E. M., Kouba, R. F., and Ray, W. H., 1971, The disposition of decoquinate-^{14}C administered orally to chickens, *J. Agr. Food Chem.* 19:1228–1233.

Crowther, A. F., Curd, F. H. S., and Rose, F. L., 1951, Synthetic antimalarials. Part XLVIII. The action of halogens on N[1]-aryldiguanides, *J. Chem. Soc.* 1780–1785.

Cuckler, A. C., Malanga, C. M., Basso, A. J., and O'Neill, R. C., 1955, Antiparasitic activity of substituted carbanilide complexes, *Science* 122:244–245.

Curd, F. H. S., and Davey, D. G., 1950, "Antrycide"—A new trypanocidal drug, *Br. J. Pharmacol.* 5:25–32.

Curd, F. H. S., and Rose, F. L., 1946, Synthetic antimalarials. Part X. Some aryldiguanide ("-biguanide") derivatives, *J. Chem. Soc.* 729–737.

Das Gupta, S. J., 1953, Preparation of sodium antimony gluconate, *Indian J. Pharm.* 15:84–85.

Datta, S., Ghosh, T. N., and Bose, A. N., 1946, Condensation of p-aminophenylstibonic acid with urea, *Sci. Cult.* 11:385; 1947, *Chem. Abstr.* 41:105h.

Davies, N. A., 1943, Production of tartar emetic with use of metallic Sb, U.S. Patent 2,335,585.

Davies, N. A., 1945, Tartar emetic, U.S. Patent 2,391,297.

Davisson, J. W., and Finlay, A. C., 1959, Catenulin, U.S. Patent 2,895,876.

Di Marco, A., and Bertazzoli, C., 1963, Pharmacology of new basic oligosaccharide antibiotics, *Antibiot. Chemother.* 11:2–20.

Downing, J. G., Hanson, M. C., and Lamb, M., Use of 5-Nitro-2-furaldehyde semicarbazone in dermatology, 1947, *J.A.M.A.* 133:299–306.

Drake, G. D., and Hayes, K. J., 1956, 3-(5-Nitro-2-furfurylideneamino)-2-oxazolidinone, U.S. Patent 2,759,931.

Duggar, B. M., 1948, Aureomycin: A product of the continuing search for new antibiotics, *Ann. N.Y. Acad. Sci.* 51:177–181; see also immediately subsequent articles.

Edwards, C., Doxycycline, 1979, in: *Pharmacological and Biochemical Properties of Drug Substances* (M. E. Goldberg, ed.), Vol. 2, pp. 305–332, American Pharmacology Association, Washington, D.C.

Elderfield, R. C., Gensler, W. J., Head, J. D., Hageman, H. A., Cremer, C. B., Wright, J. B., Holley, A. D., Williamson, B., Galbreath, J., Wiederhold, L., III, Frohardt, R., Kupchan, S. M., Williamson, T. A., and Birstein, O., 1946, Alkylaminoalkyl derivatives of 8-aminoquinoline, *J. Am. Chem. Soc.* 68:1524–1529.

Ercoli, N., 1968, Chemotherapeutic and toxicological properties of antimonyl tartrate-dimethylcysteine chelates, *Proc. Soc. Exp. Biol. Med.* 129:284–290.

Ertürk, E., Morris, J. E., Cohen, S. M., Price, J. M., and Bryan, G. T., 1970, Transplantable rat mammary tumors induced by 5-nitro-2-furaldehyde semicarbazone and by formic acid 2-[4-(5-nitro-2-furyl)-2-thiazolyl]hydrazide, *Cancer Res.* 30:1409–1412.

Evans, R. C. (ed.), 1968, Tetracycline, in: *The Technology of the Tetracyclines* Vol. 1, pp. 209–426, Quadrangle Press, New York.

Evstigneeva, R. P., Livshits, R. S., Zakharkin, L. I., Bainova, M. S., and Preobrazhenskii, N. A., 1950, Synthesis of the alkaloid emetine, *Dokl. Akad. Nauk SSSR* 75:539–542.

Fabre, J., Pitton, J. S., Kunz, J. P., Rozbroj, S., and Hungerbühler, R. M., 1966, Distribution and excretion of doxycycline in man, *Chemotherapia* 11:73–85.

Ferry, C. W., Buck, J. S., and Baltzly, R., 1955, 4,4'-Diaminodiphenylsulfone, *Org. Syn. Coll.* 3:239–241.

Festy, B., 1979, Hydroxystilbamidine, in: *Antibiotics* (F. E. Hahn, ed.), Vol. 5, part 2, pp. 223–235, Springer-Verlag, New York.

Feyns, L. V., and Grady, L. T., 1981, Emetine hydrochloride, in: *Analytical Profiles of Drug Substances* (K. Florey, ed.), Vol. 10, pp. 289–335, Academic Press, New York.

Fieser, L. F., Schirmer, J. P., Archer, S., Lorenz, R. R., and Pfaffenbach, P. I., 1967, Naphthoquinone antimalarials. XXIX. 2-Hydroxy-3-(ω-cyclohexylalkyl)-1,4-naphthoquinones, *J. Med. Chem.* 10:513–517.

Fischer, R., and Hirt, R., 1965, Polybasic compounds, Br. Patent 1,007,334.

Fourneau, E., Trefouel, J., Trefouel, Mme, J., and Vallee, J., 1924, Chemotherapeutic research in the series "Bayer 205," *Ann. Inst. Pasteur* 38:81–114.

Freiberg, L. A., Egan, R. S., and Washburn, W. H., 1974, The synthesis of 9-epi-leucomycin A₃. The revised configurational assignment of C-9 in natural leicomycin A₃, *J. Org. Chem.* 39:2474–2475; see also references cited therein.

Friedheim, E. A. H., 1944, Trypanocidal and spirochetocidal arsenicals derived from s-triazine, *J. Am. Chem. Soc.* 66:1775–1778.

Friedheim, E. A. H., 1953, Heterocyclic organometallic compounds, U.S. Patent 2,659,723.

Friedheim, E. A. H., 1956, Therapeutic organometallic compounds of antimony and sulfur, U.S. Patent 2,772,303.

Frohardt, R. P., Haskell, T. H., Ehrlich, J., and Knudsen, M. P., 1959, Paromomycin, U.S. Patent 2,916,485.

Fromm, E., and Wittmann, J., 1908, Derivatives of *p*-nitrothiophenol, *Ber.* 41:2264–2273.

Fukayama, T., Akasaka, K., Karanewsky, D. S., Wang, C.-L. J., Schmid, G., and Kishi, Y., 1979, Total synthesis of monensin. 3. Stereocontrolled total synthesis of monensin, *J. Am. Chem. Soc.* 101:262.

Gailliot, P., 1952, N^1-*p*-Chlorophenyl-N^5-isopropylbiguanide, Fr. Patent 1,001,548.

Gaillot, M., 1934, Composition and solubility of acriflavine and some other derivatives of 2,8-diaminoacridine used in therapeutics, *Q. J. Pharm. Pharmacol.* 7:63–75.

Gasparini, G. 1971, Kelfizina, a low dosage sulfanilamide, *Veterinaria (Milan)* 20:302–309.

Gasparini, G., and Pignatelli, P., 1972, Pharmacology of aminosidine, *Veterinaria (Milan)* 21:7–17.

Geze, M., Blanchard, P., Fourrey, J. L., and Robert-Gero, M., 1983, Synthesis of sinefungin and its C-6' epimer, *J. Am. Chem. Soc.* 105:7638–7640.

Gibaldi, M., 1967, Pharmacokinetics of absorption and elimination of doxycycline in man, *Chemotherapia* 12:265–271.

Giraldi, P. N., and Mariotti, V., 1968, *N*-Tertiary-aminoalkylene 4- or 5-nitroimidazoles, U.S. Patent 3,399,193.

Giraldi, P. N., Tosolini, G. P., Dradi, E., Nannini, G., Longo, R., Meinardi, G., Monti, G., and de Carneri, I., 1971, Studies on antiprotozoals—III. Isolation, identification and quantitative determination in humans of the metabolites of a new trichomonacidal agent, *Biochem. Pharmacol.* 20:339–349.

Gold, W., Stout, H. A., Pagano, J. F., and Donovick, R., 1956, Amphotericins A and B, antifungal antibiotics produced by a streptomycete, in: *Antibiotic Annual 1955–1956* (H. Welch and M. Marti-Ibañez, eds.), pp. 579–586, Medical Encyclopedia Inc., New York.

Goldenthal, E. I., 1971, Compilation of LD_{50} values in newborn and adult animals, *Toxicol. Appl. Pharmacol.* 18:185–207.

Gönnert, R. 1972, Nifurtimox: Causal treatment of Chagas' disease, *Arzneimittelforsch.* 22:1563; see pp. 1564–1642 for related articles.

Gray, J. E., Weaver, R. N., Bollert, J. A., and Feenstra, E. S., 1972, Oral toxicity of clindamycin in laboratory animals, *Toxicol. Appl. Pharmacol.* 21:516–531.

Grimme, W., and Schmitz, H., 1954, On derivatives of 4-amino-salicyclic acid. II. Communication, *Ber.* 87:179–186.

Grollman, A. P., and Jarkovsky, Z., 1975, Emetine and related alkaloids, in: *Antibiotics* (J. W. Corcoran and F. E. Hahn, eds.), Vol. 3, pp. 420–435, Springer-Verlag, New York.

Hahn, F. E., 1975, Chloroquine (Resochin), in: *Antibiotics* (J. W. Corcoran and F. E. Hahn, eds.), Vol. 3, pp. 58–78, Springer-Verlag, New York.

Hahn, F. E., 1979, Quinine, in: *Antibiotics* (F. E. Hahn, ed.), Vol. 5, part 2, pp. 353–362, Springer-Verlag, New York.

Hamill, R. L., and Hoehn, M. M., 1971, *Abstracts of the Eleventh Interscience Conference on Antimicrobial Agents and Chemotherapy*, p. 21.

Haney, M. E., Jr., and Hoehn, M. M., 1967, Monensin, a new biologically active compound. I. Discovery and isolation, in: *Proceedings of the Seventh Interscience Conference on Antimicrobial Agents and Chemotherapy, Chicago, October 25–27, 1967* (G. L. Hobby, ed.), pp. 349–352, American Society for Microbiology, Ann Arbor, Michigan.

Hartman, G. D., Biffar, S. E., Weinstock, L. H., and Tull, R., 1978, New synthesis of a 9-substituted adenine, *J. Org. Chem.* 43:960–961.

Haskelberg, L., 1947, Derivatives of 6-nitro- and 6-aminoquinoline, *J. Org. Chem.* 12:434.

Haskell, T. H., French, J. C., and Bartz, Q. R., 1959*a*, Paromomycin. I. Paromamine, a glycoside of D-glucosamine, *J. Am. Chem. Soc.* 81:3480–3482.

Haskell, T. H., French, J. C., and Bartz, Q. R., 1959*b*, Paromomycin. II. Paromobiosamine, a diaminohexosyl-D-ribose. *J. Am. Chem. Soc.* 81:3482.

Herlinger, H., Mayer, K. H., Petersen, S., and Bock, M., 1964, 5-Nitrofurfurylideneamino derivatives, Ger. Patent 1,170,957.

Hoff, D. R., Rooney, C. S., and Carlson, J. A., 1967, Substituted alkylimidazol-2-yl carbamates, Neth. Patent 6,609,552.

Hoffer, M., and Mitrovic, M., 1968, 1-Methyl-2-isopropyl-5-nitroimidazole, Brit. Patent 1,119,636.

Hoffman, K., 1972, Toxicological investigations on the tolerability of Nifurtimox, *Arzneimittelforsch.* 22:1590–1603.

Hollingshead, R. G. W., 1954–1956, *Oxine and Its Derivatives*, Vols. I–IV, Butterworths, London.

Holz, R. W., 1979, Polyene antibiotics: Nystatin, amphotericin B, and filipin, in: *Antibiotics* (F. E. Hahn, ed.), Vol. 5, part 2, pp. 313–340, Springer-Verlag, New York.

Hong, D. D., 1976, Chloroquine analogs, in: *Analytical Profiles of Drug Substances* (K. Florey, ed.), Vol. 5, pp. 61–85, Academic Press, New York.

Hoogerheide, J. G., and Wyka, B. E., 1982, Clotrimazole, in: *Analytical Profiles of Drug Substances* (K. Florey, ed.), Vol.,11 pp. 225–255, Academic Press, New York; see also a series of articles, 1972, *Arznemittelforsch.* 22:1260–1299.

Hudson, A. T., 1984, Lapinone, menoctone, hydroxyquinolinequinones and similar structures, in: *Antimalarial Drugs*, Volume II (W. Peters and W. H. G. Richards, eds.), *Handbook of Experimental Pharmacology*, Volume 68, pp. 343–361, Springer-Verlag, New York.

Ings, R. M. J., Law, G. L., and Parnell, E. W., 1966, The metabolism of metronidazole (1-2'-hydroxyethyl-2-methyl-5-nitroimidazole), *Biochem. Pharmacol.* 15:515–519.

Jacob, R. M., Régnier, G. L., and Crisan, C., 1960, Nitroimidazoles and acyl derivatives, U.S. Patent 2,944,061.

Jacobs, W. A., and Heidelberger, M., 1919, Aromatic arsenic compounds. II. The amides and alkyl amides of N-arylglycine arsonic acids, *J. Am. Chem. Soc.* 41:1587–1590.

Jacobs, W. A., Heidelberger, M., and Rolf, I. P., 1918, Nitro- and aminoarylarsonic acids, *J. Am. Chem. Soc.* 40:1580–1590.

Jauch, R., Griesser, E., and Oesterhelt, G., 1980, Metabolism of Ro 21-5998 (mefloquin) in the rat, *Arzneimittelforsch.* 30:60–67.

Kaji, A. and Ryoji, M., 1979, Tetracycline, in: *Antibiotics* (F. E. Hahn, ed.), Vol. 5, part 1, pp. 304–328, Springer-Verlag, New York.

Kano, H., Nishimura, H., Nakajima, K., and Ogata, K., 1959, Sulfonamides, U.S. Patent 2,888,455.

Kerr, K. B., Cavett, J. W., and Thompson, O. L., 1963, The toxicity of an organic arsenical, 3-nitro-4-hydroxyphenylarsonic acid. Acute and subacute toxicity, *Toxicol. Appl. Pharmacol.* 5:507–525.

Kishi, Y., Hatakeyama, S., and Lewis, M. D., 1982, Total synthesis of polyether antibiotics narasin and salinomycin, in: *Frontiers in Chemistry, Plenary Keynote Lecture, Twenty-eighth IUPAC Congress* (K. J. Laidler, ed.), pp. 287–304, Pergamon, Oxford.

Kouba, R. F., Craine, E. M., and Ray, W. H., 1971, The presence of residues in the tissues of rats receiving decoquinate orally, *J. Agr. Food Chem.* 19:1234–1237.

Ledet, A. E., Duncan, J. R., Buck, W. B., and Ramsey, F. K., 1973, Clinical, toxicological, and pathological aspects of arsanilic acid poisoning in swine, *Clin. Toxicol.* 6:439–457.

LePecq, J.-B., 1971, Use of ethidium bromide for separation and determination of nucleic acids of various conformational forms and measurement of their associated enzymes, in: *Methods of Biochemical Analysis* (D. Glick, ed.), Vol. 20, pp. 41–48, Wiley–Interscience, New York.

Lewers, W. W., and Lowry, A., 1925, Comparative study of azo dyes made with H acid and acetyl-H acid, *Ind. Eng. Chem.* 17:1289–1290.

Lewis, W. L., and Cheetham, H. C., 1941, Arsanilic acid, in: *Organic Synthesis Coll.* Vol. 1, 2nd ed. (H. Gilman, ed.), Vol. 1, pp. 70–73, Wiley, New York.

Lin, D. C., and Kun, E., 1973, Mode of action of the antibiotic X-537A on mitochondrial glutamate oxidation, *Biochem. Biophys. Res. Commun.* 50:820–825.

Lira, E. P., Barker, W. M., and McCrae, R. C., 1972, 6-Amino-9-(2,6-dichlorobenzyl)purine N'-oxide for treatment of coccidiosis, Fr. Patent 2,128,600.

Liu, C.-M., Prosser, B., and Westley, J., 1981, Antibiotic X-14868A, B, C, and D, U. S. Patent 4,278,663.

Magerlein, B. J., Birkenmeyer, R. D., and Kagan, F., 1967, Chemical modification of lincomycin, in: *Proceedings of the Sixth Interscience Conference on Antimicrobial Agents and Chemotherapy, Philadelphia, October 26–28, 1966* (G. L. Hobby, ed.), pp. 727–736, American Society for Microbiology, Ann Arbor, Michigan.

Manius, G. J., 1978, Trimethoprim, in: *Analytical Profiles of Drug Substances* (K. Florey, ed.), Vol. 7, pp. 445–475, Academic Press, New York.

Manske, R. H. F., Ledingham, A. E., and Ashford, W. R., 1949, The preparation of quinolines by a modified Skraup reaction, *Can. J. Res.* 27F:359–367.

Marusich, W. L., Ogrinz, E. F., and Mitrovic, M., 1970, Toxicity and safety studies with the antihistomonal agent, ipronidazole, in turkeys, *J. Poultry Sci.* 49:92–98.

McChesney, E. W. and Hoppe, J. O., 1950, Absorption, excretion, and toxicity of bismuthoxy-*p*-*N*-glycolylarsanilate (Milibis) following oral administration, *Proc. Soc. Exp. Biol. Med.* 73:326–330.

McGookin, A., Swift, S. R., and Tittensor, E., 1940, Orientation problems. III. 4,6-Dinitro-*o*-toluidine, *J. Soc. Chem. Ind.* 59:92–94.

Mechlinski, W., Schaffer, C. P., Ganis, P., and Avitable, G., 1970, Structure and absolute configuration of the polyene macrolide antibiotic amphotericin B, *Tetrahedron Lett.* 3873–3876.

Mietzsch, F., and Mauss, H., 1934, Acridine derivatives, Ger. Patent 553,072.

Miller, M. W., Howes, H. L., Kasubick, R. V., and English, A. R., 1970, Alkylation of 2-methyl-5-nitroimidazole. Some potent antiprotozoal agents, *J. Med. Chem.* 13:849–852.

Miyazaki, Y., Suguwara, H., Nagatsu, J., and Shibuya, M., 1972, Salinomycin from streptomyces, Japan, Patent 72 25392.

Miyazaki, Y., Shibuya, M., Suguwara, H., Kawaguchi, O., Hirose, C., Nagatsu, J., and Esumi, S., 1974, Salinomycin, a new polyether antibiotic, *J. Antibiot.* 27:814–821.

Mock, G. A., and Moffat, J. G., 1982, An approach to the total synthesis of sinefungin, *Nucleic Acids Res.* 10:6223–6234.

Modest, E. J., 1956, Chemical and biological studies on 1,2-dihydro-*s*-triazines. II. Three component systems, *J. Org. Chem.* 21:1–13.

Modest, E. J., Foley, G. E., Pechet, M. M., and Farber, S., 1952, A series of new, biologically significant dihydrotriazines, *J. Am. Chem. Soc.* 74:855–856.

Morris, J. E., Price, J. M., Lalich, J. J., and Stein, R. J., 1969, The carcinogenic activity of some 5-nitrofuran derivatives in the rat, *Cancer Res.* 29:2145–2156.

Muxfeldt, H., Haas, G., Hardtmann, G., Kathawala, F., Mooberry, J. B., and Vedejs, E., 1979, Tetracyclines. 9. Total synthesis of *dl*-terramycin, *J. Am. Chem. Soc.* 101:689–690.

Nakata, T., Schmid, G., Vranesic, B., Okigawa, M., Smith-Palmer, T., and Kishi, Y., 1978, A total synthesis of lasalocid A, *J. Am. Chem. Soc.* 100:2933–2935.

Nakatsu, H., and Kawase, S., 1956, Preparation of carbarsone, *Annu. Rep. Takamine Lab.* 8:44–47.

Newberry, G., and Easson, A. P. T., 1946a, Soluble diamine salts, U.S. Patent 2,394,003.

Newberry, G., and Easson, A. P. T., 1946b, Soluble amidine salts, U.S. Patent 2,410,796.

Newton, B. A., 1975, Berenil: A trypanocide with selective activity against extranuclear DNA, in: *Antibiotics* (J. W. Corcoran and F. E. Hahn, eds.), Vol. 3, pp. 34–47, Springer-Verlag, New York.

Nord, C. E., and Phillips, I. (eds.), 1982, Anaerobic infections: The role of tinidazole, *J. Antimicrob. Chemother.* (Suppl. A) 10:1–184.

Ohnmacht, C. J., Patel, Á. R., and Lutz, R. E. 1971, Antimalarials. 7. Bis(trifluoromethyl)-α-(2-piperidyl)-4-quinolinemethanols, *J. Med. Chem.* 14:926–928.

Olenick, J. G., 1975a, Suramin, in: *Antibiotics* (J. W. Corcoran and F. E. Hahn, eds.), Vol. 3, pp. 699–703, Springer-Verlag, New York.

Olenick, J. G., 1975b, Primaquine, in: *Antibiotics* (J. W. Corcoran and F. E. Hahn, eds.), Vol. 3, pp. 516–520, Springer-Verlag, New York.

Orzech, C. E., Nash, N. G., and Daley, R. D., 1976, Dapsone, in: *Analytical Profiles of Drug Substances* (K. Florey, ed.), Vol. 5, pp. 87–114, Academic Press, New York.

Oxley, P., Bristow, N. W., Williams, G. A. H., Woolfe, G., and Wilmhurst, E. C., 1959, Derivatives of acetanilide, U.S. Patent 2,912,438.

Papesch, V., and Burtner, R. R., 1936, 5,7-Diiodo-8-hydroxyquinoline, *J. Am. Chem. Soc.* 58:1314.

Petering, H. G., Buskirk, H. H., and Underwood, G. E., 1964, The anti-tumor activity of 2-keto-3-ethoxybutyraldehyde bis(thiosemicarbazone) and related compounds, *Cancer Res.* 24:367–372.

Pfeiffer, P., and Schmitz, E., 1949, Constitution of tartar emetic, *Pharmazie* 4:451.

Phillips, J. P., 1956, The reactions of 8-quinolinol, *Chem. Rev.* 56:271–297.

Plempel, M., Bartmann, K., Büchel, K. H., and Regel, E., 1970, BAY b 5097, a new orally applicable antifungal substance with broad-spectrum activity, in: *Proceedings of the Ninth Interscience Conference on Antimicrobial Agents and Chemotherapy, Washington, D.C., October 27–29, 1969* (G. L. Hobby, ed.), pp. 271–274, American Society for Microbiology, Bethesda, Maryland.

Plisek, K., Dvorak, M., Bohumil, S., and Blazek, K., 1971, Examination of toxic effects of metichlorpindol, *Vet. Spofa* 12:111–125; *Chem. Abstr.* 74:138780p.

Raaflaub, J., and Ziegler, W. H., 1979, Single-dose pharmacokinetics of the trypanosomicide benznidazole in man, *Arzneimittelforsch.* 29:1611–1614.

Rabe, P., and Marschall, O., 1911, Fluorescence phenomena in Cinchona alkaloids, *Liebigs Annalen der Chemie* 382:362–364.

Radomski, J. L., Hagan, E. C., Fuyat, H. N., and Nelson, A. A., 1952, The pharmacology of ipacac, *J. Pharmacol. Exp. Ther.* 104:421–426.

Raiziss, G. W., Clemence, L. W., Severac, M., and Moetsch, J. C., 1939, Chemistry and chemotherapy of 4,4'-diaminodiphenylsulfone, 4-amino-4'-hydroxy-diphenylsulfone, and related compounds, *J. Am. Chem. Soc.* 61:2763–2765.

Regna, P. P., and Solomons, I. A., 1950, The chemical and physical properties of terramycin, *Ann. N.Y. Acad. Sci.* 53:221–237; see also associated articles.

Regna, P. P., Solomons, I. A., Murai, K., Timreck, A. E., Brunings, K. J., and Lazier, W. A., 1951, The isolation and general properties of terramycin and terramycin salts, *J. Am. Chem. Soc.* 73:4211–4215.

Roblin, R. O., Jr., Williams, J. H., Winnek, P. S., and English, J. P., 1940, Chemotherapy. II. Some sulfanilamido heterocycles, *J. Am. Chem. Soc.* 62:2002–2005.

Rogers, G. S., Belloff, G. B., Paul, M. F., Yurchenco, J. A., and Gever, G., 1956, Furazolidone, a new antimicrobial nitrofuran. A review of laboratory and clinical data, *Antibiot. Chemother.* 6:231–242.

Rogers, E. F., Clark, R. F., Pessolano, A. A., Becker, H. J., Leanza, W. J., Sarett, L. H., Cuckler, A. C., McManus, E., Garzillo, M., Malanga, C., Ott, W. H., Dickenson, A. M., and Van Iderstine, A., 1960, Antiparasitic drugs. III. Thiamine-reversible coccidiostats, *J. Am. Chem. Soc.* 82:2974–2975.

Roth, B., Aig, E., Lane, K., and Rauckman, B. S., 1980a, 2,4-Diamino-5-benzylpyrimidines and analogs as antibacterial agents. 4. 6-Substituted trimethoprim derivatives from phenolic Mannich intermediates. Application to the synthesis of trimethoprim and 3,5-dialkylbenzyl analogs, *J. Med. Chem.* 23:535–541.

Roth, B., Strelitz, J. Z., and Rauckman, B. S., 1980b, 2,4-Diamino-5-benzylpyrimidines and analogs as antibacterial agents. 2. C-Alkylation of pyrimidines with Mannich bases and application to the synthesis of trimethoprim and analogs, *J. Med. Chem.* 23:379–384.

Rudy, B. C., and Senkowski, B. Z., 1973, Sulfamethoxazole, in: *Analytical Profiles of Drug Substances* (K. Florey, ed.), Vol. 2, pp. 467–486, Academic Press, New York.

Russel, P. B., and Hitchings, G. H., 1951, 2,4-Diaminopyrimidines as antimalarials. III. 5-Aryl-derivatives, *J. Am. Chem. Soc.* 73:3763–3770.

Schmidt, H., 1930, Antimony in drug synthesis, *Angew, Chem.* 43:963–970.

Schmidt, L. H., Hughes, H. B., and Smith, C. C., 1947, On the pharmacology of N_1-para-chlorophenyl-N_5-isopropylbiguanide (Paludrine), *J. Pharmacol. Exp. Ther.* 90:233.

Schönhöfer, F., and Henecka, H., 1933, Urea and thiourea derivatives, Ger. Patent 583,207.

Schwartzman, G., Wayland, L., Alexander, T., Furnkranz, K., and Selzer, G., and the USASRG, 1979, Chlortetracycline hydrochloride, in: *Analytical Profiles of Drug Substances* (K. Florey, ed.), Vol. 8, pp. 101–137, Academic Press, New York.

Seki, T., Segawa, T., Komatsu, T., and Nakagome, T., 1965, Biological properties of 4-sulfanilamido-3,6-dimethoxypyridazine (CS-61)—A new sulfonamide, *Arzneimittelforsch.* 15:1441–1445.

Sheverdina, N. I., Abramova, L. V., Paleeva, I. E., and Kocheshkov, K. A., 1962, Preparation of dibutyltin organic salts, *Khim. Prom.* 10:707–708; 1963, *Chem. Abstr.* 59:8776f.

Skraup, Z. H., 1880, A synthesis of quinolines, *Monatshefte für Chemie* 1:316–318.

Skraup, Z. H., 1882, Synthetic studies in the quinoline series. IV. Communication, *Monatshefte für Chemie* 3:531–569.

Slack, R., Stickings, C. E., and Barber, H. J., 1946, Amidine salts, Br. Patent 575,145.

Smith, G. N., 1964, Pathways for the metabolism of 3,5-dinitro-*o*-toluamide (Zoalene) in chickens, *Anal. Biochem.* 7:461–471.

Smith, G. N., 1969, The metabolism of ^{36}Cl-clopidol (3,5-dichloro-2,6-dimethyl-4-pyridinol) in chickens, *Poultry Sci.* 48:420–436.

Smith, G. N., and Watson, B. L., 1969, The metabolism of ^{36}Cl-clopidol (3,5-dichloro-2,6-dimethyl-4-pyridinol) in rats, *Poultry Sci.* 48:436–443.

Smith, G. N., Thiegs, B. J., and Ludwig, P. D., 1963, Identification of the metabolites of 3,5-dinitro-*o*-toluamide-C^{14} (Zoalene) in chicken tissues, *J. Agr. Food Chem.* 11:253–256.

Sous, H., Krüpe, W., Osterloh, G., and Mückter, H., 1958, Antibiotic drugs with medium range of action erythromycin, oleandomycin, novobiocin, and spiramycin in experimental investigations, *Arzneimittelforsch.* 8:386–390.

Stark, W. M., 1969, Monensin, a new biologically active compound produced by a fermentation process, in: *Fermentation Advances, Papers Third International Fermentation Symposium* (D. Perlman, ed.), pp. 517–540, Academic Press, New York.

Stempel, A., and Westley, J. W., 1971, Antibiotics by culturing streptomyces organisms, Ger. Patent 2,040,998.

Stenbuck, P., and Hood, H. M., 1962, 2,4-Diamino-5-benzylpyrimidines, U.S. Patent 3,049,544.

Stevenson, G. T., 1965, Pyridinols employed in animal husbandry, U.S. Patent 3,206,358.

Stickings, R. W. E., 1928, Heterocyclic compounds containing arsenic. IV. Carbamido derivatives of arylarsonic acids, *J. Chem. Soc.* 3131–3134.

Stillman, W. B., and Scott, A. B., 1947, Substituted nitrofurans, U.S. Patent 2,416,234.

Stober, H., and DeWitte, W., 1982, Sulfadiazine, in: *Analytical Profiles of Drug Substances* (K. Florey, ed.), Vol. 11, pp. 523–551, Academic Press, New York.

Surrey, A. R., and Hammer, H. F., 1946, Some substituted 4-aminoquinoline derivatives, *J. Am. Chem. Soc.* 68:113–116.

Surrey, A. R., and Hammer, H. F., 1950, The preparation of 7-chloro-4-(4-N-ethyl-N-hydroxyethylamino)-1-(methylbutylamino)quinoline and related compounds. *J. Am. Chem. Soc.* 72:1814–1815.

Taylor, J. A., Jr., Migliardi, J. R., and Schach von Wittenau, M., 1970, Tinidazole and metronidazole pharmacokinetics in man and mouse, in: *Proceedings of the Ninth Interscience Conference on Antimicrobial Agents and Chemotherapy Washington D.C., 9 October 27–28, 1969,* (G. L. Hobby, ed.), pp. 267–270, American Society for Microbiology, Bethesda, Maryland.

Tettenborn, Von D., 1972, Acute toxicity and local tolerance of clotrimazole, *Arzneimittelforsch.* 22:1272–1276.

Tomcufcik, A. S., 1970, Substituted bis(benzylideneamino)guanidines and salts, Ger. Patent 1,933,112.

Ungar, J., and Robinson, F. A., 1944, Investigation of the antibacterial and toxic action of certain acridine derivatives, *J. Pharmacol. Exp. Ther.* 80:217–232.

Van Tamelen, E. E., Placeway, C., Schiemenz, G. P., and Wright, I. G., 1969, The total synthesis of *dl*-ajmalicine and emetine, *J. Am. Chem. Soc.* 91:7359–7371.

von Büchel, K. H., Draber, W., Regel, E., and Plempel, M., 1972, Synthesen und Eigenschaften von Clotrimazol und weiteren antimykotischen 1-Triphenylmethylimidazolen, *Arzneimittelforsch* 22:1260–1272.

von Duhm, B., Maul, W., Medenwald, H., Patzschke, K., Wegner, L. A., and ObersteLehn, H., 1972, Pharmakokinetik nach topischer Anwendung von Bisphenyl-(2-chlorophenyl)-1-imidazolyl-methan-[^{14}C], *Arzneimittelforsch.* 22:1276–1280.

von Wittenau, M. S., Beereboom, J. J., Blackwood, R. K., and Stephens, C. R., 1962, 6-Deoxytetracyclines. III. Stereochemistry at C.6, *J. Am. Chem. Soc.* 84:2645–2647.

Voogd, C. E., Van der Stel, J. J., and Jacobs, J. J. J. A. A., 1979, The mutagenic action of several nitroimidazoles and some imidazoles, *Mutat. Res.* 66:207–221.

Waletzky, E., Berkelhammer, and Kantor, S., 1967, Quinazolones for treating coccidiosis, U.S. Patent 3,320,124.

Waring, M., 1975, Ethidium and propidium, in: *Antibiotics* (J. W. Corcoran and F. E. Hahn, eds.), Vol. 3, pp. 141–165, Springer-Verlag, New York.

Watkins, T. I., 1952, Trypanocides of the phenanthridine series. Part I. The effect of changing the quaternary grouping in dimidium, *J. Chem. Soc.* 3059–3064.

Watkins, T. I., 1958, Trypanocides of the phenanthridine series. Part II. Pyrimidinyl-phenanthridines, *J. Chem. Soc.* 1443–1450.

Watson, E. J., 1965, Ethyl 6,7-diisobutoxy-4-hydroxyquinoline-3-carboxylate, Belg. Patent 659,237.

Wearly, L. L., and Anthony, G. D., 1976, Metronidazole, in: *Analytical Profiles of Drug Substances* (K. Florey, ed.), Vol. 5, pp. 327–344, Academic Press, New York.

Weijlard, J., Tishler, M., and Erickson, A. E., 1944, Sulfaquinoxaline and some related compounds, *J. Am. Chem. Soc.* 66:1957–1959.

Weiss, P. J., Andrew, M. L., and Wright, W. W., 1957, Solubility of antibiotics in twenty-four solvents: Use in analysis, *Antibiot. Chemother.* 7:374–377.

Westley, J. W., 1978, Antibiotics (Polyether), in: Kirk-Othmer *Encyclopedia of Chemical Technology*, (M. Grayson, ed.), 3rd ed., p. 61, Wiley–Interscience, New York.

Windholz, M., Budavari, S., Blumetti, R. F., and Otterbein, E. S. (eds.), 1983, *The Merck Index*, 10th ed., Merck & Co., Rahway, New Jersey.

Wolfe, A. D., 1975, Quinacrine and other acridines, in: *Antibiotics* (J. W. Corcoran and F. E. Hahn, eds.), Vol. 3, pp. 203–233, Springer-Verlag, New York.

Woodward, R. B., and Doering, W. E., 1944, The total synthesis of quinine, *J. Am. Chem. Soc.* 66:849.

Wragg, W. R., Washbourne, K., Brown, K. N., and Hill, J., 1958, Metamidium: A new trypanocidal drug, *Nature (Lond.)* 182:1005–1006.

Wu, D. L., and DuBois, K. P., 1970, Mechanism of the toxic action of diaminodiphenylsulfone (DDS) to mammals, *Arch. Int. Pharmacodyn. Ther.* 183:36–45.

Yamamoto, K., Hirose, K., Eigyo, M., Jyoyama, H., and Naito, Y., 1973, Sulfamethoxazole and trimethoprim. Pharmacological studies on sulfamethoxazole, trimethoprim, and their mixture. I. *Chemotherapy (Tokyo)* 21:187–196.

Yurchenco, J. A., Yurchenco, M. C., and Piepoli, C. R., 1953, Antimicrobial properties of Furoxone, 3-(5-nitro-2-furfurylideneamino)-2-oxazolidinone, *Antibiot. Chemother.* 3:1035–1039.

Zulalian, J., Champagne, D. A., Wayne, R. S., and Blinn, R. C., 1972a, Isolation and identification of the major metabolites of robenidene [1,3-bis(p-chlorobenzylideneamino)guanidine hydrochloride] in the chicken, *Abstracts of Papers, One Hundred Sixty-Third American Chemical Society Meeting, Boston, PEST 12.*

Zulalian, J., Gatterdam, P. E., and Boyd, J. E., 1972b, Fate of robenidene [1,3-bis(p-chlorobenzylideneamino)guanidine hydrochloride] in the rat, *Abstracts of Papers, American Chemical Society Meeting, Boston, PEST 13.*

3

Protozoan Infections of Man

Malaria

TIMOTHY G. GEARY and JAMES B. JENSEN

1. INTRODUCTION

The history of antimalarial chemotherapy is discussed briefly in Chapter 1. A number of excellent reviews of the subject are available (Peters, 1970, 1974, 1980; Thompson and Werbel, 1972; WHO, 1973; Pratt, 1977; Rozman and Canfield, 1979; Richards, 1979; Bruce-Chwatt, 1980, 1981; Rollo, 1980; Dietrich and Kern, 1981; Wyler, 1983; Rieckmann, 1983; Ellis and Chiodini, 1984; Peters and Richards, 1984). The intention of the present chapter is to provide succinct coverage of the clinical pharmacology of currently useful antimalarial drugs as well as some guidelines for their deployment in therapy. Comprehensive descriptions of the disease can be found in any good medical or parasitological text.

All the pathology and symptoms of malaria are related to the asexual blood stages of *Plasmodium* spp. After the clearance of blood-stage parasites by chemotherapy, malaria may recur. There are two types of recurrence: relapse and recrudescence. Relapse is seen only in *P. vivax* and *P. ovale* infections and represents reinfection from an activated hypnozoite (latent exoerythrocytic stage). Recrudescence is seen with *P. falciparum,* in which parasites reappear in the blood after clearance, and represents either inadequate therapy or drug resistance, since the liver is cleared within 1 month of infection (see Chapter 9). Therapy and immunity can combine to reduce *P. malariae* parasitemias to undetectable levels; the infection may become apparent even 50 years after exposure, but this is not a true recrudescence.

Drugs can affect these stages selectively: some eliminate developing exoerythrocytic schizonts (tissue schizontocides), some are effective against hypnozoites (latent exoerythrocytic stages) and some against asexual erythrocytic stages (blood

TIMOTHY G. GEARY and JAMES B. JENSEN • Department of Microbiology and Public Health, Michigan State University, East Lansing, Michigan 48824.

schizontocides), some are gametocytocidal, and others can sterilize the gametocytes or otherwise act as sporontocidal drugs. The type of infection will thus naturally affect the selection of chemotherapy; *P. vivax* or *P. ovale* infections require the use of a drug effective against hypnozoites, while *P. falciparum* or *P. malariae* infections do not. The addition of gametocytocidal or sporontocidal drugs to a standard therapeutic regimen may help decrease the spread of drug-resistant strains. No drugs currently available are effective against sporozoites.

2. GOALS OF MALARIA CHEMOTHERAPY

2.1. Prophylaxis

Nonimmune persons venturing into areas in which malaria transmission occurs should be protected against possible infection by taking antimalarial drugs on a regular basis. Generally, this preventive measure entails taking a drug effective against asexual blood stages that will provide a radical cure of *falciparum* and *malariae* malaria if therapy is continued after exposure for a period sufficient to ensure that all exoerythrocytic schizonts have matured and burst. These drugs only provide a suppressive cure of *vivax* and *ovale* malaria; after termination of therapy, parasites may appear in the bloodstream. Radical cure is then achieved with a combination of a blood schizontocide with a tissue schizontocide, which are also causal prophylactics. Toxicity and drug resistance are the major limits to prophylaxis.

2.2. Cure of Acute Malarial Attacks

Treatment is required for malaria in both nonimmune and semiimmune individuals, although the impetus for immediate treatment is perhaps less dramatic in these cases, depending on the clinical status. Cure of *falciparum* and *malariae* malaria can be achieved through the use of blood schizontocides; for *vivax* and *ovale* attacks, a tissue schizontocide should be added. Again, toxicity and drug resistance are the major constraints of this chemotherapy, although in developing countries, problems of economics and drug availability may predominate.

2.3. Malaria Eradication Programs

There can be no question that vector control is the optimal route for eradication of malaria. Such programs are currently unable to check the resurgence of malaria, however, because of mosquito resistance, the potential toxicity of alternative insecticides, the lack of necessary infrastructure (i.e., roads and airstrips) and of trained personnel in malarious regions, high cost, and low levels of available financial support for large-scale efforts. Many drug administration programs have been used in conjunction with attempts at vector control with great initial success that unfortunately has not been maintained. Prospects for an antimalarial vaccine are dim, for little is understood about immunity to *P. falciparum* in humans, which may vary genetically and apparently involves both humoral and cell-mediated immunity (cf. Jensen *et al.*, 1983, 1984; Cox, 1984). In addition, *P. falciparum* possesses impressive antigenic diversity among geographically distinct strains (McBride *et al.*, 1982; Schofield *et al.*, 1982; Brown *et al.*, 1983; Vernes *et al.*, 1984; Knowles *et al.*, 1984*b*). Any vaccine will have to establish long-term effectiveness (as yet unattained), broad coverage against all strains, good stability to overcome problems of storage and distribution, and low cost. It is unlikely that these objectives will be met in the near future. It must always be remembered that populations whose immunity has waned following malaria eradication programs have been devastated by the reintroduction of malaria after a number of years. It is therefore desirable that no malaria eradication program involving vaccines be implemented unless it can guarantee that *P. falciparum* will not be reintroduced; in Africa, in particular, this seems difficult.

Chemotherapy alone is not sufficient to eradicate malaria. Drug resistance, drug-delivery problems, and cost argue against this possibility. Although eradication can be achieved in small, isolated areas that do not suffer from importation of malaria cases or of infected mosquitos, for the time being, at least, chemotherapy can only play a major role in preventing and treating malaria. Even so, it is becoming increasingly difficult to meet this goal (see Chapter 9).

3. ANTIMALARIALS AND THEIR USES

3.1. 8-Aminoquinolines: Primaquine

Only two compounds of this intensely studied group are currently available: primaquine and its congener, quinocide. Quinocide offers no therapeutic advantages and is more toxic. Primaquine is by far the most important and will be the focus of this discussion; it is also readily available. For recent reviews see Carson (1984), Sweeney (1984*a*).

3.1.1. Spectrum of Action

Primaquine affects all mammalian stages of malaria parasites. Killing of exoerythrocytic stages and gametocytes is the most important, and these actions provide the clinical rationale for use. Asexual erythrocytic stages of *P. falciparum* are killed *in vitro* by primaquine concentrations of about $0.5-1.0$ μM (IC_{50}) (T. G. Geary and J. B. Jensen, unpublished observation). It is not clear how *in vitro* and *in vivo* sensitivity are related, but blood levels of 1 μM primaquine are achieved 1 hr after primaquine administration. However, the pharmacokinetics are unfavorable, and concentrations drop with a half-life ($t_{\frac{1}{2}}$) of about 6 hr, so that drug levels sufficient to exert profound effects against erythrocytic schizonts are not maintained during routine therapy. Administration of primaquine in doses sufficient to reduce circulating parasitemia is accompanied by unacceptable host toxicity. An active metabolite is apparently the lethal species (cf. Grewal, 1981).

3.1.2. Indications

Clinically, the use of primaquine is restricted to four conditions: (1) prophylaxis against all malaria species since, by killing the liver stages, the drug prevents the progression of the infection to blood stages; (2) in conjunction with a blood schizontocide, in mass drug administration programs since, by killing gametocytes, it prevents transmission; (3) most commonly, in conjunction with chloroquine to effect a radical cure of *vivax* and *ovale* malaria, since it kills the hypnozoites and prevents relapses; and (4) along with other drugs for the treatment of multiply drug-resistant *falciparum* malaria. Again, by killing gametocytes, primaquine will reduce the spread of these strains. This should be an especially strong consideration in areas in which transmission is high and such strains are rare.

For practical purposes, primaquine is not used for prophylaxis, since the risk of toxicity outweighs the advantage of radical (as opposed to suppressive) cure of *vivax* malaria. Similarly, its use in mass drug administration programs is restricted to small, isolated areas, where the chances of eradication are good and close clinical supervision is possible. The predominant use of primaquine is for the radical cure of malaria attacks caused by *P. vivax* or *P. ovale*.

3.1.3. Pharmacokinetics

Primaquine is well absorbed after oral administration. A single dose is essentially completely eliminated after 24 hr. It is extensively metabolized, and the metabolites show rapid renal excretion. Blood levels achieved vary considerably among individuals and are not well correlated with efficacy or the hemolytic toxicity (see Rollo, 1980).

3.1.4. Toxicity

Primaquine is generally nontoxic in most patients given small doses; the ratio between the maximally tolerated dose and minimally effective dose in humans is 10. The primary toxicity in most individuals is gastrointestinal (GI) and is dose related. Complaints include abdominal cramping, epigastric distress, nausea and anorexia, and headache. Particularly at higher doses, cyanosis and methemoglobinomia may be seen. Leukopenia, granulocytopenia, and even agranulocytosis are rare manifestations usually seen only after significant overdosage. All these effects are reversible once the drug is discontinued.

The most important toxicity of primaquine occurs in individuals who are genetically deficient in glucose 6-phosphate dehydrogenase ($G6PD^-$). This condition occurs in about 10% of American blacks and to a variable extent in African, Mediterranean, and Middle Eastern populations. The trait is believed to be protective for malaria; its incidence, like that of sickle cell hemoglobin, follows the original geographic distribution of *P. falciparum*. The erythrocytes of affected individuals lack the ability to respond to oxidant stress, by generating reducing equivalents (as NADPH) *via* the pentose phosphate shunt. When faced with oxidant stress (e.g., primaquine and its active metabolites), G6PD⁻ red cells lose reduced glutathione and undergo oxidation of important SH groups on hemoglobin and enzymes; also, the damage caused by membrane oxidation leads to mechanical fragility and lysis.

G6PD deficiency is an X-linked trait, and hemolysis is seen to a variable extent in heterozygous females; variable penetrance has been invoked to explain the lower than expected frequency of hemolysis seen in these individuals. The extent of hemolysis is dose dependent. At low doses, the hemolysis is self-limiting because older red cells are the primary targets; as they are lysed, hematopoiesis increases and younger, resistant red cells replace the lysed cells. Nonetheless, primaquine treatment in G6PD⁻ individuals requires supervision, including urine observation, hematocrit determination, and peripheral blood counts. Several simple tests for G6PD⁻ trait have been developed and should be used if possible before primaquine therapy is initiated in at-risk individuals.

3.1.5. Contraindications

Hemolysis should be expected in G6PD⁻ patients; this is not a contraindication but a precaution. Primaquine is contraindicated in conditions predisposing to granulocytopenia and should not be given with other agents that depress the myeloid elements of bone marrow or that are hemolytic in G6PD⁻ individuals. It should not be administered during the first trimester of pregnancy; rather, to achieve a suppressive cure of *P. vivax* chloroquine should be given and primaquine reserved for radical cure later in pregnancy or after delivery.

3.1.6. Dosage

Standard treatment of *P. vivax* malaria includes a daily dose of 15 mg primaquine base orally for 14 days; during an initial attack or a relapse with circulating parasites, this is administered with a standard regimen of chloroquine. During the latent period between relapses, primaquine alone will effect a radical cure. This regimen has a relapse rate of less than 3%, with little or no required medical supervision. Shorter periods of treatment may not be effective, and full compliance is required. This schedule is usually well tolerated even in G6PD⁻ individuals, who will often show only a mild, self-limiting hemolytic anemia. However, this schedule is not sufficient to cure some *vivax* cases contracted in the southwest Pacific (Chesson strain), which are not as sensitive to primaquine. Daily doses of 30–45 mg primaquine base for 14 days are effective but often toxic. The recommended regimen instead for these cases is 45 mg primaquine plus 300 mg chloroquine in a weekly oral dose for 8 weeks; the relapse rate will be less than 10%. Increasing the primaquine dose to 60 mg lowers this figure below 6% and is still well tolerated. Reduction in dose or in length of treatment will increase the relapse rate and, although compliance for 8 weeks may be difficult to achieve (particularly since the patient will feel well), it is the regimen of choice. A single oral dose of 45 mg primaquine base is toxic to gametocytes of *P. falciparum* and effectively prevents further transmission.

3.2. Quinine

The cinchona alkaloid quinine represents the first classic antimalarial drug (see Chapter 1). It was largely replaced by chloroquine and other synthetic compounds that are more efficacious and less toxic; however, with increasing resistance to these compounds (see Chapter 9), quinine has returned to occupy an extremely important niche in malaria chemotherapy. Resistance to quinine, still rare, is a potentially devastating problem. Quinine is still extracted from natural sources; synthetic pathways are available but expensive. Thus, preparations of quinine may vary in purity. Other cinchona alkaloids have antimalarial activity, but quinine is the most important. However, its dextroisomer, quinidine, can also serve as a useful antimalarial. For a recent review see Hofheinz and Merkli (1984).

3.2.1. Spectrum of Action

Quinine is ineffective as a causal prophylactic; it cannot effect a radical cure of *vivax* or *ovale* malaria because the drug has no effect on sporozoites or on exoerythrocytic stages. It is extremely effective against asexual erythrocytic stages. Quinine has gametocytocidal effects against *P. vivax, P. ovale,* and *P. malariae* but is much less toxic to gametocytes of *P. falciparum,* displaying modest efficacy against immature but little action against mature gametocytes of this species. Quinine is less potent than chloroquine *in vitro* (Geary and Jensen, 1983a) and is less efficacious *in vivo.*

3.2.2. Indications

Currently, quinine has only two uses: (1) the treatment of acute severe *falciparum* malaria with parasitemias (in nonimmune patients) >2%, cerebral malaria, hyperpyrexia, or other desperate symptoms, or (2) the cure of acute attacks of multiply drug-resistant strains of *falciparum* malaria.

3.2.3. Pharmacokinetics

Quinine is available for oral, intravenous, or intramuscular administration as the hydrochloride and sulfate salts. Orally, quinine is extremely bitter and may stimulate vomiting; the unpleasant taste may reduce patient compliance. Consequently, quinine is often given with fruit juices or honey to conceal the taste. Sweetened preparations are available but are more expensive. Oral therapy is always to be preferred, although seriously ill patients may require initial intravenous treatment for rapid onset of action; in these cases, oral therapy should replace the intravenous route as soon as possible. In the rare case in which oral administration is impossible (the patient is in a coma) or a lack of intravenous equipment or of trained personnel precludes the intravenous route, quinine can be given intramuscularly, with caution. The solution must be sterile and at neutral pH, and the optimum site of injection is 6–7.5 cm below the center of the iliac crest, given deeply into the gluteal muscles. Intravenously, the drug must be given very slowly in a large volume of physiological saline, with vital signs carefully monitored.

Quinine is rapidly and completely absorbed after oral dosing. Peak plasma levels are reached 1–3 hr after an oral dose. The drug is 70% bound to plasma proteins but does not accumulate in the body. The plasma $t\frac{1}{2}$ is about 10 hr (range 5–15 hr), and little drug is detected in the serum after 48 hr. Quinine is extensively metabolized by hydroxylation in the liver, and <5% is excreted unchanged. Plasma concentrations in the range of 2–5 mg/liter reduce *vivax* parasitemia, but must be >5 mg/liter to eliminate *P. vivax* and even higher for *P. falciparum*. Standard dose regimens result in plateau concentrations of 4–7 mg/liter. This value is increased significantly by fever; high temperatures impair the metabolism of the drug in the liver. Blood levels >7 mg/liter are commonly associated with toxicity.

3.2.4. Toxicity

Quinine has the lowest therapeutic index of any currently available antimalarial and causes a variety of dose-dependent toxic effects. Nonetheless, some specificity against malaria parasites does occur, and toxicity is generally seen at blood levels at least slightly higher than those required for antimalarial efficacy.

A variety of other pharmacological effects are observed at antimalarial doses (see Rollo, 1980). Quinine exerts a minor analgesic and antipyretic effect on the central nervous system (CNS). There is a modest curarelike effect on skeletal muscle that may decrease shaking and tremor during malaria attacks. Quinine causes uterine muscles to contract during labor, and overdoses can induce abortion; the two effects may not be related. Quinine has little effect on the heart in antimalarial doses, but in overdoses its actions resemble its dextroisomer, quinidine. Quinine is a long-lasting local anesthetic and is a marked local irritant.

Intramuscular injections of the drug may be very painful and may cause sterile abscesses. Intravenous injections can cause thrombosis of the injected vein. Taken orally, the drug often causes gastric distress, including nausea, vomiting, and diarrhea; toxic doses further stimulate nausea and vomiting *via* a CNS effect.

The most common toxicity consists of a constellation of symptoms termed "cinchonism," including tinnitus, decreased hearing acuity, nausea, headache, and visual disturbances. These effects may be observed in routine therapy and are generally reversible, although some residual optic or otic damage may remain after high doses. Increased dosage or prolonged therapy may increase these symptoms and extend the toxicity to the CNS, cardiovascular system, and skin. Hearing and vision are quite sensitive. Effects on the 8th nerve impair balance as well. Optic damage can be severe and may be mediated by both vascular and neural injury. Quinine poisoning (8 g can be fatal) is reflected in CNS involvement, and death may result from respiratory collapse.

During intravenous administration, an excessive rate of infusion or overdosage may result in moderate to marked hypotension and progress to shock due to vasodilation and direct cardiac depression. Rarer effects of quinine include renal damage leading to anuria and uremia, acute hemolytic anemia, hypoprothrombinemia, agranulocytosis, and drug-associated immune thrombocytopenia (Christie *et al.*, 1985). Some patients are hypersensitive to quinine and will show cinchonism after initial or low doses; other symptoms in such individuals may include flushing, pruritis, rashes, fever, and dyspnea, with extreme flushing and intense pruritis most common. Quinine-induced asthma and hemoglobinuria are rare signs of hypersensitivity. The drug may cause hemolysis in $G6PD^-$ individuals.

3.2.5. Contraindications

Quinine may exacerbate myasthenia gravis because of its effects on skeletal muscles. It should not be given to patients who show an idiosyncratic reaction to it. The drug should be stopped immediately if hemolysis occurs and should be given cautiously to patients who have previously suffered blackwater fever. If possible, quinine therapy should be avoided in patients with tinnitus or optic neuritis. In patients with atrial fibrillation, caution must be exercised, since quinine, like quinidine, can generate a paradoxical ventricular tachycardia. If possible, quinine should be avoided in pregnancy.

3.2.6. Dosage

Quinine is usually given in conjunction with tetracyclines, clindamycin, or an antifolate-PABA antagonist combination. This is because quinine is very effective at reducing parasitemia, but it often fails to completely eliminate the parasites. For uncomplicated, multiply drug-resistant cases, the therapy of choice is oral quinine 1.8–2.0 g/day in divided doses for the first 2 days, followed by 1.2–1.3 g/day in divided doses for 5–7 additional days, for a total dose of 9.6–14.0 g over 7–10 days. Some clinicians recommend maintaining the initial dose schedule for 7 days. Recommended combinations of tetracyclines and clindamycin with quinine treatment are quinine 600 mg 3 times/day for 5–7 days, followed by either tetracycline, 250 mg 4 times/day for 7 days, or doxycycline, 200 mg on day 6 followed by 100 mg/day for 6 days, or minocycline 200 mg initially followed by 100 mg tiwce daily for 6 days. With clindamycin, quinine is given 600 mg 3 times daily for 3 days followed by 5 mg/kg clindamycin twice daily for 5 days.

For severely ill patients, quinine must be given immediately. The intravenous route is recommended initially in such patients, although the oral route should be adopted as soon as possible. The iv drip should contain 500 ml saline–glucose, plasma, or dextran. The initial adult dose is 500–1000 mg quinine HCl (or diHCl), and the infusion should take at least 1–2 hr, up to 4 hr. The infusion can be repeated within 24 hr, but the total daily dose must not exceed 2 g. The volume and dose must be adjusted in pediatric cases proportionally to weight (Section 3.14). If no iv setups are available,

250–500-mg doses of quinine HCl can be given by syringe in 20 ml saline–glucose using a small-bore needle. The infusion must last at least 10 min. Recently, the use of a loading dose has been recommended (White *et al.*, 1983*b*). If trained personnel and proper iv equipment are unavailable, quinine can be given intramuscularly in single doses of up to 1 g (not more than 2 g/day), given the restrictions cited above.

It is interesting to note that quinidine is also an effective treatment for *falciparum* malaria. Given in dosage schedules similar to those of quinine, both intravenously and orally, this drug can cure even severe cases (White *et al.*, 1981; Ris *et al.*, 1983). Although quinidine is more cardiotoxic than quinine (White *et al.*, 1983*a*), it can be used safely. In areas where quinine is not readily available, quinidine may prove a valuable and life-saving drug.

3.3. Mefloquine

Mefloquine is a 4-quinoline methanol chemically related to quinine; it has recently become commercially available, but not in the United States, in a fixed-dose combination with Fansidar (Section 3.10). The preclinical data have been summarized (Sweeney, 1981, 1984*b*; WHO, 1981), and more recent clinical trials are available as well (Danis *et al.*, 1982; Harinasuta *et al.*, 1983, 1985; de Souza, 1983*a,b*; Ekue *et al.*, 1983; Lapierre *et al.*, 1983).

3.3.1. Spectrum of Action

Mefloquine resembles quinine in its spectrum of action, ineffective against sporozoites and exoerythrocytic stages but exhibiting extremely high activity against asexual erythrocytic stages. Gametocytocidal activity is like that with quinine. Mefloquine is much more potent than quinine against *P. falciparum in vitro* (Geary and Jensen, 1983*a*) and, like chloroquine, is fully efficacious. Most importantly, single-dose therapy is sufficient for cure. Reports of mefloquine resistance (see Chapter 9) are ominous, since this is the last new compound that can reasonably be expected to become commercially available for the next few years.

3.3.2. Indications

Mefloquine is reserved for the treatment of multiply drug-resistant cases of *falciparum* malaria. The drug apparently does not act as quickly as quinine in severely ill patients (time to negative blood films is 50–100 hr) and may not supplant it for this use, although it may completely replace the older drug for the treatment of uncomplicated drug-resistant infections. Mefloquine has been marketed with Fansidar in an attempt to reduce the development of parasite resistance. As the drug becomes more widely available, despite its cost, it will no doubt come to be used casually. Since resistance to Fansidar is already widespread, the probability that mefloquine resistance will eventually occur is high; indeed, it has already been detected in areas in which the drug has never been used (see Chapter 9). Cross-resistance in quinine-resistant strains has also been observed (S. Hoffman, personal communication). This is indeed a somber prospect, and physicians are urged to reserve the drug for cases in which it is truly necessary to prolong its current usefulness.

3.3.3. Pharmacokinetics

In tablet form, mefloquine is slowly and variably absorbed from the GI tract; administration as an aqueous suspension improves this situation. The peak blood concentration of 0.8 mg/liter is delayed until 36 hr after dosing with 1 g. The $t_{\frac{1}{2}}$ is about 14 days but is highly variable. Studies of infection and examination of volunteer sera *in vitro* show effective blood levels to be present at least 30 days after an initial dose.

Mefloquine is 99% bound to serum proteins. Some metabolism occurs in the liver, and the drug and its metabolites are excreted primarily in the feces. Enterohepatic circulation is one factor that generates the lengthy $t_{\frac{1}{2}}$. A carboxylic acid derivative, inactive as an antimalarial, reaches relatively high plasma levels and, as it retains the toxicity of the parent drug, may be responsible for the side effects.

3.3.4. Toxicity

Mefloquine does not cause serious problems in humans. Doses of 0.5 g weekly for 1 year produced no toxic consequences in healthy volunteers. Observed side effects have been mild and transient, including dizziness, nausea, vomiting, and diarrhea. Sinus bradycardia has occurred in up to 7% of patients beginning 4–7 days post-treatment, with pulse rates returning to normal within 2 weeks of the dose. No evidence of myocardial toxicity has been found. In rare instances, psychiatric symptoms have been reported, occurring during the second week after therapy and including disorientation, hallucination, and impaired consciousness. All were reversible.

3.3.5. Contraindications

For lack of data, mefloquine should be avoided during pregnancy if possible. In long-term animal studies, retinal and epididymal lesions have been observed; on the basis of these findings alone, mefloquine should not be used for long-term prophylaxis.

3.3.6. Dosage

Mefloquine is currently available in Europe in combination with Fansidar (Fansimef). Two tablet sizes are available, one containing 250 mg mefloquine, 25 mg pyrimethamine, and 500 mg sulfadoxine, and another with one-half these amounts. The typical treatment is 500 mg mefloquine, 50 mg pyrimethamine, and 100 mg sulfadoxine on two successive days. In the United States, this preparation will not be marketed. Instead, approval for mefloquine alone (Lariam) is expected within a year or so. The drug will probably be marketed in 250-mg (base) tablets. Treatment will consist of a single dose of 1000 mg, which has produced a 100% cure in field studies; 750-mg and 500-mg treatment as single-dose therapy resulted in ~6% failure rates and, since the highest dose is safe and well tolerated, it is recommended.

3.4. 4-Aminoquinolines: Chloroquine, Amodiaquine, Amopyroquine, and Hydroxychloroquine

This discussion focuses on the prototype, chloroquine. Few significant differences exist in clinical pharmacology among the members of this class. A recent review is available (McChesney and Fitch, 1984). Chloroquine (CQ) was the mainstay of malaria chemotherapy globally for nearly 20 years. The drug's low expense, low toxicity, and high efficacy in combination with the use of vector control programs led to impressive gains against malaria during the 1950s and 1960s. The development and spread of CQ resistance greatly eroded this achievement and was partially responsible for the return of P. falciparum to cleared areas. Resistance has progressed over much of the world to a severe extent (see Chapter 9) with the exception of continental Africa where, until recently, CQ-resistant infections had only been reported in nonimmune travelers or expatriates. Considering the low cost, efficacy, and safety, CQ was nearly an ideal antimalarial, and no other drug is likely to replace it as such.

3.4.1. Spectrum of Activity

The 4-aminoquinolines are not causal prophylactics; they do not provide radical cures of *vivax* malaria. They are inactive against sporozoites and exoerythrocytic schizonts and have only moderate gametocytocidal activity against P. vivax, P. ovale, and P. malariae and none against P. falciparum. They are extremely toxic to asexual blood stages of all four malarial species, although P. falciparum resistance has eroded this activity considerably. The drugs vary in potency against P. falciparum in vitro (Geary and Jensen, 1983a) and in vivo, but this is not clinically important. The drugs exert their effects primarily on the erythrocytic trophozoite and early schizont stages of P. falciparum (Yayon et al., 1983).

3.4.2. Indications

Chloroquine remains the drug of choice for the treatment of *malariae* malaria and (with primaquine) of *ovale* and *vivax* malaria. All the other 4-aminoquinolines are therapeutically equivalent, although somewhat more expensive. For *falciparum* malaria, CQ is still the drug of choice for infections that retain sensitivity to it. In such cases, it is curative. Amodiaquine is equal to CQ for this purpose and is also capable of curing some CQ-resistant strains, although generally not the most resistant types (see Chapter 9). Cross-resistance to other 4-aminoquinolines in CQ-resistant parasites is not absolute (Schmidt et al., 1977; Spencer et al., 1983; Watkins et al., 1984a; Geary and Jensen, 1983a; Knowles et al., 1984a). It is worthwhile to consider amodiaquine in R-I or R-II

CQ-resistant infections if they are not life threatening. No information is yet available on the activity of amopyroquine or hydroxychloroquine on such infections in humans, and so they cannot be similarly recommended. These drugs resolve symptoms quickly and clear parasitemias (in sensitive cases) within 48–72 hr.

Chloroquine is also used for prophylaxis; it provides suppressive control of *vivax* and *ovale* malaria and complete protection against sensitive *falciparum* and *malariae* malaria. Because of increasing CQ resistance, however, chloroquine should not be used for prophylaxis unless CQ-resistant infections will not be encountered. Some reports are available suggesting that increased doses of chloroquine can cure mildly drug-resistant strains (Hoffman *et al.*, 1984), but more work in other areas is required to confirm this finding.

3.4.3. Pharmacokinetics

These drugs are well absorbed from the GI tract after oral administration. Very little is eliminated in the feces; urinary excretion is the primary pathway. Metabolism occurs by N-deethylation in the liver, and the (bis)desethyl derivative is the major result. The drug is bound 50–60% to serum components, which are proteins (Adelusi and Salako, 1982; Walker *et al.*, 1983) and/or lipids (Geary *et al.*, 1983). The drugs accumulate markedly in tissues, especially the liver, but spleen, kidney, lung, and leukocytes also concentrate CQ 200–700-fold over plasma levels. Brain and spinal cord concentrations are an order of magnitude lower than in these tissues. These stores are largely responsible for the prolonged $t\frac{1}{2}$ of CQ, which is about 3–4 days following single or weekly prophylactic doses. The pharmacokinetics of CQ may to a certain extent be dose dependent and after daily doses the $t\frac{1}{2}$ is 6–7 days (Frisk-Holmberg *et al.*, 1979; Gustafsson *et al.*, 1983*a,b*). The extensive tissue binding also necessitates the use of initially high (or for prophylaxis, preexposure) loading doses to saturate the sites and achieve satisfactory blood levels. The drug can be detected in serum and urine for up to years following treatment.

During therapy, plasma concentrations of CQ reach >1 μM, gradually falling to 0.04 μM by the 7th day; with prolonged therapy, plateau concentrations fluctuate between 0.6 and 0.2 μM. These concentrations are fully effective against CQ-sensitive strains, although 0.04 μM approaches the IC_{50} of sensitive strains *in vitro* (Geary and Jensen, 1983*a*).

Primaquine interferes with the metabolism of CQ, leading to increased CQ serum levels and a prolonged half-life when the drugs are given simultaneously; in addition to the risk of primaquine toxicity, this fact argues against the use of the two drugs for prophylaxis.

Chloroquine is rapidly absorbed after intramuscular injections in individuals who cannot take oral medication. Intravenous use is not generally recommended. Chloroquine in suppository form is available in some areas and gives satisfactory results. Chloroquine is extremely bitter and may be poorly tolerated orally; sweetened preparations are available but expensive. Amopyroquine is also available in a parenteral formulation but amodiaquine is not; however, oral preparations of amodiaquine base are not unpleasant tasting and compliance may be much better.

3.4.4. Toxicity

Weekly prophylactic doses of CQ are virtually without toxicity, and only very rarely must the drug be stopped due to intolerance. During treatment of acute malaria attacks, mild side effects are more common. Vomiting is significant after oral CQ and supervision is needed to ensure that the drug is retained. Transient headaches, minor visual disturbances (blurring, difficulty in focusing and accommodation), dizziness, GI distress, and pruritis (Osifo, 1984) may be seen, the last two most commonly. All are transient and completely reversible with cessation of treatment. Significant toxicity is not observed unless CQ is given at high daily doses for treatment of other conditions not relevant to this discussion. In some individuals in malarious areas, CQ is routinely taken for a variety of complaints and overdosage is not uncommon. In such cases, progressive retinopathy, skin lesions, ototoxicity and even heart block may occur. Some toxic effects appear to be related to cumulative dose levels, and consumption of a total of 100 g of CQ may be associated with retinopathy. Weekly prophylaxis with CQ thus should probably not exceed 6 years. The drug may cause hemolysis in $G6PD^-$ individuals. Intramuscular injections, if overdosage occurs, may result in respiratory depression, cardiovascular collapse, convulsions, and death. The drug dosage must be carefully determined, particularly in infants and children, who are more sensitive to CQ than adults, if the intramuscular route is necessary. The toxicity of other 4-aminoquinolines, as far as is known, resembles that of CQ in humans.

3.4.5. Contraindications

Few contraindications exist for these drugs. They should be avoided in patients with hepatic disease due to high liver concentration, and also in patients with severe GI disease or neurological or blood disorders. Individuals who are sensitive to CQ may demonstrate severe pruritis and the drug should not be given. These drugs are not known to be teratogenic and can be safely used throughout pregnancy. It should always be remembered that CQ is more toxic in children.

3.4.6. Dosage

For prophylaxis, CQ administered once weekly as the phosphate or sulfate salt is suitable in areas in which CQ resistance is still relatively rare (e.g., Africa), although confident protection in nonimmunes is impossible. The dose is 300-mg CQ base, orally. Treatment should begin 2 weeks prior to exposure. Alternatively, a single dose of 600-mg base just prior to exposure is also satisfactory, with subsequent reduction to 300 mg/week. The therapy must be continued for at least 4 weeks after the termination of exposure. In areas of intense transmission, the usual dose may be doubled. Ingestion of > 100 g total should be avoided. Compliance is essential; missing one dose can result in an attack of malaria.

Chloroquine has been given with primaquine to provide curative prophylaxis against both *P. falciparum* and *P. vivax*. However, the risk of primaquine toxicity outweights the potential benefits, and this combination is not recommended for routine use. Chloroquine is also combined with pyrimethamine or proguanil for prophylaxis, particularly in areas where CQ resistance is common. The rationale is that CQ can provide protection against *P. vivax* (which the other two cannot; see below) while control of *P. falciparum* is also achieved. The dose of CQ is reduced to 150 mg, but this regimen has been questioned (Peters, 1980).

Amodiaquine prophylaxis requires 400 mg base/week, supplied as the hydrochloride or free base, the latter being tasteless and well tolerated. Hydroxychloroquine is supplied as the sulfate, and recommended weekly doses are 310 mg base or 400 mg base. The recommendations for amopyroquine are not well defined; 600 mg/week is well tolerated and effective. There is some evidence that these last two compounds are safer than amodiaquine or CQ (Thompson and Werbel, 1972).

For treatment of acute malaria attacks, oral treatment is desired unless the patient cannot swallow the drug. In adults, an immediate dose of 600 mg CQ base is given, followed 6 hr later by 300 mg base. Further 300 mg doses are given daily for the next 2 days, leading to a total of 1.5 g/3 days. If parasitemia is not cleared, additional 300-mg doses may be given daily for 4 more days. At that time, if cure has not been attained, medication should be switched. For amodiaquine, the initial dose is 600 mg base followed 6 hr later by 200 mg base, and 400 mg base daily for the next 2 days, for a total of 1.6 g/3 days. Additional 400-mg doses may be given daily for 4 days, as above, if needed. Hydroxychloroquine is administered initially at 800 mg base, followed by 400 mg 6 hr later, and 400 mg/day for the next 2 days. Amopyroquine can be administered in the same doses and schedule as chloroquine.

Hydroxychloroquine, amopyroquine, and CQ are available for parenteral therapy. Chloroquine is given as 200 mg base (250 mg HCl), one-half the dose in each buttock. The treatment may be repeated every 6 hr, but the does should not exceed 800 mg base in 24 hr. Oral treatment should begin as soon as possible. Equivalent treatments are 360 mg hydroxychloroquine base or 150 mg amopyroquine base. Chloroquine suppositories are available in some areas; the dose is usually doubled or tripled (on a milligram basis), but satisfactory results are obtained. In children, 4-aminoquinolines must be given with more caution. Oral doses should be reduced proportionately with body weight; intramuscular injections should be 5 mg/kg, 1–2 hr apart in divided injections.

3.5. Diaminopyrimidines: Pyrimethamine and Trimethoprim

These compounds have extremely useful antimalarial activity. Pyrimethamine was developed specifically for use as an antimalarial and is much more potent than trimethoprim, which is a commonly used antibiotic. If pyrimethamine is available, trimethoprim has no therapeutic advantages, and the discussion will focus on pyrimethamine. A recent review is available (Ferone, 1984).

3.5.1. Spectrum of Action

The activity of pyrimethamine is somewhat species specific. It has no action against sporozoites but has activity against exoerythrocytic stages of P. falciparum; this effect is less pronounced and incomplete against P. vivax. Pyrimethamine kills asexual erythrocytic stages of the four human malarias, but the effect is slow. Although it has no obvious effects on gametocyte number or morphology, pyrimethamine apparently sterilizes them so that sporogony in the mosquito does not occur. Less is known about trimethoprim, but it is reasonable to assume that it shares the same spectrum of activity.

3.5.2. Indications

Pyrimethamine used alone has only one indication, that of prophylaxis. It gives suppressive cures of P. falciparum when given once weekly. It is potent, inexpensive, safe, and well accepted orally. However, pyrimethamine resistance occurs readily in P. falciparum and is a significant problem in many areas (Chapter 9). It has variable effects against P. vivax and can be counted on to provide suppressive but not radical cures in prophylaxis. Even the suppressive action is somewhat unreliable, unless therapy is continued for 10 weeks past exposure. Since the drug is much more effective in combination with PABA antagonists, which are synergistic, its use alone is waning and not generally recommended.

Pyrimethamine is commonly combined in propietary formulations with sulfadoxine, sulfalene, or dapsone (see Section 3.12). These combinations are more effective and less susceptible to resistance development than is pyrimethamine alone and have been recommended for prophylaxis particularly in areas with abundant CQ resistance. However, an unexpectedly high incidence of Stevens–Johnson syndrome has recently been found in patients taking pyrimethamine–sulfadoxine combinations and chloroquine, and the use of such combinations for prophylaxis may not be advisable (Centers for Disease Control, 1985a,b). These combinations also are useful in the treatment of uncomplicated attacks of falciparum malaria, although the effect is slow. They are often given with quinine for the treatment of severely ill patients with falciparum malaria. The combinations are often effective against strains that are moderately resistant to pyrimethamine, but resistance to the combinations has been noted (Chapter 9).

The use of pyrimethamine–CQ combinations for prophylaxis in areas where both P. vivax and CQ-resistant P. falciparum occur is not advisable (Peters, 1980); since any cases of vivax malaria can be easily treated with primaquine and CQ, pyrimethamine or the combinations can be given alone for P. falciparum prophylaxis in such areas. Trimethoprim may be substituted for pyrimethamine when the latter is unavailable. Cross-resistance between the drugs is to be expected.

3.5.3. Pharmacokinetics

Pyrimethamine is well absorbed after oral dosing, and peak blood concentrations are reached 2–4 hr after administration. Levels of 10–100 μg/liter are required to affect asexual erythrocytic forms of drug-sensitive strains. Peak blood levels after a single 25-mg dose average over 200 μg/liter, and effective concentrations are maintained for at least 1 week after a single dose. The $t_{\frac{1}{2}}$ is about 4 days. Pyrimethamine is extensively bound in tissues with a large volume of distribution. The pharmacokinetics are not altered by sulfa drugs. Pyrimethamine is extensively metabolized and little is excreted unchanged. Pyrimethamine is excreted in the milk of nursing mothers, and protection of suckling infants has been observed.

3.5.4. Toxicity

At prophylactic doses, essentially no adverse effects are seen. At higher doses, symptoms of megaloblastic anemia may sometimes be observed. Similar toxicity may be seen if prophylactic doses (25 mg) are given daily. The symptoms are readily reversible by the addition of 10 mg/kg folinic acid. If prophylaxis is to be continued for longer than 6 months, or in individuals susceptible to anemia, folinic acid may be routinely added at this dose, on a weekly basis. Poisoning by pyrimethamine in children is not uncommon due to the pleasant taste, and 4–10 tablets (100–250 mg) can be extremely toxic, causing convulsions, unconsciousness, collapse, and often death. Gastric lavage, diazepam, and folinic acid are recommended in such cases.

3.5.5. Contraindications

Pyrimethamine is teratogenic in some animals and for that reason is not recommended during pregnancy. However, the drug has been widely used in humans for more than two decades, even in pregnant women, and such effects have not been reported. If the drug is necessary, the risk of malaria to the fetus is greater than the risk of pyrimethamine. Patients predisposed to folic acid deficiencies, including pregnant women, alcoholics, individuals with malabsorption syndormes, chronic GI illness, or malnutrition, should be given folinic acid (10 mg/kg) weekly during prophylaxis.

3.5.6. Dosage

Prophylactically, pyrimethamine is given alone orally in 25-mg doses once per week if there are no local cases of pyrimethamine or proguanil-resistant infections. Combinations of 25 mg pyrimethamine with sulfadoxine (500 mg), sulfalene (500 mg), or dapsone (12.5 mg pyrimethamine + 100 mg dapsone; 2 tablets/dose) are also available; one tablet per week (except as noted) is the prophylactic dose. The combinations provide prophylactic coverage even if given every 2–4 weeks. It should be noted that combinations are contraindicated in sulfa-sensitive individuals (see Section 3.12).

For treatment of acute attacks of uncomplicated CQ-resistant *falciparum* malaria, an initial dose of 50 mg pyrimethamine plus 1000 mg sulfadoxine (two Fansidar tablets) is followed 6 hr later by 25 mg pyrimethamine + 500 mg sulfadoxine (one Fansidar tablet), or 50 mg pyrimethamine + 1000 mg sulfalene (two Metakelfin tablets) followed 6 hr later by 25 mg pyrimethamine + 500 mg sulfalene. Since these drugs act slowly, such infections should, if possible, receive initial quinine therapy (600 mg three times per day for 2 days), followed by two to three doses (tablets) of Fansidar or Metakelfin. Other schedules are also possible (Bruce-Chwatt, 1981).

Fansidar is also available in ampules for injection. The volume is 2.5 ml containing 25 mg pyrimethamine and 500 mg sulfadoxine. The adult dose is two injections, given intramuscularly or intravenously (slowly). Since the drug is not rapid-acting and has no use in the treatment of unconscious severely ill patients, this route has no obvious advantages.

For timethoprim, a 500-mg dose with 1000 mg sulfalene or sulfadoxine may replace pyrimethamine. The $t\frac{1}{2}$ of trimethoprim is only about 11 hr, but this regimen is effective. The combination of trimethoprim and sulfamethoxazole (co-trimoxazole) is not as effective and is not recommended.

3.6. Biguanides (Proguanil and Chlorproguanil) and Triazines (Cycloguanil)

These drugs have a role in malaria chemotherapy like that of the diaminopyrimidines; they share a common mechanism of action (Ferone, 1984). Proguanil (chloroguanide in America) and chlorproguanil (unavailable in America) are unusual drugs in that they are inactive as administered and are converted metabolically, primarily in the liver, to the effective compounds (Watkins et al., 1984b). The active metabolite of proguanil is cycloguanil, which is also available for use, but not in the United States.

3.6.1. Spectrum of Action

The spectrum of action of these drugs is identical to that of pyrimethamine. Their action against the asexual erythrocytic stages is too slow to be useful in treating acute attacks. They are usually combined with PABA antagonists since resistance to them occurs readily, and cross-resistance between these drugs and pyrimethamine is to be expected.

3.6.2. Indications

These drugs are used for prophylaxis of *falciparum* malaria; although suppressive cures of *P. vivax* can be obtained, chloroquine is the drug of choice for this purpose. Chlorproguanil is much longer acting than proguanil, although otherwise they are very similar. Cycloguanil is available in some areas as a very long-lasting repository preparation as the pamoate (embonate) salt for prophylaxis; it has no use in acute treatment.

The use of these drugs alone has met with great resistance and cross-resistance in pyrimethamine-resistant *falciparum* malaria. Consequently, combination with PABA antagonists is becoming more common. These drugs offer no benefit over pyrimethamine in the treatment of acute *falciparum* infections; if this drug is unavailable, proguanil or chlorproguanil may be substituted for it, in conjunction with quinine, for the treatment of CQ-resistant infections.

3.6.3. Pharmacokinetics

Proguanil is slowly but completely absorbed after oral administration. At least three metabolites are formed, one of which is the active compound cycloguanil. Peak blood levels are achieved 2–4 hr after dosing, and the drug is absent after 24 hr. It is 75% bound to plasma proteins. Concentrations in red cells are six times plasma levels. In humans, 60% of a dose is excreted in urine as proguanil and 30% as cycloguanil.

Chlorproguanil is very similar to proguanil but has a much longer half-life. The active triazine metabolite has a very short half-life, and the parent drug appears to be concentrated in a tissue or protein depot and is released (and thus metabolized) slowly.

Cycloguanil is administered in deep intramuscular injections as the pamoate (also known as embonate) salt. At recommended doses of 5 mg/kg, more than 80% of the drug remains at the injection site after 2 weeks and can be detected as long as 1 year later. Protection can be obtained up to 3 months after a single injection. Plasma concentrations of 5 μg/liter are effective against drug-sensitive *P. falciparum*, whereas control of *P. vivax* requires 10–20 μg/liter. Cycloguanil has a short $t_{\frac{1}{2}}$ in blood and is excreted largely unchanged in the urine. Coadministration with PABA antagonists is not known to affect the pharmacokinetics of these compounds.

3.6.4. Toxicity

These drugs are remarkably well tolerated and are the safest antimalarials available. Injection of cycloguanil pamoate may cause local irritation, although this is rare if it is properly given. Mild induration and tenderness occur in about 10% of cases. Urticaria, rashes, and itching are also seen in 5–10% of injected patients. No significant effects attributable to folate antagonism, including teratogenicity, have been reported.

Oral doses of proguanil (100–200 mg/day) or chlorproguanil (20 mg/week) are essentially free of side effects. Some patients experience anorexia, abdominal discomfort, or nausea, which is mild and transient. Long-term use is not associated with other toxic effects.

3.6.5. Contraindications

No specific contraindications exist. If combined with sulfonamides or sulfones, these drugs should be avoided in persons sensitive to them. Resistance is widespread, and these agents should not be used alone for prophylaxis unless it is clear that resistance to them or to pyrimethamine has not been found in the relevant areas.

3.6.6. Dosage

Cycloguanil pamoate is administered at 5 mg/kg body weight for adults. The injection volume is 2–2.5 ml, given preferably in the gluteal muscles. For infants, up to 16 mg/kg has been given without ill effect.

Proguanil is given as the hydrochloride, 100–200 mg/day. Chlorproguanil is given as a 20-mg dose weekly; it has also been combined with 150 mg chloroquine base. In semi-immunes, proguanil can be given in 200-mg doses twice weekly or 300 mg once weekly. For acute attacks of uncomplicated *falciparum* malaria in the absence of other medication, proguanil may be given at an initial dose of 300–600 mg, followed by 300 mg/day for as long as needed.

3.7. PABA Antagonists: Sulfonamides and Sulfones

These drugs were initially developed as antibacterial agents but have been found to possess useful antimalarial effects, particularly those that have a long serum half-life and that are synergistic with the antimalarial antifolates. The most important of these agents include sulfadoxine, sulfalene, sulfadiazine, dapsone, and diacetyldapsone (acedapsone). (See Schaefer *et al.*, 1984 for a recent review).

3.7.1. Spectrum of Action

PABA antagonists are inactive against sporozoites and exoerythrocytic stages. They are active against asexual erythrocytic stages of *P. falciparum* but less so against other species. Onset of action is slow, and resistance develops easily when they are used alone.

3.7.2. Indications

Although these drugs are effective against *falciparum* malaria when given alone, such use is not recommended, because of drug resistance. Their use is restricted to combination chemotherapy for the prophylaxis and acute treatment of *falciparum* malaria (Section 3.10). They may also be given following quinine for acute attacks of CQ-resistant malaria, but the combinations are recommended. Acedapsone is used as a long-acting repository injection only in conjunction with cycloguanil pamoate for prophylaxis. Proguanil can be given with dapsone, 25 mg/day, as an effective combination (Black, 1973).

3.7.3. Pharmacokinetics

Dapsone is well absorbed after oral dosing, and peak serum concentrations are seen 3–6 hr after administration. The $t_{\frac{1}{2}}$ is about 28 hr. Acedapsone is insoluble and is used as an intramuscular injection. A 300-mg dose has a $t_{\frac{1}{2}}$ of 40–43 days. The monoacetylated compound is also active, as is dapsone itself, as an antimalarial. Sulfadiazine, sulfalene, and sulfadoxine are well if variably absorbed from the GI tract after oral dosing. Urinary excretion is the major route of elimination for these drugs and their acetylated or glucuronidated metabolites. Sulfalene ($t_{\frac{1}{2}} = 65$ hr) and sulfadoxine ($t_{\frac{1}{2}} = 120-200$ hr) are preferred and most commonly used. Sulfadiazine has a relatively short $t_{\frac{1}{2}}$ (~ 16 hr) which, for pharmacokinetic reasons, makes the drug suboptimal for malaria prophylaxis.

3.7.4. Toxicity

Doses employed in prophylaxis are associated with low toxicity. Side effects may occur, including skin reactions such as urticaria or GI distress. Rarely, especially in overdosages, the Stevens-Johnson syndrome may result. That this syndrome has recently been found to occur with an unexpectedly high frequency in patients taking pyrimethamine–sulfadoxine prophylactically may be due to the prolonged half-life of sulfadoxine which is also the characteristic which makes it a good antimalarial (Center for Disease Control, 1985a). Agranulocytosis has been observed, particularly with the antifolate combinations. They may precipitate hemolysis in G6PD⁻ individuals and methemoglobinemia in patients genetically deficient in NADH-methemoglobin reductase. A plethora of side effects typical of the short-acting sulfonamides could occur (see Mandell and Sande, 1980), but it should be remembered that by virtue of their long half-life, sulfadoxine and sulfalene are administered in considerably lower doses and less frequently than are those drugs used for bacterial infections. Individual hypersensitivity is not uncommon (Mandell and Sande, 1980).

For dapsone, toxicity is dose related. At standard daily doses of 25 mg, such symptoms as nausea, vomiting, headache, blurred vision, and insomnia may occur. In sensitive patients, agranulocytosis has been reported. Dapsone may induce hemolysis in G6PD⁻ individuals, especially at higher doses. Overdoses (>200 mg/day) cause anemia; dermatitis and hepatitis were observed in patients taking 100 mg/day. Acedapsone probably has similar toxicity, but one might expect it to be less severe and common because of the nature of the preparation and its pharmacokinetics.

3.7.5. Contraindications

Sulfonamides should not be given during pregnancy or to children <2 months of age because of the risk of neonatal jaundice (not reported, to our knowledge, in the field). Individuals who are sulfa sensitive should not be treated. Sulfonamides should not be used alone; in addition to questionable efficacy and easily obtained resistance, the sulfa antibiotics are still useful in many areas, and bacterial resistance could be generated. Caution should be exercised in treating G6PD⁻ individuals, and combinations with other hemolytic drugs are to be avoided. If Fansidar is to be administered for longer than 6 months, routine blood films are recommended.

3.7.6. Dosage

For prophylaxis, 12.5 mg pyrimethamine + 100 mg dapsone (Maloprim), 2 tablets prior to exposure followed by 1 tablet/week, is useful. Other regimens include 1

Fansidar tablet/week or 2 every 2 weeks; this schedule can be used for Metakelfin as well. Acedapsone is given as a 300-mg intramuscular injection with cycloguanil pamoate.

3.8. Antibiotics: Tetracyclines (Tetracycline, Doxycycline, Minocycline) and Clindamycin

The antimalarial activity of antibiotic compounds has been known for more than 30 years. The use of these drugs should be restricted in malaria chemotherapy for a variety of reasons (discussed below), but they do have an increasingly important role in the chemotherapy of multiply drug-resistant infections of P. falciparum. Rieckmann (1984) has recently reviewed the field.

3.8.1. Spectrum of Action

Tetracyclines do not affect sporozoites but do inhibit primary exoerythrocytic stages of P. falciparum. They are ineffective against hypnozoites of P. vivax. Tetracyclines are effective against asexual erythrocytic stages of P. falciparum and P. vivax. There is no apparent effect on gametocytes. The therapeutic effect is delayed; although symptoms may resolve, parasitemias change little during the first 2 days of therapy. In vitro, the effect is increased during prolonged incubation (Geary and Jensen, 1983b).

Clindamycin resembles the tetracyclines in these respects, although it is more potent in vitro (Geary and Jensen, 1983b). Their effects are highly O_2 dependent (Seaberg et al., 1984; Divo et al., 1985). Minocycline and doxycycline are more potent than tetracycline in vitro (Divo et al., 1985), probably because of their increased lipid solubility.

3.8.2. Indications

The only legitimate use of these antibiotics is in the treatment of acute attacks of multiply drug-resistant falciparum malaria, and they should be reserved for that purpose. They are effective, although slow acting, and it is imperative that this situation be maintained. Cost, toxicity, and the chance of developing resistant bacterial strains argue against the prophylactic use of these antibiotics. The tetracyclines are effective when given for falciparum malaria (Rieckmann et al., 1971; Clyde et al., 1971; Colwell et al., 1972; Willerson et al., 1972; Ponnampalan, 1981), and most common usage is after quinine therapy or recently, with amodiaquine (Noeypatimanond et al., 1983). Clindamycin is also effective when given alone (Clyde et al., 1975; Cabrera et al., 1982; Rivera et al., 1982), and we have found it so in Sudan (M. Homeida, T. G. Geary, H. M. Ali, and J. B. Jensen, unpublished observations), but is also given after quinine (Miller et al., 1974). Combinations of these drugs with chloroquine are not effective in chloroquine-resistant malaria, especially if the illness is severe (Phillips et al., 1984). In any case in which parasitemias are high or symptoms are severe, quinine treatment is an absolute requirement, and these compounds cannot replace it initially. They are not recommended for routine use.

3.8.3. Pharmacokinetics

A great deal of information is available on this subject in a variety of standard pharmacology texts. Briefly, tetracyclines are variably and incompletely absorbed following oral administration. Divalent cations or increased pH decrease this process and should be avoided (e.g., milk, antacids). Tetracyclines should be given on an empty stomach. Tetracycline reaches peak plasma levels of 3–4 μg/ml following 250-mg doses every 6 hr. The $t_{\frac{1}{2}}$ is 8–10 hr. Minocycline and doxycycline are more potent and have longer $t_{\frac{1}{2}}$ values. Doxycycline is the best absorbed. These drugs are bound to plasma proteins 50–90% and are excreted largely unchanged in urine and feces, except for doxycycline, which is excreted fecally as an inactive metabolite that has little effect on the gut flora.

Clindamycin is well absorbed after oral dosing and reaches peak serum levels 1–2 hr later of 4–8 μg/ml. The $t_{\frac{1}{2}}$ is 2–3 hr, and the drug is 60–90% bound in the plasma. It is metabolized to inactive derivatives in the liver, and patients with hepatic dysfunction have elevated drug levels. This may be important in areas in which schistosomiasis is common.

3.8.4. Toxicity

Again, these problems are well documented elsewhere. Briefly, tetracyclines may discolor teeth in growing children and can interfere with enamel and bone development. In high doses or in patients with renal impairment, or in pregnant women, tetracycline may cause hepatotoxicity. Photosensitivity, itching, and skin toxicity are common side effects. Nausea, vomiting, and diarrhea are frequent, as are abdominal discomfort and epigastric distress. These effects may be reduced by giving smaller doses more frequently, but they often disappear during treatment anyway. Minocycline or doxycycline may be given with food, since their absorption is less affected; this may ease the GI effects. Superinfection with drug-resistant bacterial strains is possible.

With clindamycin, the most serious effect is severe diarrhea and pseudomembranous colitis, which is caused by overgrowth of clindamycin-resistant *Clostridium difficile;* this complication can be fatal, although it is usually treatable with metronidazole or vancomycin. This effect occurs to a variable extent in North America but was not seen in Brazil during antimalarial treatment (R. Westerman, personal communication). Its importance in malarious regions, many of which have little experience with clindamycin, remains to be determined. Other common side effects are nausea and vomiting, cramping, and fever. Skin rashes may occur as well.

3.8.5. Contraindications

Tetracyclines should be avoided in pregnancy and in children and should not be administered to patients with renal insufficiency; in such cases, doxycycline should be considered. Clindamycin should be avoided in patients with hepatic disease and should not be given to patients taking opiates, since this may worsen the GI toxicity. If diarrhea occurs, the drug should be stopped.

3.8.6. Dosage

Quinine should be given initially at 600 mg three times daily for 5–7 days, followed by tetracycline, 250 mg four times daily for 7 days, or doxycycline, 200 mg followed by 100 mg/day for 6 days, or minocycline, 200 mg followed by 100 mg twice daily for 7 days; the antibiotics can be given alone in these schedules. Clindamycin can be given alone at 5 mg/kg twice daily for 5 days or can follow a 3-day course of quinine.

4. GUIDELINES FOR MALARIA CHEMOTHERAPY

Assuming competent diagnosis and correct speciation, malaria treatment can be conveniently divided into several types.

4.1. Treatment of P. vivax and P. ovale

The drugs of choice are primaquine and chloroquine; no others should be required or used if these are available. If primaquine is unavailable or contraindicated, relapse attacks can always be cured with chloroquine.

4.2. Treatment of P. malariae

Chloroquine is the only drug recommended and necessary.

4.3. Treatment of P. falciparum

4.3.1. Semi-immune Patients

In Africa, single-dose treatment with 600 mg CQ base or 600–800 mg amodiaquine base appears to be effective. In areas of CQ resistance, quinine (1.5–2.0) may be used in three divided doses over 1 day. Proguanil (300–500 mg) or pyrimethamine (50 mg) also may be used; in areas with extensive CQ resistance or antifolate resistance, the latter is combined with a sulfonamide. Mefloquine–Fansidar should be reserved only for quinine-resistant cases. Tetracyclines or clindamycin may also be employed.

4.3.2. Nonimmune Patients

If the infection is sensitive to CQ, this is the drug of choice. If no therapeutic benefit is obtained within 3 days, another drug should be selected. In such cases, the recommended treatment is quinine orally, followed by an antifolate–PABA antagonist combination. Tetracyclines or clindamycin may be used also. Mefloquine should be given only in quinine-resistant cases. In mild to moderate cases of CQ resistance, amodiaquine has proved effective, and an amodiaquine–tetracycline combination, given for longer than usual periods, may be of benefit.

4.3.3. Critical Infections

Intravenous quinine is the drug of choice for initial therapy in patients who are severely ill. A variety of support measures, including cooling, blood transfusions, and dexamethasone treatment of cerebral malaria, may also be indicated but are beyond the scope of this chapter. Readers are referred to Peters (1980) and Bruce-Chwatt (1981). See also the latter author for treatment of blackwater fever.

4.4. Treatment of Malaria in Children

Falciparum malaria is a deadly disease in children. Prompt, accurate diagnosis is necessary but difficult, since symptoms are highly variable. Rapid progression of the disease to desperate stages is common. Quinine is relatively better tolerated in children than in adults and has great use in these cases. By contrast, chloroquine is somewhat more toxic, particularly if injected. These are the recommendations of Bruce-Chwatt (1981). Quinine is given intravenously as 5–10 mg/kg body weight slowly in high dilution. It can be repeated 6–12 hr later, but the total dose over 24 hr should not exceed 20 mg/kg body weight at a concentration of 1 g/liter infused over a total of 2–4 hr. CQ can also be used, intravenously, at a dose of 5 mg/kg, repeated 6–8 hr later if oral administration is not possible. Intramuscular injections are dangerous in children but can be given in the buttocks as 5 mg/kg in two divided injections 1–2 hr apart; this can be repeated once within 24 hr.

As soon as possible, oral treatment is begun. Doses for all these drugs must be reduced proportionately with body weight until the age of 12–15 years. Detailed instructions are to be found in Bruce-Chwatt (1981).

4.5. Prophylaxis

The constantly changing status of drug resistance makes perfect recommendations impossible. Recent recommendations are available (Centers for Disease Control, 1985*a,b;* Stürchler, 1984), but local situations require timely adjustments in treatment, and visitors to malarious regions are urged to contact the Centers for Disease Control in Atlanta if questions exist. If the individual will only be exposed to *vivax, ovale,* or *malariae* malaria, chloroquine is the drug of choice. Any relapses after exposure has ended can easily be treated with primaquine and chloroquine.

For *falciparum* malaria, certain areas of Africa may still be safe for CQ prophylaxis, but protection cannot be guaranteed. Fansidar prophylaxis was a judicious choice for much of the world, although resistance to it is not uncommon, and reports of serious toxicity have led to a reevaluation of its role in prophylaxis (Centers for Disease Control, 1985*a,b*). In areas with a high degree of resistance to these drugs, amodiaquine might be a better choice, although much work remains to be done on this possibility. In some areas, especially the refugee camps of Southeast Asia, mefloquine is the only drug that provides protection, although tetracycline prophylaxis should be tested. A short visit may also be covered with primaquine, although this approach cannot be generally recommended. The situation is expected to deteriorate as resistance spreads.

5. FUTURE DIRECTIONS

It is clear to the present authors that, after mefloquine, no new antimalarial drugs can be reasonably expected to be marketed in the near future. Economic considerations are the primary reason, but no one can deny the urgent need for new compounds. Until these become available, more research is needed on the ability of other 4-aminoquinolines to cure CQ-resistant infections, on the use of mefloquine, on optimization of antibiotic doses and schedules, and on the search for other available antibiotics with useful antimalarial activity.

REFERENCES

Adelusi, S. A., and Salako, L. A., 1982, Protein binding of chloroquine in the presence of aspirin, *Br. J. Clin. Pharmacol.* 13:451–455.

Black, R. H., 1973, Malaria in the Australian Army in South Vietnam; successful use of a proguanil–dapsone combination for the chemoprophylaxis of chloroquine-resistant falciparum malaria, *Med. J. Aust.* 1:1265–1270.

Brown, G. H., Anders, P. F., and Knowles, G., 1983, Differential effect of immunoglobulins on the *in vitro* growth of several isolates of *Plasmodium falciparum*, *Infect. Immun.* 39:1228–1235.

Bruce-Chwatt, L. J., 1980, *Essential Malariology*, Heinemann, London.

Bruce-Chwatt, L. J. (ed.), 1981, *Chemotherapy of Malaria*, World Health Organization, Geneva.

Cabrera, B. D., Rivera, D. G., and Lara, M. T., 1982, Study on clindamycin in the treatment of falciparum malaria, *Rev. Inst. Med. Trop. Sao Paulo* (Suppl. 6) 24:62–69.

Carson, P. E., 8-Aminoquinolines, in: *Antimalarial Drugs*, Vol. II (W. Peters and W. H. G. Richards, eds.), *Handbook of Experimental Pharmacology*, Volume 68, pp. 83–121, Springer-Verlag, New York.

Centers for Disease Control, 1985a, Adverse reactions to Fansidar and updated recommendations for its use in the prevention of malaria, *Morbid. Mortal. Weekly Rep.* 33:713–714.

Centers for Disease Control, 1985b, Revised recommendations for preventing malaria in travelers to areas with chloroquine-resistant *Plasmodium falciparum*, *Morbid. Mortal. Weekly Rep.* 34:185–190.

Christie, D. J., Mullen, P. C., and Aster, R. H., 1985, Fab-mediated binding of drug-dependent antibodies to platelets in quinidine- and quinine-induced thrombocytopenia, *J. Clin Invest.* 75:310–314.

Clyde, D. R., Miller, R. M., DuPont, H. L., and Hornick, R. B., 1971, Antimalarial effects of tetracycline in man, *J. Trop. Med. Hyg.* 74:238–242.

Clyde, D. R., Gilman, R. H., and McCarthy, V. C., 1975, Antimalarial effects of clindamycin in man, *Am. J. Trop. Med. Hyg.* 24:369–370.

Colwell, E. J., Hickman, R. L., Intraprasert, R., and Tirabutan, C., 1972, Minocycline and tetracycline treatment of acute falciparum malaria in Thailand, *Am. J. Trop. Med. Hyg.* 21:144–149.

Cox, F. E. G., 1984, Malarial immunity Indonesian and Sudanese style, *Nature (Lond.)* 309:402–403.

Danis, M., Felix, H., Brucker, G., Druilhe, P., Richard-Lenoble, D., and Gentilini, M., 1982, Place de la méfloquine dans le traitement curatif et préventif du paludisme, *Pathol. Biol.* 30:589–592.

de Souza, J.-M., 1983a, A phase I clinical trial of mefloquine in Brazilian male subjects, *Bull. WHO* 61:809–814.

de Souza, J.-M., 1983b, A phase II clinical trial of mefloquine in Brazilian male subjects, *Bull. WHO* 61:815–820.

Dietrich, M., and Kern, P., 1981, Malaria, *Antibiot. Chemother.* 30:224–256.

Divo, A. A., Geary, T. G., and Jensen, J. B., 1985, Oxygen- and time-dependent effects of antibiotics and selected mitochondrial inhibitors on *Plasmodium falciparum* in culture, *Antimicrob. Agents Chemother.* 27:21–27.

Ekue, J. M. K., Ulrich, A.-M., Rwabwago-Atenyi, J., and Sheth, U. K., 1983, A double-blind comparative clinical trial of mefloquine and chloroquine in symptomatic falciparum malaria, *Bull. WHO* 61:713–718.

Ellis, C. J., and Chiodini, P. L., 1984, The treatment of falciparum malaria, *J. Antimicrob. Chemother.* 13:311–314.

Ferone, R., 1984, Dihydrofolate reductase inhibitors, in: *Antimalarial Drugs,* Vol. II (W. Peters and W. H. G. Richards, eds.), *Handbook Experimental Pharmacology,* Vol. 68, pp. 207–221, Springer-Verlag, New York.

Frisk-Holmberg, M., Bergqvist, Y., Domeij-Nyberg, B., Hellström, L., and Jansson, F., 1979, Chloroquine serum concentration and side effects: Evidence for dose-dependent kinetics, *Clin. Pharmacol. Ther.* 25:345–350.

Geary, T. G., and Jensen, J. B., 1983a, Lack of cross-resistance to 4-aminoquinolines in chloroquine-resistant *Plasmodium falciparum in vitro, J. Parasitol.* 69:97–105.

Geary, T. G., and Jensen, J. B., 1983b, Effects of antibiotics on *Plasmodium falciparum in vitro, Am. J. Trop. Med. Hyg.* 32:221–225.

Geary, T. G., Akood, M. A., and Jensen, J. B., 1983, Characterization of chloroquine binding to glass and plastic, *Am. J. Trop. Med. Hyg.* 32:19–23.

Grewal, R. S., 1981, Pharmacology of 8-aminoquinolines, *Bull. WHO* 59:397–406.

Gustafsson, L. L., Walker, O., Alván, G., Beerman, B., Estevez, F., Gleisner, L., Lindström, B., and Sjöquist, F., 1983b, Disposition of chloroquine in man after single intravenous and oral doses, *Br. J. Clin. Pharmac.* 15:471–479.

Gustafsson, L. L., Rumbo, L., Alván G., Björkman, A., Lind, L., and Walker, O., 1983a, On the question of dose-dependent chloroquine elimination of a single oral dose, *Clin. Pharmacol. Ther.* 34:383–385.

Harinasuta, T., Bunnag, D., and Wernsdorfer, W. H., 1983, A phase II clinical trial of mefloquine in patients with chloroquine-resistant falciparum malaria in Thailand, *Bull. WHO* 61:299–305.

Harinasuta, T., Lasserre, R., Bunnag, D., Leimer, R., and Vinijanont, S., 1985, Trials of mefloquine in vivax and of mefloquine plus "Fansidar" in faliparum malaria, *Lancet* I:885–888.

Hoffman, S. L., Masber, S., Hussein, P. R., Soewerta, A., Haran, S., Marwoto, H. A., Campbell, J. R., Smrkovski, L., Purnomo, and Wiady, I., 1984, Absence of malaria mortality in villagers with chloroquine-resistant *Plasmodium falciparum* treated with chloroquine, *Trans. R. Soc. Trop. Med. Hyg.* 78:175–178.

Hofheinz, W., and Merkli, B., 1984, Quinine and quinine analogs, in: *Antimalarial Drugs,* Vol. II (W. Peters and W. H. G. Richards, eds.), *Handbook Experimental Pharmacology,* Vol. 68, pp. 61–81, Springer-Verlag, New York.

Jensen, J. B., Boland, M. T., Allan, J. S., Carlin, J. M., Vande Waa, J. A., Divo, A. A., and Akood, M. A. S., 1983, Association between human serum-induced crisis forms in cultured *Plasmodium falciparum* and clinical immunity to malaria in Sudan, *Infect. Immun.* 41:1302–1311.

Jensen, J. B., Hoffman, S. L., Boland, M. T., Akood, M. A. S., Laughlin, L. W., Kurniawan, L., and Marwoto, H. A., 1984, Comparison of immunity to malaria in Sudan and Indonesia: Crisis-form versus merozoite-invasion inhibition, *Proc. Natl. Acad. Sci. U.S.A.* 81:922–925.

Knowles, G., Davidson, W. L., Jolley, D., and Alpers, M. P., 1984a, The relationship between the *in vitro* response of *Plasmodium falciparum* to chloroquine, quinine and mefloquine, *Trans. R. Soc. Trop. Med. Hyg.* 78:146–150.

Knowles, G., Davidson, W. L., McBride, J. S., and Jolley, D., 1984b, Antigenic diversity found in isolates of *Plasmodium falciparum* from Papua New Guinea by using monoclonal antibodies, *Am. J. Trop. Med. Hyg.* 33:204–211.

Lapierre, J., Devant, J., Coquelin, B., Faurant, C., and Galal, A. A., 1983, Bilan d'une expérience de chimioprophylaxie du paludisme par la méfloquine au Cambodge, *Bull. Sôc. Pathol. Exp.* 76:357–363.

Mandell, G. L., and Sande, M. A., 1980, Sulfonamides, trimethoprim-sulfamethoxazole, and urinary tract antiseptics, in: *The Pharmacological Basis of Therapeutics,* 6th ed. (A. G. Gilman, L. S. Goodman, and A. Gilman, eds.), pp. 1106–1125, Macmillan, New York.

McBride, J. S., Walliker, D., and Morgan, G., 1982, Antigenic diversity in the human malaria parasite *Plasmodium falciparum, Science* 217:254–257.

McChesney, E. W., and Fitch, C. D., 1984, 4-Aminoquinolines, in: *Antimalarial Drugs*, Vol. II (W. Peters and W. H. G. Richards, eds.), *Handbook of Experimental Pharmacology*, Vol. 68, pp. 3–60, Springer-Verlag, New York.

McLarty, D. G., Jaatinen, M., Murru, M., Aubert, B., Webber, R. H., Kihamia, C. H., Kumano, M., and Magnuson, L. W., 1984, Chemoprophylaxis of malaria in non-immune residents in Dar Es Salaam, Tanzania, *Lancet* II:656–659.

Miller, L. H., Glew, R. H., Wyler, D. J., Howard, W. A., Contacos, P. G., and Neva, F. A., 1974, Evaluation of clindamycin in combination with quinine against multidrug-resistant strains of *Plasmodium falciparum*, *Am. J. Trop. Med. Hyg.* 23:565–569.

Noeypatimanand, S., Malikul, S., Benjapong, W., Duriyananda, D., and Ungkasrithongkul, M., 1983, Treatment of *Plasmodium falciparum* malaria with a combination of amodiaquine and tetracycline in Central Thailand, *Trans. R. Soc. Trop. Med. Hyg.* 77:338–340.

Osifo, N. G., 1984, Chloroquine-induced puritis among patients with malaria, *Arch. Dermatol.* 120:80–82.

Peters, W., 1970, *Chemotherapy and Drug Resistance in Malaria*, Academic Press, London and New York.

Peters, W., 1974, Recent advances in antimalarial chemotherapy and drug resistance, in: *Advances in Parasitology* (B. Dawes, ed.), Vol. 12, pp. 69–114, Academic Press, London and New York.

Peters, W., 1980, Chemotherapy of malaria, in: *Malaria*, (J. P. Kreier, ed.), Vol. 1, pp. 145–283, Academic Press, New York and London.

Peters, W., and Richards, W. H. G. (eds.), 1984, *Antimalarial Drugs*, Vols. I and II (*Handbook of Experimental Pharmacology*, Vol. 68, Springer-Verlag, New York).

Ponnampalan, J. T., 1981, Doxycycline in the treatment of falciparum malaria among aborigine children in West Malaysia, *Trans. R. Soc. Trop. Med. Hyg.* 75:372–377.

Pratt, W. B., 1977, *Chemotherapy of Infection*, Oxford Univeristy Press, New York.

Richards, W. H. G., 1979, Some promising leads in experimental antimalarial drugs, in: *Advances in Pharmacology and Therapeutics* (M. Adolphe, ed.), Vol. 10, pp. 71–112, Pergamon Press, Oxford and New York.

Rieckmann, K. H., 1983, *Falciparum* malaria: The urgent need for safe and effective drugs, *Annu. Rev. Med.* 34:321–335.

Rieckmann, K. H., 1984, Antibiotics, in: *Antimalarial Drugs*, Vol. II (W. Peters and W. H. G. Richards, eds.), *Handbook of Experimental Pharmacology*, Vol. 68, pp. 443–470, Springer-Verlag, New York.

Rieckmann, K. H., Powell, R. D., McNamara, J. V., Willerson, D. Jr., Koss, L., Frischer, H., and Carson, P. E., 1971, Effects of tetracycline against chloroquine-resistant and chloroquine-sensitive *Plasmodium falciparum*, *Am. J. Trop. Med. Hyg.* 20:811–815.

Ris, H. B., Stabel, E., Pittet, J. F., and Friedman, M., 1983, Das Antiarrhythmikum Chinidin als Alternative in der Behandlung der schweren Falciparum-Malaria, *Schweiz, Med. Wochenschr.* 113:254–258.

Rivera, D. G., Cabrera, B. D., and Lara, N. T., 1982, Treatment of falciparum malaria with clindamycin, *Rev. Inst. Med. Trop. Sao Paulo* (Suppl. 6) 24:70–75.

Rollo, I. M., 1980, Drugs used in the chemotherapy of malaria, in: *The Pharmacological Basis of Therapeutics*, 6th ed. (A. G. Gilman, L. S. Goodman, and A. Gilman, eds.), pp. 1038–1060, Macmillan, New York.

Rozman, R. S., and Canfield, C. J., 1979, New experimental antimalarial drugs. *Adv. Pharmacol. Chemother.* 16:1–43.

Schmidt, L. H., Vaughan, D., Mueller, D., Crosby, R., and Hamilton, R., 1977, Activities of various 4-aminoquinolines against infections with chloroquine-resistant strains of *Plasmodium falciparum*, *Antimicrob. Agents Chemother.* 11:826–843.

Schofield, L., Saul, A., Myler, P., and Kidson, C., 1982, Antigenic differences among isolates of *Plasmodium falciparum* demonstrated by monoclonal antibodies, *Infect. Immun.* 38:893–897.

Scholer, H. J., Leiner, R., and Richie, R., 1984, Sulphonamides and sulphones, in: *Antimalarial Drugs*, Vol. II (W. Peters and W. H. G. Richards, eds.), *Handbook of Experimental Pharmacology*, Vol. 68, pp. 123–206, Springer-Verlag, New York.

Seaberg, L. S., Parquette, A. R., Gluzman, I. Y., Phillips, G. W., Jr., Brodasky, T. F., and Krogstad, D. J., 1984, Clindamycin activity against chloroquine-resistant *Plasmodium falciparum*, *J. Infect. Dis.* 150:904–911.

Spencer, H. C., Kipingor, T., Agure, R., Koech, D. K., and Chulay, J. D., 1983, *Plasmodium falciparum* in Kisumu, Kenya: differences in sensitivity to amodiaquine and chloroquine *in vitro*, *J. Inf. Dis.* 148:732–736.

Sturchler, D., 1984, Malaria prophylaxis in travellers: the current position, *Experentia* 40:1357–1362.

Sweeney, T. R., 1981, The present status of malaria chemotherapy: Mefloquine, a novel antimalarial, *Med. Res. Rev.* 1:281–301.

Sweeney, T. R., 1984a, 8-Aminoquinolines, in *Antimalarial Drugs*, Vol. II (W. Peters and W. H. G. Richards, eds.), *Handbook of Experimental Pharmacology*, Vol. 68, pp. 267–324, Springer-Verlag, New York.

Thompson, P. E., and Werbel, L. M., 1972, *Antimalarial Agents. Chemistry and Pharmacology*, Academic Press, New York.

Vernes, A., Haynes, J. D., Tapchaisri, P., Williams, J. L., Dutoit, E., and Diggs, C. L., 1984, *Plasmodium falciparum* strain-specific human antibody inhibits merozoite invasion of erythrocytes, *Am. J. Trop. Med. Hyg.* 33:197–203.

Walker, O., Birkett, D. J., Alván, G., Gustafsson, L. L., and Sjöqvist, F., 1983, Characterization of chloroquine plasma protein binding in man, *Br. J. Clin. Pharmacol.* 15:375–377.

Watkins, W. M., Spencer, H. C., Kariuki, D. M., Sixsmith, D. G., Boriga, D. A., Kipingor, T., and Koech, D. K., 1984a, Effectiveness of amodiaquine as a treatment for chloroquine-resistant *Plasmodium falciparum* infections in Kenya, *Lancet* I:357–359.

Watkins, W. M., Sixsmith, D. G., and Chulay, J. D., 1984b, The activity of proguanil and its metabolites, cycloguanil and p-chlorophenylbiguanide, against *Plasmodium falciparum in vitro*, *Ann. Trop. Med. Parasitol.* 78:273–278.

White, N. J., Looareesuwan, S., Warrell, D. A., Bunnag, D., Changsuphajaisiddhi, T., and Harinasuta, T., 1981, Quinidine in falciparum malaria, *Lancet* 2:1069–1071.

White, N. J., Looareesuwan, S., and Warrell, D. A., 1983a, Quinine and quinidine: A comparison of EKG effects during the treatment of malaria, *J. Cardiovasc. Pharmacol.* 5:173–175.

White, N. J., Looareesuwan, S., Warrell, D. A., Warrell, M. J., Chanthavanich, P., Bunnay, D., and Harinasuta, T., 1983b, Quinine loading dose in cerebral malaria, *Am. J. Trop. Med. Hyg.* 32:1–5.

WHO, 1973, *Chemotherapy of Malaria and Resistance to Antimalarials*, WHO Technical Report Series No. 529, World Health Organization, Geneva.

WHO, 1981, Development of mefloquine as an antimalarial drug, *Bull. WHO* 61:169–183.

Willerson, D., Jr., Rieckmann, K. H., Carson, P. E., and Frischer, H., 1972, Effects of minocycline against chloroquine-resistant falciparum malaria, *Am. J. Trop. Med. Hyg.* 21:857–863.

Wyler, D. J., 1983, Malaria—resurgence, resistance, and research, *New Eng. J. Med.* 308:875–878, 934–940.

Yayon, A., Vande Waa, J. A., Yayon, M., Geary, T. G., and Jensen, J. B., 1983, Stage-dependent effects of chloroquine on *Plasmodium falciparum in vitro*, *J. Protozool.* 30:642–649.

4

Protozoan Infections of Man

American Trypanosomiasis and Leishmaniasis

PATRICK B. McGREEVY and PHILIP D. MARSDEN

1. INTRODUCTION

The genera *Leishmania* and *Trypanosoma* are characterized by intra- and interspecific diversity, which occurs at all levels of organization, ranging from basic metabolism and morphology to pathology and epidemiology. This chapter focuses on the clinical aspects of treatment and emphasizes variations in parasite virulence and variations in the human response to infection as they relate to a particular chemotherapeutic strategy. For detailed life histories of these parasites or a summary of experimental therapeutics, consult a general reference (Molyneaux and Ashford, 1983; Cancado and Brener, 1979; WHO, 1979a, 1984; Peters and Killick-Kendrick, 1985; Steck, 1972).

Trypanosomiasis and leishmaniasis usually cause chronic debilitating diseases. In general, treatment is substandard and often requires hospitalization for the delivery of toxic drugs over long periods. In Brasilia, the course of treatment for mucosal leishmaniasis can cost $4000 (U.S.) excluding salaries, laboratory support, and drugs. The financial impact on the patient and family would be catastrophic without support from the public sector.

The inadequacy of chemotherapy is related to the fact that trypanosomiasis and leishmaniasis are diseases of rural subsistence farmers in developing tropical countries. Medical service in rural communities is often inadequate because of the inequitable distribution of health resources in favor of urban centers; this problem is particularly acute in the developing world. To be useful in this environment, a drug must be

PATRICK B. McGREEVY • Department of Parasitology, Division of Experimental Therapeutics, Walter Reed Army Institute of Research, Walter Reed Army Medical Center, Washington, D.C. 20307.   PHILIP D. MARSDEN • Nucleo de Medicina Tropical e Nutricao, Faculdade de Ciencias de Saude, Universidade de Brasilia, Brasilia DF 70,000, Brazil.

inexpensive, have a long shelf life without refrigeration, and be given by paramedics orally, without side effects.

In addition to these practical considerations, each trypanosomatid parasite has unique properties that make it an evasive target for potential chemotherapeutic agents and a formidable challenge to the pharmacologist and medicinal chemist. For example, the ability of African trypanosomes to infect the CNS limits the number of potential drugs for advanced disease to those which pass the blood-brain barrier (see Chapter 5). American trypanosomes are intracellular parasites in a variety of tissues, and the activity of a circulating compound depends on its ability to cross the vascular endothelium and cell membranes to this cytoplasmic compartment. *Leishmania* infect the phagolysosomes of macrophages, and circulating compounds must travel to this compartment and resist digestion by lysosomal enzymes in order to maintain their activity. These practical and theoretical factors contribute to the high cost of drug development and account for the sad fact that this is the only area of modern medicine where heavy metal therapy, a mainstay of nineteenth-century medicine, still plays an important role.

2. AMERICAN TRYPANOSOMIASIS (CHAGAS' DISEASE)

The chemotherapeutic targets in Chagas' disease are the circulating trypomastigotes and the tissue amastigotes. *Trypanosoma cruzi* is not a homogeneous species, and there are geographic strains which vary in tissue tropism, response to chemotherapy and biochemical parameters such as electrophoretic profiles of isoenzymes and peptides. The value of a particular drug depends on its activity against both the amastigote and trypomastigote stages of all geographic strains.

2.1. Nifurtimox and Benznidazole

Two drugs are currently used for Chagas' disease, i.e., nifurtimox (Lampit, Bayer 2502) and benznidazole (Rochagan, Ro7-1051, Radinil). Both have high activity against both trypomastigotes and amastigotes. Neither drug is licensed in the United States, but nifurtimox is available from the Centers for Disease Control (CDC), Atlanta, Georgia.

Nifurtimox, a nitrofuran, is an oral drug given three times a day after meals at a daily dose of 8–10 mg/kg (Macedo, 1982). Although treatment can extend for 120 days, it is just as effective when given for 60 days. Nifurtimox is readily absorbed and rapidly metabolized with a peak plasma concentration at 1–3 hr, which declines to 0 by 24 hr. Animal studies have revealed a number of metabolites that have no particular tissue tropism and are excreted in urine. It is not known whether the parent compound or its metabolites are active.

Benznidazole, a nitroimidazole, is given orally at a daily dose of 5–7 mg/kg for 30–120 days (Macedo, 1982). It is rapidly absorbed and distributed through the body tissues, metabolites being excreted in the urine.

2.1.1. Toxicity and Hypersensitivity

Both drugs can produce gastric upset and consequent weight loss, skin rashes, peripheral neuritis, and bone marrow depression. They are also carcinogenic in animals when given in high doses, but no such patient effect has been described.

In one study using nifurtimox, all patients had weight loss, 70% had anorexia, and 33% had peripheral neuritis during treatment at 7–8 mg/kg per day for 60 days (C. A. N. Silveira, unpublished data). Peripheral neuritis and psychosis depend on the dose of nifurtimox and usually occur at the end of high-dose treatment (15–20 mg/kg per day). Fortunately, these serious side effects are reversible if the drug is stopped. Nifurtimox, like any nitrofuran, will cause hemolytic anemia in glucose 6-phosphate dehydrogenase (G6PD) -deficient individuals.

Benznidazole causes erythematous light sensitive skin rashes in half of the patients and these can be severe (Boainain, 1979). It can also cause a marked thrombocytopenia in man and depresses thymus-dependent immune functions in rabbits (Teixeira *et al.*, 1983).

2.1.2. Strain Variation

There is marked variation in efficacy of chemotherapy in different geographical areas. Studies in both acute and chronic Chagas' disease show that patients from central Brazil are relatively unresponsive to nifurtimox as compared with patients from Chile and Argentina (Cancado and Brener, 1979; Brener, 1979). Regarding chronic patients in central Brazil, xenodiagnosis is usually negative during nifurtimox treatment, but it converts to positive in 60–70% of the patients over a 4-year period. Post-treatment serodiagnosis usually remains positive in chronic patients, suggesting that parasites persist even when xenodiagnosis is negative. In the same geographical area, benznidazole produced similar results and sterilized the blood of only 40% of chronic patients. These partial effects are difficult to interpret, but resistance to both compounds has been induced in the laboratory.

2.2. Clinical Strategy

There is a clear indication for the use of either drug for acute Chagas' disease to minimize parasitic invasion of vital tissues. Good results are achieved within a few days of treatment, as indicated by the disappearance of circulating trypanosomes, remission of signs and symptoms, and occasional reversion to a serologically negative condition. However, in central Brazil most patients are not cured, as evidenced by the demonstration of parasites by xenodiagnosis on follow-up, several years later.

Nifurtimox and benznidazole are often prescribed for chronically infected patients, especially if they have a positive xenodiagnosis. It is not clear, however, whether treatment actually benefits these patients. Although treatment suppresses parasitemia it certainly fails to cure some (perhaps all) of the patients as circulating trypomastigotes are often detected years later by xenodiagnosis. Available data on the clinical response of patients with chronic infection to treatment do not suggest that therapy halts the progress of ECG abnormalities, the first signs of cardiomyopathy. In one short-term study over 18 months using 7.5 mg/kg per day nifurtimox and 5–6 mg/kg per day benznidazole for 60–90 days, no difference was found in ECG evolution between treated and control groups. It must be noted that only 78% of these patients completed the designated course of therapy, because of side effects (C. A. N. Silveira, unpublished data). Owing to questionable parasitological results, uncertain clinical benefit, and side effects, neither drug is recommended for treatment of patients with chronic infection. Symptomatic treatment is the only alternative, but the delivery of digitalis, diuretics, pacemakers, and emergency services for cardiomyopathies, and surgery for mega-esophagus and megacolon is too expensive and logistically impractical to carry out in rural endemic areas.

2.2.1. Evaluation of Treatment

The effect of therapy on acute disease is measured by the remission of signs and symptoms, decline in antibody titer, and the elimination of parasitemia. Low concentrations of circulating parasites are difficult to detect, and monthly xenodiagnosis or blood culture is required.

2.3. The Future

Recently another nitroimidazole [2-amino-5-(1-methyl-5-nitro-2-imidazo-lyl)-1,3,4 thiadiazole] has shown remarkable efficacy in mice, curing 89% of cases with a single dose. It is also active against strains that are resistant to nifurtimox and 2-nitroimidazole derivatives (Filardi and Brener, 1982). Trypomastigotes are cleared from the bloodstream in 6 hr and destruction of amastigotes occurs in 18–36 hr (Almeida Maria et al., 1984). This drug has gone to limited human trial.

Unlike the situation in leishmaniasis and African trypanosomiasis, the immediate solution to Chagas' disease is not new treatment measures, but rather control of domiciliated vector bugs (Marsden, 1983). Brzail has mounted the largest attack in its history against house-dwelling bugs, using residual insecticides, funded by the National Health Insurance Program (Fiusa Lima, 1983). Only in this way will the burden of chronic chagasic cardiomyopathy and megasyndrome be lifted from the struggling hospital services. The children infected this year will be patients in hospitals in the twenty-first century; even if immediate control were possible, Brazil would still be left with 6 million infected people. New less toxic drugs that can be given over a shorter period are needed. In addition, ways of assessing the effects of such drugs in chronically infected patients, other than laborious xenodiagnosis, are required.

3. LEISHMANIASIS

The chemotherapeutic target in leishmaniasis is the tissue amastigote, which is found in phagolysosomes of macrophages. There are more that a dozen subspecies of *Leishmania* that produce either cutaneous, mucosal, or visceral disease in man.

3.1. Pentavalent Antimonials

Meglumine antimoniate (Glucantime) and sodium stibogluconate (Pentostam) are the first-line drugs for the treatment of leishmaniasis. These drugs are not licensed in the United States, but Pentostam is available from the CDC, Atlanta, Georgia.

The precise chemical structures of these drugs are unknown, and quality control is maintained through chemical analysis for pentavalent antimony (Sb^v) and other physicochemical measurements. Sb^v, rather than the sugar component of these drugs, is lethal to amastigotes, but the mechanism of action is unknown. Sodium stibogluconate contains 100 mg Sb^v/ml and meglumine antimoniate contains 85 mg Sb^v/ml. The efficacy and toxicity of both drugs are similar on a Sb^v-per kg basis, and it is surprising that the manufacturers recommend different dosages. For Pentostam, the Wellcome Foundation Ltd., Beckenham, England, recommends that adults (60 kg) be given intravenous or intramuscular injections of Sb^v, 10 mg/kg per day, for 7–10 days and that two to three cycles be separated with 10-day rest intervals if additional treatment is necessary. For Glucantime, Rhodia S. A., Sao Paulo, Brazil, recommends that adults be given intramuscular injections of Sb^v, 17–28 mg/kg per day, for 10–20 days, followed by a 15-day rest interval and a second cycle if needed. These divergent recommendations indicate that optimal doses are still not defined.

Pharmacokinetic data on Pentostam and Glucantime given at 10 mg Sb^v/kg per day up to 600 mg per person per day for 10 days show that peak blood levels of Sb^v of $\leqslant$ 100 mg/liter occur 15 min after intravenous injection, while levels of Sb^v of 10 mg/liter occur 1–2 hr after intramuscular injection (WHO, 1982). The half-life of Sb^v in blood after treatment with Pentostam or Glucantime is only 2 hr (WHO, 1982; Chulay et al., 1983b), and 81–97% of Sb^v delivered as Pentostam is excreted during the first 6–8 hr (Rees et al., 1980). There is a slight accumulation of Sb^v in the tissues after daily injections of Pentostam or Glucantime, as blood levels of Sb^v increase from 0.05 mg/liter at 24 hr after the first dose to 0.1–0.3 mg/liter at 24 hr after the ninth dose. These observations imply that a dose of 10 mg Sb^v/kg can be given more than once a day and that rest periods are not necessary.

These pharmacokinetic principles have been applied by Chulay et al. (1983b), who compared the efficacy of three treatment schedules for visceral leishmaniasis: 10 mg Sb^v/kg qd for 30 days, 10 mg Sb^v/kg bid for 15 days, and 10 mg Sb^v/kg tid for 10 days. Although the total dose was the same, 300 mg Sb^v/kg, the disappearance of parasites from splenic aspirates was accelerated in the group given three injections per day—the dosage schedule designed to sustain high levels of Sb^v in the tissues.

3.1.1. Toxicity and Hypersensitivity

The initial phases of Sb^v treatment are usually well tolerated. Injection volumes of Pentostam and Glucantime range from 6–21 ml, depending on the dose of Sb^v, and they are usually given by slow intravenous injection of undiluted drug. Venous thrombosis has been associated with Pentostam; this complication can be controlled by delivering the drug in 50 ml of diluent. In the absence of medical personnel in rural villages, these large volumes of Sb^v are injected intramuscularly by a friend—a painful injection that occasionally causes abscesses and often leads to default on dosage.

Immediate toxic effects and hypersensitivity reactions are very rare. Regarding toxic effects, we have seen a patient given an initial intravenous dose of Pentostam at 17 mg Sb^v/kg in whom shock developed, along with marked sweating, dizziness, and hypotension. For this reason, we advise a small test dose before beginning therapy. As an additional precaution, patients treated in a field clinic should rest for half an hour before walking home. Regarding hypersensitivity reactions, care must be given to patients with advanced mucosal disease at the beginning of therapy. Sometimes the granulomata enlarge and erythema appears in affected facial areas with bleeding from lesion sites—a type of Jarish Herxheimer reaction (Rocha *et al.*, 1980). Edema at the laryngeal level can be fatal if airway obstruction occurs and tracheostomy equipment is not available. We manage these side effects by simply suspending treatment for a few days and have found corticosteroids unnecessary. These complications do not recur on resumption of treatment.

Objective clinical laboratory abnormalities occur in one-third of patients receiving Pentostam at 10 mg Sb^v/kg per day for 10 days, including thrombophlebitis and induration at the site of injection (18% of patients) and transient elevations of alanine aminotransferase (13%), lactic dehydrogenose (7%), aspartate aminotransferase (5%), triglycerides (5%), creatine phosphokinase (3%), and alkaline phosphatase (2%) (Chulay *et al.*, 1985*a*). Minor side effects occur in about 25% of patients taking 10–20 mg Sb^v/day; in order of decreasing frequency they include arthralgia, myalgia, anorexia, nausea, headache, and vomiting. Less frequent symptoms are epigastric discomfort, heartburn, itching, fever, weakness, dizziness, palpitations, insomnia, and nervousness (Sampaio, 1984). An occasional patient given these moderate doses suffers from more serious effects. After 20 mg/kg per day Sb^v for 8 days, one patient was unable to raise her arms because of shoulder pain; this symptom returned after a rest period when her treatment was switched from Pentostam to Glucantime. On a third treatment attempt, this symptom returned after the first injection of Pentostam.

Worrisome toxic effects, although rare, are seen in unresponsive cases when treatment is being given near the toxicity limit for extended periods. For example, a nonresponding patient with mucosal leishmaniasis who was given Sb^v, 20 mg/kg per day for 85 days showed evidence of arthritis of one wrist and shoulder, an inverted T wave on ECG, raised transaminases with tender hepatomegaly, and a renal tubular defect (Marsden *et al.*, 1985).

Renal changes are usually assessed by monitoring urea and creatinine levels during treatment, and it is rare to see elevation. However, urinary concentration tests show that in spite of normal glomerular function, a tubular defect is induced by daily doses of Sb^v, 20–30 mg/kg (Veiga *et al.*, 1983). Of eight patients studied longitudinally after Sb^v-induced tubular malfunction, five recovered normal concentrating functions within a month of cessation of therapy (Veiga *et al.*, 1985). The toxicity of Sb^v in the tubule is complex, influencing antidiuretic hormone (ADH) function as well as cell respiration (Gagliardi *et al.*, 1985).

Electrocardiographic changes are dose related and one of the main reasons for the care with which Sb^v is delivered (Chulay *et al.*, 1985*b*). After treatment with Glucantime at 28 mg/kg per day Sb^v for 10 days, repeated three times with rest intervals of 10 days, 40% of patients had abnormal ECG (Sampaio *et al.*, 1980). The rare sudden death may be the result of severe dysrhythmias such as ventricular fibrillations.

Typical side effects of heavy metals are not common with Sb^v. Skin reactions are rare and minor, usually an erythema with pruritis. However, in one series of 80 patients treated with Glucantime at 28 mg Sb^v/day there were two cases of herpes zoster, a known complication of heavy metal therapy (Sampaio *et al.*, 1980).

3.2. Second-Line Drugs

Pentamidine is a second-line drug for the treatment of mucosal and diffuse cutaneous leishmaniasis caused by *L. aethiopica* and for unresponsive and relapse cases of visceral leishmaniasis (see Section 3.4.3). For visceral leishmaniasis, the World Health Organization (WHO, 1982) recommends intramuscular injections at 4 mg/kg per day given three times per week for 5–25 weeks or longer, depending on the response. Pentamidine cured 81 of 82 cases of antimony-resistant disease in India (Jha, 1983). Patients with *L. aethiopica* should be treated with 2–4 mg/kg at weekly intervals for 3 months or beyond the time that parasites are no longer detected in smears and cultures of cutaneous lesions (WHO, 1983; Bryceson, 1970). Severe toxicity, including hypotension and collapse, may follow intravenous injection of pentamidine, so careful intramuscular injections with aspiration are required. Cumulative effects are abdominal pain, weakness, nausea, vomiting, nephrotoxicity, abnormal liver function, and altered carbohydrate metabolism, including hypoglycemia, hyperglycemia, and diabetes mellitus (Walzer *et al.*, 1974; Bouchard *et al.*, 1982).

Amphotericin B is a second-line drug for unresponsive and relapse cases of visceral leishmaniasis and the usual choice for mucosal leishmaniasis in South America. The World Health Organization (WHO, 1982) recommends intravenous infusions given in 500 ml of 5–10% glucose solution over several hours. The initial dose of 5–10 mg should be increased by 5–10 mg/day until a level of 0.5–1 mg/kg is reached. The latter dose is continued on alternate days until a total of 1–3 g is given, the exact amount depending on the response. Amphotericin B causes serious nephrotoxicity in addition to other side effects: local thrombophlebitis, anorexia, nausea, vomiting, fever, chills, and anemia. This drug is unsuitable for outpatient treatment.

3.3. Clinical Strategy for Cutaneous and Mucosal Disease

3.3.1. Local Treatment

In the Old World, it is safe to give local treatment to patients with limited cutaneous leishmaniasis caused by *L. tropica* and *L. major* because the lesions heal spontaneously within a few months without metastasis. A variety of physical treatments have been used: surigcal excision (Azab *et al.*, 1983), cryotherapy (Bassiouny *et al.*,

1982), and heat (Neva *et al.*, 1984). Local medicinal treatments have included berberine, Glucantime, tartar emetic, and quinacrine (Steck, 1972; Duperrat *et al.*, 1966; Elkerton, 1944). All these treatments appeared to accelerate healing, but firm conclusions cannot be made because the study groups were small and efficacy was not compared with nontreated groups or with groups given standard systemic therapy with Sb^v.

In the New World, local treatment should not be used alone for lesions caused by the *L. braziliensis* complex because these parasites can disseminate and cause mucosal disease. However, the combination of local and systemic therapy might be useful if it permits a reduction of the dosage of systemic Sb^v and facilitates closure of lesions that resist conventional parenteral treatment. Encouraging results for the treatment of lesions caused by *L. braziliensis panamensis* were recently reported by Solano *et al.* (1984), who cured all of 45 patients with one to four infusions of Glucantime. The efficacy of local heat therapy is variable and may be related to the thermosensitivity of the infecting species of *Leishmania*. Heat therapy healed diffuse cutaneous lesions caused by *L. mexicana* ssp. but had no effect on cutaneous lesions caused by *L. tropica* or *L. braziliensis* (Neva *et al.*, 1984). Cryotherapy did not accelerate healing of lesions caused by *L. braziliensis* (Llanos-Cuentas *et al.*, 1983).

Topical preparations are currently under evaluation. Creams containing 15% solutions of berberine, paromomycin, Glucantime, Pentostam, tartar emetic, and antimony chloride applied twice a day for 10 days are active against cutaneous ulcers caused by *L. braziliensis panamensis* in the African White-Tailed Rat, *Mystromys albicaudatus*. Although primary ulcers heal within 30 days after the beginning of treatment, viable amastigotes persist beneath normal skin and ulcers reappear around day 60 (McGreevy *et al.*, unpublished observations). Similar results were obtained in BALB/c mice infected with *L. major*, using topical preparations of paromomycin (El-On *et al.*, 1984).

3.3.2. Systemic Treatment

Absolute indications for the systemic treatment of cutaneous leishmaniasis are (1) cosmetic considerations, (2) evidence of immunosuppression, (3) persistence of a lesion for more than 6 months, or (4) infection with a species noted for persistence or metastasis. While the need for systemic Sb^v is usually obvious, the selection of treatment regimens is complicated and depends on the species of parasite, lesion size, anatomical site, risk of dissemination, immunological status, and practical considerations.

In the Old World, the recommended regimen for *L. tropica* and *L. major* is a dose of 10–20 mg Sb^v/kg per day (maximum dose 850 mg/day) given daily for 10–30 days according to the clinical and parasitological response (WHO, 1983). As patients with recidivans leishmaniasis caused by *L. tropica* or *L. major* respond poorly to Sb^v and often relapse, treatment with Sb^v should continue beyond 30 days or until the lesions heal (WHO, 1983). Second-line drugs and local therapy may be required in difficult cases. Patients with post-kala-azar dermal leishmaniasis respond initially to treatment with Sb^v, but more than 50% of them relapse and additional treatment or a second-line drug is required (Thakur, 1984). For simple cutaneous lesions caused by *L. aethiopica*, Chulay

·*et al.* (1983*a*) used Pentostam at 18–20 mg Sb^v/kg twice daily for 30 days, with success. Diffuse cutaneous leishmaniasis caused by *L. aethiopica* fails to respond to treatment with Sb^v, and Bryceson (1970) recommends pentamidine as a first-line drug.

There are few well-controlled studies on American cutaneous leishmaniasis on which to base recommendations for treatment. For example, Chulay *et al.* (1985*a*) and Oster *et al.* (1985) found that Pentostam at 600 mg Sb^v/day per person (about 8 mg/kg) for 10 consecutive days cured 10 of 12 patients with either *L. chagasi*, *L. mexicana* spp., *L. mexicana amazonensis*, or other species of the *mexicana* complex. However, this treatent failed to cure 10 of 14 patients with *L. braziliensis braziliensis* or *L. braziliensis panamensis*. Continuing studies in Brazil suggest that Glucantime given at the rate of 17 mg Sb^v/kg per day for 10 days is inadequate for simple cutaneous leishmaniasis caused by *L. braziliensis braziliensis* infections (J. M. Costa, unpublished data), while two series of treatment at 28 mg Sb^v/kg per day for 10 days, which approaches the level of toxicity, gives satisfactory results (Llanos-Cuentas, 1984).

In American cutaneous leishmaniasis, there is an obvious association between the size and location of the lesion and the difficulty in treatment. Regarding size, there is an inverse relationship between the area of a lesion and the therapeutic response to Sb^v in humans infected with *L. braziliensis* spp. (Llanos-Cuentas, 1984; Chulay *et al.*, 1985*a*). This observation has been confirmed experimentally using *L. braziliensis panamensis* in rodents (McGreevy, unpublished observations). Regarding site, lesions caused by *L. braziliensis braziliensis* on the pretibial surface of the leg are frequently slow to heal with Glucantime and often require extended treatment (Llanos-Cuentas, 1984). The poor response of these lesions may relate to circulatory and immunological deficiencies in this part of the leg (Jones and Sanders, 1983; Hall *et al.*, 1969).

3.3.3. Mucosal Leishmaniasis

Patients with mucosal leishmaniasis caused by *L. braziliensis braziliensis* are most difficult to treat; the frustrations associated with their management are clearly expressed by Rocha *et al.* (1980) and Sampaio *et al.* (1980). On the basis of past experience, these workers treated 51 hospitalized mucosal patients with subtoxic levels of Glucantime at 28 mg Sb^v/kg per day for 10 consecutive days, repeated three times with rest intervals. Only 29 patients completed the treatment. It was possible to examine nine of these patients a year later, and three of them had relapsed.

In an effort to optimize treatment, Sampaio (1984) compared three schedules of Glucantime for the treatment in mucosal disease: (1) 28 mg/kg per day Sb^v for 10 days repeated on three occasions with 15-day rest intervals; (2) 10 mg/kg per day Sb^v for 30 days, and (3) 20 mg/kg per day Sb^v, for a mean of 30 days with prolongation if necessary for complete healing. The latter schedule was the most effective, curing 11 of 12 patients, based on a mean follow-up period of 7 months; this schedule is the current recommendation for the treatment of mucosal disease. The maximum continuous therapy at 20 mg/kg per day Sb^v was 85 days, with a successful result (Marsden *et al.*, 1985). Side effects indicating temporary cessation of therapy were T-wave inversion, marked slowing of conduction or dysrhythmias on ECG, and a rise in blood urea, creatinine, or transaminases.

3.3.4. Post-treatment Evaluation for Cutaneous and Mucosal Disease

Parasitological, histological, clinical, and immunological criteria are used to evaluate post-treatment prognosis (WHO, 1979b). The detection of living parasites after treatment using parasitological and histological techniques constitutes solid evidence of drug failure but is rarely performed. Unfortunately, amastigotes of some speices of *Leishmania* such as *L. braziliensis braziliensis* are difficult to demonstrate before treatment and rarely detected after treatment. Histology requires patient consent for biopsy and usually produces inconclusive results because pathological changes are difficult to interpret.

Clinical cure is still the best method to evaluate post-treatment prognosis; it is defined as the complete resolution of initial lesions with the formation of scars without satellite nodules or induration. Mucosal lesions require careful examination with nasal speculum and retronasal and laryngoscopic mirrors in good light with biopsy of suspicious areas. The key factor is follow-up, which should be at least 1 year and preferably longer in relapsing forms of the disease. The leishmanin skin test has little value in the evaluation of cure for cutaneous leichmaniasis except in diffuse cutaneous disease, for which the development of a strong delayed response during therapy is a favorable sign. Repeated examinations for circulating antibodies over 6–12 months may reveal a significant decline in titer, indicating successful treatment. Nevertheless, some patients still develop late mucosal recurrence with reappearance of these antibodies.

3.4. Clinical Strategy for Visceral Disease

3.4.1. Systemic Treatment

Wide variations in the susceptibility of *L. donovani* to Sb^v throughout its geographical range have forced clinicians to tailor drug doses and regimens to fit their local situations. The World Health Organization recommends an initial dose of 20 mg Sb^v/kg per day or a maximum of 850 mg/day for 20 days but that therapy be adjusted to meet local needs by extending it 2 weeks beyond the day of anticipated parasitological cure (WHO, 1982).

3.4.2. Post-treatment Evaluation for Visceral Leishmaniasis

Cure should be evaluated on clinical, parasitological and immunological criteria. The normalization of anemia, thrombocytopenia, leukopenia, hepatosplenomegaly, elevated serum gammaglobulin, weight loss, and the development of a positive leishmanin skin test are signs of successful therapy. A reduction in the number of amastigotes in splenic aspirates correlate well with clinical response (Chulay *et al.*, 1983b). Post-treatment follow-up should be conducted after 3 months, and later if possible.

3.4.3. Drug Failure

The failure of Sb^v to cure visceral leishmaniasis is expressed clinically as either primary unresponsiveness, relapse visceral leishmaniasis, or secondary unresponsiveness

(WHO, 1982). Primary unresponsiveness occurs when there is no clinical or parasitological improvement after initial treatment with Sb^v. Some 2–8% of patients with visceral leishmaniasis demonstrate primary unresponsiveness; this group should be retreated with Sb^v at higher doses for longer periods or given a second-line drug.

Relapse visceral leishmaniasis follows an initial treatment and apparent cure. Relapse is often associated with an inadequate dose and can be minimized by using the recommended schedule of 20 mg/kg per day Sb^v. This schedule was used to treat an epidemic in Bihar, India, and only 0.5% of 603 patients relapsed after initial cure (Thakur, 1984).

Relapse leishmaniasis is particularly difficult to cure, and some 40% of these patients fail a second course of treatment if repeated at the initial regimen—a phenomenon called secondary unresponsiveness. These patients must be given higher doses of Sb^v for longer periods until amastigotes can no longer be detected in splenic aspirates or be given a second-line drug. Unresponsiveness may be an expression of drug resistance (see Chapter 10).

REFERENCES

Almeida Maria, T., Filardi, L. S., and Brener, Z., 1984, Alteracoes ultra-estruturais dos estagios intracelulares e efeito sobre as formas sanguineas induzidas in vivo pelo 2-amino-5-(1-methyl-5-nitro-2-imidazolyl)-1,2,3-thiadiazole, *Rev. Soc. Brasil. Med. Trop.* 17:89–93.

Azab, A. S., Kamal, M. S., El Haggar, M. S., Metawaa, B. A., and Hindawy, D. S., 1983, Early surgical treatment of cutaneous leishmaniasis, *J. Dermatol. Surg. Oncol.* 9:1007–1012.

Bassiouny, A., El Meshad, M., Talaat, M., Kutty, K., and Metawaa, B., 1982, Cryosurgery in cutaneous leishmaniasis. *Br. J. Dermatol.* 107:467–474.

Boainain, E., 1979, Tratamento etiologico da doenca de Chagas na fase cronica, *Rev. Goiana Med.* 25:1–60.

Bouchard, P. H., Sai, P., Reach, G., Caubarrere, I., Ganeval, D., and Assan, R., 1982, Diabetes mellitus following pentamidine-induced hypoglycemia in humans, *Diabetes* 31:40–45.

Brener, S., 1979, Present status of chemotherapy and chemoprophylaxis of human trypansomiasis in the western hemisphere, *Pharmacol. Ther.* 7:71–90.

Bryceson, A. D. M., 1970, Diffuse cutaneous leishmaniasis in Ethiopia: II. Treatment, *Trans. R. Soc. Trop. Med. Hyg.* 64:369–379.

Cancado, J. R., and Brener, Z., 1979, Terapeutica, in: *Trypanosoma cruzi. Doenca de Chagas* (Z. Brener and Z. Andrade, eds.), pp. 362–424, Guanabara Koogan, Rio de Janeiro.

Chulay, J. D., Anzeze, E. M., Koech, D. K., and Bryceson, A. D. M., 1983a, High-dose sodium stibogluconate treatment of cutaneous leishmaniasis in Kenya, *Trans. R. Soc. Trop. Med. Hyg.* 77:717–721.

Chulay, J. D., Bhatt, S. M., Muigai, R., Ho, M., Gachihi, G., Were, J. B. O., Chunge, C., and Bryceson, A. D. M., 1983b, A comparison of three dosage regimens of sodium stibogluconate in the treatment of visceral leishmaniasis in Kenya, *J. Infect. Dis.* 148:148–155.

Chulay, J. D., Oster, C. N., McGreevy, P. B., Kreutzer, R. D., and Hendricks, L. D., 1985a, American cutaneous leishmaniasis: Clinical presentation and problems of patient management, *J. Inf. Dis.* (manuscript submitted).

Chulay, J. D., Spencer, H. C., and Mugambi, M., 1985b, Electrocardiographic changes during treatment of leishmaniasis with pentavalent antimony (Sodium Stibogluconate), *Am. J. Trop. Med. Hyg.* 34:702–709.

Duperrat, B., Puissant, A., Fisher, R., Badillet, G., and Mascaro, J. H., 1966, Leishmaniose cutanée plurifocale traitée par glucantime intralésionnelle, *Bull. Soc. Fr. Dermatol. Syph.* 73:219–220.

Elkerton, L. E., 1944, Oriental sore. Atebrin treatment. *Indian Med. Gaz.* 79:519–521.

El-On, J., Jacobs, G. P., Witztum, E., and Greenblatt, C. L., 1984, Development of topical treatment for cutaneous leishmaniasis caused by *Leishmania major* in experimental animals, *Antimicrob. Agents Chemother.* 26:745–751.

Filardi, L. S., and Brener, Z., 1982, A nitroimidazole-thiadiazole derivative with curative action in experimental *Trypanosoma cruzi* infections, *Ann. Trop. Med. Parasitol.* 76:293–297.

Fiusa Lima, J. T., 1983, Boost in the programme for the control of Chagas' disease in Brasil, *Rev. Soc. Brasil. Med. Trop.* 16:128–129.

Gagliardi, A. R. T., Veiga, J. P. R., Rosa, T. T., and Marsden, P. D., 1985, Pentavalent antimony inhibition of water transport by the toad bladder, *Bras. J. Med. e. Biol. Res.* (in press).

Hall, J. G., Smith, M. E., Edwards, P. A., and Shooter, K. V., 1969, The low concentration of macroglobulin antibodies in peripheral lymph, *Immunology* 16:773–778.

Jha, T. K., 1983, Evaluation of diamidine compounds (pentamidine isethionate) in the treatment of resistant cases of Kala-azar occurring in North Bihar, India, *Trans. R. Soc. Trop. Med. Hyg.* 97:167–170.

Jones, B. M., and Sanders, R., 1983, Pretibial injuries: A common pitfall, *Br. Med. J.* 286:502.

Llanos-Cuentas, E. A., 1984, Estudo clinico evolutivo de leishmaniose en area endemica de *Leishmania braziliensis braziliensis* en Tres Bracos Bahia, Masters thesis, University of Brasilia.

Llanos-Cuentas, E. A., Marsden, P. D., Torre, D., and Barreto, A. C., 1983, Attempts using cryotherapy to achieve more rapid healing in patients with cutaneous leishmaniasis due to *L. braziliensis braziliensis*, *Rev. Soc. Brasil. Med. Trop.* 16:85–89.

Macedo, V., 1982, Chagas's disease (American trypanosomiasis), in: *Cecil Textbook of Medicine 16th edition* (J. B. Wyngaarden and L. H. Smith, eds.), pp. 1728–1731, W. B. Saunders, Philadelphia.

Marsden, P. D., 1983, The transmission of *Trypanosoma cruzi* infection to man and its control, in: *Human Ecology and Infectious Diseases* (N. A. Croll and J. H. Cross, eds.), pp. 253–289, Academic Press, New York.

Marsden, P. D., Sampaio, R. N. R., Carvalho, E. M., Veiga, J. P. T, Costa, J. L. M., and Llanos-Cuentas, E. A., 1985, High continuous antimony therapy in two patients with unresponsive mucosal leishmaniasis, *Am. J. Trop. Med. Hyg.* 34:710–713.

Molyneaux, D. H., and Ashford, R. W., 1983, *The Biology of Trypanosoma and Leishmania, Parasites of Man and Domestic Animals*, Taylor and Francis, London.

Neva, F. A., Petersen, E. A., Corsey, R., Bogaert, D. H., and Martinez, D., 1984, Observations on local heat treatment for cutaneous leishmaniasis, *Am. J. Trop. Med. Hyg.* 33:800–804.

Oster, C. N., Chulay, J. D., Hendricks, L. D., Pamplin, C. L., Ballou, W. R., Berman, J. D., Takafuji, E. T., Tramont, E. C., and Canfield, C. J., 1985, American cutaneous leishmaniasis: A comparison of three sodium stibogluconate treatment schedules, *Am. J. Trop. Med. Hyg.* 34:856–860.

Peters, W., and Killick-Kendrick, R., 1985, *The Leishmaniases in Biology and Medicine*, Academic Press, London (in press).

Rees, P. H., Keating, M. I., Kager, P. A., and Hochmeyer, W. T., 1980, Renal clearance of pentavalent antimony (sodium stibogluconate), *Lancet* 2:226–229.

Rocha, R. A. A., Sampaio, R. N., Guerra, M., Magalhaes, A., Cuba, C. C., Barreto, A. C., and Marsden, P. D., 1980, Apparent Glucantime failure in five patients with mucocutaneous leishmaniasis, *J. Trop. Med. Hyg.* 83:131–139.

Sampaio, R. N. R., 1984, Tratamento hospitalar de leishmaniose cutaneo-mucosa, Masters thesis, Universidade Federal de Belo Horizonte.

Sampaio, R. N. R., Rocha, R. A. A., Marsden, P. D., Cuba, C. C., Barreto, A. C., 1980, Leishmaniose tegumentar americana: Casuistica do Hospital escola da UnB, *Ann. Brasil Dermatol.* 55:69–76.

Solano, E., Hidalgo, H. and Zeledon, R., 1984, Tratamiento exitoso de la leishmaniasis por Leishmania brasiliensis panamensis con Glucantime, *Med. Cutan. Iber. Lat. Am.* 12:19–24.

Steck, E. A., 1972, *The Chemotherapy of Protozoan Diseases*, Vols. I–IV. Division of Medicinal Chemistry, Walter Reed Army Institute of Research, Washington, D.C.

Teixeira, A. R. L., Jabur, E., Cordoba, J. C., Souto Maior, I. C., and Solorzano, E., 1983, Alteracao da resposta imune mediada por celulas durante o tratamento com benzonidazol, *Rev. Soc. Brasil. Med. Trop.* 16:11–22.

Thakur, C. P., 1984, Epidemiological, clinical and therapeutic features of Bihar kala-azar (including post kala-azar dermal leishmaniasis), *Trans. R. Soc. Trop. Med. Hyg.* 78:391–398.

Veiga, J. P. R., Wolff, E. R., Sampaio, R. N., and Marsden, P. D., 1983, Renal tubular dysfunction in patients with mucocutaneous leishmaniasis treated with pentavalent antimonials, *Lancet* 2:569.

Veiga, J. P. R., Rosa, T. T., Kimachi, T., Wolff, E. R., Sampaio, R. N., Gagliardi, R. T., Junqueira, L. F., Costa, J. M. L., and Marsden, P. D., 1985, Funcao renal en patientes com leishmaniose mucocutaneo tratados com antimonias pentavalentes, *Rev. Inst. Med. Trop. Sao Paulo* (in press).

Walzer, P. D., Perl, D. P., Krogstad, D. J., Rawson, P. G., and Schultz, M. G., 1974, *Pneumocystis carinii* pneumonia in the United States. Epidemiologic, diagnostic, and clinical features, *Ann. Intern. Med.* 80:83–93.

WHO, 1979a, The African Trypanosomiases, *WHO Tech. Rep. Ser. 635,* 96 pp.

WHO, 1979b, Report of the workshop on the chemotherapy of mucocutaneous leishmaniasis, *WHO Offset Publ.* TDR/LEISH/MCL/79.3, 19 pp.

WHO, 1982, Report of the informal meeting of the chemotherapy of visceral leishmaniasis, *WHO Offset Publ.* TDR/CHEMLEISH/VL/82.3, 19 pp.

WHO, 1983, Report of the workshop on chemotherapy of old world cutaneous leishmaniasis, *WHO Offset Publ.* TDR/LEISH/CL-JER/83.3, 19 pp.

WHO, 1984, The Leishmaniases, *WHO Tech. Rep. Ser. 701,* 140 pp.

5

Protozoan Infections of Man

African Trypanosomiasis

ROBERT S. REW

1. INTRODUCTION

Human sleeping sickness is caused by one of two subspecies of *Trypanosoma brucei: T. b. gambiense* the causative agent of Gambian sleeping sickness and *T. b. rhodesiense* the causative agent of Rhodesian sleeping sickness. Gambian sleeping sickness is characterized by 100% mortality of untreated cases, neurological symptoms being expressed gradually and death occurring at least 2 years after infection, low parasitemia, and a life cycle based on transmission between tsetse fly and man. Rhodesian sleeping sickness, too, is characterized by 100% mortality of untreated cases, but with rapid onset of neurological symptoms, high parasitemia, and a zoonotic life cycle (involving tsetse fly and wild animals) that man shares only as an occasional host.

Treatment of African trypanosomiasis has a long history dating back to 1905 with the discovery of phenyl-arsenical, atoxyl. Since that time, the control of human African sleeping sickness has rested on two additional arsenicals, one naphthylamine sulfonic acid, and one diamidine, all discovered before 1950. These available compounds have severe toxicity problems, and only the arsenicals pass the blood-brain barrier in large enough concentrations to be active against parasites within the central nervous system (CNS). In short, no safe effective treatment of African trypanosomiasis in man is currently available. However, many new compounds or combinations provide hope for a brighter future for the treatment of this disease.

2. EXPERIMENTAL MODELS

2.1. In Vitro

Before 1977, trypanosome cultivation was limited to short-term survival of bloodstream forms, or growth systems that permitted growth of the procyclic forms found in

---

ROBERT S. REW • Merck Sharp & Dohme Research Laboratories, Rahway, New Jersey 07065.

the vector's gut. Trypanocidal compounds could be detected following separation of parasites from host blood cells and exposure to drugs at 37°C for up to 24 hr; however, "trypanostatic" compounds could not be detected in this system, since no division occurred. Use of procyclic forms for screening purposes does not appear to be relevant, since the metabolism of these forms is quite different from that found in the mammalian host.

A major breakthrough in the cultivation of bloodstream forms was reported by Hirumi *et al.* (1977). The use of fibroblast monolayers with an overlay of RPMI medium with HEPES buffer and 20% serum at 37°C provided a system that permitted survival and multiplication of bloodstream forms. This work and additional improvements by Brun *et al.* (1979) have provided a system for screening trypanocidal as well as trypanostatic compounds.

Certain pitfalls of *in vitro* screening have been seen when such methods are applied to trypanocidal testing. Typically the pentavalent arsenicals which are active *in vivo* are not active *in vitro*, whereas trivalent arsenicals that are active *in vitro* and *in vivo* show greater host toxicity. Host metabolism of pentavalent to trivalent arsenicals appears necessary for trypanocidal activity.

Second, acriflavine and other fluorescent compounds are active *in vitro* by virtue of the induction of photosensitivity (Jancso, 1931, 1932). *In vivo*-treated trypanosomes that are removed from the host for examination are also affected even though these dyes have intrinsic trypanocidal activity only at their toxic levels. Interestingly, certain acriflavine-resistant strains of trypanosomes are cross-resistant to the phenyl-arsenicals.

2.2. In Vivo

Two types of screens should be considered for use as *in vivo* models: (1) general, and (2) specialty (i.e., CNS or prophylactic activity). General screens typically use mice or rats, in some cases using immunosuppression or nursing animals to enhance the parasitemias. Recently the Gambian pouched rat (Evans, 1981), the mountain vole (Seed and Negus, 1970), and deer mice (Stevens and Moulton, 1977) have also been used to study pathology, immunology, or drug efficacy of *T. brucei* infections (for a comprehensive review, see Murray and Jennings, 1983). Unfortunately, either incomplete information or drug sensitivity patterns inconsistent with human sleeping sickness restrict the predictive value of these models for drug screening.

General screening procedures are done in a laboratory-adapted strain of parasite and host, the hosts being inoculated with blood containing trypanosomes and examined 1 day later for presence of the trypanosomes. The maximum tolerated dose of the drug (which may be determined simultaneously) is injected into the host and trypanosome counts are made on the blood for the next 7 days, then every other day for 30 days (see Hawking, 1963, for detailed procedures). Alternatively, duration of host life can be used to compare infected-treated and infected-untreated controls; this procedure is labor saving but sacrifices a certain amount of reliability.

Specialty screens should be used as a follow-up for actives coming through the general screen. Recent field isolates or drug-resistant isolates of trypanosomes should be utilized to determine more precisely the activity of the test compound. In addition, tests should be made for activity against trypanosomes in CNS and other tissues. Chronic mouse, rabbit, or monkey systems in which infections have reached the CNS, or in which trypanosomes have been inoculated directly into CNS, may be used. Alternatively, direct measures of drug concentration in cerebrospinal fluid (CSF) can be indicative of activity.

Recently, Murray and Jennings (1983) showed that the mouse TREU 667 model infected with *T. brucei* MERB 2D2 has a drug sensitivity pattern that is consistent with human sleeping sickness. Berenil, a drug that is only effective prior to CNS involvement, blocks relapses completely on day 3 following infection, but has lost all its activity by day 21, a time when the parasites have invaded the CNS.

Prophylactic activity can be tested by inoculating trypanosomes on a weekly basis into separate groups of mice treated simultaneously with the candidate drug. Re-inoculation of the same mice may result in nonvalid results due to induction of partial immunity.

3. CURRENTLY AVAILABLE DRUGS

Two classes of compounds can be identified on the basis of their biological activity: drugs active against both CNS and bloodstream forms (i.e., arsenicals) and drugs active only against bloodstream forms (i.e., sulfonic acid and diamidines). CNS activity of the arsenicals is present by virtue of their ability to cross the blood-brain barrier. Because of this property, arsenicals are effective even when neurological symptoms are present; unfortunately, this same property confers neurotoxicity on the arsenicals with primary consequence on the optic nerve.

It is desirable to assess the stage of infection by examination of cerebrospinal fluid (CSF) before treatment. If the CSF contains more than 5 cells/ml or has an elevated protein level, then an arsenical should be used. However, pentamidine may be used if no CNS symptoms are involved and suramin may effect a cure in very early nervous system involvement. A raised CSF cell count or protein content, in the absence of a more obvious cause, in a patient from an endemic area should justify chemotherapy even in the absence of demonstrable parasites.

3.1. CNS- and Bloodstream-Active Drugs

3.1.1. Tryparsamide

Tryparsamide is a pentavalent arsenical first described by Jacobs and Heidelberger (1919). This compound is practically inactive *in vitro* but active *in vivo* with a minimum effective dose for *T. brucei* in mice of 200 mg/kg sc or iv. A 1–6-hr delay occurs before trypanosomes disappear from blood, probably due to the time required for conversion to the trivalent form. Following intravenous injection in rabbits, 88–95% of the tryparsamide disappears from the blood in 1 hr, and 99% in 3–4 hr (Launoy and Fleury,

1937). In man following intravenous injection, trypanocide activity reaches a maximum after 24 hr during which time 70% of the drug is excreted in the urine unchanged. Peak CSF concentration is seen at 20 hr (Hawking, 1940a). Tryparsamide has been used primarily against late stage *T. b. gambiense* infections. It is given intravenously in doses of 2–3 g/patient/week for 10–12 doses. In advanced *T. b. rhodesiense* infections with CNS involvement, tryparsamide is given together with suramin. Toxicity to tryparsamide in man is primarily optic atrophy and blindness. Occasionally, nervous symptoms, loss of appetite, diarrhea, renal damage, and death are seen, thereby limiting the usefulness of tryparsamide.

3.1.2. Melarsoprol

Melarsoprol (Mel B) is a trivalent arsenical that was introduced by Friedheim (Friedheim, 1949). This compound is active *in vitro*, penetrates the blood-brain barrier, and is the drug of choice against the meningoencephalitic stage of Rhodesian or Gambian trypanosomiasis because of its reduced toxicity as compared to tryparsamide. Peak serum melarsoprol following three successive daily intravenous injections was seen at 6 hr at which time only about 1% of the drug was found in the CSF (Hawking, 1962). Plasma drug concentrations had decreased by 60–70% in hours, and it was undetectable in a few days. Melarsoprol is administered intravenously to adults at a dose of 3.6 mg/kg per day for 3 days, or children at 1.8 mg/kg per day for 3 days. The 3-day regimen is repeated after a 10-day interval. Dosages may need to be adjusted downward if cell counts or total protein are high in the CSF. Even though melarsoprol is less toxic than tryparsamide, complications such as jaundice, diarrhea, and conjunctival infection may occur. In about 1% of Mel B treatments, reactive encephalopathy develops (Hawking, 1963) with headache, tremor, speech difficulty, hyperpyrexia, convulsions, coma, and 5–10% deaths (WHO, 1979).

3.2. Bloodstream-Active Drugs

3.2.1. Suramin

Suramin, a naphthylamine sulfonic acid that was introduced in 1920, is very effective in early stages of *T. b. rhodesiense* and *T. b. gambiense* infections. However, since it is unable to penetrate the blood-brain barrier, it has no effect on disease progression after CNS invasion. *In vitro* activity of suramin is low, requiring high dosages (4 mM) and long time periods (>6 hr). Trypanocidal activity *in vivo* is seen after a 24-hr delay. Suramin is administered intravenously, binds to blood proteins and is detectable for long periods. In man, 4×1-g doses over a 3-day period resulted in 150–340 mg/liter 1 day after the final dose and 5 mg/liter 200 days later (Hawking, 1940b). Clinically suramin is given intravenously in adults at a dosage of 1 g repeated weekly for a total of 5 weeks. An initial dose of 200 mg is given 24–48 hr prior to the first 1-g dose to test for tolerance. Because of the long half-life, suramin also acts prophylactically.

Idiosyncratic reactions occur in 0.1–0.3% of the population with symptoms including nausea, vomiting, circulatory collapse, and loss of consciousness (Rollo,

1980). Risk is increased in concomitant onchocerciasis (WHO, 1979). A variety of untoward reactions are seen with suramin, especially in malnourished individuals or in patients with renal damage. These reactions include optic atrophy and blindness (Thylefors and Rolland, 1979), adrenal insufficiency (Wells *et al.*, 1937), nephrotoxicity (Chesterman, 1924), and hemolytic anemia, rash, and agranulocytosis (Rollo, 1980).

3.2.2. Pentamidine

Pentamidine is an aromatic diamidine, the trypanocidal activity of which was demonstrated by Lourie and York (1939). It has efficacy and excretion properties similar to those of suramin but has reduced toxicity. Pentamidine is very active *in vitro* (2.5 mg/ml) (Hawking, 1963). A single intramuscular injection of pentamidine provides up to 6 months of prophylaxis against *T. b. gambiense* in man. Pentamidine is fairly well absorbed from an intramuscular injection site. Little drug is detectable in the blood; however, it can be detected in liver and kidney for months (Launoy *et al.*, 1960). The prophylactic dosage of pentamidine is 300 mg intramuscularly every 3–6 months. Trypanosomal infections prior to CNS involvement are treated with 150–300 mg mg/day intramuscularly for 7–15 days. Toxicity with pentamidine treatment is rare, although hypotensive responses, vomiting, and abdominal discomfort may occur after the injection. Waalkes *et al.* (1970) have reported nephrotoxicity; hypoglycemia and hyperglycemia have also been reported (Rollo, 1980).

4. EXPERIMENTAL TRYPANOCIDAL DRUGS

Trypanocidal drugs currently under investigation provide us with a wide array of compounds with many different modes of action (see Chapter 9) and, in some cases, reduced toxicity. Interestingly, even though only one new compound by itself is active against CNS forms of *T. brucei*, combinations of drugs seem to act synergistically to overcome that weakness.

4.1. Nitrofurans

Nitrofurazone has been found active against late-stage Rhodesian and Gambian trypanosomiasis, but unpredictable efficacy and toxicity limit its usefulness (Apted, 1980). It is currently the only drug of value in arsenical-insensitive infections. Polyneuropathy, hemolytic anemia (linked to G6PD deficiency), headache, GI disturbances, skin reactions, mental excitement, and weight loss have all been recorded as toxic reactions to nitrofurazone (Apted, 1980).

4.2. Bloodstream-Active Drugs

4.2.1. Phenothiazines

Phenothiazines have been shown to be active *in vitro* against *T. brucei* at micromolar concentrations, inhibiting motility and damaging the cell rapidly (Seebeck and

Gehr, 1983). In addition, these compounds are concentrated in the CNS without toxicity (Cann and Hinman, 1975), indicating possible usage against CNS forms.

4.2.2. DFMO

α-Difluoromethylornithine (DFMO) is a potent inhibitor of polyamine biosynthesis. This compound is remarkably nontoxic and has been shown to eliminate bloodstream forms of *T. b. brucei* and *T. b. rhodesiense* in mice (Bacchi *et al.*, 1980; McCann *et al.*, 1981).

4.2.3. Bleomycin

Bleomycin is an antibiotic with a glycopeptide backbone. It is active *in vitro* (Ono and Nakabayashi, 1980) and in *T. b. brucei*-infected mice at 7 mg/kg (Nathan *et al.*, 1981). Bleomycin has some accumulative toxicity in man, and death from pulmonary fibrosis and edema has been reported in 1% of patients given extended treatment (Pratt and Ruddon, 1979).

4.2.4. Sinefungin

Sinefungin is an antifungal antibiotic nucleoside containing an ornithine residue. Treatment of *T. b. brucei* in mice with 3×5 mg/kg effected cures that did not show relapse before 2 months (Dube *et al.*, 1983).

4.2.5. 5-Nitroimidazoles

One of the 5-nitroimidazoles, designated L-611,744, was effective in clearing bloodstream *T. brucei* from infected mice at dosages as low as 4×20 mg/kg, but could not effectively stop relapse at doses as high as 4×250 mg/kg (Jennings *et al.*, 1984; Murray and Jennings, 1983).

4.3. Combination Therapy

Several studies have recently demonstrated synergism between trypanocidal drugs, in which activity of compounds effective against bloodstream forms only when given individually, was extended to include activity against CNS forms when given together. In addition, this synergism generally permitted the use of lower dosages of the drugs, decreasing toxic reactions.

4.3.1. SHAM–Glycerol

Benzyhydroxamic acid, more commonly called SHAM, is not lethal *in vitro* or *in vivo*, but inhibits O_2 uptake of *T. brucei in vitro* (Opperdoes *et al.*, 1976). Interestingly, this did not translate to a lethal effect as the parasite shifted its metabolism to counteract the effect. However, a SHAM–glycerol combination was then used to overcome the metabolic shift of the parasite (Clarkson and Brohn, 1976). SHAM–glycerol is active in combination against bloodstream forms, but only at enormously high dosage (SHAM, 500 mg/kg plus glycerol, 5 g/kg). SHAM is neurotoxic at these high levels and is excreted very rapidly (Evans, 1981). Theoretically, though, if more active slowly metabolized compounds of this mode of action could be found, the selective toxicity for the metabolic pathway involved should be valuable.

4.3.2. Bleomycin-DFMO

Bleomycin-DFMO, when used in combination against *T. b. brucei,* was completely effective in a mouse model with CNS involvement. The bleomycin dosages were 3.5–7.0 mg/kg per day for 3 days, and DFMO dosages were 2–4 g/kg per day for 14 days in water. Neither drug given singly was active at 7.0 mg/kg per day for 6 days (bleomycin) or 4 g/kg per day for 14 days (DFMO) in curing infected mice with CNS involvement (Clarkson *et al.,* 1983).

4.3.3. DFMO-Suramin

DFMO-suramin, when given as DFMO (4 g/kg per day for 7–14 days in water) and suramin (20 mg/kg i.v.), was 90–100% effective against *T. b. brucei*-infected mice with CNS involvement. Again, neither was effective singly (Clarkson *et al.,* 1984).

4.3.4. 5-Nitroimidazole-Suramin

The combination of L-611,744 (4 × 10 mg/kg) and suramin (1 × 20 mg/kg) was effective against *T. brucei* in mice with CNS involvement. As in previous combinations, neither drug was effective against such infections when given singly (Jennings *et al.,* 1984).

4.3.5. Others

A number of other synergistic combinations have been reported to extend trypanocidal activity to CNS activity or to reduce toxicity, including berenil-5-nitroimidazole (Jennings *et al.,* 1980), suramin-pentamidine (Guimaraes and Lourie, 1951), suramin-tryparsamide, suramin-puromycin, and suramin-berenil (Williamson *et al.,* 1982). The explanations for the synergy to include CNS activity are not entirely clear or consistent. They include drug resistance, drug hypersensitivity, insensitive cryptic amastigotes that produce trypamastigotes sensitive to the second compound, and accumulation of critical drug concentrations in the CSF. The fact that synergy can be shown *in vitro* and *in vivo* makes this an intriguing problem.

REFERENCES

Apted, F. I. C., 1980, Present status of chemotherapy and chemoprophylaxis of human trypanosomiasis in the eastern hemisphere, *Pharmacol. Ther.* 11:391–413.

Bacchi, C. J., Nathan, H. C., Hutner, S. H., McCann, P. P., and Sjoerdsma, A., 1980, Polyamine metabolism: A potential therapeutic target in trypanosomes, *Science* 210:332–334.

Brun, R., Jenni, L., Tanner, M., Schonenberger, M., and Schell, K. F., 1979, Cultivation of vertebrate infective forms derived from metacyclic forms of pleomorphic *Trypanosoma brucei* stocks, *Acta Trop.* 36:387–390.

Cann, J. R., and Hinman, N. D., 1975, Interaction of chlorpromazine with brain microtubule subunit protein, *Mol. Pharmacol.* 11:256–267.

Chesterman, C., 1924, Therapeutic effect of "Bayer 205" in trypanosomiasis of the central nervous system, *Trans. R. Soc. Trop. Med. Hyg.* 18:311–317.

Clarkson, A. B., Jr., and Brohn, F., 1976, Trypanosomiasis. An approach to chemotherapy by the inhibition of carbohydrate metabolism, *Science* 194:204–206.

Clarkson, A. B., Jr., Bacchi, C. J., Mellow, G. H., Nathan, H. C., McCann, P. P., and Sjoerdsma, A., 1983, Efficacy of combinations of difluoromethylornithine and bleomycin in a mouse model of central nervous system, African trypanosomiasis, *Proc. Natl. Acad. Sci. U.S.A.* 80:5729–5733.

Clarkson, A. B., Jr., Bienen, E. J., Bacchi, C. J., McCann, P. P., Nathan, H. C., Hutner, S. H., and Sjoerdsma A., 1984, New drug combination for experimental late-stage African trypanosomiasis: DL-alpha-difluoromethylornithine (DFMO) with suramin, *Am. J. Trop. Med. Hyg.* 33:1073–1077.

Dube, D. K., Mpimbaza, G., Allison, A. C., Lederer, E., and Rovis, L., 1983, Antitrypanosomal activity of sinefungin, *Am. J. Trop. Med. Hyg.* 32:31–33.

Evans, D. A., 1981, African trypanosomes, in: *Antibiotics and Chemotherapy* (H. Schonfeld, ed.), Vol. 30, pp. 272–287, Karger, Basel.

Friedheim, E. A. H., 1949, Mel B in the treatment of human trypanosomiasis, *Am. J. Trop. Med.* 29:173–180.

Guimaraes, J. L., and Lourie, E. M., 1951, The inhibition of some pharmacological actions of pentamidine by suramin, *Brit. J. Pharmacol.* 6:514–530.

Hawking, F., 1940a, Trypanocidal activity and arsenic content of the cerebrospinal fluid of sleeping-sickness patients after the administration of tryparsamide, *Trans. R. Soc. Trop. Med. Hyg.* 34:269–280.

Hawking, F., 1940b, Concentration of Bayer 205 (Germain) in human blood and cerebrospinal fluid after treatment, *Trans. R. Soc. Trop. Med. Hyg.* 34:37–52.

Hawking, F., 1962, The concentration of melarsoprol (Mel B) and Mel W in plasma and cerebrospinal fluid estimated by bioassay with trypanosomes *in vitro*, *Trans. R. Soc. Trop. Hyg.* 56:354–363.

Hawking, F., 1963, Chemotherapy of trypanosomiasis, in: *Experimental Chemotherapy* (R. J. Schnitzer and F. Hawking, eds.), Vol. 1, pp. 129–256, Academic Press, New York.

Hirumi, H., Doyle, J. J., and Hirumi, K., 1977, African trypanosomes. *In vitro* cultivation of animal-infective *Trypanosoma brucei*, *Science* 196:992–994.

Jacobs, W. A., and Heidelberger, M., 1919, Chemotherapy of trypanosome and spirochete infections. Chemical Series I. N-phenylglycineamide-p-arsonic acid, *J. Exp. Med.* 30:411–415.

Jancso, N. von, 1931, Photobiologische Studien in der Chemotherapie. I. Lichtempfindliche Trypanosomen in Trypaflavinbehandelten Tieven, *Zentr. Bakteriol. Parasitenk.* 122:388–392.

Jancso, N. von, 1932, Mechanismus der Arzneifestigkeit bei Protozoen: Sur Frage der Parasitotropie chemotherapeutischer Mittel, *Zentr. Bakteriol. Parasitenk.* 124:167–176.

Jennings, F. W., Urquhart, G. M., Murray, P. K., and Miller, B. M., 1980, "Berenil" and nitroimidazole combinations in the treatment of *Trypanosoma brucei* infection with central nervous system involvement, *Int. J. Parasitol.* 10:27–32.

Jennings, F. W., Urquhart, G. M., Murray, P. K., and Miller, B. M., 1984, The use of 2-substituted 5-nitroimidazoles in the treatment of chronic murine *Trypanosoma brucei* infections with central nervous system involvement, *Z. Parasitenkd.* 70:691–697.

Launoy, L., and Fleury, O., 1937, Sur la vitesse d'élimination hors du courant sanguin, de l'arsenic injecté par voie veineuse, sous forme de tryparsamide, à des lapins normaux ou infectés par *Trypanosoma annamense*, *Bull. Soc. Pathol. Exot.* 30:315–318.

Launoy, L., Guillot, M., and Jonchere, H., 1960, Storage and elimination of pentamidine in mice and white rats, *Ann. Pharm. Fr.* 18:273–284, 424–439.

Lourie, E. M., and York, W., 1939, Studies in chemotherapy. XXI. The trypanocidal action of certain aromatic amidines, *Ann. Trop. Med. Parasitol.* 33:289–304.

McCann, P. P., Bacchi, C. J., Hanson, S. L., Cain, G. D., Nathan, H. C., Hutner, S. H., and Sjoerdsma, A., 1981, Effect on parasitic protozoa of alpha-difluoromethylornithine, an inhibitor of ornithine decarboxylase, in: *Advances in Polyamine Research* (C. M. Calderera, V. Zuppia, and U. Bachrach, eds.), Vol. 3, pp. 97–110, Raven Press, New York.

Murray, P. K., and Jennings, F. W., 1983, African trypanosomiasis: Chemotherapy in rodent models of sleeping sickness, in: *Animal Models for Experimental Bacterial and Parasitic Infections* (G. Keusch and I. Waldstrom, eds.), pp. 343–354, Elsevier North-Holland, Amsterdam.

Nathan, H. C., Bacchi, C. J., Sakai, T. T., Rescigno, D., Stumpf, D., and Hutner, S. H., 1981, Bleomycin-induced life prolongation of mice infected with *Trypanosoma brucei brucei* EATRO 110, *Trans. R. Soc. Trop. Med. Hyg.* 75:394–398.

Ono, T., and Nakabayashi, T., 1980, Studies on the effect of bleomycin on *Trypanosoma gambiense*, *Biken J.* 23:143–155.

Opperdoes, F. R., Aarsen, P. N., van der Meer, C., and Borst, P., 1976, *Trypanosoma brucei:* An evaluation of salicylhydroxamic acid as a trypanocidal drug, *Exp. Parasitol.* 40:198–205.

Pratt, W., and Ruddon, R. W., 1979, The antibiotics, in: *Anticancer Drugs* (W. Pratt and R. W. Ruddon, eds.), pp. 148–194, Oxford University Press, London.

Rollo, I., 1980, Miscellaneous drugs used in the treatment of protozoal infections, in: *The Pharmacological Basis of Therapeutics* (A. G. Gilman, L. S. Goodman, and A. Gilman, eds.), pp. 1070–1079, Macmillan, New York.

Seebeck, T., and Gehr, P., 1983, Trypanocidal action of neuroleptic phenothiazines in *Trypanosoma brucei*, *Mol. Biochem. Parasitol.* 9:197–208.

Seed, J., and Negus, N. C., 1970, Susceptibility of *Microtus montanus* to infection by *Trypanosoma gambiense*, *Lab. Anim. Care* 20:657–661.

Stevens, D. R., and Moulton, J. E., 1977, Experimental meningoencephalitis in *T. b. brucei* infections of deer mice, *Acta Neuropathol.* 38:173–180.

Thylefors, B., and Rolland, A., 1979, The risk of optic atrophy following suramin treatment of ocular onchocerciasis, *Bull. WHO* 57:479–480.

Waalkes, T. P., Denham, C., and DeVita, V. T., 1970, Pentamidine: Clinical pharmacological correlations in man and mice, *Clin. Pharmacol. Ther.* 11:505–512.

Wells, H., Humphreys, E., and Work, E., 1937, Significance of the increased frequency of selective cortical necrosis of adrenal, *J.A.M.A.* 109:490–493.

WHO, 1979, *The African Trypanosomiases*, Technical Report Series 635, pp. 1–96, World Health Organization, Geneva.

Williamson, J., March, J. C., and Scott-Finnigan, T. J., 1982, Drug synergy in experimental African trypanosomiasis, *Tropenmed. Parasitol.* 33:76–82.

6

Protozoan Infections of Man

Other Infections

JOSEPH A. KOVACS and HENRY MASUR

1. INTRODUCTION

The choice of the optimal chemotherapy for the protozoan infections covered in this chapter deserves particular attention by physicians because of the potentially life-threatening nature of some of these diseases such as pneumocystosis, toxoplasmosis, and amebiasis, and because of the large numbers of individuals with clinical diseases caused by pathogens such as *Giardia lamblia, Entamoeba histolytica,* and *Trichomonas vaginalis.* The initial therapeutic decision that must be made is whether treatment needs to be instituted. Some of the manifestations of certain protozoan disease are almost always mild and self-limiting, such as cryptosporidiosis or lymphadenopathic toxoplasmosis in the immunocompetent host. In other situations, therapy is probably not warranted because the protozoan infection is producing no clinical illness and the likelihood of immediate reinfection is high, e.g., asymptomatic *Entamoeba histolytica* cyst passers in a high-risk endemic population.

If therapy is warranted in a particular clinical and epidemiological setting, the choice of agents must be made on the basis of documented experiences that are not always easy to compare. The definition of the clinical entity being treated is often imprecise, making it difficult to know with certainty whether the diarrheal syndrome was true dysentery as opposed to a more modest diarrheal illness. Parameters of response are often measured on the basis of subjective evaluation rather than by objective criteria. The duration and thoroughness of follow-up management is also variable, leading to uncertainty as to whether therapy is actually effective in curing patients or is merely suppressing disease. True cures of these protozoal diseases are ideally determined by

JOSEPH A. KOVACS and HENRY MASUR • Critical Care Medicine Department, Clinical Center, National Institutes of Health, Bethesda, Maryland 20205.

scrupulous parasitological follow-up as well as clinical assessments. Many studies do not specify the number of follow-up examinations and use techniques involving less than optimal sensitivity. For instance, culture of *Trichomonas vaginalis* is much more sensitive than wet mounts (Hager *et al.*, 1980). Thus, it can be somewhat misleading to compare trials when the clinical and parasitological assessments are not equivalent.

A chapter of this length cannot provide an exhaustive review of the literature. The studies cited are reasonable trials that support the approach to disease entities taken by these authors, as summarized in Table I. For certain diseases, particularly amebiasis, a variety of therapeutic regimens can be successfully used; however, each must be carefully chosen according to the extent and severity of the illness, as well as any special conditions that might affect patient management, such as age, immunological status, pregnancy, heart disease, eye disease, hepatic dysfunction, or renal insufficiency. Very few drugs effective against protozoal diseases are known to be safe in pregnancy. For patients who fail the initial regimen (as opposed to those who are reinfected), there are rarely guidelines for how to proceed: in some cases a second, identical course is given; in other cases, an alternative regimen is administered or several effective drugs are given concurrently.

2. ENTAMOEBA HISTOLYTICA

2.1. Clinical Considerations

Amebiasis consists of a spectrum of clinical processes that include asymptomatic carriers, mild bowel disease, dysentery, and extraintestinal disease, particularly liver abscesses. The therapy of amebiasis has been greatly simplified by the development of both oral and parenteral forms of metronidazole, a safe and effective drug that is active against all forms of *E. histolytica*. Metronidazole can have an important role in the treatment of any form of amebiasis, yet there remain a number of important roles for other drugs as part of initial therapeutic regimens and as alternatives for patients who fail metronidazole-containing treatment protocols or who cannot tolerate metronidazole. For example, emetine and dehydroemetine are still highly useful drugs for initial therapy of patients with life-threatening bowel or liver disease. Diloxanide furoate is preferred by many authorities for the treatment of patients with mild or asymptomatic bowel disease, because of the low incidence of significant adverse reactions (Wolfe, 1973).

The precise regimen that is best for the treatment of a specific syndrome depends on clinical considerations. Because several useful drugs are available, authorities recommend a number of different regimens: one approach to the therapy of specific syndromes is offered in Table I. In assessing the drugs discussed below, it is important to be reminded that a true cure of intestinal amebiasis must be documented by repeated stool examinations for several months—a criterion that is not always used in studies and that is difficult to demand in endemic areas in which reinfection is common.

2.2. Individual Agents

2.2.1. Metronidazole and Tinidazole

Metronidazole is a central drug in the treatment of amebiasis because of its efficacy for luminal and tissue organisms and its activity against cysts and trophozoites. For asymptomatic cyst passers, metronidazole is a relatively effective drug. When 750 mg p.o. three times/day is given for 10 days, cure rates of 85% (17 of 20 patients) (Kanani and Knight, 1972) and of 94% (47 of 50 patients) (Pehrson and Bengtsson, 1984) have been achieved. Five-day courses using the same dose are less effective, with cure rates of 63–79% (Kanani and Knight, 1972; Spillman et al., 1976).

For the treatment of dysentery, metronidazole is also very effective as a single agent. Powell et al. (1966) followed patients with dysentery by periodic sigmoidoscopy with inspection for ulcers and examination for ameba: when 800 mg three times/day for 10 days was administered, 88% of 25 patients were cured. In another series in a nonendemic area in which 89 patients with diarrhea, including dysentery, were treated with the same regimen, an 85% cure was achieved (Pehrson and Bengtsson, 1984). Smaller studies have shown that higher doses for fewer days can be effective: a single 2.4-g dose cured 75% of 20 patients with dysentery; two daily doses of 2.4 g cured 87% of 30 patients (Powell et al., 1969).

For the treatment of amebic liver abscess, metronidazole as a single agent is also quite effective: 800 mg three times/day for 10 days cured 100% of 11 patients (Powell et al., 1966) and 94% of 36 patients (Cohen and Reynolds, 1975) when clinical parameters were assessed. Smaller doses may be less effective: only 65% of 20 patients were cured by 400 mg given three times/day for 10 days (Datta et al., 1974), although 98% of 105 patients were cured in another study in which variable low-dose, short-term regimens were used (Powell et al., 1969). Thus, metronidazole administered in a regimen of 750–800 mg three times/day for 10 days is the standard regimen, alone or in combination with other drugs, for all forms of amebiasis against which other schedules must be judged.

Metronidazole is a relatively well-tolerated drug that is available in an oral or parenteral form. Life-threatening adverse reactions are very unusual, but annoying adverse effects are common. The latter processes include nausea, vomiting, diarrhea, numbness and tingling of extremities, bitter taste in mouth, disulfiramlike reactions to alcohol, as well as dizziness, ataxia, and neutropenia (Finegold, 1980). Animal and bacterial studies suggest that metronidazole may be mutagenic and carcinogenic (Roe, 1983).

Tinidazole, only available outside the United States, appears to be quite effective for treating various forms of amebiasis for abbreviated periods. In one study a single daily dose of tinidazole (mean 63 mg/kg) for three consecutive days cured 93% of 30 children with dysentery (Scragg et al., 1976); in another study, a course of 800 mg three times/day for 5 days cured 92% of 24 adults with liver abscess (Hatchuel, 1975). Evidence to date suggests that tinidazole may not be as effective for the treatment of asymptomatic cyst passers (Spillmann *et al.*, 1976). Adverse reactions to tinidazole are similar to those for metronidazole.

2.2.2. Iodoquinol

Iodoquinol is a substituted 5-hydroxyquinolone. When a dose of 650 mg is given three times/day for 20 days, asymptomatic cyst passers are cured in about 75% of cases (Most, 1960). This same regimen is standard therapy for eradicating cysts in any patient in whom active bowel disease has been treated initially with a drug such as metronidazole that exhibits good activity against invasive trophzoites but less activity against cysts (especially when given for less than 10 days).

Adverse reactions are relatively mild and include rash, headache, and nausea. Subacute myelooptic neuropathy has been associated with a related compound, iodochlorohydroxyquin, but not with iodoquinol (Oakley, 1973). Blindness has been associated with long courses (2–11 months) of iodoquinol (given to treat chronic gastrointestinal disorders in children) but not with 20-day courses (Fleisher *et al.*, 1974).

2.2.3. Diloxanide Furoate

Diloxanide furoate is a substituted acetanilide that has been an effective agent in patients with mild disease when 500 mg is given three times/day for 10 days. Cures have been reported in 64 of 77 patients (83%), in 105 of 110 patients (95%), and in 73 of 85 patients (86%) with mild or asymptomatic infection (Wolfe, 1973; Woodruff and Bell, 1967; Botero, 1964). Patients with dysentery treated with diloxanide have had less impressive cure rates, ranging from 17 of 25 patients (68%) in one series to 17 of 22 patients (77%) in another series (Botero, 1964; Woodruff and Bell, 1967). Diloxanide furoate is a well-tolerated drug, with anorexia, nausea, diarrhea, and particularly flatulence common complaints (Wolfe, 1973).

2.2.4. Paromomycin

Paromomycin is a poorly absorbed aminoglycoside that has been useful in treating patients with asymptomatic or mild bowel disease. The usual dose is 25–35 mg/kg per day in three divided doses (1.5–2.0 g/day). Cure rates of 83–95% have been reported with variable duration of therapy, usually 5–10 days (Woodruff and Bell, 1967; Simon *et al.*, 1967; Forsyth, 1962). Adverse reactions are mild, with GI disturbances occurring in 15–20% of patients (Simon *et al.*, 1967).

2.2.5. Tetracycline

Tetracyclines are useful indirect amebicides that can provide immediate amelioration in up to 97% of patients with acute dysentery, but relapse rates are high (Powell, 1971). The usual dose is 250–500 mg four times/day for 5–10 days. In one study, 187 of 215 patients (87%) were free of ulcers and ameba after therapy, but 18% of patients relapsed within 1 month, presumably because of incomplete therapy rather than reinfection (Powell, 1967a). If ulcers have not healed sigmoidoscopically at the end of therapy, evidence of persistent disease can be found after 1 month in a very high percentage of patients, including 11 of 13 such patients (85%) in one series (Powell, 1967a). Tetracyclines can cause diarrhea, epigastric burning, monilial infections, hepatotoxicity, and discoloration of teeth.

2.2.6. Emetine and Dehydroemetine

Emetine and dehydroemetine are parenteral alkaloid drugs that have been important in treating serious gastrointestinal and extraintestinal disease. Emetine is given intramuscularly in a dose of 1 mg/kg (maximum daily dose, 60 mg) for up to 10 days. Dehydroemetine, a synthetic derivative of emetine, is given in daily intramuscular doses of 1.0–1.5 mg/kg (maximum daily dose, 90 mg) also for up to 10 days. Both drugs are valuable primarily as tissue amebicides; they have very little intraluminal activity. They are principally used in combination with other drugs: as single agents only 3 of 10 patients with dysentery were cured by either drug in one study (Powell et al., 1962).

For amebic liver abscess, either emetine or dehydroemetine is very effective; in a comparative trial each agent cured 22 of 25 patients (88%) after a 10-day course (Powell et al., 1965). Combining a 10-day course of emetine or dehydroemetine with 1 month of chloroquine can achieve cure rates of greater than 95% (Powell et al., 1967). Because of inadequate efficacy of these drugs in intestinal disease, treatment with the above regimen is standardly given in conjunction with an active intraluminal agent and, if dysentery is present, with tetracycline. In life-threatening disease (e.g., perforated bowel), most authorities recommend simultaneous administration of emetine or dehydroemetine, until the patient stabilizes, plus intravenous metronidazole, to be followed by an active intraluminal agent, although clinical studies are lacking (Knight, 1980).

Emetine and dehydroemetine are associated with considerable toxicity, since these drugs can persist in the body for a long time and accumulate. Hypotension, precordial pain, tachycardia, and dyspnea may be seen. Electrocardiographic (ECG) abnormalities, primarily T-wave flattening or inversion, are found in 25–50% of cases (Powell, 1967b). Also common are a local reaction at the injection site, nausea, vomiting, and diarrhea. Dehydroemetine is excreted more rapidly than emetine and seems to be less toxic.

2.2.7. Chloroquine

Chloroquine, a 4-aminoquinoline derivative, is an effective agent for the treatment of liver abscesses but has no role in the treatment of intestinal disease. If chloroquine is to be used successfully as a single agent to cure a liver abscess, prolonged courses must be given such as 500 mg/day for 10 weeks (Cohen and Reynolds, 1975). Alternative shorter courses (4 weeks) can be given in conjunction with emetine (10 days), and cure rates may exceed 95% (Powell *et al.*, 1967).

Adverse reactions to chloroquine are described in Chapter 3 (malaria). The prolonged courses used in amebic disease can be associated with lichenoid skin eruptions, diplopia, blurred vision, and hair bleaching. A major and irreversible complication of prolonged therapy is a retinopathy characterized by loss of central visual acuity.

3. *NAEGLERIA* AND *ACANTHAMOEBA* SPECIES

3.1. Clinical Considerations

Naegleria can cause a primary amebic meningoencephalitis that is almost invariably fatal. Survival of documented cases has only been reported with a few patients, making comparative assessments of drug therapy impossible. *Acanthamoeba* can cause a granulomatous amebic encephalitis as well as keratitis; documentation of successful therapy is minimal.

3.2. Specific Agents

3.2.1. Amphotericin B

Four patients with primary amebic meningoencephalitis caused by *Naegleria* survived following a course of amphotericin B given systemically (1.0–1.5 mg/kg per day for 10 days) and in two cases, intrathecally (1.0–1.5 mg/day for 10 days) (Seidel *et al.*, 1982; Apley *et al.*, 1970; Anderson and Jamieson, 1972). One patient also received rifampin and miconazole. A mouse model has confirmed the efficacy of amphotericin B (Thong *et al.*, 1979). The literature provides some suggestion that rifampin, tetracycline, and miconazole may provide some synergy with amphotericin B (Seidel *et al.*, 1982; Thong *et al.*, 1979).

Amphotericin B is a toxic drug that can be associated with impressive fever, chills, hypotension, renal tubular defects, azotemia, bone marrow depression, nausea, vomiting, thrombophlebitis, and rash. After a 1-mg test dose, the full dose should be infused over 2–4 hr in 250 ml of dextrose in water. Premedication with acetaminophen (650 mg) and diphenyldramine (25–50 mg po or iv) is almost universally needed. Hydrocortisone (25–100 mg iv) may be needed in the infusion to minimize chills and fever; hydrocortisone may also need to be added to the intrathecal drug.

3.2.2. Other Agents

No patient has been successfully treated for *Acanthamoeba* disease of the central nervous system (CNS), although *in vitro* studies suggest that polymyxin B and pentamidine have some activity (Duma and Finley, 1976). Animal experiments have not clearly shown the therapeutic value of any agent. One patient with *Acanthamoeba castellani* keratitis was cured by a combination of pimaricin and several other agents (Ma *et al.*, 1981).

4. GIARDIA LAMBLIA

4.1. Clinical Considerations

Giardia lamblia infections in nonendemic areas need to be treated regardless of patient symptomatology in order to prevent person-to-person spread. In endemic areas the treatment of asymptomatic carriers may be unwarranted in terms of expense and toxicity. Analysis of drug trials is particularly difficult in giardiasis because finding the organism in infected individuals can be quite difficult. Multiple stool examinations prior to therapy may be necessary before the organism is found, and even these may fail, requiring small bowel aspiration or biopsy. Thus, after treatment, negative stools may not accurately assess the efficacy of the drug.

4.2. Individual Agents

4.2.1. Quinacrine Hydrochloride

Quinacrine (daily adult dose, 100 mg three times/day for 7 days) has been reported to be highly effective in eradicating organisms: cure rates of 95% were recorded in one series of more than 100 patients, with at least three negative stools evaluated 1 month post-therapy (Wolfe, 1975). Some smaller studies have reported lower cure rates (Wright *et al.*, 1977).

Quinacrine therapy is often associated with adverse reactions. A reversible psychosis can occur in up to 1.5% of patients (Wolfe, 1975). Yellow discoloration of the skin, sclera, or urine is reportedly not common at the doses recommended for giardiasis, but this can be recognized particularly in children (Craft *et al.*, 1981). Headache, GI disturbance, and rash have also been reported.

4.2.2. Metronidazole and Other Nitroimidazoles

Metronidazole, 250 mg three times/day for 7 days (not approved for this infection in the United States), has been reported to cure giardiasis in 60–95% of cases when symptoms were assessed and three stools obtained during the month following therapy (Bassily *et al.*, 1970; Levi *et al.*, 1977; Khambatta, 1971). Single-dose therapy using 1.6–2.4 g of metronidazole has yielded less favorable results; in one study, 50% of 26 patients, all of whom initially ceased to excrete cysts, developed recurrent symptoms and positive stool examinations 1–8 weeks after therapy (Jokipii and Jokipii, 1979). A 3-day regimen of 2 g/day (given as a single dose) has been more effective, with 91% of 22 patients in one study cured by clinical and parasitological criteria (Wright *et al.*, 1977).

Tinidazole, given as one single dose of 1.5–2.0 g (not available in the United States), appears to be highly effective; in one series 90% of 50 patients were cured (Jokipii and Jokipii, 1982).

Adverse reactions to metronidazole have been described (Section 2). It should be noted that more nausea, cramps, and diarrhea are associated with high doses (1.5–2.0 g) given for 1–3 days as compared with the longer courses at lower doses.

4.2.3. Furazolidone

Furazolidone has been a popular agent for the treatment of giardiasis, primarily in children, because it is available in a suspension suitable for administration to children. When this drug is administered (100 mg four times/day in adults and 1.25–2 mg/kg four times/day in children) for 7–10 days, cure rates of 80–89% have been reported in adults and children (Craft et al., 1981; Bassily et al., 1970). In one series of children under 5 years of age the response rate for furazolidone was higher (17/19, 89%) than for quinacrine (9/14, 64%) (Craft et al., 1981).

Furazolidone therapy has been associated with nausea, vomiting, rash, discoloration of the urine, hemolytic anemia in G6PD deficient individuals, as well as with a disulfuran-like reaction to alcohol. Furazolidone has also induced mammary tumors in rats (Wolfe, 1978).

4.2.4. Paromomycin

Paromomycin, 1.5–1.75 g/day in divided doses for 7 days, is a poorly absorbed aminoglycoside that has been used as an oral agent to treat several patients with giardiasis, including pregnant women (Kreutner et al., 1981). Patients who fail to respond to initial antigiardia therapy may respond to retreatment with the original drug or treatment with one of the alternatives outlined above. Refractory cases may respond to combination therapy (Smith et al., 1982). None of the standard drugs for the treatment of Giardia lamblia has been clearly documented to be safe during pregnancy. While paromomycin offers an attractive alternative, since it is poorly absorbed, experience with it is limited.

5. TRICHOMONAS VAGINALIS

5.1. Clinical Considerations

For epidemiological reasons, asymptomatic as well as symptomatic patients with Trichomonas vaginalis infections should receive therapy. To minimize reinfection, sexual partners should be treated as well. Assessment of therapy is based on elimination of organisms seen on wet mounts as well as on eradication of symptoms. Although culture techniques are more sensitive in documenting persistent infection, this mode of assessment has been used only in recent studies. Reinfection by sexual partners confounds accurate determination of drug efficacy.

5.2. Individual Agents

5.2.1. Metronidazole and Tinidazole

Treatment of *Trichomonas* vaginitis with metronidazole (200–250 mg three times/day) for 7 days has been reported to eliminate the organism and to bring symptomatic relief in 85–95% of patients in several series. Among 83 patients with both wet-mount and culture follow-up, 76 (92%) were cured in one study (Hager *et al.*, 1980). In a group of 496 prisoners in whom good compliance and low risk of infection seemed relatively certain (Keighly, 1971), 98% were cured.

Single-dose therapy using a 2-g oral dose has resulted in cure rates of 84–97%, but reduction to a single 1-g oral dose resulted in lower cure rates; only 55% of 77 patients were cured as assessed by wet mounts and culture (Austin *et al.*, 1982; Underhill and Peck, 1979; Lossick, 1980). Tinidazole (not available in the United States) appears at least as effective as metronidazole: in a summary of more than 1000 cases from several studies treated with a one-time 2-g dose, a parasitological cure rate of 95% was reported (Sawyer *et al.*, 1976). Single-dose therapy with either agent appears to be particularly useful in treating male sexual contacts: in a placebo-controlled study of tinidazole, cure rates in women at 2-month follow-up increased from 73% (45/62) to 92% (56/61) when sexual partners were treated simultaneously (Lyng and Christensen, 1981).

Treatment failures occur due to metronidazole resistance, but the importance of such resistance epidemiologically is uncertain. Treatment failures often respond to repeat courses of metronidazole in conventional doses, although dose escalation may be necessary in some patients (Muller *et al.*, 1980). Local measures such as douches may be helpful.

The adverse reactions caused by metronidazole have been discussed (Section 2). The relatively low doses used with *Trichomonas* are associated with fewer, less severe toxic effects than the high doses used with amebiasis. Single doses of 2 g are associated with more GI effects, especially nausea and vomiting, than are the longer courses with lower doses. Because metronidazole is potentially mutagenic and carcinogenic, its use is not considered to be safe in pregnant women, especially during the first trimester.

6. DIENTAMOEBA FRAGILIS

6.1. Clinical Considerations

Dientamoeba fragilis is often present in stool, but it rarely appears to produce diarrhea. In a few patients, particularly children, large quantities of this organism are present, and eradication of the organism correlates with clinical improvement.

6.2. Individual Agents

Iodoquinol, tetracycline, and paromomycin have been used successfully in a few cases using doses similar to those for *Entamoeba histolytica* (Simon *et al.*, 1967; Spencer *et al.*, 1979).

7. BALANTIDIUM COLI

7.1. Clinical Considerations

Because *Balantidium coli* infections are less frequent than other protozoal diseases of the gastrointestinal tract, there has been less information in the literature on the efficacy of treatment.

7.2. Individual Agents

7.2.1. Metronidazole and Other Nitroimidazoles

All 20 patients in one study treated with metronidazole 0.5–1.25 g/day in three divided doses for 5–10 days and followed for up to 20 months were reported to have parasitological cures (Garcia-Laverde and DeBonilla, 1975). In another study, however, only two of five similarly treated patients improved (Beasley and Walzer, 1972). A related compound, nitrimidazine (not available in the United States) was effective in 12 of 17 children when 500 mg/day was given for 5 days (Botero, 1973). Patients remained asymptomatic and free of parasites during 1 month of follow-up evaluation.

7.2.2. Tetracycline or Iodoquinol

Tetracycline (0.75–2.0 g/day in divided doses) effectively cured 9 of 10 patients followed with multiple stools over 3–5 months (Hoekenga, 1953). Individual case reports suggest that iodoquinol (650 mg, three to four times/day for 20 days) is effective (Beasley and Walzer, 1972).

8. CRYPTOSPORIDIUM

8.1. Clinical Considerations

Cryptosporidium has only recently been recognized as a human pathogen. Most infections appear to clear spontaneously and require no therapy. Chronic, debilitating diarrhea can occur, primarily in patients with acquired immunodeficiency syndrome (AIDS), and less frequently in other immunocompromised patients. Because special techniques such as sucrose flotation are needed to detect the organism in stool specimens, diagnosis as well as assessment of therapy required special expertise.

8.2. Individual Agents

No drug has been shown to be consistently effective against *Cryptosporidium*, although most agents with antiprotozoan activity have been tried (Centers for Disease Control, 1982). Spiramycin, a macrolide antibiotic with anti-*Toxoplasma* activity, has been reported to be effective when given in a dose of 1 g three times/day for 1–16 weeks (Portnoy *et al.*, 1984; Collier *et al.*, 1984). Of 11 patients (nine with AIDS), six had complete resolution of diarrhea and four had symptomatic improvement. In six patients therapy resulted in parasitological cure, although symptoms occasionally persisted. Discontinuation of immunosuppressive therapy probably hastens resolution of infection.

In three patients with overwhelming cryptosporidiosis, amprolium has been tried; there was an indication that high and toxic dosages (33 mg/kg, increasing to 200 mg/kg per day) had a suppressive effect on diarrhea and oocyst excretion in one of them (Sloper *et al.*, 1982; Pitlik *et al.*, 1983; Veldhuyzen van Zanten *et al.*, 1984). Neither the efficacy nor the safety of this drug has been established in human coccidial infections.

9. TOXOPLASMA GONDII

9.1. Clinical Considerations

Toxocplasma gondii can cause systemic infection in immunocompetent or immunosuppressed individuals; however, only a small fraction of humans develop clinically important or symptomatic disease for which treatment needs to be considered. Studies of drug efficacy in man have been difficult to interpret for three primary reasons: (1) the frequency of diagnosed cases is rare at most centers, (2) systemic or ocular disease has such variable natural histories that small studies are uninterpretable, and (3) there is no practical microbiologic technique for assessing viability of organisms in human patients. Conceptually, it is important to recognize that both the folic acid antagonists and the macrolides are probably inhibitory and not microbicidal and thus are likely to be active against the tachyzoites but not the cysts. Current information on drug therapy is based on animal work, *in vitro* data, and anecdotes.

9.2. Individual Agents

9.2.1. Sulfa Drugs and Pyrimethamine

In vitro studies suggest that parasite multiplication or uracil uptake by *T. gondii* cannot be inhibited by clinically relevant levels of sulfa drugs alone, but that the addition of trimethroprim or pyrimethamine can produce synergy (Grossman *et al.*, 1978). In experimentally infected mice given various drug regimens in their diets, sulfamethazine appeared to be more potent than sulfadiazine, which was more potent than sulfisoxazole, although blood levels were not measured (Eyles and Coleman, 1953;

Eyles and Coleman, 1955a). Pyrimethamine has been shown in the mouse model to be synergistic with sulfa drugs (Eyles and Coleman, 1955b).

The standard therapy for humans with clinically serious disease is sulfadiazine 1 g four times daily (100 mg/kg for infants) given orally plus pyrimethamine 75 mg orally as an initial dose followed by 25 mg/day (1 mg/kg for infants). Treatment is continued for at least 6 weeks. Patients with severe disease and immunoincompetent patients (especially those with AIDS) may require considerably longer courses, since cessation of therapy following clinical improvement may result in prompt relapse (Wong et al., 1984). Pyrimethamine is not available in a parenteral form. Pyrimethamine and sulfadiazine are probably more effective than the trimethoprim–sulfamethoxazole combination. The toxicity of pyrimethamine is primarily inhibition of folic acid metabolism and resultant thrombocytopenia, leukopenia, and anemia. These can be prevented or treated in some cases with the administration of folinic acid (leucovorin calcium) 10 mg iv or po several times weekly (Frenkel et al., 1960). Gastrointestinal distress and headache also occur.

9.2.2. Clindamycin and Spiramycin

Clindamycin and spiramycin are macrolide antimicrobial agents advocated for the treatment of retinochoroiditis and congenital disease, respectively. Convincing animal and human data are, however, sparse. Direct inoculation of toxoplasma into rabbit retinas has been used to study the effectiveness of clindamycin therapy; data suggest that clindamycin is useful (Tabbara et al., 1974). Two reports in humans support the use of oral or subconjunctival clindamycin to treat retinochoroiditis (Ferguson, 1981; Tabbara and O'Connor, 1980).

Spiramycin has been shown to be equally efficacious as sulfa and pyrimethamine in the treatment of congenitally infected mice (Beverly et al., 1973). The drug is popular in Europe as a nonteratogenic agent for therapy of pregnant women with toxoplasmosis acquired during pregnancy. Studies have not been controlled, so its efficacy is unproven.

If these macrolides are to be used, doses in adults might be clindamycin 300 mg four times daily or spiramycin 100 mg/kg per day in two to four divided doses. Toxicity includes pseudomembranous colitis, diarrhea, and nausea. Duration of therapy for optimal effect is unknown.

9.2.3. Trimethoprim–Sulfamethoxazole

In vitro studies have suggested that sulfamethoxazole in combination with trimethoprim can inhibit metabolism or multiplication of trophozoites (Grossman et al., 1978). Anecdotal experience in humans reports success using this drug combination, but these studies have been uncontrolled (Norrby et al., 1975). At this point, there seems to be no in vitro, animal, or clinical data to suggest that trimethoprim–sulfamethoxazole should be used in preference to sulfadiazine and pyrimethamine.

10. ISOSPORA BELLI

10.1. Clinical Considerations

Isospora belli infection will often clear spontaneously. Only heavy and persistent infections require treatment. Such cases are so unusual that there is little available literature for guidance.

10.2. Individual Agents

Trimethoprim–sulfamethoxazole (160 mg trimethoprim and 800 mg sulfamethoxazole four times daily for 10 days, then twice/day for 3 weeks) (Westerman and Christensen, 1979) or pyrimethamine (75 mg/day) plus sulfadiazine (1 g four times/day) for 3 weeks followed by an additional 4 weeks at one-half that dosage (Trier *et al.*, 1974) have been reported to be successful. Weekly sulfadoxine (1500 mg) and pyrimethamine (75 mg) can also be effective (Piens *et al.*, 1981). Adverse reactions for these drugs are described in Sections 9 and 12.

In a patient with severe *I. belli* diarrhea, the oral administration of amprolium (10 mg/kg, increasing to 90 mg/kg per day) was followed by prompt clinical relief (Veldhuyzen van Zanten *et al.*, 1984). Neither the efficacy nor the safety of this drug has been established.

11. SARCOCYSTIS SPECIES

11.1. Clinical Considerations

Although occasional case reports describing disease associated with *Sarcocystis* species have appeared, infection appears to be primarily asymptomatic and discovered only incidentally. Therapy is usually unnecessary, and reports of effective therapy are lacking.

12. PNEUMOCYSTIS CARINII

12.1. Clinical Considerations

Clinically significant *Pneumocystis carinii* pneumonia occurs almost exclusively in immunocompromised patients, especially patients with AIDS, leukemia, and lymphoma. Without therapy, death is inevitable in these patients. Because *Pneumocystis* cannot be grown reproducibly *in vitro,* efficacy of drugs has been evaluated systematically in the rodent model as well as by clinical improvement and survival in man. Although serial bronchoscopic biopsies are being used to evaluate histopathological response to therapy in patients with AIDS, published data in this regard are limited.

12.2. Individual Agents

12.2.1. Pentamidine

Pentamidine has been used effectively since 1958 for the treatment of pneumocystis pneumonia. It is available in the United States as the isethionate salt; in other countries a methylsulfonate salt is also available. Although efficacy was originally suggested by human experience, pentamidine has subsequently been shown to be effective in cortisone-treated rats. Following the original demonstration by Frenkel *et al.* (1966), Kluge *et al.* (1978) gave 20 mg/kg per day to rats and found that *Pneumocystis* was present in 13 of 29 treated animals, as compared with 21 of 28 control animals, although Hughes *et al.* (1974) were able to show only minimal efficacy when using the same dose three times weekly.

In humans, pentamidine was the only widely used agent from 1958 until the late 1970s. Two large series from the CDC suggested that the recovery rate for patients treated with 4 mg/kg per day intramuscularly for 2 weeks was 42%, but if the patient survived long enough to receive nine or more daily doses, survival was 63% (Western *et al.*, 1970; Walzer *et al.*, 1974). Currently, a 2-week course is recommended, but longer courses may be necessary for patients with AIDS.

Clinically important adverse reactions occur in about 47% of patients and include pain, inflammation, and sterile abscess at the injection site; hypotension; azotemia; hypoglycemia and hyperglycemia; liver function abnormality; thrombocytopenia or leukopenia; hypocalcemia; and rash (Walzer *et al.*, 1974). The drug was originally reported to cause profound hypotension when given intravenously. Subsequent investigations, not yet confirmed, suggest that slow administration of 4 mg/kg diluted in 100 ml of 5% dextrose given over 1–2 hr is safe. Azotemia occurs in at least 25% of patients.

12.2.2. Sulfadiazine and Pyrimethamine

The rat model suggests that sulfadiazine used as a single agent has some effect against *Pneumocystis* but that pyrimethamine as a single agent has no effect. When the drugs are combined, however, only two of nine rats were found to have pneumocystis pneumonia in one study compared with 16 of 16 controls (Frenkel *et al.*, 1966). Several humans have been treated successfully with sulfadiazine and pyrimethamine in doses similar to those suggested for *Toxoplasma* (where toxicity is also discussed) (Kirby *et al.*, 1971), but the popularity of trimethoprim–sulfamethoxazole has limited further trials.

12.2.3. Trimethoprim–Sulfamethoxazole

In the rat model, trimethoprim–sulfamethoxazole (T/S) is more effective than pentamidine: in one study, 6 of 15 T/S-treated rats developed pneumocystis compared with 13 of 15 pentamidine-treated rats and all of 15 controls (Hughes *et al.*, 1974). A subsequent study confirmed this (Kluge *et al.*, 1978). Trimethoprim alone does not appear to be effective, however, in this model.

In humans, numerous reports attest to the efficacy of 2-week courses with T/S given either orally or intravenously in a dose of sulfamethoxazole 100 mg/kg per day and trimethoprim 20 mg/kg per day, in three to four divided doses, with a total trimethoprim dose usually not exceeding 960 mg/day (Winston *et al.*, 1980; Sattler and Remington, 1981). As with pentamidine, AIDS patients may need longer courses. Peak serum levels, which appear to correlate with successful outcome, are sulfamethoxazole 100–150, μg/ml, and trimethoprim, 4–10 μg/ml (Winston *et al.*, 1980). In seriously ill patients, in whom failure to achieve adequate serum levels may be fatal, intravenous administration is preferable.

The relative efficacy of T/S and pentamidine has been well studied only in children, in whom a controlled study of 50 patients demonstrated comparable efficacy for the two drugs but considerably more toxicity with pentamidine (Hughes *et al.*, 1978). In adults, there is no convincing data for superior efficacy of either drug (Kovacs *et al.*, 1984). T/S is currently considered the drug of choice for treatment of pneumocystis pneumonia. In patients who do not tolerate T/S or who fail to respond after 5–10 days of therapy, pentamidine can be added or substituted. There are no data in humans on the relative usefulness of two-drug therapy compared with one drug.

Adverse reactions to T/S in most patient populations occur in fewer than 10% of patients and include hypersensitivity, crystalluria, and marrow aplasia. The latter can occasionally be reversed by administration of folinic acid (leucovorin calcium) 10 mg IV several times weekly. Patients with AIDS have an unusually high frequency of rash, neutropenia, liver function abnormalities, and nausea while receiving T/S (Kovacs *et al.*, 1984).

12.2.4. Other Drugs

Dapsone appears to exhibit activity against *Pneumocystis* in studies using the rat model (Hughes and Smith, 1984), but human studies to date are only anecdotal. No other agent with impressive antipneumocystis activity has been identified.

12.2.5. Prophylaxis

Certain patient populations have such a high risk of acquiring *Pneumocystis* that prophylaxis would be desirable. In the rat model and in humans, prophylaxis is only effective when given continuously during immunosuppression; a short course before or during immunosuppression only delays the onset of pneumocystic pneumonia if it has any effect at all (Wolff and Baehner, 1978). In the rat model, T/S prophylaxis is highly effective; pentamidine has not been as thoroughly tested. In humans, only T/S has been examined: sulfamethoxazole 20 mg/kg per day and trimethoprim 4 mg/kg per day in two equal doses was completely effective in children (Hughes *et al.*, 1977). The same dose given 2 consecutive days each week may also be effective.

13. *BABESIA* SPECIES

13.1. Clinical Considerations

The natural history of *Babesia* infections is sufficiently unpredictable to make interpretation of small therapeutic trials uncertain. Moreover, many reports follow the parasitemia by examining the peripheral smear, yet hamster inoculations are a more sensitive assessment of parasite eradication. At this juncture, however, recommendations for drug therapy must be based on a few, well-studied patients plus studies in the hamster model.

13.1.1. Chloroquine

In hamsters and mice, chloroquine fails to have any effect on degree of parasitemia (Miller *et al.*, 1978). Although patients have responded clinically while receiving chloroquine, no clear relationship between parasitemia and symptomatic improvement was documented; amelioration of symptoms may have been related to anti-inflammatory properties of chloroquine or the unpredictable natural history of the disease (Ruebush *et al.*, 1977).

13.1.2. Pentamidine

Aromatic diamidines, including pentamidine isethionate, have been successful in decreasing parasitemia in some animal models though parasitemia has not been eradicated. Several humans have been treated with daily pentamidine (4 mg/kg per day im) with parallel results: symptomatic improvement and reduction in parasitemia were noted during the first 5 days, but hamster inoculation could still succeed in isolating the organism (Francioli *et al.*, 1981).

13.1.3. Clindamycin and Quinine

Clindamycin alone, or clindamycin plus quinine, have been successful in reducing parasitemia in hamsters (Rowin *et al.*, 1982). Parasitemia did not recur after cessation of therapy, unlike the situation with aromatic diamidines. Quinine alone had no effect, but its addition to clindamycin produced a faster and more substantial decrease in parasitemia. For unexplained reasons, oral quinine was more effective than intravenous.

One human has been reported cured of *Babesia* with clindamycin 20 mg/kg per day and quinine 25 mg/kg per day, given for 7 days (Wittner *et al.*, 1982). No recurrence was found. At this point, parenteral clindamycin and oral quinine appear to be the therapy of choice for clinically significant babesiosis.

REFERENCES

Anderson, K., and Jamieson, A., 1972, Primary amoebic meningoencephalitis, *Lancet* 1:902–903.

Apley, J., Clarke, S. K. R., Roome, A. P. C. H., Sandry, S. A., Saygi, G., Silk, B., and Warhurst, D. C., Primary amoebic meningoencephalitis in Britain, 1970, *Br. Med. J.* 1:596–599.

Austin, T. V., Smith, E. A., Darwish, R., Ralph, E. D., and Pattison, F. L. M., 1982, Metronidazole in a single dose for the treatment of trichomoniasis, *Br. J. Vener Dis.* 58:121–123.

Bassily, S., Farid, Z., Mikhail, J. W., Kent, D. C., and Lehman, J. S., 1970, The treatment of *Giardia lamblia* infection with mepacrine, metronidazole, and furazolidone, *J. Trop. Med. Hyg.* 73:15–18.

Beasley, J. W., and Walzer, P. D., 1972, Ineffectiveness of metronidazole in treatment of *Balantidium coli* infections, *Trans. R. Soc. Trop. Med. Hyg.* 63:152.

Beverly, J. K. A., Freeman, A. P., Henry, L., and Whelan, J. P. F., 1973, Prevention of pathological changes in experimental congenital toxoplasma infections, *Lyon Med.* 230:491–498.

Botero, D., 1964, Treatment of acute and chronic intestinal amoebiasis with entamide furoate, *Trans. R. Soc. Trop. Med. Hyg.* 58:419–421.

Botero, D., 1973, Effectiveness of nitrimidazine in treatment of *Balantidium coli* infections, *Trans. R. Soc. Trop. Med. Hyg.* 67:145.

Centers for Disease Control, 1982, Cryptosporidiosis: Assessment of chemotherapy of males with acquired immunodeficiency syndrome (AIDS), *M.M.W.R.* 31:589–592.

Cohen, H. G., and Reynolds, T. B., 1975, Comparison of metronidazole and chloroquine for the treatment of amoebic liver abscess, *Gastroenterology* 69:35–41.

Collier, A. C., Miller, R. A., and Meyers, J. D., 1984, Cryptosporidiosis after marrow transplanation: Person-to-person transmission and treatment with spiramycin, *Ann. Intern. Med.* 101:205–206.

Craft, C. J., Murphy, T., and Nelson, J. D., 1981, Furazolidone and quinacrine. Comparative study of therapy of giardiasis in children, *Am. J. Dis. Child.* 135:164–66.

Datta, D. V., Singh, A. K., and Chhuttani, P. N., 1974, Treatment of amebic liver abscess with emetine hydrochloride, niridazole, and metronidazole. A controlled clinical trial, *Am. J. Trop. Med. Hyg.* 23:586–589.

Duma, R. J., and Finley, R., 1976, In vitro susceptibility of pathogenic *Naegleria* and *Acanthamoeba* species to a variety of therapeutic agents, *Antimicrob. Ag. Chemother.* 10:370–376.

Eyles, D. E., and Coleman, N., 1953, The relative activity of the common sulfonamides against experimental toxoplasmosis in the mouse, *Am. J. Trop. Med.* 2:54–63.

Eyles, D. E.,and Coleman, N., 1955a, The effect of sulfadimetine, sulfisoxazole, and sulfapyrazine against mouse toxoplasmosis, *Antibiot Chemother.* 5:525–528.

Eyles, D. E., and Coleman, N., 1955b, An evaluation of the curative effects of pyrimethamine and sulfadiazine, alone and in combination, on experimental mouse toxoplasmosis, *Antibiot. Chemother.* 5:529–539.

Ferguson, J. G., 1981, Clindamycin therapy for toxoplasmosis, *Ann. Ophthalmol.* 13:95–100.

Finegold, S. M., 1980, Metronidazole, *Ann. Intern. Med.* 93:585–587.

Fleisher, D. I., Hepler, R. S., and Landau, J. W., 1974, Blindness during diiodohydroxyquin therapy: A case report, *Pediatrics* 54:106–108.

Forsyth, D. M., 1962, The treatment of amoebiasis: A field study of various methods, *Trans. R. Soc. Trop. Med. Hyg.* 56:400–403.

Francioli, P. B., Keithly, J. S., Jones, T. C., Brandstetter, R. D., and Wolf, D. J., 1981, Response of Babesiosis to pentamidine therapy, *Ann Intern Med.* 94:326–330.

Frenkel, J. K., Weber, R. W., and Lunde, M. N., 1960, Acute toxoplasmosis: Effective treatment with pyrimethamine, sulfadiazine, leucovorin calcium, and yeast, *J.A.M.A.* 173:1471–1476.

Frenkel, J. K., Good, J. T., and Shultz, J. A., 1966, Latent pneumocystis infection of rats, relapse, and chemotherapy, *Lab. Invest.* 15:1559–1577.

Garcia-Laverde, A., and De Bonilla, L., 1975, Clinical trials with metronidazole in human balantidiasis, *Am. J. Trop. Med. Hyg.* 24:781–783.

Grossman, P. L., and Remington, J. S., The effects of trimethoprim and sulfamethoxazole on *Toxoplasma gondii* in vitro and in vivo, 1979, *Am. J. Trop. Med.* 28:445–455.

Hager, W. D., Brown, S. T., Kraus, S. J., Kleris, G. S., Perkins, G. J., and Henderson, M., 1980, Metronidazole for vaginal trichomoniasis. Seven-day vs. single-dose regimens, *J.A.M.A.* 244:1219–1220.

Hatchuel, W., 1975, Tinidazole for the treatment of amoebic liver abscess, *S. Afr. Med. J.* 49:1879–1881.

Hoekenga, M. T., 1953, Terramycin treatment of balantidiasis in Honduras, *Am. J. Trop. Med. Hyg.* 2:271–272.

Hughes, W. T., and Smith, B. L., 1984, Efficacy of biaminodiphenylsulfone murine *Pneumocystis carinii* pneumonites, *Antimicrob. Agents Chemother.* 26:436–440.

Hughes, W. T., McNabb, P. C., Makres, T. D., and Feldman, S., 1974, Efficacy of trimethoprim and sulfamethoxazole in the prevention and treatment of *Pneumocystis carinii* pneumonitis, *Antimicrob. Agents Chemother.* 5:289–293.

Hughes, W. T., Kuhn, S., Chaudhary, S., Feldman, S., Verzosa, M., Aur, R. J. A., Pratt, C., and George, S. L., 1977, Successful chemoprophylaxis for *Pneumocystis carinii* pneumonitis, *N. Engl. J. Med.* 297:1419–1426.

Hughes, W. T., Felman, S., Chaudhary, S. C., Ossi, M. G., Cox, F., and Sanyal, S. K., 1978, Comparison of pentamidine isethionate with trimethoprim-sulfamethoxazole in the threatment of *Pneumocystis carinii* pneumonia, *J. Pediatr.* 92:285–292.

Jokipii, L., and Jokipii, A. M. M., 1979, Single-dose metronidazole and tinidazole as therapy for glardiasis: Success rates, side effects, and drug absorption and elimination, *J. Infect. Dis.* 140:984–988.

Jokipii, L., and Jokipii, A. M. M., 1982, Treatment of giardiasis: Comparative evaluation of ornidazole and tinidazole as a single oral dose, *Gastroenterology* 83:399–404.

Kanani, S. R., and Knight, R., 1972, Experiences with the use of metronidazole in the treatment of non-dysenteric intestinal amoebiasis, *Trans. R. Soc. Trop. Med. Hyg.* 66:244–249.

Keighley, E. E., 1971, Trichomoniasis in a close community: One hundred percent followup, *Br. Med. J.* 1:207–209.

Khambatta, R. B., 1971, Metronidazole in giardiasis, *Ann. Trop. Med. Parasitol.* 65:487–489.

Kirby, H. B., Kenamore, B., and Guckian, J. C., 1971, *Pneumocystis carinii* pneumonia treated with pyrimethamine and sulfadiazine, *Ann. Intern. Med.* 75:505–509.

Kluge, R. M., Spaulding, D. M., and Spain, A. J., 1978, Combination of pentamidine and trimethoprim-sulfamethoxazole in the therapy of *Pneumocystis carinii* pneumonia in rats, *Antimicrob. Agents Chemother.* 13:975–978.

Knight, R., 1980, The chemotherapy of amoebiasis, *J. Antimicrob. Chemother.* 6:577–593.

Kovacs, J. A., Hiemenz, J. W., Macher, A. M., Stover, D., Murray, H. W., Shelhamer, J., Lane, H. C., Urmacher, C., Honig, C., Longo, D. L., Parker, M. M., Natanson, C., Parrillo, J. E., Fauci, A. S., Pizzo, P. A., and Masur, H., 1984, *Pneumocystis carinii* pneumonia: A comparison between patients with the acquired immunodeficiency syndrome and patients with other immunodeficiencies, *Ann. Intern. Med.* 100:663–671.

Kreutner, A. K., Del Bene, V. E., and Amstey, M. S., 1981, Giardiasis in pregnancy, *Am. J. Obstet. Gynecol.* 140:895–899.

Levi, G. C., deAvila, C. A., and Neto, V. A., 1977, Efficacy of various drugs for treatment of giardiasis, *Am. J. Trop. Med. Hyg.* 26:564–565.

Lossick, J. G., 1980, Single-dose metronidazole treatment for vaginal trichomoniasis, *Obstet. Gynecol.* 56:508–510.

Lyng, J., and Christensen, J., 1981, A double-blind study of the value of treatment with a single dose of tinidazole of partners of females with trichomoniasis, *Acta Obstet. Gynecol. Scand.* 60:199–201.

Ma, P., Willaert, E., Juechter, K. B., and Stevens, A. R., 1981, A case of keratitis due to *Acanthamoeba* in New York, New York, and features in 10 cases, *J. Infect Dis.* 143:662–667.

Miller, L. H., Neva, F. A., and Gill, F., 1978, Failure of chloroquine in human babesiosis (*Babesia microti*); case report and chemotherapeutic trials in hamsters, *Ann. Intern. Med.* 88:200–202.

Most, H., 1960, Treatment of amebiasis, *N. Engl. J. Med.* 262:513–514.

Muller, M., Meingassner, J. G., Miller, W. A., and Ledger, W. J., 1980, Three metronidazole-resistant strains of *Trichomonas vaginalis* from the United States, *Am. J. Obstet Gynecol.* 138:808–812.

Nguyen, B. T., Stadtsbaeder, S., and Horvat, F., 1978, Comparative effect of trimethoprim and pyrimethamine, alone and in combination with a sulfonamide, on *Toxoplasma gondii:* in vitro and in vivo studies, in: *Current Chemotherapy: Proceedings of the Tenth International Congress of Chemotherapy*, (W. Siegentheler and R. Luthy, eds.), Vol. 1, pp. 137–140, American Society for Microbiology, Washington, D.C.

Norrby, R., Eilard, T., Svedhem, A., and Lycke, E., 1975, Treatment of toxoplasmosis with trimethoprim-sulfamethoxazole, *Scand. J. Infect. Dis.* 7:72–75.

Oakley, G. P., 1973, The neurotoxicity of the halogenated hydroxyquinolines, *J.AM.A.* 225:395–397.

Pehrson, P. O., and Bengtsson, E., 1984, A long term follow up study of amoebiasis treated with metronidazole, *Scand. J. Infect. Dis.* 16:195–198.

Piens, M. A., Excler, J. L., and Roux, M., 1981, Une cause rare et peu connue de diarrhée: L'isosporose humaine, *Lyon Med.* 245:123–128.

Pitlik, S. D., Fainstein, V., Garza, D., Guard, L., Bolivar, R., Rios, A., Hopfer, R. L., and Mansell, P. A., 1983, Human cryptosporidiosis: Spectrum of disease. Arch. Intern. Med. 143:2269–2275.

Portnoy, D., Whiteside, M. E., Buckley, E., and MacLeod, C. L., 1984, Treatment of intestinal cryptosporidiosis with spiramycin, Ann. Intern. Med. 101:202–204.

Powell, S. J., 1967a, Short-term follow-up studies in amoebic dysentery, Trans. R. Soc. Trop. Med. Hyg. 61:765–769.

Powell, S. J., 1967b, The cardiotoxicity of systemic amebicides. A comparative electrocardiographic study, Am. J. Trop. Med. Hyg. 16:447–450.

Powell, S. J., 1971, Therapy of amebiasis, Bull. N.Y. Acad. Med. 47:469–477.

Powell, S. J., McLeod, I., Wilmot, A. J., and Elsdon-Dew, R., 1962, Dehydroemetine in amebic dysentery and amebic liver abscess, Am. J. Trop. Med. Hyg. 5:607–609.

Powell, S. J., Wilmot, A. J., MacLeod, I. N., and Elsdon-Dew, R., 1965, Dehydroemetine in the treatment of amoebic liver abscess, Ann. Trop. Med. Parasitol. 59:208–209.

Powell, S. J., MacLeod, I., Wilmot, A. J., and Elsdon-Dew, R., 1966, Metronidazole in amoebic dysentery and amoebic liver abscess, Lancet 2:1329–1331.

Powell, S. J., Wilmot, A. J., MacLeod, N., and Elsdon-Dew, R., 1967, A comparative trial of dehydroemetine and emetine hydrochloride in identical dosage in amoebic liver abscess, Ann. Trop. Med. Parasitol. 61:26–28.

Powell, S. J., Wilmot, A. J., and Elsdon-Dew, R., 1969, Single and low dosage regimens of metronidazole in amoebic dysentery and amoebic liver disease, Ann. Trop. Med. Parasitol. 63:139–142.

Roe, F. J. C., 1983, Toxicologic evaluation of metronidazole with particular reference to carcinogenic, mutagenic, and teratogenic potential, Surgery, 93:158–164.

Rowin, K. S., Tanewitz, H. B., and Wittner, M., 1982, Therapy of experimental babesiosis, Ann. Intern. Med. 97:556–558.

Ruebush, T. K., Cassaday, P. B., Marsh, H. J., Lisker, S. A., Voorhees, D. B., Mahoney, E. B., and Healy, G. R., 1977, Human babesiosis on Nantucket Island: Clinical features, Ann. Intern. Med. 86:6–9.

Sattler, F. R., and Remington, J. S., 1981, Intravenous trimethoprim-sulfamethoxazole therapy for Pneumocystis carinii pneumonia, Am. J. Med. 70:1215–1221.

Sawyer, P. R., Brogden, R. N., Pinder, R. M., Speight, T. M., and Avery, G. S., 1976, Tinidazole: A review of its antiprotozoal activity and therapeutic efficacy, Drugs 11:423–440.

Scragg, J. N., Rubidge, C. J., and Proctor, E. M., 1976, Tinidazole in treatment of acute amebic dysentery in children, Arch. Dis. Child. 51:385–387.

Seidel, J. S., Harmatz, P., Visvesvara, G. S., Cohen, A., Edwards, J., and Turner, J., 1982, Successful treatment of primary amebic meningoencephalitis, N. Engl. J. Med. 306:346–348.

Simon, M., Shookhoff, H. B., Terner, H., Weingarten, B., and Parker, J. G., 1967, Paromomycin in the treatment of intestinal amebiasis: A short course of therapy, Am. J. Gastroenterol. 48:504–511.

Sloper, K. S., Dourmashkin, R. R., Bird, R. B., Slvain, G., and Webster, A. D., 1982, Chronic malabsorption due to cryptosporidiosis in a child with immunoglobulin deficiency, Gut 23:80–82.

Smith, P. D., Gillin, F. D., Spira, W. M., and Nash, T. E., 1982, Chronic giardiasis: Studies on drug sensitivity, toxin production, and host immune response, Gastroenterology 83:797–803.

Spencer, M. J., Garcia, L. S., and Chapin, M. R., 1979, Dientamoeba Fragilis. An intestinal pathogen in children?, Am. J. Dis. Child. 133:390–393.

Spillmann, R., Ayala, S. C., and DeSanchez, C. E., 1976, Double-blind test of metronidazole and tinidazole in the treatment of asymptomatic Entamoeba histolytica and Entamoeba hartmanii carriers, Am. J. Trop. Med. Hyg. 25:549–551.

Tabbara, K. F., and O'Connor, G. R., 1980, Treatment of ocular toxoplasmosis with clindamycin and sulfadiazine, Ophthalmology 87:129–134.

Tabbara, K. F., Nozik, R. A., and O'Connor, G. R., 1974, Clindamycin effects on experimental ocular toxoplasmosis in the rabbit, Arch. Ophthalmol. 92:244–247.

Thong, Y. H., Rowan-Kelly, B., and Ferrante, A., 1979, Treatment of experimental Naegleria meningoencephalitis with a combination of amphotericin B and rifamycin, Scand. J. Infect. Dis. 11:151–153.

Trier, J. S., Moxey, P. C., Schimmel, E. M., and Robles, E., 1974, Chronic intestinal coccidiosis in man: Intestinal morphology and response to treatment, Gastroenterology 66:923–935.

Underhill, R. A., and Peck, J. E., 1974, Causes of therapeutic failure after treatment of trichomonal vaginitis with metronidazole: Comparison of single dose treatment with a standard regimen, *Br. J. Clin. Pract.* 28:134–136.

Veldhuyzen van Zanten, S. J. O., Lange, J. M. A., Saurwein, H. P., Rijpstra, A. C., Laarman, J. J., Rietra, P. J. G. M., and Danner, S. A., 1984, Amprolium for coccidiosis in AIDS. *Lancet* 2:345–346.

Walzer, P. D., Perl, D. P., Krogstad, D. J., Rawson, P. G., and Schultz, M. G., 1974, *Pneumocystis carinii* pneumonia in the United States: Epidemiologic, diagnostic, and clinical features, *Ann. Intern. Med.* 80:83–93.

Westerman, E. L., and Christensen, R. P., 1979, Chronic *Isospora belli* infection treated with co-trimoxazole, *Ann. Intern. Med.* 91:413–414.

Western, K. A., Perera, D. R., and Schultz, M. G., 1970, Pentamidine isethionate in the treatment of *Pneumocystis carinii* pneumonia, *Ann. Intern. Med.* 73:695–702.

Winston, D. J., Lau, W. K., Gale, R. P., and Young, L. S., 1980, Trimethoprim-sulfamethoxazole for the treatment of *Pneumocystis carinii* pneumonia, *Ann. Intern. Med.* 92:762–769.

Wittner, M., Rowin, K. S., Tanowitz, H. B., Hobbs, J. F., Saltzman, S., Wenz, B., Hirsch, R., Chisholm, E., and Healy, G. R., 1982, Successful chemotherapy of transfusion babesiosis, *Ann. Intern. Med.* 96:601–604.

Wolfe, M. S., 1973, Nondysenteric intestinal amebiasis. Treatment with diloxanide furoate, *J.A.M.A.* 224:1601–1604.

Wolfe, M. S., 1975, Giardiasis, *J.AM.A.* 233:1362–1365.

Wolfe, M. S., 1978, Gierdiasis, *N. Engl. J. Med.* 298:319–321.

Wolff, L. J., and Baehner, R. L., 1978, Delayed development of pneunumocystis pneumonia following administration of short-term high-dose trimethoprim-sulfamethoxazole, *Am. J. Dis. Child.* 132:525–526.

Wong, B., Gold, J. W. M., Brown, A. E., Lange, M., Fried, R., Grieco, M., Mildvan, D., Girou, J., Tapper, M. L., Lerner, C. W., and Armstrong, D., 1984, Central nervous system toxoplasmosis in homosexual men and parenteral drug abusers, *Ann. Intern. Med.* 100:36–42.

Woodruff, A. W., and Bell, S., 1967, The evaluation of amoebicides, *Trans. R. Soc. Trop. Med. Hyg.* 61:435–439.

Wright, S. G., Tomkins, A. M., and Ridley, D. S., 1977, Giardiasis: Clinical and therapeutic aspects, *Gut* 18:343–350.

7

Protozoan Infections of Domestic Animals

Coccidian and Related Infections

L. R. McDOUGALD

1. INTRODUCTION

Among parasitic diseases of domestic animals, few have the widespread importance ascribed to the coccidia. Historically, poultry were most vulnerable to coccidiosis, because large numbers of birds were reared in confinement. Most domestic animals are susceptible to coccidiosis; wherever young animals are gathered together in close quarters, such as in lambing or calving sheds or around watering or feeding facilities, there is likely to be some prevalence of coccidiosis. Most of the economic damage can be done to chickens by this disease before the clinical signs are recognized, making prevention more important than treatment of sick animals. Thus, the practice of giving medication in the feed as a prophylactic measure is well accepted in the poultry industry. The cost of prophylactic medication has been estimated at more than $280 million worldwide. Despite this expenditure, losses to coccidiosis in poultry continue; drugs are not completely effective, drug resistance sometimes becomes a problem, and the drug may be inadvertently omitted because of erroneous feed-mill operation. More new drugs and alternative control measures are always needed to maintain good control of this important disease.

The parasites causing coccidiosis and related diseases are Sporozoa of the phylum Apicomplexa, mostly *Eimeria* or *Isospora,* which in one stage (the zoite) possess a characteristic apical complex. Essentially all aspects of the taxonomy, biology, and pathology of *Coccidia* were reviewed by Pellerdy (1974) and Long (1982).

L. R. McDOUGALD • Department of Poultry Science, University of Georgia, Athens, Georgia 30602.

2. EVOLUTION OF PRESENT-DAY CHEMOTHERAPEUTIC PRACTICES IN COCCIDIOSIS CONTROL

Prior to 1939 there were no known drugs active against coccidiosis. Treatments consisted of buttermilk, antiseptics, borax, and other materials with no proven chemotherapeutic value. Sulfur, when given in large amounts (4% of the feed), had some beneficial effect, but the first drug with demonstrated effectiveness against coccidiosis was sulfanilamide (Levine, 1939). The early sulfonamides were very expensive and fairly toxic. During the late 1940s the principle of continuous medication with lower levels of the drugs was suggested (Grumbles *et al.*, 1948), and the first commercial drugs, nitrophenide and sulfaquinoxaline, were available for use in chickens. The superiority of the preventive approach over the treatment method with this disease was quickly recognized and has been widely accepted to this day. Treatment drugs are available and are used whenever necessary, but the primary means of dealing with coccidiosis continues to be prevention. Some of the drugs enjoyed more commercial success than others. The extent to which some drugs were used in the United States was illustrated by McDougald and Reid (1983), who noted that the demand for drugs grew as the poultry industry expanded, except that the monetary inflation of the 1970s caused a faster rate of growth in the market.

3. METHODS OF DRUG TESTING

3.1. Laboratory Trials

Anticoccidial drugs can be tested in many ways, but with the advantage that most laboratory models use the target parasite and the target animal. Eimerian coccidia can be grown *in vitro* in chick embryos and in cultured cells. Both systems are used for testing or screening of experimental compounds for possible activity, with the advantage of economy and the small amount of experimental compound needed for each test. Generally, compounds that are active in chickens will be active *in vitro*, but those active *in vitro* are not necessarily active in the chicken. In a few rare instances, e.g., arprinocid, the compound must be metabolized to an active form in the bird (Wang and Simashkevich, 1980). Such compounds are rarely active *in vitro*.

Laboratory tests *in vivo* are usually designed in batteries of cages containing 5–10 chicks aged 10–14 days. The chicks are fed diets containing the test compounds for 1 or 2 days and are then orally inoculated with infective oocysts of *E. tenella* or other coccidia. Demonstration of efficacy against other species of coccidia is important to determine the spectrum of activity once activity against *E. tenella* is established. The tests are terminated 5–14 days postinoculation, with measurement of weight gain and feed consumption. At necropsy, the intestinal lesions are examined and assigned a score on a scale of 0–4 (Johnson and Reid, 1970). The effectiveness of a drug is directly related to improvement in weight gain of infected birds and to the reduction of lesion scores. Feed consumption and weight gain can be measures of the control of coccidiosis or may reflect the toxicity of the test compound. The extent of diarrhea caused by an infection can sometimes be estimated and is called a droppings score (Jeffers, 1974). Methods of drug screening were reviewed by Ryley and Betts (1973).

In recent years, the testing of drugs under simulated natural conditions has become well accepted. The floor-pen test is conducted in houses divided into small pens, so that several treatments can be replicated 4–10 times. Day-old chicks are started on litter and reared to market size, usually with *ad libitum* feeding. Coccidiosis infections are induced by one of several means, with oocysts (1) mixed directly into the feed and water; (2) spread on the litter; or (3) given to seeder birds that are introduced into the pens in suspended cages, contaminating the litter with their fecal droppings (Mitchell and Scoggins, 1970; Brewer and Kowalski, 1970). Evaluation of the efficacy of drugs in these tests is similar to that of laboratory tests: Birds are removed 7–14 days postexposure and are killed to permit examination of their intestinal lesions (Johnson and Reid, 1970). All the birds are weighed by group, usually on day 25 or 28 and at termination of the trial. Coccidiosis usually has a maximum effect on weight gain 7 days postexposure, but this lost gain will also be reflected in reduced final weights. Sometimes measurement of skin or blood pigmentation is used, since coccidiosis tends to cause loss of xanthophylls.

3.2. Field Trials

There are many difficulties in conducting a true field trial with a new anticoccidial agent. The many factors affecting actual growth and performance of chickens under commercial conditions negate the accuracy and significance of most field trials (Kilgore, 1970). The only true field trials are conducted by large poultry or livestock producers, who are in a position to produce literally millions of chickens on one product, in comparison with a similar number of chickens on another product. Most so-called field trials could more accurately be termed demonstrations, of the type used solely for customer conviction, and have little scientific merit.

4. CHARACTERISTICS OF DRUGS AND THEIR LIMITATIONS

4.1. Spectrum of Activity

There are at least six economically important species of coccidia in commercial poultry. In cattle, sheep, and goats there are many others. Drugs are first tested for activity against chicken coccidia because the broiler market constitutes their largest application. Early drugs generally had a more limited spectrum of activity than did present-day drugs. Farmers could easily recognize the devastating bloody cecal coccidiosis (*E. tenella*) and intestinal coccidiosis (*E. necatrix*) and required drugs to control these species. In modern poultry operations, the effect of other species can be measured in lost weight gain, pigmentation, and poor feed conversion. Diagnosticians are now better trained, and there is more general awareness of the importance of the species of coccidia. A general estimate of the spectrum of activity of some drugs is given in Table I.

4.2. Specific Activity

Most of the drugs used commercially had optimal activity at 100–125 ppm in the feed. A few were used at 250 ppm or even higher, but the costs of drugs at such high use levels becomes prohibitive. A few drugs are used at 50–75 ppm, and others are active at even lower levels. Halofuginone is used at 3 ppm; prinicin, a new ionophore, is used at 5 ppm, and some experimental drugs are active at less than 1 ppm. The use level of some drugs is summarized in Table II.

4.3. Clinical versus Static Mode of Action

Early drugs were called coccidiostats because they appeared to arrest the development of coccidia without killing them. Other drugs appeared to be lethal in their action. Most drugs have both properties, depending on the conditions of use. The most cidal drugs are nicarbazin and the ionophores; the quinolones are the most static, and other drugs appear to be intermediate (Reid et al., 1969).

4.4. Stage in the Life Cycle Most Sensitive to the Drug

Most drugs act principally against a particular stage in the life cycle of coccidia, usually the sporozoite or early asexual stages. The ionophores, quinolones and clopidol, act mostly against the early stages, while amprolium, nicarbazin, stenorol, and arprinocid act against later asexual stages (Reid, 1972, 1973; Joyner and Norton, 1977;

Table 1. Spectrum of Activity of Some Anticoccidial Drugs[a,b]

| Drug | Activity against each species of Eimeria | | | | |
	E. acervulina	E. maxima	E. necatrix	E. tenella	E. brunetti
Amprolium	−	+ +	+ +	+ + +	−
Robenidine	+ + +	+ + +	+ + +	+ + +	+ + +
Monensin	+ + +	+ + +	+ + +	+ +	+ + +
Ethopabate	+ + +	−	−	−	−
Sulfaquinoxaline	+ + +		+ +	+	
Zoalene	+	+ +	+ +	+ +	+
Lasalocid	+	+ + +	+ + +	+ + +	+ + +

[a]General pattern of efficacy; may not apply in specific instances. −, no activity; +, low activity; + +, moderate activity; + + +, strong activity.
[b]Data compiled from various sources.

Ruff *et al.*, 1978). A few drugs, such as arprinocid, amprolium, or sulfas, have some action against the sexual stages of coccidia, resulting in fewer or defective oocysts.

5. LIMITATIONS IN THE USE OF ANTICOCCIDIAL DRUGS

The perfect drug has not been discovered. All drugs have some features that have limited their use. In some cases, these features have seriously shortened the life of the drug; in other cases not.

5.1. Toxicity

When drugs are given continuously in the feed, an important consideration is the subacute toxicity or even palatability. Also, errors in feed compounding may expose the animal to higher than recommended doses of a drug. During the 1950s and 1960s, the successful drugs had a wide margin of safety. Amprolium and zoalene (DOT), the most popular drugs of the period, could be fed at two or three times the recommended dose without causing serious harm to the animals. More recently, the drugs in common use have a much narrower safety margin (Keshavarz and McDougald, 1982) but are better accepted because of improvements in the capabilities of the feed industry. Drugs that depress weight gain of the animal cannot be well accepted in an industry that depends on so narrow a margin of profit, unless other important benefits are realized.

5.2. Drug-Resistance Potential

Coccidia are able to develop resistance to some drugs more easily than others. Some drugs have had very short commercial lives because drug resistance was recognized within a few months of their introduction. One drug, glycarbylamide, was withdrawn within a month of its introduction because of preexisting resistant lines of coccidia. The quinolones, extremely potent anticoccidial agents, fell quickly to resistance. All drugs have permitted resistance sooner or later, but they differ greatly; ionophores have been used for more than 12 years in the United States, and only recently have strains of reduced sensitivity become a problem in some areas (Mathis *et al.*, 1984a). The potential of a new class of drugs to facilitate resistance should be investigated very early in the development process. Drug resistance was reviewed extensively by Chapman (1978, 1982a) and is discussed further in Chapter 9.

5.3. Drug Residues

Regulations of the Food and Drug Administration (FDA) of the U.S. government, or of similar agencies in other countries, make certain requirements of drugs as regards the occurrence and disappearance of residues of the drug from edible tissues of the animal prior to slaughter for human consumption. In the United States, the drug must be withdrawn for 2 days longer than is required for residues to be eliminated, or

Table II. *Drugs Currently Used for the Prevention of Coccidiosis in Chickens*

Generic name	Trade name	Manufacturer	Dose	Date available	Remarks
Amprolium	Amprol, Amprolmix, Amprol Plus, Amprol Hi E, Pancoxin, Pancoxin Plus	Merck	0.0125%	1961	Amprolium and its combinations used widely in many forms, very safe; effectiveness seriously limited by drug resistance; also weak against some species; popular in pullet and breeder programs
Arprinocid	Arpocox	Merck	0.006%	1979	Highly effective initially, but effectiveness quickly limited by drug resistance; future uncertain
Clopidol, meticlorpindol clopindol	Coyden	Dow	0.0125%	1968	Well tolerated, but weak against *E. acervulina*; rapid drug resistance
Decoquinate	Deccox	May and Baker, Hess and Clark, Rhone-Polenc	30	1971	Excellent efficacy, broad spectrum and well tolerated, but rapid drug resistance
Dinitolmide	DOT, Zoalene	Dow, Salsbury	125	1962	Widely used and inexpensive; limited activity against some species, widespread resistance
Ethopabate	Amprol Plus	Merck	4–40	1963	Used in combinations with amprolium to extend spectrum of activity to upper intestinal *Coccidia*
Halofuginone	Stenorol	Roussell UCLAF	3	1980	Good efficacy, broad spectrum, well tolerated, but rapid resistance in some instances
Lasalocid	Avatec	Hoffman-LaRoche	75–125	1974	Ionophore, good efficacy and well tolerated; weak against *E. acervulina*, causes excess water excretion and wet litter
Monensin	Coban, Monelan, Elancoban	Eli Lilly	80–121	1971	The first ionophore, widely used for more than 13 years: still the drug of choice; many side effects, but very well accepted, slow-developing drug resistance; many field isolates causing problems

Drug	Trade names	Level	Company	Year	Comments
Narasin	Monteban	70	Eli Lilly	1983	Ionophore, but not as effective as monensin or salinomycin; introduced with much fanfare but little acceptance in Europe
Nicarbazin	Nicarb, Nicrazin	125	Merck	1955	Highly efficacious, broad-spectrum activity, very little resistance despite its use for many years; many side effects (toxic to layers, depresses growth); interaction with heat stress, depresses growth); still recognized as the best alternative to the ionophores today
Prinicin	Cygro	5(?)	Cyanamid	1984	Ionophore, extremely potent; efficacious against all important coccidia, well tolerated at use level; incomplete cross-resistance with monensin-tolerant field isolates
Robenidine	Robenz, Cycostat	33	Cyanamid	1972	Excellent broad-spectrum activity, well tolerated, some problems with drug resistance; limited use to shuttle programs
Roxarsone	3-Nitro, Nitro-10	50	Salsbury, Rhone-Poulenc	1951	Originally used as drug for coccidiosis, an arsenical used mostly for growth promotion; weakly efficacious against some *Coccidia*, contributes to action of other anticoccidial drugs when used in combination
Salinomycin	Biocox Coxistac Saccox Usten	45–66 50–60 60 50–60	A. H. Robins Pfizer Hoechst Kaken	1983 1978 1983 1979	Ionophore, widely used, some advantages over monensin because of differences in action against certain species, some difference in potency, side effects similar to those with monensin; so far the only serious competitor to monensin; drug tolerance patterns following monensin closely, although not complete cross-resistance
Sulfadimethoxine	Rofenaid	125	Hoffman-LaRoche	1971	Used mostly for antibacterial activity
Sulfaquinoxaline	SQ, Sulquin	150–250	Merck		Widely used for treatment of coccidiosis, limited effectiveness against cecal coccidia; some drug resistance because of its long-term use; depresses weight and has other side effects

extensive tests must be done to demonstrate the safety of the residue. Basically, the establishment of an analytical end point is *de facto* declaration that residues smaller than the limits of sensitivity of the assay are safe. In the European Common Market (EEC) a slightly different approach is used, with the emphasis placed in definition of the toxicity or risk of a residue. Even so, there has been a movement in some European countries toward mandatory withdrawal of all drugs several days prior to slaughter.

5.4. Limitations in the Technology of Feed Manufacture or Other Means of Drug Delivery

Individual administration of medicines to poultry is physically and economically impossible because of the large scale of the poultry industry and the cost of labor. Incorporation of drugs in the feed has been well accepted for more than 30 years. The principal strength of feed medication is quality control from a single location, where samples can be retained for assay routinely. The ability of feed manufacturers to mix feeds adequately with drugs as dilute as 1 ppm has been well established. Water medication is used where immediate treatment of disease is required, although it is considered less accurate and less dependable than feed medication. Water consumption of sick animals is more variable than feed consumption, and the devices used to disperse medications in drinking water are sometimes unreliable. Many drugs cannot be manufactured in water-soluble form.

5.5. Interference of Anticoccidial Drugs with Other Medicaments

Occasionally there is an interaction between drugs used for different purposes. One recent example is the interference between the polyether ionophore anticoccidial drugs and tiamulin, a macrolide antibiotic used for treatment of *Mycoplasma* infections (Meingassner *et al.*, 1979). When monensin or salinomycin is fed at the same time that tiamulin is given in the water or feed, the toxicity of the ionophores is intensified, probably because of interference with the metabolism and excretion of the ionophores by the P450 system in the liver. Other ionophores may not interact in this way.

5.6. Side Effects, Subclinical Toxicity, and Other Effects of Drugs

Drugs are suspected of causing many conditions in practical use, some of which can be proved to be related to the drug and others attributable to other causes. For example, roxarsone and other arsenical drugs cause transient paralysis of the legs in cold weather. If not withdrawn for 3 days, robenidine will leave an undesirable taste in edible tissues, especially the liver. Sulfaquinoxaline may cause hemorrhagic enteritis because of antagonism of vitamin K. In hot weather, nicarbazin will cause excessive death losses from heat stress. In many cases it is impossible to devise laboratory experiments to reproduce a side effect or condition because the exact conditions in commercial poultry houses cannot be duplicated. The behavior of animals in large houses is rarely taken into consideration, yet it may influence the toleration of drugs by poultry or other animals.

6. DRUGS USED IN THE PREVENTION OF COCCIDIOSIS IN POULTRY

6.1. Drugs Used in Broiler Chickens

Because of the large potential market, anticoccidial drugs are usually developed first for use in broilers. Despite the availability of drugs, the actual use of drugs is confined to two or three major products at any time (McDougald and Reid, 1983). After the immediate success of monensin (introduced in 1971), the ionophores were considered the standard for anticoccidial drugs. Today, other ionophores are available, including lasalocid, salinomycin, and narasin, and others are soon to be available. Most of the other available drugs are not used because of widespread drug resistance or limited spectrum of activity. The ionophores have been phenomenally free from drug resistance, even though they have been used more widely and intensively than any other class of drug. Even so, there has been a gradual reduction in sensitivity of coccidia exposed to the ionophores in commercial use (Mathis and McDougald, 1982, 1984; Mathis et al., 1984a,b; Chapman, 1979, 1982b; Voeten and Jansen, 1983). Despite the increasing frequency of coccidia showing reduced sensitivity to ionophores, there is no clear alternative to their use. Poultrymen are increasingly turning to shuttle programs and other management programs in attempting to deal with the increasing incidence of clinical and subclinical coccidiosis. As of this writing, there is no drug under active development that promises to replace the ionophores in overall effectiveness of reliability. The use of drugs to control coccidiosis was reviewed extensively by McDougald (1982) and Ryley and Betts (1973).

6.2. Drugs for Layer Pullets and Other Poultry

Chickens intended as layers or breeders are considered differently than are broilers, for regulatory purposes. Consequently, the newer drugs are usually not available for such uses. Amprolium and zoalene have been the most commonly used in layer or breeder pullets, but these drugs have been used for many years, and drug resistance has limited their effectiveness on many farms (Mathis et al., 1984b; Chapman, 1982a). Monensin is available for layer pullets but not for breeders. Since breeder chickens are kept on litter during production, they must be made immune to coccidia. In most instances, the grower uses a regimen of reducing drug levels to permit increasing exposure to coccidia. In this program, the chickens become immune to coccidiosis through gradually increasing exposure. Unfortunately, the important species of coccidia are not always present, and the drugs do not always work. Alternative programs are badly needed for this application.

Coccidiosis in turkeys is mostly a problem of young birds (Warren et al., 1963). Anticoccidial drugs are used for about 8 weeks; then attention is turned to protection against blackhead disease. The main drugs available for turkeys are amprolium and sulfaquinoxaline. A combination of nitromide and butynorate has also been used. Outside the United States, other drugs can be used by veterinary prescription. Monensin is used sometimes at 60–90 ppm.

No drugs are approved in the United States for use in guinea fowl, quail, or other game birds, although coccidiosis is not considered a frequent problem in such birds. In occasional outbreaks, amprolium or sulfaquinoxaline are used for treatment.

7. TREATMENT OF CLINICAL COCCIDIOSIS

7.1. Poultry

While most effort is directed toward prevention in poultry, outbreaks occur and require treatment. Three classes of drugs are available: (1) the sulfonamides, (2) the potentiated sulfonamides, and (3) amprolium. These drugs are available in water-soluble form, and are usually administered by means of a proportioning device installed in the water system of the poultry house. The potentiated sulfonamides are a combination of a sulfonamide with a 2,4-diaminopyrimidine, which acts at a different step in folate metabolism (see review of synergism in McDougald, 1982). Despite the use of these drugs for many years, recent surveys found these drugs effective except where the spectrum of activity was limited (Mitrovic and Schildknecht, 1973; Mathis et al., 1984b). The treatment drugs act relatively late in the development cycle of coccidia, accounting for effectiveness against established infections.

7.2. Mammalian Coccidiosis

The sparse literature on treatment of coccidiosis in cattle, sheep, goats, rabbits, dogs, cats, and other mammals was reviewed by McDougald (1982). In recent years, the availability of decoquinate, monensin, and lasalocid in cattle and sheep has contributed significantly to reducing losses to coccidiosis in young animals and in feedlots.

8. CRYPTOSPORIDOSIS IN DOMESTIC ANIMALS

Although little known until recently, the etiological agent of cryptosporidosis is now established as a coccidianlike organism, because of its apical complex. Although several species of Cryptosporidium have been named, their lack of host specificity casts doubts on the validity of most of them. Cryptosporidosis in humans is normally a nuisance, except in immune-compromised individuals, such as victims of acquired immune deficiency syndrome (AIDS). Cryptosporidium is reportedly widespread in animals and was recently diagnosed as a cause of respiratory infections in commercial turkeys (Fischer et al., 1975; Hoerr et al., 1978) and chickens (Dhillon et al., 1981).

8.1. Chemotherapy of Cryptosporidosis

There is no known chemotherapeutic agent active against Cryptosporidium. None of these agents known to cure other coccidian or protozoan infections has been effective.

9. *TOXOPLASMA* AND *SARCOCYSTIS* IN DOMESTIC ANIMALS

Both *Toxoplasma* and *Sarcocystis* infections are widespread in domestic animals (Fayer and Reid, 1982) and appear to be most important in pregnant animals. Abortion is common in sheep, cattle, and pigs, which are often infected with *Sarcocystis*. Control or therapy is difficult because of a lack of suitable drugs. The search for drugs active against these parasites has largely been limited to drugs known to be active against other parasites, such as sulfonamides. Amprolium (100 mg/kg for 30 days) reportedly reduces damage in cattle from *S. cruzi*. Sulfadiazine (73 mg/kg) combined with pyrimethamine (0.44 mg/kg) reduces acute toxoplasmosis in laboratory animals (reviewed by Frenkel, 1971; Dubey, 1977).

REFERENCES

Brewer, R. N., and Kowalski, L. M., 1970. Coccidiosis: Evaluation of anticoccidial drugs in floor-pen trials, *Exp. Parasitol.* 28:64–71.

Chapman, H. D., 1978, Drug resistance in coccidia, in: *Avian Coccidiosis* (P. L. Long, K. N. Boorman, and B. M. Freeman, eds.), *Thirteenth Poultry Science Symposium*, pp. 387–412, British Poultry Science, Ltd., Edinburgh.

Chapman, H. D., 1979, Studies on the sensitivity of recent field isolates of *E. maxima* to monensin, *Avian Pathol.* 8:181–186.

Chapman, H. D., 1982a, Anticoccidial drug resistance, in: *The Biology of the Coccidia* (P. L. Long, ed.), pp. 429–452, University Park Press, Baltimore.

Chapman, H. D., 1982b, The sensitivity of field isolates of *Eimeria acervulina* type to monensin, *Vet. Parasitol.* 9:179–183.

Dhillon, A. S., Thacker, H. L., Dietzel, A. V., and Winterfield, R. W., 1981, Respiratory Cryptosporidosis in broiler chickens, *Avian Dis.* 25:747–752.

Dubey, J. P., 1977, *Toxoplasma, Hammondia, Besnoitia, Sarcocystis* and other tissue cyst-forming coccidia of man and animals, in: *Parasitic Protozoa* (J. P. Kreier, ed.), pp. 102–238, Academic Press, New York.

Fayer, R., and Reid, W. M., 1982, Control of coccidiosis, in: *The Biology of the Coccidia* (P. L. Long, ed.), pp. 453–488, University Park Press, Baltimore.

Fletcher, O. J., Munnell, J. F., and Page, R. K., 1975, Cryptosporidosis in the bursa of Fabricius of chickens, *Avian Dis.* 19:630–639.

Frenkel, J. K., 1971, Toxoplasmosis: Mechanism of infection, laboratory diagnosis and management, *Curr. Top. Pathol.* 54:28–75.

Grumbles, L. C., Delaplane, J. P., and Higgins, T. C., 1948, Continuous feeding of low concentrations of sulfaquinoxaline for the control of coccidiosis in poultry, *Poultry Sci.* 27:605–608.

Hoerr, F. J., Ranck, F. M., Jr., and Hastings, T. F., 1978, Respiratory Cryptosporidosis in turkeys, *J. Am. Vet. Med. Assoc.* 173:1591–1593.

Jeffers, T. K., 1974, *Eimeria acervulina* and *E. maxima:* Incidence and anticoccidial drug resistance of isolants in major broiler-producing areas, *Avian Dis.* 18:331–342.

Johnson, J. K., and Reid, W. M., 1970, Anticoccidial drugs: Lesion scoring techniques in battery and floor-pen experiments with chickens, *Exp. Parasitol.* 28:30–36.

Joyner, L. P., and Norton, C. C., 1977, The anticoccidial effects of amprolium, dinitolmide and monensin against *Eimeria maxima, E. brunetti* and *E. acervulina* with particular reference to oocyst sporulation, *Parasitology* 75:155–164.

Keshavarz, K., and McDougald, L. R., 1982, Anticoccidial drugs: Growth and performance depressing effects in young chickens, *Poultry Sci.* 61:699–705.

Kilgore, R. L., 1970, Coccidiosis: Problems involved in obtaining reliable field data, *Exp. Parasitol.* 28:118–121.

Levine, N. D., 1939, The effect of sulfanilamide on the course of experimental avian coccidiosis, *Cornell Vet.* 29:309–320.

Long, P. L., ed., 1982, *The Biology of the Coccidia,* University Park Press, Baltimore, 502 pp.

Mathis, G. F., and McDougald, L. R., 1982, Drug responsiveness of field isolates of chicken coccidia, *Poultry Sci.* 61:38–45.

Mathis, G. F., McDougald, L. R., and McMurray, B., 1984a, Drug sensitivity of coccidia from broiler breeder pullets and from broilers in the same integrated company, *Avian Dis.* 28:453–459.

Mathis, G. F., McDougald, L. R., and McMurray, B., 1984b, Effectiveness of therapeutic anticoccidial drugs against recently isolated coccidia, *Poultry Sci.* 63:1149–1153.

McDougald, L. R., 1982, Chemotherapy of coccidiosis, in: *The Biology of the Coccidia* (P. L. Long, ed.), pp. 373–428, University Park Press, Baltimore.

McDougald, L. R., and Reid, W. M., 1983, New anticoccidial drugs: Better things to come or "endangered species"?, *Feedstuffs* August 15, 55:23–24.

Meingassner, J. G., Schmook, F. P., Czok, R., and Mieth, H., 1979, Enhancement of the anticoccidial activity of polyether antibodies in chickens by tiamulin, *Poultry Sci.* 58:308–313.

Mitchell, G. A., and Scoggins, R. W., 1970, Avian *Eimeria* infection technique: Suspended seeder cage, *Exp. Parasitol.* 28:87–89.

Mitrovic, M., and Schildknecht, E. G., 1973, Comparative chemotherapeutic efficacy of Agribon® (sulfadimethoxine) and other agents against coccidiosis in chickens and turkeys, *Poultry Sci.* 52:1253–1260.

Pellerdy, L. P., 1974, *Coccidia and Coccidiosis,* Akademiai Kiado, Budapest.

Reid, W. M., 1972, Anticoccidials used in the poultry industry: Time of action against the coccidial life cycle, *Folia Vet. Lat.* 2:641–667.

Reid, W. M., 1973, Anticoccidials: Differences in day of peak activity against *Eimeria tenella,* in: *Proceedings of the Symposium on Coccidia and Related Organisms,* pp. 119–134, University of Guelph, Guelph, Ontario.

Reid, W. M., Taylor, E. M., and Johnson, J. K., 1969, A technique for demonstration of coccidiostatic activity of anticoccidial agents, *Trans. Am. Microsc. Soc.* 88:148–159.

Ruff, M. D., Reid, W. M., Dykstra, D. D., and Johnson, J. K., 1978, Efficacy of arprinocid against coccidiosis of broilers in battery and floor pen trials, *Avian Dis.* 22:32–41.

Ryley, J. F., and Betts, M. J., 1973, Chemotherapy of chicken coccidiosis, *Adv. Pharmacol. Chemother.* 2:221–293.

Voeten, A. C., and Jansen, B. A. P., 1983, The monitoring and evalution of coccidiostats in broilers, *Arch. Gefluegelkd.* 47:181–185.

Wang, C. C., and Simashkevich, P. M., 1980, A comparative study of the biological activities of arprinocid and arprinocid-1-N-oxide, *Biochem. Parasitol.* 1:335–345.

Warren, E. W., Ball, S. J., and Fagg, J. R., 1963, Age resistance by turkeys to *Eimeria meleagrimitis* Tyzzer, 1929, *Nature (Lond.)* 200:238–240.

8

Hemoprotozoan Infections of Domestic Animals

Trypanosomiasis, Babesiosis, Theileriosis, and Anaplasmosis

KENNETH L. KUTTLER and JULIUS P. KREIER

1. INTRODUCTION

Arthropod-transmitted hemoparasitic diseases, caused by *Trypanosoma, Babesia, Theileria,* and *Anaplasma,* occur throughout the world but are frequently of greatest importance in the tropics and subtropics, where conditions are favorable to the maintenance of vector populations. Vector control and chemotherapy are the primary defenses against these disease agents. Vaccines that prevent these infections have yet to be developed. The attenuated or live vaccines described for anaplasmosis, babesiosis, and theileriosis often depend on specific therapy to reduce the severity of infection while allowing the development of a premunizing immunity (Kuttler, 1979; Todorovic, 1974; Radley, 1981). Chemotherapy, chemoimmunization, and chemoprophylaxis thus comtinue to play an important role in hemoparasitic disease management and prevention. Even so, chemotherapy is not without problems; drug-resistant microorganisms arise, drug residues in tissues of food animals may be detected and prompt removal of the drug from its approved status, and the cost of drugs may be too high for use by poor farmers. The expense and difficulty in developing new replacement compounds for those no longer used for one reason or another are also a serious problem in the world today.

2. EXPERIMENTAL METHODS

Experimental rodent models are available for most of the pathogenic trypanosomes that lend themselves to drug-screening trials. Although useful, the need persists for

KENNETH L. KUTTLER • U.S. Department of Agriculture, Agricultural Research Service, Hemoparasitic Diseases Research Unit, Washington State University, Pullman, Washington 99164. JULIUS P. KREIER • Department of Microbiology, Ohio State University, Columbus, Ohio 43210.

trials with the primary host because of such factors as host tolerance, tissue residues, and differences in drug susceptibility among the many pathogenic trypanosomes.

Until the development of methods for the *in vitro* growth of *Theileria*, treatment trials were limited to inducing infection followed by treatment of the infected animals at various time intervals. The expense and time required for such trials severely limited the number of compounds that could be tested. The *in vitro* cultivation of *T. parva* macroschizonts in lymphoblasts (Malmquist *et al.*, 1970) contributed to the development of screening techniques that led to the discovery of the more effective quinone compounds (McHardy *et al.*, 1976). These techniques continue to provide the method of choice for screening potentially new compounds.

The absence of suitable *in vitro* methods of growth for *Anaplasma* and the *Babesias* (except for *B. bovis* and *B. divergens*) has created problems in mass screening of compounds for therapeutic efficacy. Most preliminary experimental drug trials designed to evaluate drug efficacy for anaplasmosis are conducted using splenectomized calves. In these cases, infection is induced and treatment given at the onset of parasitemia and the course of infection among the treated and nontreated (or placebo group) calves compared. Drug efficacy is usually determined using parameters such as packed cell volume (PCV), percentage drop in PCV, parasitemia, rate of recovery, and survivability.

A unique treatment consideration for anaplasmosis is the need in some circumstances to remove clinically nonapparent carrier infections. These trials are expensive and time consuming, requiring lengthy observation following treatment. To ensure that the infection has been entirely eliminated, subinoculation of blood from the treated cow to a susceptible splenectomized calf is usually required. The disappearance of a serological response, as measured by complement fixation, is presumptive evidence of a successful treatment program but cannot be relied on.

The same basic methods are used to evaluate drugs with potential babesiacidal activity. In addition to these methods, some rodent and tissue-culture models can be used. *Babesia rodhaini* infections in mice have been used to screen potential babesiacidal compounds (Beveridge, 1953; Lucas, 1960). Caution is recommended in such trials, since results can be misleading. An example is that diminazene, while highly effective against *B. bigemina* and *B. bovis*, is not equally as effective against *B. rodhaini* (Kuttler, 1981). The recent development of tissue-culture techniques for the *in vitro* propagation of *B. bovis* (Erp *et al.*, 1978; Levy and Ristic, 1980), the adaptation of *B. divergens* to the Mongolian gerbil (Lewis and Williams, 1979), and its growth on tissue cultures (Vayrynen and Tuomi, 1982) provide additional models for evaluating drug efficacy. It has been found that babesiacidal drugs will inhibit the uptake of tritiated purines such as hypoxanthine (Irvin and Young, 1977, 1979). This *in vitro* technique should prove a valuable asset in future drug-screening programs.

3. TRYPANOSOMIASIS

3.1. *Clinical Importance of Chemotherapy and Chemoprophylaxis*

In the absence of effective vaccines, and because of the limitations of vector control, chemotherapy and chemoprophylaxis (Table I) remain the major defenses against trypanosomiasis of livestock.

Table 1. Chemotherapy of Trypanosomiasis in Domestic Animals

Compound class	Generic name	Trade name	Treatment data	
			Dose and route (mg/kg)	Susceptible trypanosomes
Quinoline pyrimidine	Quinapyramine dimethyl sulfate or chloride[a]	Antrycide sulfate or Antrycide prosalt	5.0 sc	vivax, congolense, brucei, equiperdum, simiae (?) evansi
Phenanthridine	Homidium chloride or bromide[b]	Ethidium bromide, Ethidium chloride, Novidium chloride, Barbidium	1.0 im	vivax, congolense, brucei
Aromatic diamidine	Diminazene aceturate[c]	Berenil, Ganaseg	3.5–7.0 im	vivax, congolense, brucei, evansi
Phenanthridine aromatic amidine	Isometamidium chloride[b]	Samorin Trypamidium	0.5–2.0 im	vivax, congolense
Sulfonated naphthylamine	Suramin[d]	Moranyl, Nagarol, Antrypol, Bayer 205, Naphuride, Germanin	7.0–10.0 iv	evansi, brucei, equiperdum
Phenanthridine pyrimidine	Pyrithidium bromide[e]	Prothidium	2.0 im	vivax, congolense

[a]ICI Ltd. Wilmslow, England.
[b]May and Baker, Ltd. Dagenham, England.
[c]Farbwerke Hoechst Ag. Frankfurt, W. Germany.
[d]Bayer Co. Leverkusen, W. Germany.
[e]Boots Pure Drug Co., Ltd. Nottingham, England.

Effective treatment of trypanosomiasis is frequently limited by the rapid development of drug resistance, by toxicity, and by the damaging cutaneous necrosis produced by some of the trypanocidal agents in use (Aliu, 1981; Leach and Roberts, 1981). The absence of any new commercially available compounds since 1955 has led to reliance on the same drugs, in turn exacerbating the resistance problem (Williamson, 1979). Treatment—symptomatic, curative, and preventive—still relies on the use of six basic compounds: quinapyramine, homidium, pyrithidium, isometamidium, diminazene, and suramin. Because of the problems associated with drug resistance, these compounds are often used in sequence and in combination with reasonable success (Aliu, 1981).

3.2. Trypanosoma brucei, T. evansi, and T. simiae

Quinapyramine remains the most effective drug for the treatment of T. brucei and T. evansi in horses, even though it is poorly tolerated. Quinapyramine as a complex with suramin has shown good prophylactic properties for horses, with periods of protection of 6–29 months, depending on the dose level and the severity of challenge (Gill and Malhotra, 1971). The drug of choice in T. evansi infections in camels is also quinapyramine; however, suramin given at the level of 7–10 mg/kg iv is usually effective, although there are some drug-resistant strains. Suramin-resistant strains of T. evansi are usually sensitive to quinapyramine (Aliu, 1981). Dogs infected with T. brucei are successfully treated with quinapyramine (5 mg/kg), diminazene (7 mg/kg sc), or suramin (7–10 mg/kg iv). Left untreated, this infection in dogs is often fatal. Swine infected with T. brucei may be treated successfully with either homidium or quinapyramine, but T. simiae infections proceed so rapidly that treatment is often ineffective (Williamson, 1979). Trypanosoma simiae in swine may be prevented by prophylactic administration of isometamidium (12.5–35 mg/kg), or quinapyramine (7.5 mg/kg sc) plus diminazene (5 mg/kg sc) (Aliu, 1981).

3.3. T. vivax and T. congolense

Trypanosoma vivax and T. congolense infections in cattle can be treated successfully with isometamidium or with diminazene, and often with both. If these compounds are used properly, the problem of drug resistance is greatly reduced (Wilson et al., 1975). When trypanosomes are encountered, the entire herd should be considered for treatment, as the infection is probably not limited to sick animals or to those with positive blood smears. In tsetse areas, regular periodic treatment is often required. Over a 20-year period, one successful program involved the prophylactic injection of quinapyramine (antrycide pro-salt) to each animal every 2 months. After 7 years, because of the fear of drug resistance, this was replaced by diminazene (Berenil) given at monthly intervals for 3 years. After this, isometamidium (Samorin) was given every 3 months for 3 years and then diminazene for a year, with an alternating pattern back to isometamidium and diminazene (Ford and Blaser, 1971). Infections that relapse after treatment should always be treated with a different drug than that initially used. At present, alternate treatments with isometamidium and diminazene are preferred.

Isometamidium has been successfully used to treat the *T. vivax* infections in sheep and cattle that occur in Venezuela. These infections, which occur in the absence of tsetse, are probably transmitted by horse flies. Isometamidium is reportedly well tolerated and treatment has protected animals for 118–195 days (Toro *et al.*, 1983). The infection of cattle with *T. brucei* is usually mild, but if treatment is indicated either quinapyramine or diminazene is effective.

3.4. New Compounds of Potential Value

Many new treatments use combinations of drugs, including one or more of the basic trypanocidal compounds. Isometamidium is very irritating, often producing ulcerative skin or muscle lesions (Williamson, 1979). A marked decrease in local and systemic reactions is noted when the isometamidium (2 mg/kg) is complexed with the polyanion dextransulfate (Aliu and Sannusi, 1979). Other promising new compounds and combinations include diminazene plus potassium aluminum sulfate (Toure *et al.*, 1979); nitroimidazoles (Cuckler *et al.*, 1970); Berenil and nitroimidazole combinations (Jennings *et al.*, 1980); suramin–tryparsamide complex (Gill, 1971); salichydroxamic acid (Evans and Holland, 1978); DAPI, a diamidine derivative (Dann *et al.*, 1971); sinefungin (Dube *et al.*, 1983); and bleomycin (Tadasuke and Nakabayashi, 1980). Large-scale drug-screening procedures have demonstrated potentially useful trypanocidal activity in a group of benzyl and triphenyl phosphonium salts (Kinnamon *et al.*, 1979). It has also been found that some antitumor drugs have antitrypanosomal activity (Kinnamon *et al.*, 1980). The terephthalanilides given at low doses were the most active.

Even though there have been no new commercially available trypanocides introduced during the past 20 years, there has been considerable progress in the basic understanding of trypanosomal biology, which should aid the search for chemotherapeutic agents and perhaps put it on a more rational basis.

4. BABESIOSIS

4.1. Clinical Importance of Chemotherapy and Chemoprophylaxis

In the treatment of babesiosis, drug selection and dosage are determined by the objectives of treatment. Different drugs and dosages are chosen to moderate clinical signs, to eliminate the infectious organism, or to prevent infection. The compound selected and its dose are also influenced by the *Babesia* species causing the infection, the drug tolerance of the vertebrate being treated, and the purpose of treatment. The large number of *Babesia* species, with their distinctive hosts, complicates the selection of appropriate babesiacidal compounds.

As the result of a successful *Boophilus* tick-eradication program, bovine babesiosis does not occur in the United States (Graham and Hourrigan, 1977). In most areas of the world, however, ticks have not been eradicated, and the disease persists (McCosker,

1981), controlled by a variety of measures, including chemotherapy and chemoprophylaxis.

Numerous chemical compounds, some of which are listed in Table II, have been used in the treatment of babesiosis with varying degrees of success. In addition to the use of babesiacidal compounds, supportive treatment should not be overlooked. If specific and effective chemotherapy is given early in the course of infection before the onset of severe anemia or nervous system disorders, recovery without supportive treatment is the rule. If delayed, however, supportive treatment including blood transfusions, fluids, vitamins, hematinics, and good nourishment becomes essential to survival (Kuttler, 1981).

Therapy of babesiosis is usually concerned with moderating clinical signs. Some of the babesiacidal drugs are so effective that one treatment will eliminate the causative agent. Such treatment is desirable in that reservoirs of infection are eliminated, but it may be undesirable if the animal is to be kept in an endemic zone in which reexposure is likely to occur (DeVos, 1979). Elimination of infection by treatment is usually followed by a period of immunity, but this eventually wanes, rendering the animal susceptible to reinfection (Lewis *et al.*, 1981).

Most of the babesiacidal compounds are toxic to the host, so caution is required in their use, and it is necessary to stay within the tolerance levels of each species of animal. Drug-resistant babesias can be developed experimentally and probably occur in nature, but this problem has not yet evolved as a major constraint in treating babesiosis as it has for trypanosomiasis (Dalgliesh and Stewart, 1977).

The large babesias such as *B. bigemina*, *B. canis*, and *B. caballi* respond more readily to treatment, frequently at lower drug doses than their smaller counterparts, *B. bovis*, *B. gibsoni*, and *B. equi*.

4.2. Treatment of Cattle Babesias

Trypan blue was probably the first compound used successfully to treat cattle babesiosis (Theiler, 1912). An intravenous injection at the rate of 2–3 mg/kg body weight is effective against *B. bigemina* but is ineffective against *B. bovis* (Rees, 1934). This compound has the disadvantage of producing discoloration of the animal's flesh and body secretions. If injected extravascularly, it is highly irritating and may produce tissue sloughing. It is also effective against *B. caballi* and not *B. equi* of horses and against *B. canis* of dogs. Its use is usually limited to dogs, and then only under special circumstances (Moore, 1979).

The quinoline derivatives for many years were the drugs of choice for the treatment of bovine babesiosis (Kuttler, 1981). These drugs, however, have a low therapeutic index and may produce transient side effects including excessive salivation, rapid and labored breathing, frequent urination, and general restlessness. Such reactions usually disappear in about an hour and may be moderated by atropine (Eyre, 1967).

Quinuronium is used successfully in the treatment of either *B. bigemina* or *B. bovis* at the rate of 1 mg/kg given once or twice with a 24-hr interval between doses (Barnett, 1965). This treatment is also effective against the disease caused by *B. divergens* (Purnell

Table II. Chemotherapy of Babesiosis in Domestic Animals

Compound class	Generic name	Trade name	Treatment data	
			Dose and route mg/kg	Susceptible Babesia species
Azonaphthalene dyes	Trypan blue	Congo blue, Niagara blue, Trypan blue	2.0–3.0 iv	bigemina, caballi, canis
Acridine derivatives	Acriflavine hydro-chloride[a]	Gonacrine	2.2 iv	bigemina, bovis
Quinoline derivatives	Quinuronium sulfate[b]	Acaprin, Akiron, Pirevan, Piroplasmin, Babesan[c]	1.0–2.0 sc or im	bigemina, bovis, divergens, caballi, motasi
Diamidine derivatives Aromatic	Diminazene diaceturate[d]	Berenil,[d] Ganaseg[e]	3.0–7.0 im	bigemina, bovis, divergens, ovata, caballi, equi, motasi, perroncitoi, canis, gibsoni
	Pentamidine isethio-nate[a]	Lomidine	2.0–16.0 sc or im	bigemina, canis, gibsoni
	Phenamidine isethio-nate[a]	Lomadine	8.0–13.0 sc	bigemina, caballi, canis, gibsoni
Carbanilide	Amicarbalide diisethio-nate[a]	Diampron	5.0–10.0 im	bigemina, bovis, divergens, caballi, ovata
	Imidocarb dipropionate[f] (and dihydrochloride)	Imizol	1.0–5.0 sc or im	bigemina, bovis, caballi, equi, canis, motasi, ovis divergens

[a]May and Baker Ltd., Dagenham, England.
[b]Bayer Co., Leverkusen, W. Germany.
[c]Imperial Chemical Industries Ltd., Macclesfield, England.
[d]Farbwerke Hoechst Ag., Frankfurt, W. Germany.
[e]Squibb Mathieson, E.R. Squibb & Sons de Mexico, Mexico.
[f]Burroughs Wellcome Co. Ltd., London, England.

et al., 1981); however, it does not eliminate infection. A relatively insoluble salt of quinuronium given as a 1-g implant will prevent *B. bovis* and *B. divergens* infections for over 21 days (Newton and O'Sullivan, 1969; Ryley, 1964). Quinuronium may be used to treat *B. canis* infections, but it is not recommended for *B. gibsoni* infections (Groves and Dennis, 1972).

Although acridine derivatives are effective, they appear to have been largely replaced by the diamidine derivatives. Acriflavine is reportedly effective against both *B. bigemina* and *B. bovis* at the rate of 2.2 mg/kg given as a 5% solution intravenously (Riek, 1968).

A wide variety of diamidine derivatives have proved effective and safe in the treatment of babesiosis. Probably the most commonly used compounds are diminazene, imidocarb, amicarbalide, phenamidine, and pentamidine (Barnett, 1965).

Diminazene is one of the compounds most commonly used to treat babesiosis in domestic animals. It is effective against *B. bigemina*, *B. bovis*, *B. ovata*, and *B. divergens* in cattle and is used usually in a dose range of 3–5 mg/kg im (Kuttler, 1981; Barnett, 1965). In horses, *B. caballi* is susceptible to diminazene at 5 mg/kg given twice within a 24-hr interval between doses (Kirkham, 1969), but 6–12 mg/kg given twice with a 24-hr interval between doses is required for therapy of *B. equi* (Singh *et al.*, 1980*a*). Treatment at 6 mg/kg will not eliminate *B. equi*, and relapses following treatment at this dose level can be expected; however, doses of 12 mg/kg given two times with a 24-hr interval between doses has been reported to eliminate infection (Singh *et al.*, 1980*a*). In dogs, administration of as little as 2.5–3.5 mg/kg diminazene has been successful in treating *B. canis* infection, but 5–7 mg/kg is required for treatment of *B. gibsoni* infection (Moore, 1979; Dennig *et al.*, 1980). Administration of diminazene at 4–5 mg/kg is reported to eliminate *B. canis* in some instances. Diminazene administered at 7.5–10 mg/kg has been observed to produce severe CNS disorders in dogs, including nystagmus, ataxia, extensor rigidity, opisthotonus, coma, and even death (Farwell *et al.*, 1982). Toxicity can be minimized by extending the time interval in which the drug is given.

Pentamidine, at 0.5–2.0 mg/kg sc usually brings about clinical recovery of cattle acutely infected with *B. bigemina*. As much as 5 mg/kg, however, failed to eliminate carrier infections. For this reason, pentamidine has been recommended for use in chemoimmunization procedures in which induction of carrier infections, while avoiding severe clinical reactions, is desirable (Pipano *et al.*, 1979).

Phenamidine has been used with success to treat infections with the large babesias, *B. bigemina*, *B. caballi*, and *B. canis* (Aliu, 1983). Levels of 8–13 mg/kg im are generally required. Two doses of phenamidine at 10 and 5 mg/kg, given 3 days apart, were reported to be effective against *B. gibsoni* infection (Ruff *et al.*, 1973).

Amicarbalide was shown to be active against *B. divergens* infection (Beveridge *et al.*, 1960). It is also effective against *B. bigemina* and *B. bovis* in cattle at the level of 10 mg/kg im (Aliu, 1983). Two doses of 8.8 mg/kg im at 24-hr intervals eliminated *B. caballi* infections of horses, but 11 mg/kg im given four times at 24- and 48-hr intervals did not eliminate *B. equi* infections. Only four of eight horses became free of *B. equi* infection when treated by injection of 22 mg/kg daily for 7 days (Taylor *et al.*, 1972).

Imidocarb, a diamidine of the carbanilide series, has recently been found effective in the treatment and prevention of babesiosis (Kuttler, 1981; Todorovic et al., 1973). The early formulation using the dihydrochloride salt has been replaced by a dipropionate formulation. In cattle, imidocarb is used safely for the treatment of B. bigemina, B. bovis, and B. divergens at 1–3 mg/kg sc or im. Imidocarb is not recommended for intravenous use. Imidocarb at 1–3 mg/kg generally eliminates the infection. The simultaneous administration of 0.15 mg/kg imidocarb and live attenuated B. bovis vaccine has allowed carrier infection without serious clinical signs to develop (Taylor and McHardy, 1979). Imidocarb at 2 mg/kg was effective for 6–8 weeks in preventing clinical babesiosis due to B. divergens, and clinical babesiosis due to B. bigemina for up to 61 days (Haigh and Hagan, 1974). This prophylactic effect has been used to protect cattle being shipped from Babesia-free areas to endemic zones of the tropics. Treatment given a group of 44 Charolais Babesia-free heifers with 2.8 mg/kg imidocarb before movement into a Babesia-endemic zone prevented clinical babesiosis and death, even though 70% showed serological evidence of infection 130 days after entering the endemic area (Day and Kuttler, 1975). Imidocarb is slowly metabolized, resulting in persistent tissue levels (Aliu et al., 1977). For this reason, its use is restricted in some countries to animals not used for human consumption. It is also toxic under some conditions notwithstanding a generally high therapeutic index for Babesia. Transient side effects of excessive salivation, lacrimation, increased frequency of defecation, and rapid breathing may be noticed for 30–40 min after injection. Fatal toxicosis in cattle may result when doses in excess of 15 mg/kg are given. Death attributable to imidocarb is associated with renal hyperemia and enlargement, pulmonary congestion, edema, hydrothorax, and hydroperitoneum. Renal lesions induced consist mainly of severe cellular necrosis in the proximal convoluted tubules (Adams et al., 1980).

4.3. Treatment of Other Babesias of Domestic Animals

Babesiosis in horses, caused by both B. equi and B. caballi, may be treated with imidocarb. One injection of 2 mg/kg is usually sufficient to bring about a clinical remission of infection due to B. caballi, and two injections 24 hr apart will usually clear up the infection (Frerichs and Holbrook, 1974). Babesia equi is more refractory to treatment, usually requiring two doses of 5 mg/kg 48 hr apart (Singh et al., 1980a). This treatment schedule reportedly cures B. equi carrier infection, but the usual treatment to cure infection is to give four doses of 4 mg/kg at 72-hr intervals (Frerichs et al., 1973). This latter procedure was reported to clear B. equi infections in 13 of 14 horses. Transient toxic side effects are seen in horses, so that the 4-mg/kg dose is usually divided, the second half-dose being given 30–40 min after the initial. The transient side effects consist of extreme restlessness, sweating, and signs of abdominal pain. Imidocarb is the compound of choice for eliminating B. equi infection. Imidocarb (3–5 mg/kg) has been used to treat B. canis infections in dogs, and there is some indication that it has prophylactic activity as well (Euzeby et al., 1980). Babesia ovis infection in sheep was relatively resistant to imidocarb given as a single treatment (2 mg/kg sc), but three treatments of 2 mg/kg sc proved successful (Michael and Refaii, 1982).

It is possible that overreliance on these highly effective babesiacidal drugs has led to some neglect of supportive and symptomatic treatment. With the increasing numbers of babesiosis cases occurring in companion animals, greater emphasis is being given to supportive treatment, and the extrapolation of these techniques to large food-producing animals is indicated in selected cases and should probably receive greater attention in the future.

5. THEILERIOSIS

5.1. Clinical Importance of Cattle Theilerias

Theileria parva (East Coast fever), *Theileria annulata* (tropical theileriosis, Mediterranean Coast fever), *Theileria mutans* (tzaneen disease), and *T. lawrencei* (corridor disease) are pathogenic *Theileria*, which are responsible for losses of cattle. Until only a few years ago, there was no effective specific treatment for acute theileriosis other than symptomatic and supportive therapy. Aliu (1983) describes trials of various chemotherapeutic compounds that did not show activity against theileriosis. The aminoquinolines, first reported by Neitz (1950), appeared to be effective against the intraerythrocytic piroplasms but were not effective against the schizonts. Pyrimethamine has limited antitheilerial activity, which is enhanced by combining it with sulfonamides or chloroquine. Even so, it is not sufficiently active for use as a specific therapeutic agent for theileriosis (Wilde, 1967).

5.2. Tetracyclines in the Chemoprophylaxis and Treatment of Cattle

The tetracyclines were probably the first compounds to be used successfully in treating theileriosis caused by *T. parva*, but they are primarily effective prophylactically, and then only in large dosages. Chlortetracycline given at the rate of 10 mg/kg iv daily after tick exposure and until schizonts began to decrease in numbers prevented fatal infection (Neitz, 1953). Given orally both chlortetracycline daily at 1.5 mg/kg for 28 days after exposure and oxytetracycline daily at 10–15 mg/kg for 28 days were effective in preventing death (Brocklesby and Bailey, 1962; Neitz, 1957). The number of treatments required following *T. parva* infection has been reduced as improved tetracycline formulations have been developed. Methods of chemoimmunization have been developed in which infective *T. parva* stabilates were inoculated followed by injections of oxytetracycline at 5–10 mg/kg for 4–6 days. This treatment allowed the development of immunity without the serious clinical manifestations of theileriosis seen in controls (Radley et al., 1975a–c). The introduction of a new, long-acting oxytetracycline formulation (LA 200) has permitted a reduction in the number of treatments to a single injection of 20 mg/kg given im on the day of stabilate exposure (Brown et al., 1977a,b; Radley et al., 1979).

It is generally accepted that the tetracyclines have only limited value as therapeutic agents for theileriosis caused by *T. parva*, but a recent report does indicate some

Table III. Chemotherapy of Theileriosis in Domestic Animals

Compound class	Generic name	Trade name	Dose and route (mg/kg)	Regimen
				Treatment data
Tetracyclines	Oxytetracycline[a]	Liquamycin 50 mg/ml (Terramycin)	5–15 iv	4–6 times daily after initial exposure, or early in infection
		Long-acting terramycin LA 200, 200 mg/ml	20.0 im	1–2 times after initial exposure
	Chlortetracycline[b]	Aureomycin	1.5 orally	Daily for 28 days
	Rolitetracycline[c]	Reverin	4.0 im	4 times daily, beginning on day of exposure
Naphthoquinones	Menoctone[d]		10.0 im or iv	Curative: 1 time
	993 C[c]		20.0 im	Curative: 1 time
Quinazolinones	Halofuginone lactate[c]	Stenorol	1.2 orally	Curative: 1 time

[a]Pfizer Inc., New York, N.Y.
[b]American Cyanimide, Pearl River, N.Y.
[c]Farbwerke Hoechst Ag., Frankfurt, W. Germany.
[d]Sterling Winthrop, New York, N.Y.
[e]Burroughs Wellcome & Co., Ltd., London, England.

therapeutic efficacy (Brown et al., 1977b). Treatment at 10 mg/kg for 5 days, beginning at the onset of fever, was found to be ineffective. Treatment of 15 mg/kg for 5 days, when started on the first day schizonts were seen in the lymph nodes, protected 9 of 10 cattle from death. The therapeutic efficacy of the tetracyclines should be viewed with caution, as conflicting results have been reported (Dolan, 1981).

Tetracyclines display both therapeutic and prophylactic activity against theileriosis caused by T. annulata (Pipano et al., 1981). Rolitetracycline was found to moderate clinical infection when administered daily for 4 days at 4 mg/kg im beginning on the day of stabilate inoculation (Jagdish et al., 1980). Cattle were immune to further challenge with T. annulata. Similar results were observed following a single injection of the long-acting oxytetracycline formulation (LA 200) at 20 mg/kg im (Khanna et al., 1983). Oxytetracycline used therapeutically at 10–15 mg/kg per day iv for 4–6 days beginning on the day of patency prevented death (Singh et al., 1980b). The combination of diminazene and oxytetracline at 10 mg and 15 mg/kg, respectively, given two times with a 3-day interval between doses, proved effective in treating patent infections caused by T. annulata (Tripathy, 1981).

5.3. New Agents in the Chemotherapy of Cattle

In 1976, McHardy et al. discovered that an antimalarial compound, a hydroxyalkylated naphthoquinone called menoctone, had a marked effect on both T. parva and T. annulata in vitro. In subsequent clinical trials, menoctone has proved highly effective in treating acute theileriosis (T. parva) (McHardy and Rae, 1981). One injection of 10 mg/kg im or iv effectively controlled the disease process when given as late as 4 days after the disease became apparent. The intramuscular route was preferred over the intravenous, and oral administration proved ineffective. Because of the expense and limited supply of menoctone, a search for a reasonable alternative was made. A closely related analogue designated 993C was identified that also had a high level of therapeutic activity (McHardy, 1979). A single intramuscular injection of 993C at 20 mg/kg (in 20% dimethylsulfoxide and 80% corn oil), or two injections of 10 mg/kg each, with a 48-hr interval between doses, had a therapeutic efficacy for infection with T. parva roughly comparable to that of menoctone. Treatment rapidly reduces the fever and produces a marked degeneration of macroschizonts. Cattle treated prophylactically neither became infected nor developed a serological response and were fully susceptible to a later T. parva challenge. Cattle with established T. annulata infections given 993C in clinical trials recovered. In these trials, 993C was administered at 20 mg/kg im 3 days after the appearance of schizonts and the development of fever (Gill et al., 1981).

The anticoccidial compound, halofuginone, has in recent years also been shown to possess marked antitheilerial activity (Schein and Voigt, 1979, 1981). Cattle showing active clinical infections of both T. parva and T. annulata recovered after treatment with halofuginone (1–2 mg/kg given orally), whereas untreated controls died. Within 12 hr the fever was gone and within 24 hr schizont degeneration was evident. Activity of halofuginone against T. parva and T. lawrencei was confirmed by Uilenberg et al. (1980). Treatment did not produce as marked an effect on T. mutans as on T. annulata.

In the former, treatment caused only a temporary reduction in parasitemia. There is a narrow tolerance range for halofuginone. Oral administration of 2 mg/kg produced a transient diarrhea, and at ≥ 3 mg/kg more severe toxic effects are detected, including profuse diarrhea, cachexia, conjunctivitis, and subnormal temperature. At doses of 5 mg/kg, severe intestinal hemorrhage and bloody diarrhea developed and death sometimes occurred. The insoluble hydrobromide of halofuginone has been replaced by the water-soluble lactate, which is somewhat better tolerated. Halofuginone does not appear to be active against *Theileria* in the incubation stages of infection.

Comparisons between 993C and halofuginone confirm the activity of these two compounds but suggest greater activity of 993C, at least in the dosages tested (Morgan and McHardy, 1982). Halofuginone was active against *T. lawrencei;* however, it was less effective than were previous trials with *T. parva* (DeVos and Roos, 1983).

Other anticoccidial compounds, the ionophores, such as monensin and lasalocid, have exhibited some *in vitro* activity against *Theileria* (Dolan, 1981; McHardy and Rae, 1982). The relatively recent discovery of menoctone, 993C, and halofuginone has renewed the hope that successful chemotherapy may be developed for theileriosis. No evidence of tolerance by *Theileria* for these drugs has been seen, but this could be attributable in part to the newness of these compounds. Over a period of time, drug resistance could occur, necessitating the continued search for new and effective compounds.

6. ANAPLASMOSIS

6.1. *Tetracyclines in the Treatment of Anaplasmosis*

Before the development of tetracyclines, treatment of acute anaplasmosis was symptomatic and was designed to moderate the clinical manifestations of infection and to reduce death losses with no thought of clearing or eliminating infection. The procedures commonly used included blood transfusions, administration of hematinics, providing good feed, water, and care to avoid physical stress, and other problems. Although these techniques were often ineffective used alone, they are not without merit and are now often unwisely neglected because of the efficacy and availability of specific chemotherapeutic compounds.

The specific activity of chlortetracycline for anaplasmosis was reported by Foote *et al.* (1951). The parenteral administration of oxytetracycline (intramuscularly or intravenously), or tetracycline hydrochloride (intravenously) at 6.6–11 mg/kg of body weight is recommended for the treatment of acute anaplasmosis. Depending on individual circumstances, one to three treatments may be required. The degree of success is enhanced by early treatment of acute infections. If treatment is given before the packed cell volume drops below 15%, recovery is the rule (Kuttler, 1980).

A relatively new oxytetracycline formulation containing 200 mg/ml (long-acting terramycin, LA 200) has recently been introduced. In a study comparing the latter formulation with one containing 50 mg/ml (Liquamycin T-50), a single intramuscular

Table IV. Chemotherapy of Anaplasmosis (Anaplasma marginale) in Domestic Animals

Compound class	Generic name	Trade name	Dose and route (mg/kg)	Treatment data — Regimen
Tetracycline	Oxytetracycline[a]	Liquamycin (50 mg/ml)	11 im or iv	Therapeutic: 1–3 times as indicated
			11 im or iv	Curative: daily 10–12 times
		Terramycin LA (200 mg/ml)	20 im	Therapeutic: 1–2 times as indicated
			20 im	Curative: 4 times, 3-day interval
	Chlortetracycline[b]	Aureomycin	11 orally	Curative: daily for 45–60 days
			1.1 orally	Prophylactic and possibly curative daily for 120 days
	Tetracycline hydrochloride[b]	Polyotic	11 im or iv	Therapeutic: 1–3 times as indicated
			11 im or iv	Curative: Daily, for 10–12 days
Diamidine (carbanilide)	Imidocarb dipropionate[c]	Imizol	3–5.0 sc or im	Therapeutic: 1 time
			5.0 sc or im	Curative: 3 times at 24- or 48-hr interval
Dithiosemicarbazone	Gloxazone[c]	Gloxazone, 356C61	4.0 sc or im	Curative: 2 times at 14-day interval
		Gloxazone + Liquamycin	5 iv	Therapeutic: 1–2 times at 24-hr interval
			5 Gloxazone iv and	Curative: 3 times at 24- or 48-hr interval
			11 Liquamycin iv	

[a]Pfizer, Inc. New York, N.Y.
[b]American Cyanimide Co., Pearl River, N.Y.
[c]Buroughs Wellcome Co., Ltd., London, England.

injection of LA 200 at 20 mg/kg appeared to be equivalent to three daily intramuscular injections of 10 mg/kg of T-50 (Kuttler and Simpson, 1978). This new formulation (LA 200) is reported to produce sustained blood concentrations of oxytetracycline (Roby and Simpson, 1978) and generally is the drug of choice in treating acute anaplasmosis. Other tetracyclines, such as doxycycline and minocycline, are also useful for treating anaplasmosis (Kuttler and Simpson, 1978; Mazzola and Kuttler, 1981).

Much larger amounts of these tetracyclines given over an extended period of time are usually required to eliminate infection. Oral chlortetracycline fed at the rate of 11 mg/kg per day for 45–60 days reportedly eliminates carrier infection (Roby et al., 1970; Brock et al., 1959). Although a very effective approach, it has the disadvantage of being time consuming and expensive. The cattle are usually confined during the feeding period. If good pasture is available, the consumption of chlortetracycline may be sporadic, hence ineffective. Chlortetracycline orally at levels as low as 2.2–5.5 mg/kg per day for 60 days, and 1.1 mg/kg per day for 120 days has been reported to eliminate carrier infections (Franklin et al., 1965, 1966, 1967).

Administration of oxytetracycline (50-mg/ml formulation) or tetracycline hydrochloride (at 11 mg/kg per day im or iv for 10–14 days) eliminated the carrier state (Pearson et al., 1957; Splitter and Miller, 1953). The treatment can be modified by doubling the daily dosage to 22 mg/kg and reducing the number of daily injections to five (Magonigle et al., 1975). The LA 200 formulation, injected twice (20 mg/kg im) with a 7-day interval between injections, was reported to eliminate carrier infection (Roby et al., 1978). More recent studies suggest that four injections of LA 200 (20 mg/kg im) at 3-day intervals, would probably be more reliable and is now usually recommended (Magonigle and Newby, 1982). Even this higher dose will not always eliminate infection under field conditions where there is continuing arthropod transmission (Kuttler et al., 1980). Recent studies indicate that two, three, or four treatments with LA 200 (20 mg/kg) failed to clear infection when the treatments were given during the prepatent period or to carrier cows that had recently been reexposed (Kuttler, 1983; Lincoln et al., 1980).

6.2. Other Compounds in the Treatment of Anaplasmosis

Two additional compounds, α-dithiosemicarbazone (Gloxazone) and imidocarb dipropionate (Imizol) have been described as effective against acute anaplasmosis (Barrett et al., 1965; Hart et al., 1971; Kuttler, 1971). A single injection of imidocarb (3–5 mg/kg sc or im) will usually suffice to cure acute anaplasmosis if given early in the course of infection. Dithiosemicarbazone is effective at 5 mg/kg iv. Both compounds were described as superior to oxytetracycline in moderating the course of experimentally induced infections in adult cattle (Kuttler and Todorovic, 1973). Neither of these compounds is approved for use in the United States. The use of dithiosemicarbazone has been discontinued because of toxicity, but imidocarb is used in most areas of the world other than the United States for the treatment of anaplasmosis and babesiosis.

Both dithiosemicarbazone and imidocarb are effective in eliminating *Anaplasma* infections. Dithiosemicarbazone given daily for 10 days (5 mg/kg iv) eliminated *Ana-*

plasma but was associated with severe delayed drug toxicosis (Adams and Kuttler, 1970). When combined with intravenous oxytetracycline (5 mg/kg dithiosemicarbazone + 11 mg/kg oxytetracycline) given daily for 3 days, eliminated *Anaplasma* without apparent toxicity (Kuttler, 1972). Imidocarb at 4.0 mg/kg sc or im, given twice with a 14-day interval between treatments or administered daily for 3 days at 5 mg/kg, eliminated infection (Roby and Mazzola, 1972; Kuttler, 1971).

The elimination of carrier infection by treatment is followed by a period of immunity that lasts for periods of up to 1 year in the absence of infection (Roby *et al.*, 1974). Presumably this noninfectious immunity will eventually wane, leaving the animal once again fully susceptible, but the duration and level of immunity following treatment is yet to be determined. The therapeutic and curative treatments of anaplasmosis are important aspects of control programs that will probably be in use for years to come and will play an important role in any future eradication efforts.

7. CONCLUSIONS

Chemotherapy and chemoprophylaxis remain the principal defense against trypanosomiasis. The rapid development of drug resistance to available compounds by trypanosomes gives rise for concern about the future. The judicious use of available drugs is still the most commonly used method of reducing losses caused by trypanosomiasis.

The currently available vaccines for babesiosis and anaplasmosis, other than those producing premunition, produce only partial protection for a limited period of time. Treatment remains important in current control strategies. Chemoimmunization and chemoprophylaxis are areas that merit further investigation in the control of anaplasmosis and babesiosis.

All currently used procedures for immunizing cattle against theileriosis involve chemotherapy. The recent discoveries of the chemotherapeutically active compounds menoctone, 993C, and halofuginone represent significant contributions to the treatment and control of theileriosis.

REFERENCES

Adams, L. G., and Kuttler, K. L., 1970, Toxicity of alpha-ethoxyethylglyoxal dithiosemicarbazone in cattle, *Am. J. Vet. Res.* 31:1493–1495.

Adams, L. G., Corrier, D. E., and Williams, J. D., 1980, A study of the toxicity of imidocarb dipropionate in cattle, *Res. Vet. Sci.* 28:172–177.

Aliu, Y. O., 1981, Approach to effective chemotherapy and chemoprophylaxis of animal trypanosomiasis in Nigeria, in: *Proceedings of the First National Conference on Tsetse and Trypanosomiasis Research in Nigeria, Kaduna, Nigeria, August 10–12, 1981* (A. A. Ilemobade, ed.), pp. 194–228, Shereef Salan Press, Zaria, Nigeria.

Aliu, Y. O., 1983, Tick-borne diseases of domestic animals in Nigeria: Current treatment procedures, *Vet. Bull.* 53:233–251.

Aliu, Y. O., and Sannusi, A., 1979, Isometamidium–dextran complex: Therapeutic activity against *Trypanosoma vivax* infection in Zebu cattle, *J. Vet. Pharmacol. Ther.* 2:265–274.

Aliu, Y. O., Davis, R. H., Camp, B. J., and Kuttler, K. L., 1977, Absorption, distribution, and excretion of imidocarb dipropionate in sheep, *Am. J. Vet. Res.* 38:2001–2006.

Barnett, S. F., 1965, The chemotherapy of *Babesia bigemina* infection in cattle, *Res. Vet. Sci.* 6:397–415.

Barrett, P. A., Beveridge, E., Bradley, P. L., Brown, C. G. D., Bushby, S. R. M., Clarke, M. L., Neal, R. A., Smith, R., and Wilde, J. K. H., 1965, Biological activities of some α-dithiosemicarbazones,*Nature (Lond.)* 206:1340–1341.

Beveridge, E., 1953, *Babesia rodhaini:* A useful organism for the testing of drugs designed for the treatment of piroplasmosis, *Ann. Trop. Med. Parasitol.* 47:134.

Beveridge, C. G. L., Thwaite, J. W., and Shepherd, G., 1960, A field trial of amicarbalide—A new babesicide, *Vet. Rec.* 72:383–386.

Brock, W. E., Pearson, C. C., and Kliewer, I. O., 1959, Anaplasmosis control by test and subsequent treatment with chlortetracycline, *Proc. U.S. Livestock San. Assoc.* 62:66–70.

Brocklesby, D. W., and Bailey, K. P., 1962, Oxytetracycline hydrochloride in East Coast fever (*Theileria parva* infection), *Br. Vet. J.* 118:81–85.

Brown, C. G. D., Radley, D. E., Burridge, M. J., and Cunningham, M. P., 1977a, The use of tetracyclines in the chemotherapy of experimental East Coast fever (*Theileria parva* infection of cattle), *Tropenmed. Parasitol.* 28:513–520.

Brown, C. G. D., Radley, D. E., Cunningham, M. P., Kirimi, I. M., Morzaria, S. P., and Musoke, A. J., 1977b, Immunization against East Coast fever (*Theileria parva* infection of cattle) by infection and treatment; chemoprophylaxis with N-pyrrolidinomethyl tetracycline, *Tropenmed. Parasitol.* 28:342–348.

Cuckler, A. C., Malanga, C. M., and Conroy, J., 1970, Therapeutic efficacy of new nitroimidazoles for experimental trichomoniasis, amebiasis, and trypanosomiasis, *Am. J. Trop. Med. Hyg.* 19:916–925.

Dalgliesh, R. J., and Stewart, N. P., 1977, Tolerance to imidocarb induced experimentally in tick-transmitted *Babesia argentina, Aust. Vet. J.* 53:176–180.

Dann, O., Walker, P. J., Kaddu, J., and Watts, J. M. A., 1971, Preliminary observations on the chemotherapeutic activity of three new diamidines, *Trans. R. Soc. Trop. Med. Hyg.* 65:266.

Day, W. C., and Kuttler, K. L., 1975, Animal health considerations involved in the movement of U.S. cattle to Haiti, *Southwest Vet.* 28:229–232.

Dennig, Von H. K., Centurier, C., Gobel, E., and Weiland, G., 1980, Ein Beitrag zur Babesiose des Hundes und ihrer Bedeutung in der Bundesrepublik Deutschland und Berlin-West, *Berl. Munch. Tierarztl. Wochenschr.* 93:373–379.

DeVos, A. J., 1979, Epidemiology and control of bovine babesiosis in South Africa,*J. South Afr. Vet. Assoc.* 50:357–362.

DeVos, A. J., and Roos, J. A., 1983, Chemotherapy of *Theileria parva lawrencei* infection in cattle with halofuginone, *Onderstepoort J. Vet. Res.* 50:33–35.

Dolan, T. T., 1981, Progress in the chemotherapy of theileriosis, in: *Advances in the Control of Theileriosis* (A. D. Irvin, M. P. Cunningham, and A. S. Young, eds.), pp. 186–208, Martinus Nijhoff, The Hague.

Dube, D. K., Mpimbaza, G., Allison, A. C., Lederer, E., and Rovis, L., 1983, Antitrypanosomal activity of sinefungin, *Am. J. Med. Hyg.* 32:31–33.

Erp, E. E., Gravely, S. M., Smith, R. D., Ristic, M., Osorno, B. M., and Carson, C. A., 1978, Growth of *Babesia bovis* in bovine erythrocyte cultures. *Am. J. Trop. Med. Hyg.* 27:1061–1064.

Euzeby, J., Moreau, Y., Chauve, C., Gevrey, J., and Gauthey, M., 1980, Experimentation des propriétés antipiroplasmiques de l'Imidocarb sur *Babesia canis*, agent de la piroplasmose canine en Europe, *Bull. Acad. Vet. Fr.* 53:475–480.

Evans, D. A., and Holland, M. F., 1978, Effective treatment of *Trypanosoma vivax* with salicylhydroxamic acid (SHAM), *Trans. R. Soc. Trop. Med. Hyg.* 72:203–204.

Eyre, P., 1967, Some pharmacodynamic effects of the babesicidal agents quinuronium and amicarbalide,*J. Pharm. Pharmacol.* 19:509–519.

Farwell, G. E., LeGrand, E. K., and Cobb, C. C., 1982, Clinical observations on *Babesia gibsoni* and *Babesia canis* infections in dogs,*J. Am. Vet. Med. Assoc.* 180:507–511.

Foote, L. E., Farley, H., and Gallagher, B., 1951, The use of aureomycin in anaplasmosis, *North Am. Vet.* 32:547–549.

Ford, J., and Blaser, E., 1971, Some aspects of cattle raising under prophylactic treatment against trypanosomiasis on the Mkwaja ranch, Tanzania, *Acta Trop.* 28:69–79.

Franklin, T. E., Huff, J. W., and Grumbles, L. C., 1965, Chlortetracycline for elimination of anaplasmosis in carrier cattle, *J. Am. Vet. Med. Assoc.* 147:353–356.

Franklin, T. E., Cook, R. W., and Anderson, D. J., 1966, Feeding chlortetracycline to range cattle to eliminate the carrier state of anaplasmosis, *Proc. U.S. Livestock San. Assoc.* 66:85–90.

Franklin, T. E., Cook, R. W., Anderson, D. J., and Kuttler, K. L., 1967, Medium and low level feeding of chlortetracycline with comparisons of anaplasmosis CF and CA tests, *Southwest Vet.* 20:101–104.

Frerichs, W. M., Allen, P. C., and Holbrook, A. A., 1973, Equine piroplasmosis (*Babesia equi*): Therapeutic trials of imidocarb dihydrochloride in horses and donkeys, *Vet. Rec.* 93:73–75.

Frerichs, W. M., and Holbrook, A. A., 1974, Treatment of equine piroplasmosis (*B. caballi*) with imidocarb dipropionate, *Vet. Rec.* 95:188–189.

Gill, B. S., 1971, Study of chemotherapeutic susceptibility of *Trypanosoma evansi* to some arsenicals and suramin–tryparsamide complex, *Acta. Vet. Brno* 40:209–214.

Gill, B. S., and Malhotra, M. N., 1971, Chemoprophylaxis of *Trypanosoma evansi* infections in ponies, *Trop. Anim. Health Prod.* 3:199–202.

Gill, B. S., Bhattacharyulu, Y., Singh, A., Kaur, D., and Gill, H. S., 1981, Chemotherapy against *Theileria annulata*, in: *Advances in the Control of Theileriosis* (A. D. Irvin, M. P. Cunningham, and A. S. Young, eds.), pp. 218–222, Martinus Nijhoff, The Hague.

Graham, O. H., and Hourrigan, J. L., 1977, Eradication programs for the arthropod parasites of livestock, *J. Med. Entomol.* 13:629–658.

Groves, M. G., and Dennis, G. L., 1972, *Babesia gibsoni:* Field and laboratory studies of canine infections, *Exp. Parasitol.* 31:153–159.

Haigh, A. J. B., and Hagan, D. H., 1974, Evaluation of imidocarb dihydrochloride against redwater disease in cattle in Eire, *Vet. Rec.* 94:56–69.

Hart, C. B., Roy-Smith, F., Berger, J., Simpson, R. M., and McHardy, N., 1971, Imidocarb for control of babesiosis and anaplasmosis, in: *Proceedings of the Nineteenth World Veterinary Congress August 1971, Mexico City, Mexico* Vol. 2, 616 pp.

Irvin, A. D., and Young, E. R., 1977, Possible *in vitro* test for screening drugs for activity against *Babesia* and other blood protozoa, *Nature (Lond.)* 169:407–409.

Irvin, A. D., and Young, E. R., 1979, Further studies on the uptake of tritiated nucleic acid precursors by *Babesia* spp. of cattle and mice, *Int. J. Parasitol.* 9:109–114.

Jagdish, S., Singh, D. K., and Gautam, O. P., 1980, Chemoprophylactic immunization against bovine tropical theileriosis, *Ind. Vet. J.* 57:177–178.

Jennings, F. W., Urquhart, G. M., Murray, P. K., and Miller, B. M., 1980, Berenil and nitroimidazole combinations in the treatment of *Trypanosoma brucei* infection with central nervous system involvement, *Int. J. Parasitol.* 10:27–32.

Khanna, B. M., Dhar, S., and Gautam, O. P., 1983, Immunization against bovine tropical theileriosis by using the infection and treatment method, *Ind. Vet. J.* 60:257–261.

Kinnamon, K. E., Steck, E. A., and Rane, D. S., 1979, A new chemical series active against African trypanosomes: Benzyltriphenylphosphonium salts, *J. Med. Chem.* 22:452–455.

Kinnamon, K. E., Steck, E. A., and Rane, D. S., 1980, Anticancer agents and antitrypanosomiasis activity in mice, *J. Natl. Cancer Inst.* 64:391–394.

Kirkham, W. W., 1969, The treatment of equine babesiosis, *J. Am. Vet. Med. Assoc.* 155:457–460.

Kuttler, K. L., 1971, Promising therapeutic agents for the elimination of *Anaplasma marginale* in the carrier animal, *Proc. Annu. Mtg. U.S. Anim. Hlth. Assoc.* 75:92–98.

Kuttler, K. L., 1972, Combined treatment with a dithiosemicarbazone and oxytetracycline to eliminate *Anaplasma marginale* infection in splenectomized calves, *Res. Vet. Sci.* 13:536–539.

Kuttler, K. L., 1979, Current anaplasmosis control techniques being used in the United States, *J. South Afr. Vet. Assoc.* 50:314–320.

Kuttler, K. L., 1980, Pharmacotherapeutics of drugs used in treatment of anaplasmosis and babesiosis, *J. Am. Vet. Med. Assoc.* 176:1103–1108.

Kuttler, K. L., 1981, Chemotherapy of babesiosis: A review, in: *Babesiosis,* (M. Ristic and J. P. Kreier, eds.), pp. 65–85, Academic Press, New York.

Kuttler, K. L., 1983, The influence of a second *Anaplasma* exposure on the success of treatment to eliminate *Anaplasma* carrier infections in cattle, *Am. J. Vet. Res.* 44:882–883.

Kuttler, K. L., and Simpson, J. E., 1978, Relative efficacy of two oxytetracycline formulations and doxycycline in the treatment of acute anaplasmosis in splenectomized calves, *Am. J. Vet. Res.* 39:347–349.

Kuttler, K. L., and Todorovic, R. A., 1973, Techniques of premunization for the control of anaplasmosis, in: *Proceedings of the Sixth National Anaplasmosis Conference,* pp. 106–112, Heritage Press, Stillwater, Oklahoma.

Kuttler, K. L., Johnson, L. W., and Simpson, J. E., 1980, The elimination of *Anaplasma marginale* by chemotherapy under field and laboratory conditions, *Proc. U.S. Anim. Hlth. Assoc.* 84:73–82.

Leach, T. M., and Roberts, C. J., 1981, Present status of chemotherapy and chemoprophylaxis of animal trypanosomiasis in the Eastern Hemisphere, *Pharmacol. Ther.* 13:91–147.

Levy, M. G., and Ristic, M., 1980, Continuous cultivation in a microaerophilous stationary phase culture, *Science* 207:1218–1220.

Lewis, D., and Williams, H., 1979, Infection of the Mongolian gerbil with the cattle piroplasm, *Babesia divergens, Nature (Lond.)* 278:170–171.

Lewis, D., Purnell, R. E., Francis, M. A., and Young, E. R., 1981, The effect of treatment with imidocarb diproprionate on the course of *Babesia divergens* infections in splenectomized calves and on their subsequent immunity to homologous challenge, *J. Comp. Pathol.* 91:285–292.

Lincoln, S. D., Eckblad, W. P., and Magonigle, R. A., 1980, Bovine anaplasmosis: Clinical, hematologic, and serologic manifestations in cows given a long-acting oxytetracycline formulation in the prepatent period, *Am. J. Vet. Res.* 43:1360–1362.

Lucas, J. M. S., 1960, The chemotherapy of experimental babesiosis in mice and splenectomized calves, *Res. Vet. Sci.* 1:218–225.

Magonigle, R. A., and Newby, R. J., 1982, Elimination of naturally acquired chronic *Anaplasma marginale* infections with a long-acting oxytetracycline injectable, *Am. J. Vet. Res.* 43:2170–2172.

Magonigle, R. A., Renshaw, H. W., Vaughan, H. W., Stauber, E. H., and Frank, F. W., 1975, Effect of five daily intravenous treatments with oxytetracline hydrochloride on the carrier status of bovine anaplasmosis, *J. Am. Vet. Med. Assoc.* 167:1080–1083.

Malmquist, W. A., Nyindo, M. B. A., and Brown, C. G. D., 1970, East Coast Fever: Cultivation *in vitro* of bovine spleen cell lines infected and transformed by *Theileria parva, Trop. Anim. Hlth. Prod.* 2:139.

Mazzola, V., and Kuttler, K. L., 1981, The effects of minocycline on the acute and carrier phases of *Anaplasma marginale* in experimentally infected splenectomized cattle, in: *Proceedings of the Seventh National Anaplasmosis Conference, Mississippi State University, Mississippi, October 1981,* pp. 577–588.

McCosker, P. J., 1981, The global importance of babesiosis, in: *Babesiosis* (M. Ristic and J. P. Kreier, eds.), pp. 1–24, Academic Press, New York.

McHardy, N., 1979, Experimental therapy of theileriosis, *J. South Afr. Vet. Assoc.* 50:321–322.

McHardy, N., and Rae, D. G., 1981, Treatment of stabilate-induced East Coast fever with menoctone, *Trop. Anim. Health Prod.* 13:227–239.

McHardy, N., and Rae, D. G., 1982, Antitheilerial activity of the coccidiostat monensin, *Trop. Anim. Health Prod.* 14:13–14.

McHardy, N., Haigh, A. J. B., and Doland, T. T., 1976, Chemotherapy of *Theileria parva* infection, *Nature (Lond.)* 261:698–699.

Michael, S. A., and Refaii, A. H., 1982, The effect of imidocarb dipropionate on *Babesia ovis* infection in sheep, *Trop. Anim. Hlth. Prod.* 14:1–2.

Moore, D. J., 1979, Therapeutic implications of *Babesia canis* infection in dogs, *J. South Afr. Vet. Assoc.* 50:346–352.

Morgan, D. W. T., and McHardy, N., 1982, Comparison of the antitheilerial effect of Welcome 993C and halofuginone, *Res. Vet. Sci.* 32:84–88.

Neitz, W. O., 1950, The specific action of pamaquin on the haemotropic parasites of *Theileria parva, South Afr. J. Sci.* 46:218–219.

Neitz, W. O., 1953, Aureomycin in *Theileria parva* infection, *Nature (Lond.)* 171:34–35.

Neitz, W. O., 1957, Theileriosis, gonderiosis, and cytauxzoonosis: A review, *Onderstepoort J. Vet. Res.* 27:275–430.

Newton, L. G., and O'Sullivan, P. J., 1969, Chemoprophylaxis in *Babesia argentina* infection in cattle, *Aust. Vet. J.* 45:404–407.

Pearson, C. C., Brock, W. E., and Kliewer, I. O., 1957, A study of tetracycline dosage in cattle which are anaplasmosis carriers, *J. Am. Vet. Med. Assoc.* 130:290–292.

Pipano, E., Jeruhan, I., and Frank, M., 1979, Pentamidine in chemoimmunization of cattle against *Babesia bigemina* infections, *Trop. Anim. Hlth. Prod.* 11:13–16.

Pipano, E., Samish, M., Kriegel, Y., and Yeruham, I., 1981, Immunization of Friesian cattle against *Theileria annulata* by the infection-treatment method, *Br. Vet. J.* 137:416–420.

Purnell, R. E., Lewis, D., and Young, E. R., 1981, Quinuronium sulphate for the treatment of *Babesia divergens* infections of splenectomized calves, *Vet. Rec.* 108:538–539.

Radley, D. E., 1981, Infection and treatment method of immunization against theileriosis, in: *Advances in the Control of Theileriosis* (A. D. Irvin, M. P. Cunningham, and A. S. Young, eds.), pp. 227–237, Martinus Nijhoff, The Hague.

Radley, D. E., Brown, C. G. D., Burridge, M. J., Cunningham, M. P., Kirimi, I. M., Purnell, R. E., and Young, A. S., 1975a, East Coast fever: 1. Chemoprophylactic immunization of cattle against *Theileria parva* (Muguga) and five theilerial strains, *Vet. Parasitol.* 1:35–41.

Radley, D. E., Brown, C. G. D., Cunningham, M. P., Kimber, C. D., Musisi, F. L., Payne, R. C., Purnell, R. E., Stagg, S. M., and Young, A. S., 1975b, East Coast fever: Chemoprophylactic immunization of cattle using oxytetracycline and a combination of theilerial strains, *Vet. Parasitol.* 1:51–60.

Radley, D. E., Young, A. S., Brown, C. G. D., Burridge, M. J., Cunningham, M. P., Musisi, F. L., and Purnell, R. E., 1975c, East Coast fever: Cross-immunity trials with a Kenya strain of *Theileria lawrencei*, *Vet. Parasitol.* 1:43–50.

Radley, D. E., Young, A. S., Grootenhuis, J. G., Cunningham, M. P., Dolan, T. T., and Morzaria, S. P., 1979, Further studies on the immunization of cattle against *Theileria lawrencei* by infection and chemoprophylaxis, *Vet. Parasitol.* 5:117–128.

Rees, C. W., 1934, Characteristics of the piroplasms *Babesia argentina* and *Babesia bigemina* in the United States, *J. Agr. Res.* 48:427–438.

Riek, R. F., 1968, Babesiosis, in: *Infectious Blood Diseases of Man and Animals* (D. Weinman and M. Ristic, eds.), pp. 219–268, Academic Press, New York.

Roby, T. O., and Mazzola, V., 1972, Elimination of the carrier state of bovine anaplasmosis with imidocarb, *Am. J. Vet. Res.* 33:1931–1933.

Roby, T. O., and Simpson, J. E., 1978, Blood levels of oxytetracycline after the use of a long-acting formulation to eliminate the carrier state of bovine anaplasmosis, *Proc. Annu. Conv. Am. Assoc. Bovine Pract.* 11:92–93.

Roby, T. O., Amerault, R. E., and McCallon, B. R., 1970, Progress in control of bovine anaplasmosis, *Proc. U.S. Livestock San. Assoc.* 74:122–128.

Roby, T. O., Amerault, R. E., Mazzola, V., Rose, J. E., and Ilemobade, A., 1974, Immunity in bovine anaplasmosis after elimination of *Anaplasma marginale* infections with imidocarb, *Am. J. Vet. Res.* 35:993–995.

Roby, T. O., Simpson, J. E., and Amerault, T. E., 1978, Elimination of the carrier state of bovine anaplasmosis with long-acting oxytetracycline, *Am. J. Vet. Res.* 39:1115–1116.

Ruff, M. D., Fowler, J. L., Fernan, R. C., and Matsuda, K., 1973, Action of certain antiprotozoal compounds against *Babesia gibsoni* in dogs, *Am. J. Vet. Res.* 34:641–645.

Ryley, J. F., 1964, A chemoprophylactic approach to babesiosis, *Res. Vet. Sci.* 5:411–418.

Schein, E., and Voigt, W. P., 1979, Chemotherapy of bovine theileriosis with halofuginone, Short communication, *Acta Trop.* 36:391–394.

Schein, E., and Voigt, W. P., 1981, Chemotherapy of theileriosis in cattle, in: *Advances in the Control of Theileriosis* (A. D. Irvin, M. P. Cunningham, and A. S. Young, eds.), pp. 212–214, Martinus Nijhoff, The Hague.

Singh, B., Banerjee, D. P., and Gautam, O. P., 1980a, Comparative efficacy of diminazene diaceturate and imidocarb dipropionate against *B. equi* infections in donkeys, *Vet. Parasitol.* 7:173–179.

Singh, B., Samad, A., Anantwar, L. G., and Bhonsle, V. G., 1980*b*, Chemotherapeutic activity of oxytetracycline against clinical cases of *Theileria annulata* infection in exotic and cross-bred cattle, *Ind. Vet. J.* 57:849–852.

Splitter, E. J., and Miller, J. G., 1953, The apparent eradication of the anaplasmosis carrier state with antibiotics, *Vet. Med.* 48:486–488.

Tadasuke, O., and Nakabayashi, T., 1980, Therapeutic effect of bleomycin on experimental infection of mice with *Trypanosoma gambiense* and *Trypanosoma evansi*, *Biken J.* 23:205–209.

Taylor, R. J., and McHardy, N., 1979, Preliminary observations on the combined use of imidocarb and *Babesia* blood vaccine in cattle, *J. South Afr. Vet. Assoc.* 50:326–329.

Taylor, W. M., Simpson, C. F., and Martin, F. G., 1972, Certain aspects of toxicity of an amicarbalide formulation to ponies, *Am. J. Vet. Res.* 33:533–541.

Theiler, A., 1912, The treatment of Redwater in cattle with trypan blue, *Vet. J.* 68:64–73.

Todorovic, R. A., 1974, Bovine babesiosis: Its diagnosis and control, *Am. J. Vet. Res.* 35:1045–1052.

Todorovic, R. A., Vizcaino, O. G., Gonzalez, E. F., and Adams, L. G., 1973, Chemoprophylaxis (Imidocarb) against *Babesia bigemina* and *Babesia argentina* infections, *Am. J. Vet. Res.* 34:1153–1161.

Toro, M., Leon, E., Lopez, R., Pallota, F., Garcia, J. A., and Ruiz, A., 1983, Effect of isometamidium on infections by *Trypanosoma vivax* and *T. evansi* in experimentally infected animals, *Vet. Parasitol.* 13:35–43.

Toure, S. M., Kebe, B., and Seye, M., 1979, Evaluation of the treatment of experimental trypanosomiasis by a compound with a base of diminazene aceturate and potassium aluminium sulphate, in: *Fifteenth Meeting of the International Science Council for Trypanosomiasis Research and Control, Banjul, the Gambia, 1977*, pp. 395–402, Eleza Services for OAU/STRC, Nairobi, Kenya.

Tripathy, S. B., 1981, Observations on treatment of bovine theileriasis, *Ind. Vet. J.* 58:66–71.

Uilenberg, G., Jongejan, F., Perie, N. M., and Franssen, F. F. J., 1980, Chimiothérapie des theilerioses bovines par un anticoccidien, l'halofuginone, Note préliminaire, *Rev. Elev. Med. Vet. Pays. Trop.* 33:33–43.

Vayrynen, R., and Tuomi, J., 1982, Continuous *in vitro* cultivation of *Babesia divergens*, *Acta Vet. Scand.* 23:471–472.

Wilde, J. K. H., 1967, East Coast fever, *Adv. Vet. Sci.* 11:207–259.

Williamson, J., 1979, Present situation of research for new trypanocidal drugs, in: *Report of the Expert Consultation on Research on Trypanosomiasis, Appendix XII: FAO, Rome 1–5 October 1979*, pp. 90–96, United Nations FAO, Rome.

Wilson, A. J., LeRoux, J. G., Paris, J., Davidson, C. R., and Gray, A. R., 1975, Observations on a herd of beef cattle maintained in a tsetse area. I. Assessment of chemotherapy as a method for the control of trypanosomiasis, *Trop. Anim. Hlth. Prod.* 7:187–199.

9

Modes of Action of Antiprotozoal Agents

DOUGLAS L. LOOKER, J. JOSEPH MARR, and RONALD L. STOTISH

1. INTRODUCTION

There are relatively few antiprotozoal agents compared with the many antibiotics available for the treatment of bacterial infections. Similarities in host and eukaryotic parasite metabolism have made development of specific chemotherapeutic agents difficult and have necessitated the use of agents that often exhibit limited specificity for the parasite and excessive toxicity to the host. This chapter examines the mechanisms by which antiprotozoal agents exert their effects. Information on modes of action of several antiprotozoals is lacking either because little research has been undertaken to define the mechanisms or because primary and secondary drug effects have been difficult to differentiate.

Although currently used antiprotozoal agents often have low specificity and high toxicity, the future holds promise for the development of superior drugs. Ongoing research in the areas of protozoan biochemistry and physiology seeks to define differences between host and parasite metabolism that may be exploited. Such research offers a promise for the development of antiprotozoal agents that are exquisitly targeted. At the end of this chapter metabolic differences are discussed that may be future targets for chemotherapy.

2. MODES OF ACTION OF ANTIPROTOZOAL AGENTS

2.1. Malaria

Drugs currently used for the treatment of malaria include 4- and 8-amino-quinolines, quinine, and dihydrofolate reductase inhibitors, the latter often in com-

DOUGLAS L. LOOKER and J. JOSEPH MARR • Division of Infectious Disease, University of Colorado Health Sciences Center, Denver, Colorado 80262. RONALD L. STOTISH • Merck Institute for Therapeutic Research, Rahway, New Jersey 07065. *Present address* for R.L.S.: Department of Chemotherapy and Immunology, American Cyanamid, Princeton, New Jersey 08540.

bination with p-aminobenzoic acid (PABA) analogues. Two modes of action have been proposed for the aminoquinolines. Chloroquine (CQ) binds to ferriprotoporphyrin IX (FP), a malarial degradation product of hemoglobin present in the food vacuole of the parasite (Chou et al., 1980). FP alone is lytic for malaria, but complexation with CQ increases its lytic properties (Fitch et al., 1982; Dutta and Fitch, 1983). Malarial parasites apparently must sequester FP to prevent autolysis. CQ treatment results in the formation of an FP–CQ complex that may divert FP from its site of sequestration and cause lysis of the parasite (Fitch et al., 1982). This mechanism explains CQ resistance in Plasmodium berghei, which does not synthesize FP. However, CQ-resistant P. falciparum contains FP, suggesting that FP must be sequestered to the extent that it is unable to bind CQ if this mechanism is correct. An alternative mechanism proposes that aminoquinolines exert their effects by alkalinization of the malarial food vacuole. Malarial parasites generate a pH gradient between the cytoplasm and food vacuole by use of a Na^+, K^+-ATPase proton pump common to eukaryotic cells (Warhurst and Thomas, 1978). CQ at physiological pH is nonprotonated and membrane permeable. Diffusion into the acidic food vacuole protonates CQ, which becomes membrane impermeable. Accumulation of the protonated drug alkalinizes the food vacuole and reduces the activity of lysosomal enzymes that require an acidic pH. Inhibition of lysosomal proteases decreases hemoglobin digestion and starves the parasite for amino acids (Homewood et al., 1972). Excessive food vacuole alkalinization may also increase the permeability of the vacuole membrane and release lysosomal hydrolyases into the cytoplasm. Electron microscopic studies of CQ-treated P. falciparum revealed swelling of primary lysosomes and endocytic vesicles within the food vacuole that contain undigested hemoglobin, suggesting that lysosomal enzyme activity is inhibited (Yayon and Ginsberg, 1983). If this mechanism of CQ toxicity is correct, CQ resistance could be related to reduced acidity of the food vacuole and decreased CQ incorporation. Reduced vacuole acidity would explain the lack of visible FP within the vacuole, since pigment clumping is pH dependent (Warhurst and Thomas, 1978). Alternatively, the lipid content of the food vacuole may be modified in CQ-resistant malaria such that CQ diffusion into the vacuole is reduced to a nontoxic level. Further research should determine which of the proposed mechanisms accounts for the antimalarial action of aminoquinolines. Quinine has been used for centuries in the treatment of malaria. Its mode of action has not been well studied, but it is presumed to be the same as that of the aminoquinolines.

Dihydrofolate (DHF) reductase inhibitors are also used in the treatment of malaria, often in combination with PABA analogues (sulfonamides). The mode of action of these folate biosynthesis inhibitors was reviewed by Hitchings and Burchall (1965) and is presented in Fig. 1. Sulfonamides inhibit the synthesis of dihydropteroic acid from pteridines, PABA, and glutamate; 2,4-diaminopyrimidines inhibit the reduction of dihydrofolate to tetrahydrofolate (THF) by dihydrofolate reductase. Inhibition of THF synthesis prevents conversion of uracil to thymine. Thymine is required for DNA synthesis.

The modes of action of the diaminopyrimidines pyrimethamine and trimethoprim have been examined in the plasmodia. Ferone et al. (1969) partially purified the DHF

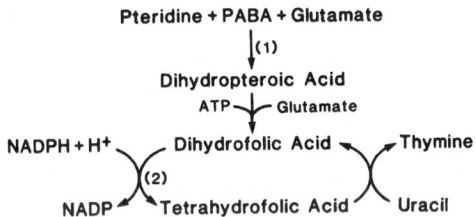

Figure 1. Folate metabolism in malarial parasite. (1) PABA analogues, such as the sulfonamides, inhibit synthesis of dihydropteroic acid from PABA and pteridine. (2) Diaminopyrimidines inhibit synthesis of tetrahydrofolic acid from dihydrofolic acid and thereby prevent the synthesis of thymine required for DNA synthesis.

reductase of *P. berghei* and determined the concentration of pyrimethamine which inhibited 50% of the enzyme activity (IC_{50}) to be 0.5 nM. DHF reductase from *P. knowlesi* has an IC_{50} of 1 nM. In comparison, the purified enzyme from rat liver has an IC_{50} of 700 nM, which gives a therapeutic index of 700–1400. The IC_{50} of trimethoprim for the malarial enzyme is approximately 100-fold higher than that of pyrimethamine, but trimethoprim still has a therapeutic index of approximately 3700. Thus, diaminopyrimidines can be highly selective for the malarial enzyme (Hitchings, 1971). Inhibition of malarial DHF reductase should result in inhibition of DNA synthesis because of the lack of thymine. However, Gutteridge and Trigg (1971) found that, at 1 nM, a concentration of pyrimethamine toxic to *P. knowlesi in vivo*, there is no inhibition of incorporation of radiolabeled adenosine, adenine, or orotic acid into DNA *in vitro*. Protein synthesis and respiration also are unaffected. Pyrimethamine also has no effect on *P. lophurae* maintained extracellularly (Trager, 1967), suggesting that extracellular plasmodia can bypass the inhibition of thymine synthesis by salvage of exogenous thymine. Intracellular plasmodia may be unable to utilize exogenous thymine because of the inability of the red blood cell to transport the pyrimidine. Other metabolic pathways utilizing THF may also be important in the mechanism of action of diaminoprimidines.

Unlike mammalian cells, which require preformed folic acid, malarial parasites synthesize DHF from pteridines, PABA, and glutamate (Ferone, 1973) (Fig. 1). Sulfonamides are therefore often used in combination with diaminopyrimidines because of the synergism that exists between the two drugs (Hitchings, 1971). DHF reductase inhibitors alone often are not sufficient to prevent THF synthesis. Accumulation of DHF can result in competition between substrate and inhibitor and permit the synthesis of some THF. The sulfonamide prevents the accumulation of DHF.

2.2. Leishmania

Pentavalent antimonials and amphotericin B are used in the treatment of leishmanial infections. Pentavalent antimonials are not effective against cultured leishmanial promastigotes, since antimonials must be reduced to the trivalent form to be toxic. After administration to humans, pentavalent antimonials are reduced to the trivalent form (Goodwin and Page, 1943). Chen (1948) proposed that trivalent antimonials inactivate sulfhydryl-containing enzymes. Bueding and Mansour (1957) determined that phosphofructokinase is inhibited in the trematode *Schistosoma mansoni*. Treatment of *L. tropica* promastigotes with trivalent antimony decreases the flow of glucose into the Krebs (TCA) cycle and causes accumulation of glycolytic byproducts and certain end products, suggesting inhibition of Krebs cycle enzymes. Thus, in *Leishmania,* antimonials appear to inhibit initial steps in glycolysis and certain enzymes of the Krebs cycle to decrease energy production by the parasite (Gutteridge and Coombs, 1977).

Amphotericin B is a second-line agent used for the treatment of antimony-resistant *Leishmania*. Studies using cholesterol bilayer membranes showed that amphotericin B greatly increases permeability of these membranes to thiourea (Lippe, 1968). The drug interacts with membrane cholesterol and its metabolites (e.g., ergosterol) to increase membrane permeability and cause the loss of low-molecular-weight components such as glucose and amino acids. Beach *et al.* (1979) identified ergosterol as a membrane component of leishmanial promastigotes.

2.3. Amoebae

Drugs commonly used against amebic infections include metronidazole, emetines, tetracycline, and iodoquinol. The mechanism of iodoquinol action is unknown. Metronidazole is a nitroimidazole compound also used in the treatment of infections caused by *Trichomonas vaginalis* and *Giardia lamblia*. The nitro group of the drug is reduced in the cytoplasm through a number of intermediates to an end product that appears to be a hydroxylamine derivative. This reduction maintains a concentration gradient across the cell membrane and permits intracellular accumulation (Ings *et al.*, 1974). Studies on metronidazole and other nitroimidazoles revealed that antitrichomonad activity and mutagenicity in *Salmonella typhimurium* correlate with the ability of the nitro group to be reduced *in vivo*. Reduction can occur nonenzymatically by chemically reduced ferridoxin or flavodoxin-type electron-transport proteins, suggesting that these proteins are responsible for reduction *in vivo* (Lindmark and Muller, 1976). Reduced metronidazole interacts with DNA and destroys its ability to serve as a template for DNA and RNA synthesis (Ings *et al.*, 1974). Binding of reduced metronidazole to DNA *in vitro* results in loss of helical structure and in strand breakage (Knight *et al.*, 1978). Using radiolabeled metronidazole reduced with sodium dithionate, LaRusso *et al.* (1977) found that reduced metronidazole covalently binds to guanine and cytosine residues. The drug also binds to protein (bovine serum albumin) but at an efficiency of one-third that of DNA.

Amebic infections can be treated with emetine hydrochlorides, inhibitors of eukaryotic protein synthesis (translation). Entner and Grollman (1973) proposed this mode of action because of a correlation between amebicidal activity and inhibition of translation by various emetines. Resistance to emetines is paralleled by resistance to cycloheximide, another inhibitor of eukaryotic protein synthesis. Entner (1979) determined that emetine binds irreversibly, but noncovalently, to the peptide-chain elongation site of the 60S ribosomal subunit. By contrast, cycloheximide binds reversibly to the 60S subunit, indicating that some unique region of the emetine molecule is responsible for its irreversibility (Fig. 2). Structural requirements for translation inhibition were further defined using isoemetine, which differs from emetine only in the bond angle of the hydrogen at the C-1 position. Isoemetine binds irreversibly to the 60S subunit but does not inhibit translation.

In mammalian cells, emetine binds to protein S14 of the 40S ribosomal subunit (Boersmer et al., 1979; Madjar et al., 1982) and prevents elongation factor 2-dependent translocation (Wasmuth et al., 1980). This mechanism was determined by comparative two-dimensional electrophoretic analyses of ribosomal proteins from emetine-resistant Chinese hamster ovary (CHO) cells (Boersmer et al., 1979). Only the S14 protein was modified in its migration compared with sensitive cells. The mRNA that codes for resistant S14 has been cloned and sequenced (Nakamichi, 1983). Emetine resistance is a result of mutation and not a post-translational modification. Similarly detailed analyses of ribosomal proteins from sensitive and resistant amebae may permit development of emetine analogues with greater specificity.

Quinacrine has been used in the treatment of amebic infections. Since it is an analogue of acridine, its mechanism of action is presumed to be the same, i.e., intercalation into DNA and inhibition of DNA and/or RNA synthesis by the induction of lesions in the macromolecule.

The amebicidal action of furazolidone is similar to that of other nitrofurans used in the treatment of *Trypanosoma cruzi*. Tetracycline is also effective in the treatment of intestinal amebiasis. The antibiotic probably eliminates intestinal bacteria that maintain the low redox potential needed for survival of amoebae.

2.4. Trypanosoma cruzi

The nitrofuran derivatives lampit (nifurtimox) are used in the treatment of *T. cruzi* infections. Nitrofurans are toxic because of their ability to form free radicals that reduce

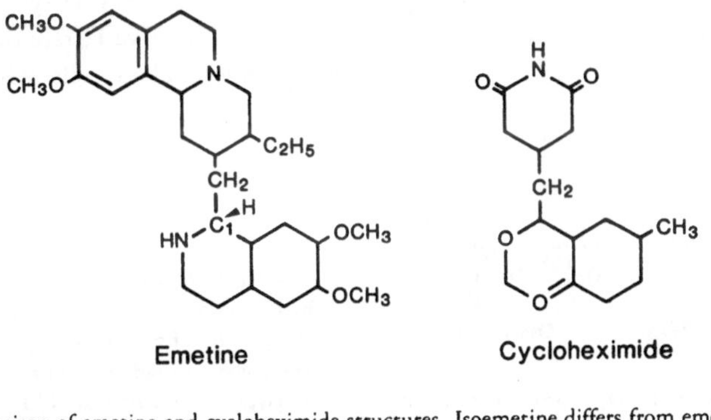

Figure 2. Comparison of emetine and cyeloheximide structures. Isoemetine differs from emetine in the bond angle of the hydrogen at C-1.

molecular oxygen (superoxide, O_2^-; hydrogen peroxide, H_2O_2; and hydroxyl radical, OH^-). *Trypanosoma cruzi* epimastigotes exposed to nifurtimox form H_2O_2. Mitochondrial fractions of epimastigotes incubated with nifurtimox and NADH or with succinate generate O_2^-. Similar results were obtained with microsomal fractions supplemented with NADPH (Docampo and Stoppani, 1979). Rat liver microsomes catalyze the reduction of nifurtimox to the nitro anion free radical. Reaction of this radical with O_2 results in formation of the nitro derivative and O_2^- (Docampo *et al.*, 1981*a*). Experiments with *T. cruzi* epimastigotes, trypamastigotes, and amastigotes and their corresponding homogenates showed similar radical formation. Since *T. cruzi* contains no glutathione peroxidase or catalase, spontaneous formation of OH^- can occur. Reaction mechanisms involved in hydroxyl radical formation are shown in Fig. 3. Hydroxyl radical may be the most damaging oxygen radical, since it causes peroxidation of lipids and DNA (Docampo *et al.*, 1981*b*). Damage to DNA by peroxidation is supported by McCalla (1983). Nitrofuran mutagenicity is increased in bacteria that lack normal DNA excision repair mechanisms. Similarly, fibroblasts from excision repair-defective xeroderma pigmentosum patients have increased nitrofuran-induced mutagenicity.

The limited selectivity of nitrofurans for *T. cruzi* may be attributable to the relative rates of formation of the free radical. Mammalian cells appear to metabolize nitrofurans, as does *T. cruzi*, although somewhat more slowly. The compounds are highly toxic to humans.

2.5. African Trypanosomes

Organic arsenicals, suramin, and diamidines are used in the treatment of African trypanosomiasis. Organic arsenicals interact with protein sulfhydryl groups such as those of carbohydrate metabolic enzymes. Flynn and Bowman (1969) showed that melarsen oxide inhibits trypanosome pyruvate kinase to prevent the synthesis of ATP and pyruvate from phosphoenolpyruvate and ADP. Bloodstream forms of the African trypanosomes lack a Krebs cycle and respiratory enzymes, indicating that mitochondrial respiration is not important. Oxygen consumption is cyanide insensitive and is mediated by a unique NAD-regenerating pathway that utilizes the enzymes *sn*-glycerol 3-phosphate oxidase and glycerol 3-phosphate dehydrogenase. These enzymes are essential for the regeneration of NAD, since trypanosomes do not have lactate dehydrogenase. Glycerol 3-phosphate oxidase is not present in mammalian cells (Gutteridge and

Figure 3. Generation of OH^- by nitrofurans. (1) Reduction of the aromatic nitrofuran ($ArNO_2$) is catalyzed by a flavin containing nitroreductase. (2) The anion free radical spontaneously reacts with O_2 to form superoxide, O_2^-. (3) Superoxide dismutase catalyzes the reaction to H_2O_2. (4) H_2O_2 spontaneously reacts with O_2^- to form hydroxyl radical, OH^-.

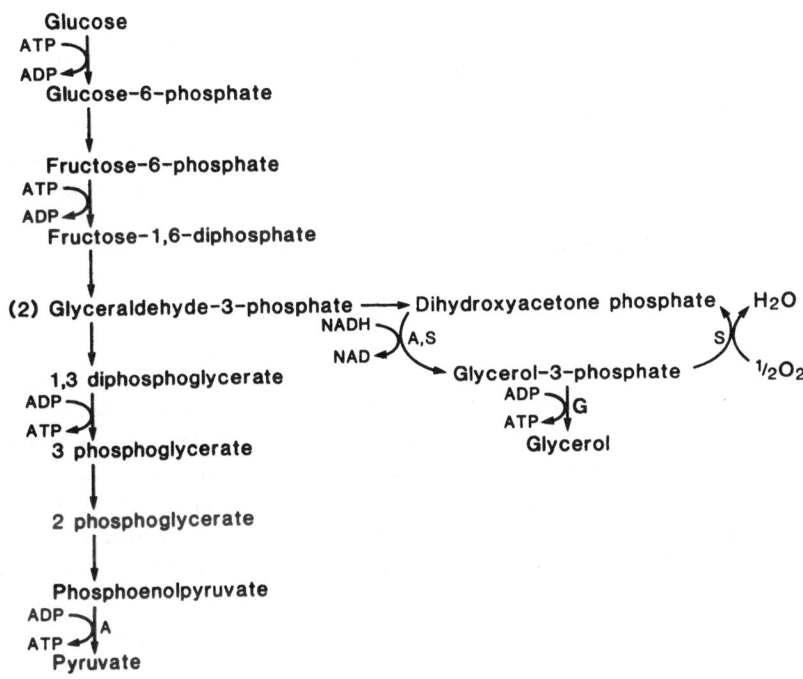

Figure 4. Glucose metabolism in African trypanosomes. (A) Arsenicals inhibit pyruvate kinase and s,n-glycerol phosphate oxidase; (S) suramin inhibits *s,n*-glycerol phosphate oxidase and *sn*-glycerol phosphate dehydrogenase; (G) glycerol inhibits glycerol kinase reaction.

Coombs, 1977) (Fig. 4). Melarsen oxide is a potent inhibitor of this enzyme (Fairlamb and Bowman, 1977). Combined inhibition of pyruvate kinase and of *sn*-glycerol 3-phosphate oxidase appears to be sufficient to kill trypanosomes. The drug may inhibit other sulfhydryl-containing enzymes as well.

Suramin inhibits *sn*-glycerol 3-phosphate oxidase and has a K_i of 4.1 μM with respect to the substrate (Fairlamb and Bowman, 1977). The drug also inhibits glycerol 3-phosphate dehydrogenase (Fairlamb and Bowman, 1980). Combined inhibition of these enzymes prevents reoxidation of NADH and decreases ATP synthesis. Suramin is incorporated into trypanosomes by endocytosis following binding to serum albumin. Degradation of the carrier complex by lysosomal proteolysis releases the drug into cytoplasm. Suramin toxicity to the host is lessened through binding to albumin and subsequent inhibition of host intralysosomal proteolysis by the albumin–drug complex. This reduces the amount of drug ultimately released into the host cell cytoplasm (Bijsterbosch *et al.*, 1982).

The diamidines pentamidine, isethionate, and berenil are also antitrypanosomal agents. Electron microscopic studies showed that the intercalation of berenil into kinetoplast DNA (kDNA) results in the formation of lampbrush chromosomes and suggests inhibition of DNA synthesis (Brack *et al.*, 1972). Nucleolar aggregation was also observed in diamidine-treated trypanosomes, suggesting inhibition of ribosomal RNA synthesis as well (Williamson *et al.*, 1975). Hentzer and Kobayasi (1977) proposed that diamidines bind primarily to DNA regions which are rich in adenine and thymine. Since kDNA is more rich in these bases than is nuclear DNA, the drug preferentially inhibits kDNA replication. After drug treatment, disintegration of kDNA begins at the periphery of the kinetoplast, where DNA replication begins. Berenil-treated *Leishmania tarentolae* have greatly reduced kDNA content (Leon *et al.*, 1977).

2.6. *Eimeria*

Eimeria infection of poultry is not chronic in the infected individual because of the self-limiting coccidial life cycle. It is an acute disease, with pathology directly related to the extent of coccidial replication. For this reason, agents that slow or prevent coccidial replication are useful in the treatment of the disease. Because of the variety of factors that can affect eukaryotic replication, there are a wide variety of structural classes that possess anticoccidial activity. This section reviews compounds that have been used commercially and that have reasonably well-understood mechanisms of action.

As early as 1946, Horton-Smith and Boyland demonstrated that the anticoccidial activities of sulfonamides were reversed by the simultaneous feeding of PABA, one of the intermediates in folate biosynthesis. Inhibition of coccidial folic acid biosynthesis by sulfonamides was substantiated by the work of Warren (1968) and Joyner (1960) suggesting that coccidia do not utilize exogenous folate. This idea was further corroborated by the observations of Rogers *et al.* (1964) with a series of 2-substituted PABA analogues. The anticoccidial effects of these compounds were antagonized by administration of PABA. The dihydropteroate synthetase of coccidia has not been studied directly, but data are available for *Plasmodium* (reviewed by Wang, 1984) showing inhibition by sulfonamides.

The action of the sulfonamides and inhibitors of dihydrofolate reductase (DHFR) such as the 2,4-diaminopyrimidine derivatives are synergistic (Lux, 1954; Joyner and Kendall, 1956), further reinforcing the idea that folate biosynthesis was affected by the sulfonamides, while the reduction of dihydrofolate was inhibited by drugs such as pyrimethamine. The inhibition of the DHFR of *Eimeria tenella* by pyrimethamine was demonstrated by Wang *et al.* (1975), and comparison with the chicken enzyme provided a rationale for the therapeutic efficacy of this compound. The chick enzyme was 12-fold less sensitive to pyrimethamine than the enzyme from *E. tenella* unsporulated occyts.

Amprolium, (1-[4-amino-2-propyl-5-pyrimidinyl)methyl]-2-picolinium chloride), is structurally related to thiamine. Since it lacks the hydroxyethyl function of thiamine, it is not phosphorylated to a thiamine pyrophosphate analogue. Polin *et al.* (1963) reported inhibition of thiamine uptake in ligated intestinal loops of birds by amprolium. Similarly, Sharma and Quastel (1965) showed amprolium to inhibit the active transport of thiamine in rat brain cortex. Direct proof of the mechanism of action came in 1980, when James demonstrated active transport of thiamine by isolated second generation schizonts of E. tenella ($K_m = 0.07$ μM). This transport was competitively inhibited by amprolium ($K_i = 7.6$ μM). The basis for the therapeutic index of amprolium became apparent in the comparison of the thiamine transport of chick epithelial cells ($K_m = 0.36$ μM) and its amprolium sensitivity ($K_i = 362.5$ μM). Considered with the established thiamine requirements of coccidia (Warren, 1968), the 50-fold greater sensitivity of the parasite transport system compared with the host established the mechanism of anticoccidial activity of amprolium. James (1980) compared a resistant and sensitive strain of coccidia and found that the K_i for amprolium increased approximately 15-fold to 115 μM in the resistant strain.

The potency and toxicity of nicarbazin make assignment of a precise mechanism of action difficult. Dougherty (1974) showed it to be a potent inhibitor of succinate-linked NAD reduction in beef heart mitochondria, so-called reverse electron flow. Wang (1978) demonstrated stoichiometric drug binding to bovine serum albumin (BSA) as well as the drug-dependent K^+ efflux from chick erythrocytes. The K^+ efflux occurred at drug concentrations of 10^{-5} M, higher than the concentration necessary for the mitochondrial effects (10^{-8} M). It may be that its activity is mediated by its potent protein binding and disruption of the microenvironment of the parasite, i.e., interacting with many protein species.

The quinoline anticoccidial agents (e.g., amquinate, buquinolate, decoquinate) were shown by Wang to inhibit cellular respiration (Wang, 1976) of E. tenella, as well as respiration in isolated mitochondria (Wang, 1975). Mitochondrial respiration of amquinate resistant cells was approximately 100-fold less sensitive to quinolones. The therapeutic index of these compounds is apparently attributable to the lack of inhibition of chicken cell respiration (Wang, 1975).

Anticoccidial hydroxynaphthoquinones also act on mitochondrial respiration. Wang (1975) found them to be potent inhibitors of succinate dehydrogenase–CoQ reductase and NADH dehydrogenase–CoQ reductase from E. tenella. Their E. tenella activity can be reversed by CoQ, in agreement with the studies conducted by Catlin et al. (1968) and by Skelton et al. (1971) in beef heart mitochondria.

Another drug possibly acting on coccidial mitochondria is robenidine. Wang et al. (1972) reported inhibition of rat liver mitochondrial oxidative phosphorylation by this drug, as well as an inhibition of ATPase. Wang (1978) reported a K^+ efflux (not coupled to H^+ influx) in chick erythrocytes exposed to robenidine ($10^{-4}–10^{-5}$ M). The effect on mitochondrial oxidative phosphorylation was observed at high drug concentration (20 mM), and there appears to be no clear-cut single mechanism of action of this drug.

The anticoccidial ionophores (monensin, lasalocid, salinomycin, narasin) mediate mono- and divalent cation transport across membranes, resulting in destruction of transmembrane electrochemical gradients or potentials. It has been suggested that these compounds act by inhibiting nutrient transport in the host cell, hence indirectly suppressing coccidial development (Wang, 1982). A recent report by Machamer and Cresswell (1984), demonstrating monensin to inhibit glycosylation, would appear to be a result of the disruption of the pH gradient rather than a primary mechanism.

A number of purine and pyrimidine analogues have good anticoccidial activity (reviewed by Wang, 1982). The precise mechanism of action of arprinocid remains uncertain, but a number of biological effects have been described. It apparently will inhibit many pyridine nucleotide-requiring enzymes (Wang et al., 1979a) as well as inhibiting the uptake of hypoxanthine and guanine in eukaryotic cells (Wang et al., 1979b; Slaughter and Barnes, 1979). In fact, there is good correlation between anticoccidial activity and inhibition of hypoxanthine uptake of infected cells.

Metabolism of arprinocid to the N-1 oxide (Jacob et al., 1978; Wolf et al., 1978) introduces another type of activity described by Wang and co-workers complicating the proposed mechanism somewhat (Wang and Simachkevich, 1980; Wang et al., 1981). The N-1 oxide is not as potent an inhibitor (as arprinocid) of the biochemical assays but is very potent both in vitro and in vivo (Wang et al., 1979a; Latter and Wilson, 1979; Wang and Simashkevich, 1980). The effects on the parasite were described by Wang et al. (1981) to include vacuolization and degeneration of intracellular membrane systems, apparently through a drug metabolism-dependent mechanism. It is thus likely that the N-1 oxide metabolite of aprinocid is the active species.

There are many compounds not described in this review that have been reported to have anticoccidial activity, a number of which have even been employed commercially. The classes of drugs selected are those for which we have the most complete information on their biochemical mechanisms. Clearly, the process of discovery will continue indefinitely as attempts are made to identify new biochemical targets and to develop more effective coccidiostats.

2.7. Other Protozoa

Tetracyclines are used in the treatment of Anaplasma, Theileria, and human Babesia infections (Hawking, 1963; Kuttler, 1983). The mechanism of action of tetracycline is presumed to be similar to that in bacteria, i.e., binding to the small ribosomal subunit inhibits binding of amino acid charged tRNA, thereby preventing elongation of the nascent peptide chain (Davis et al., 1973). Clindamycin, also used in the treatment of Babesia, is a peptidyl transferase inhibitor that binds to the large subunit of bacterial ribosomes (Davis et al., 1973). This mechanism of action is assumed to be the same in Babesia.

Animal babesial infections are treated with the substituted carbanilide, imidocarb. The structure and mechanism of action of imidocarb are similar to those of the diamidine berenil (Schmidt et al., 1969).

3. CONCLUSION

The modes of action of several antiprotozoal agents have been examined. Many of these agents are toxic. Differential toxicity of compounds such as the arsenicals and diamidines may result solely from differences in metabolic rates of parasite and host.

Bloodstream forms of African trypanosomes have a glycolytic rate 50 times that of mammalian cells and divide once every 7 hr (Wang, 1984). Inhibitors of glycolysis and DNA replication are therefore correspondingly more toxic to the parasite. Future antiprotozoal compounds may further exploit the higher rates of protozoan metabolism. Bacchi *et al.* (1980) found that α-(difluoromethyl)ornithine (DFMO), an inhibitor of ornithine decarboxylase, is effective against bloodstream African trypanosomes. Inhibition of ornithine decarboxylase prevents synthesis of polyamines required for DNA stabilization and replication. Since the short replication time of trypanosomes requires a high rate of polyamine synthesis, it is possible that DFMO treatment may eliminate the trypanosomes before host toxicity occurs.

Perhaps the most effective antiprotozoal agents of the future will be those that exploit metabolic capabilities unique to the parasite. As discussed in Section 2.5, African trypanosomes have a unique metabolic pathway for the oxidation of NADH utilizing *sn*-glycerol phosphate oxidase (Fig. 4). Salicylhydroxamic acid (SHAM) specifically inhibits this enzyme and, in combination with glycerol, can lyse trypanosome bloodstream forms (Clarkson and Brohn, 1976; Fairlamb *et al.*, 1977) *via* the following mechanism: under SHAM-induced anaerobic conditions, glycerol phosphate accumulates, since it cannot be reduced to dihydroxyacetone phosphate. ADP also accumulates as glycolysis slows from the lack of NAD. Glycerol phosphate and ADP force the reversal of glycerol kinase, resulting in synthesis of ATP and glycerol. Only one ATP is generated per glucose molecule. Addition of glycerol to bloodstream forms *in vitro* inhibits glycerol kinase so that no ATP is formed. Lysis of the trypanosomes results.

Allopurinol, (4-hydroxypyrazolo[3,4-d]pyrimidine) (HPP), a hypoxanthine analogue, and allopurinol ribonucleoside (HPPR), an inosine analogue, are effective against *Leishmania donovani* amastigotes and promastigotes (Berens *et al.*, 1980; Marr and Berens, 1977). Metabolism of these compounds differs significantly between *Leishmania* and man. Neither compound is toxic (Krenitsky *et al.*, 1980).

Leishmania, like most protozoan parasites, has no *de novo* purine synthesis, so it depends on purine salvage for survival (Marr *et al.*, 1978). HPP and HPPR are metabolized to the IMP analogue, allopurinol ribonucleoside monophosphate (HPPR-MP), by hypoxanthine-guanine phosphoribosyltransferase and purine nucleoside phosphorylase, respectively (Spector *et al.*, 1979; Nelson *et al.*, 1979a). HPPR-MP is aminated to aminopurinol ribonucleoside monophosphate (APPR-MP), an AMP analogue, by succino-AMP synthetase (SAS) and succino-AMP lyase. It is then phosphorylated to the ATP analogue and incorporated into RNA (Nelson *et al.*, 1979b). This does not occur in humans.

HPP and APP nucleotides appear to inhibit leishmanial growth by two mechanisms. As an alternate substrate, HPPR-MP competitively inhibits *L. donovani* SAS; HPPR-MP also inhibits promastigote GMP reductase. Combined inhibition of leishmanial SAS and GMP reductase should prevent synthesis of ATP from salvaged purines (Spector *et al.*, 1984). Formation of the ATP analogue APPR-TP inhibits RNA and protein synthesis in *L. donovoni* promastigotes (Looker *et al.*, 1984).

Differences in metabolism between the host and parasite described above illustrate the importance of fundamental biochemical research to chemotherapy.

REFERENCES

Bacchi, C. J., Nathan, H. C., Hutner, S. H., McCann, P. P., and Sjoerdsma, A., 1980, Polyamine metabolism: A potential therapeutic target in trypanosomes, *Science* 210:332–334.

Beach, D. H., Holz, G. G., and Anekwe, G. E., 1979, Lipids of Leishmania promastigotes, *J. Parasitol.* 65:203–216.

Berens, R. L., Marr, J. J., Nelson, D. J., and LaFon, S. W., 1980, Antileishmanial effect of allopurinol and allopurinol ribonucleoside on intracellular forms of *Leishmania donovani, Biochem. Pharmacol.* 29:2397–2398.

Bijsterbosch, M. K., Duursman, A. M., Bouma, J. M. W., and Gruber, M., 1982, Endocytosis and breakdown of mitochondrial malate dehydrogenase in the rat *in vivo, Biochem. J.* 208:61–67.

Boersmer, D., McGill, S. M., Mollenkamp, J. W., and Roufa, D. J., 1979, Emetine resistance in Chinese hamster cells is linked genetically with an altered 40S ribosomal subunit protein S20, *Proc. Natl. Acad. Sci. U.S.A.* 76:415–419.

Brack, C., Delani, E., Riou, G., and Festy, B., 1972, Molecular organization of the kinetoplast DNA of *Trypanosoma cruzi* treated with Berenil, a DNA intercalating drug, *J. Ultrastruct. Res.* 39:568–579.

Bueding, E., and Mansour, J. M., 1957, The relationship between inhibition of PFK activity and the mode of action of trivalent organic antimonials on *Shistosoma mansoni, Br. J. Pharmacol.* 12:159.

Catlin, J. C., Pardini, R. S., Daves, G. D., Heidker, J. C., and Folkers, K., 1968, New hydroxyquinones, apparent inhibitors of coenzyme Q enzyme systems, *J. Am. Chem. Soc.* 90:3572–3574.

Chen, G., 1948, Effects of arsenicals and antimonials on the activity of glycolytic enzymes in lysed preparations of *Trypanosoma equiperdium, J. Infect. Dis.* 82:226.

Chou, A. C., Chevli, R., and Fitch, C. D., 1980, Ferriprotoporphyrin IX fulfills the criteria for identification as the chloroquine receptor of malaria parasites, *Biochemistry* 19:1543–1549.

Clarkson, A. B., and Brohn, F. H., 1976, Trypanosomiasis: An approach to chemotherapy by the inhibition of carbohydrate catabolism, *Science* 194:204–206.

Davis, B. D., Dulbecco, R., Eisen, H. N., Ginsberg, H. S., Wood, W. B., and McCarty, M., 1973, *Microbiology*, 2nd ed., Harper & Row, New York.

Docampo, R., and Stoppani, A. O. M., 1979, Generation of superoxide anion and hydrogen peroxide induced by nifurtimox in *Trypanosoma cruzi, Arch. Biochem. Biophys.* 197:317–321.

Docampo, R., Mason, R. P., Motley, C., and Muniz, R. P. A., 1981a, Generation of free radicals induced by nifurtimox in mammalian tissues, *J. Biol. Chem.* 256:10930–10933.

Docampo, R., Moreno, S. N. J., Stoppani, A. O. M., Leon, W., Cruz, F. S., Villalta, F., and Muniz, R. P. A., 1981b, Mechanism of nifurtimox toxicity in different forms of *Trypanosoma cruzi, Biochem. Pharmacol.* 30:1947–1951.

Dougherty, H. W., 1974, Inhibition of mitochondrial energy transduction of carbanilides, *Fed. Proc.* 33:1657.

Dutta, P., and Fitch, C. D., 1983, Diverse membrane-active agents modify the hemolytic response to ferriprotoporphyrin IX, *J. Pharmacol. Exp. Ther.* 225:729–734.

Entner, N., 1979, Emetine binding to ribosomes of *Entamoeba histolytica*—Inhibition of protein synthesis and amebicidal action, *J. Protozool.* 26:324–328.

Entner, N., and Grollman, A. P., 1973, Inhibition of protein synthesis: A mechanism of amebicidal action of emetine and other structurally related compounds, *J. Protozool.* 20:160–163.

Fairlamb, A. H., and Bowman, I. B. R., 1977, *Trypanosoma brucei:* Suramin and other trypanocidal compounds' effects on sn-glycerol-3-phosphate oxidase, *Exp. Parasitol.* 43:353–361.

Fairlamb, A. H., and Bowman, I. B. R., 1980, Uptake of the trypanocidal drug suramin by bloodstream forms of *Trypanosoma brucei* and its effects on respiration and growth rate *in vivo, Mol. Biochem. Parasitol.* 1:315–333.

Fairlamb, A. H., Opperdoes, F. R., and Borst, P., 1977, New approach to screening drugs for activity against African trypanosomes, *Nature (Lond.)* 265:270–271.

Ferone, R., 1973, The enzymatic synthesis of dihydropteroate and dihydrofolate by *Plasmodium berghei, J. Protozool.* 20:459–464.

Ferone, R., Burchall, J. J., and Hitchings, G. H., 1969, *Plasmodium berghei* dihydrofolate reductase; isolation, properties, and inhibition by antifolates, *Mol. Pharmacol.* 5:49–59.

Fitch, C. D., Chevli, R., Banyal, H. S., Phillips, G., Pfaller, M. A., and Krogstad, D. J., 1982, Lysis of *Plasmodium falciparum* by ferriprotoporphyrin IX and a chloroquinine–ferriprotoporphyrin IX complex, *Antimicrob. Agents Chemother.* 21:819–822.

Flynn, I. W., and Bowman, I. B. R., 1969, Further studies on the mode of action of arsenicals on trypanosome pyruvate kinase, *Trans. R. Soc. Trop. Med. Hyg.* 63:121.

Goodwin, L. G., and Page, J. E., 1943, A study of the excretion of organic antimonials using a polargraphic procedure, *Biochem. J.* 37:198.

Gutteridge, W. D., and Coombs, G. H., 1977, *Biochemistry of Parasitic Protozoa*, pp. 34–42, University Park Press, Baltimore.

Gutteridge, W. E., and Trigg, P. I., 1971, Action of pyrimethamine and related drugs against *Plasmodium knowlesi in vitro*, *Parasitology* 62:431–444.

Hawking, F., 1963, Chemotherapy of anaplasmosis, in: *Experimental Chemotherapy* (R. J. Schnitzer and F. Hawking, eds.), pp. 633–639, Academic Press, New York.

Hentzer,.1, and Kobayasi, T., 1977, The ultrastructural changes of *Leishmania tropica* after treatment with pentamidine, *Ann. Trop. Med. Parasitol.* 71:157–166.

Hitchings, G. H., 1971, Folate antagonists as antibacterial and antiprotozoal agents, Part VI, Present status and future prospects for chemotherapy with folate antagonists, *Anns. N.Y. Acad. Sci.* 186:444–451.

Hitchings, G. H., and Burchall, J. J., 1965, Inhibition of folate biosynthesis and function as a basis for chemotherapy, *Adv. Enzymol.* 27:417–468.

Homewood, C. A., Warhurst, D. C., Peters, W., and Baggaley, V. C., 1972, Lysosomes, pH, and the antimalarial action of chloroquine, *Nature (Lond.)* 235:50–52.

Horton-Smith, C., and Boyland, E., 1946, Sulphonamides in the treatment of caecal coccidiosis of chickens, *Br. J. Pharmacol.* 1:139–152.

Ings, R. M. J., McFadzean, J. A., and Ormerod, W. E., 1974, The mode of action of metronidazole in *Trichomonas vaginalis* and other micro-organisms, *Biochem. Pharmacol.* 23:1421–1429.

Jacob, T. A., Buhs, R. P., Rosegay, A., Carlin, J., VandenHuevel, W. J. A., and Wolf, F. J., 1978, Identification of 6-amino-9-(2-chloro-6-fluorobenzyl)purine-1-N-oxide, a urinary metabolite of 6-amino-9-(2-chloro-6-fluorobenzyl) purine, MK-302, arprinocid, *Fed. Proc.* 37:813.

James, S., 1980, Thiamine uptake in isolated schizoats of *Eimeria tenella* and the inhibitory effects of amprolium, *Parasitology* 80:313–322.

Joyner, L. P., 1960, The relationship between toxicity and coccidiostatic efficacy of pyrimethamine and sulphonamides and their relative reversal by folic acid, *Res. Vet. Sci.* 1:2–9.

Joyner, L. P., and Kendall, S. B., 1956, Synergism in the chemotherapy of *Eimeria tenella*, *Nature (Lond.)* 176:975.

Knight, R. C., Skolimowski, I. M., and Edwards, D. I., 1978, The interaction of reduced metronidazole with DNA, *Biochem. Pharmacol.* 27:2089–2093.

Krenitsky, T. A., Koszalka, G. W., Tuttle, J. V., Adamczyk, D. L., Elion, G. B., and Marr, J. J., 1980, in: *Purine Metabolism in Man—III*, Part B (A. Rapado and R. W. E. Watts, eds.), pp. 7–12, Plenum, New York.

Kuttler, K. L., 1983, Influence of a second anaplasma exposure on the success of treatment to eliminate anaplasma carrier infections in cattle, *Am. J. Vet. Res.* 44:882–883.

LaRusso, N. F., Tomasz, M., Muller, M., and Lipman, R., 1977, Interaction of metronidazole with nucleic acids *in vitro*, *Mol. Pharmacol.* 13:872–882.

Latter, V. S., and Wilson, R. G., 1979, Factors influencing the assessment of anticoccidial activity in cell culture, *Parasitology* 79:169–175.

Leon, W., Brun, R., and Krassner, S. M., 1977, Effect of Berenil on growth, mitochondrial DNA, and respiration of *Leishmania tarentolae* promastigotes, *J. Protozool.* 24:444–448.

Lindmark, D. G., and Muller, M., 1976, Antitrichomonad action, mutagenicity, and reduction of metronidazole and other nitroimidazoles, *Antimicrob. Agents Chemother.* 10:476–482.

Lippe, C., 1968, Effects of Amphotericin B on thiourea permeability of phospholipid and cholesterol bilayer membranes, *J. Mol. Biol.* 35:635–637.

Looker, D. L., Berens, R. L., and Marr, J. J., 1984, Effects of pyrazolopyrimidines on purine and pyrimidine metabolism in Leishmania donovani, J. Cell. Biochem. (Suppl.) 7A:16.

Lux, R. E., 1954, The chemotherapy of Eimeria tenella: 1-diamino-pyrimidines and dihydrotriazines, Antibiot. Chemother. 4:971–977.

Machamer, C. E., and Cresswell, P., 1984, Monensin prevents terminal glycosylation of the N- and O-linked oligosaccharides of the HLA-DR-associated invarient chain and inhibits its dissociation from the α–β-chain complex, Proc. Natl. Acad. Sci. U.S.A. 81:1287–1291.

Madjar, J.-J., Nielsen-Smith, K., Frahm, M., and Roufa, D. J., 1982, Emetine resistance in Chinese hamster ovary cells is associated with an altered ribosomal protein S14 mRNA, Proc. Natl. Acad. Sci. U.S.A. 79:1003–1007.

Marr, J. J., and Berens, R. L., 1977, Antileishmanial effect of allopurinol II. Relationship of adenine metabolism in Leishmanial species to the action of allopurinol, J. Infect. Dis. 136:724–732.

Marr, J. J., Berens, R. L., and Nelson, D. J., Purine metabolism in Leishmania donovani and Leishmania bratiliensis, 1978, Biochem. Biophys. Acta 544:360–371.

McCalla, D. R., 1983, Mutagenicity of nitrofuron derivatives, Rev. Environ. Mutagen 5:745–765.

Nakamichi, N., Rhoads, D. D., and Roufa, D. J., 1983, The Chinese hamster cell emetine resistance gene. Analysis of cDNA and genomic sequences encoding ribosomal protein S14, J. Biol. Chem. 258:13236–13242.

Nelson, D. J., LaFon, S. W., Tuttle, J. V., Miller, W. H., Miller, R. L., Krenitsky, T. A., Elion, G. B., Berens, R. L., and Marr, J. J., 1979a, Allopurinol ribonucleoside as an antileishmanial agent, J. Biol. Chem. 25:11544–11549.

Nelson, D. J., Bugge, C. J. L., Elion, G. B., Berens, R. L., and Marr, J. J., 1979b, Metabolism of pyrazolo [3,4-d]pyrimidines in Leishmania braziliensis and L. donovani I. Allopurinol, oxipurinol, and 4-amino-pyrazolo[3,4-d]pyrimidine, J. Biol. Chem. 254:3959–3964.

Polin, D., Wynosky, E. R., and Porter, C. C., 1963, In vivo absorption of amprolium and its competition with thiamine, Proc. Soc. Exp. Biol. Med. 114:273–277.

Rogers, E. F., Clark, R. L., Becker, H. J., Pessolano, A. A., Leanza, W. J., McManus, E. C., Andriuli, F. J., and Cuckler, A. C., 1964, Antiparasitic drugs: V. Anticoccidial activity of 4-amino-2-ethoxybenzoic acid and related compounds, Proc. Exp. Biol. Med. 117:488–492.

Schmidt, G., Hirt, R., and Fisher, R., 1969, Babesicidal effect of basically substituted carbanilides. I: Activity against Babesia rodaini in mice, Res. Vet. Sci. 10:530–533.

Sharma, S. K., and Quastel, J. H., 1965, Transport and metabolism of thiamine in rat brain cortex in vitro, Biochem. J. 94:790–800.

Skelton, F. S., Bowman, C. M., Porter, T. H., and Folkers, K., 1971, New quinoline quinone inhibitors of mitochondrial reductase systems and reversal by coenzyme Q, Biochem. Biophys. Rev. Commun. 43:102–107.

Slaughter, R. S., and Barnes, E. M., Jr., 1979, Hypoxanthine transport by Chinese hamster lung fibroblasts: Kinetics and inhibition by nucleosides, Arch. Biochem. Biophys. 197:349–355.

Spector, T., Jones, T. E., and Elion, G. B., 1979, Specificity of adenylosuccinate synthetase and adenylosuccinate lyase from Leishmania donovani, J. Biol. Chem. 254:8422–8425.

Spector, T., Jones, T. E., LaFon, S. W., and Nelson, D. J., 1984, Monophosphates of formycin B and allopurinol riboside. Interaction with leishmanial and mammalian succino-AMP lyase and GMP reductase, Biochem. Pharm. 33:1611–1617.

Trager, W., 1967, The different developing intracellularly and extracellularly in vitro, Am. J. Trop. Med. Hyg. 16:15–18.

Wang, C. C., 1975, Studies of the mitochondria from Eimeria tenella and inhibition of electron transport by quinolone coccidiostats, Biochim. Biophys. Acta 396:210–219.

Wang, C. C., 1976, Inhibition of the respiration of Eimeria tenella by quinolone coccidiostats, Biochem. Pharmacol. 25:343–349.

Wang, C. C., 1978, Biochemical and nutritional aspects of coccidia, in: Avian Coccidiosis (P. L. Long, K. N. Boorman, and B. M. Freeman, eds.), pp. 135–184, British Poultry Science, Ltd., Edinburgh.

Wang, C. C., 1982, Biochemistry and physiology of coccidia, in: The Biology of the Coccidia, (P. L. Long, ed.), pp. 167–228, University Park Press, Baltimore.

Wang, C. C., 1984, Parasite enzymes as potential targets for antiparasitic chemotherapy, *J. Med. Chem.* 27:1–9.

Wang, C. C., and Simashkevich, P. M., 1980, A comparative study of the biological activities of arprinocid and arprinocid 1-N-oxide, *Mol. Biochem. Parasitol.* 1:335–345.

Wang, C. C., Stotish, R. L., and Poe, M., 1975, Dihydrofolate reductase from *Eimeria tenella:* Rationalization of the chemotherapeutic efficacy of pyrimethamine, *J. Protozool.* 22:564–568.

Wang, C. C., Simashkevich, P. M., and Stotish, R. L., 1979*a*, Mode of anticoccidial action of arprinocid, *Biochem. Pharmacol.* 28:2241–2248.

Wang, C. C., Tolman, R. L., Simashkevich, P. M., and Stotish, R. L., 1979*b*, Arprinocid, an inhibitor of hypoxanthine-guanine transport, *Biochem. Pharmacol.* 28:2241–2248.

Wang, C. C., Simashkevich, P. M., and Fan, S. S., 1981, The mechanism of anticoccidial action of arprinocid-1-N-oxide, *J. Parasitol.* 67:137–149.

Warhurst, D. C., and Thomas, S. C., 1978, The chemotherapy of rodent malaria, XXXI. *Ann. Trop. Med. Parasitol.* 72:203–211.

Warren, E. W., 1968, Vitamin requirements of the coccidia of the chicken, *Parasitology* 58:137–148.

Wasmuth, J. J., Hill, J. M., and Vock, L. S., 1980, Biochemical and genetic evidence for a new class of emetine-resistant Chinese hamster cells with alterations in the protein biosynthesis machinery, *Somat. Cell Genet.* 6:495–576.

Williamson, J., Macadam, R. F., and Dixon, H., 1975, Drug induced lesions in trypanosome fine structure: A guide to modes of trypanocidal action, *Biochem. Pharmacol.* 24:147–151.

Wolf, F. J., Steffens, J. J., Alvaro, R. F., and Jacob, T. A., 1978, Microsomal conversion of MK-302, arprinocid [6-amino-9-(2-chloro-6-fluorobenzyl) purine] to 6-amino-9-(2-chloro-6-fluorobenzyl)purine-1-N-oxide by liver microsomes from the chicken and the dog and to 2-chloro-6-fluorobenzyl alcohol by liver microsomes from the rat and mouse, *Fed. Proc.* 37:814.

Yayon, A., and Ginsburg, H., 1983, Chloroquine inhibits the degradation of endocytic vesicles in human malaria parasites, *Cell Biol. Int. Rep.* 7:895.

10

Drug Resistance in Protozoa

TIMOTHY G. GEARY, S. ALLEN EDGAR, and JAMES B. JENSEN

1. PROTOZOAL INFECTIONS OF HUMANS

Treatment failures have been recorded in the chemotherapy of protozoal diseases almost since such therapy began. Failures may have a number of causes, only one of which is true pathogen resistance to the drug. Perhaps the major obstacle to our comprehension of the problems of drug resistance is our lack of basic understanding of the biology of protozoal infections in humans. Parasites may show reduced sensitivity to chemotherapy because of hidden forms in drug-impermeable areas such as abscesses or the CNS, differences in susceptibility of the various stages of protozoan life cycles, dependence on the host immune response of drug efficacy, individual variations in pharmacokinetics, inadequate dosing, oxygen dependence of some drugs, or simply inherent variations among strains or species of parasites in drug sensitivity. This last factor is especially important for drugs that are effective only when given at or near the maximally tolerated dose.

True drug resistance can be defined as a stable genotypic variant, selected from a normally sensitive population by drug exposure, that has the ability to survive and even multiply in the presence of normally effective drug concentrations. Every population contains individuals having a range of drug sensitivity distributed in a Poisson fashion, and different strains or closely related species may show inherent profound differences in drug sensitivity. These are not examples of true drug resistance, although they may be of considerable clinical importance, any more than gram-negative bacteria can be considered "resistant" to penicillin G. As Peters (1974a) noted, we must differentiate resistance to therapy attributable to drug failure or innate insensitivity from true selected drug resistance. Although our present understanding of drug resistance in

TIMOTHY G. GEARY and JAMES B. JENSEN • Department of Microbiology and Public Health, Michigan State University, East Lansing, Michigan 48824.   S. ALLEN EDGAR • Department of Poultry Science, Auburn University, Auburn, Alabama 36849.

bacteria is far greater than that in protozoa, the advent of successful *in vitro* culture techniques for most protozoal pathogens may be expected to lead to rapid advances (cf. Jensen, 1983) (*vide infra*).

1.1. Toxoplasma gondii

Treatment failures occur in these infections, but no evidence is available suggesting drug resistance as the cause. Strain differences in sensitivity have been described (Oshima and Hoshino, 1977). It is likely that cyst forms are relatively insensitive to available drugs by virtue of their inaccessability and low metabolic rate. Experimentally induced resistance to sulfonamides (Sanders and Midved, 1971; Lai *et al.*, 1974) and to other drugs (cf. Pfefferkorn and Pfefferkorn, 1978) is of uncertain relevance to human disease.

1.2. Entamoeba histolytica

Recent reviews of the chemotherapy of amebiasis indicate that treatment failures are not uncommon in this disease but that no evidence is yet available demonstrating drug-resistant parasites to be the cause (Biagi, 1981; Neal, 1983). Some of the useful drugs have effects that are more or less limited to parasites in tissues or in the intestinal lumen, undoubtedly accounting for some reports of failure (Biagi, 1981). Ameba in abscesses may sometimes be difficult to treat because of poor drug penetration. Biagi (1981) summarized data on local drug concentrations necessary to produce amebicidal effects in different sites. Differences in invasiveness among *E. histolytica* strains may thus cause apparent resistance to metronidazole (Sargeaunt and Williams, 1978; Sargeaunt *et al.*, 1982; Pehrson and Bengtsson, 1983). Other explanations for treatment failures include the insensitivity of cyst stages (Bakshi *et al.*, 1978) and inactivation of drugs (particularly metronidazole) by gut flora (Ralph and Clark, 1978). Species differences in sensitivity also exist (cf. Chacin-Bonilla, 1980) that might lead to assumptions of drug resistance in improperly diagnosed cases.

It has proved difficult to create drug-resistant strains *in vitro* (Neal, 1983), and currently no proof of true clinical drug resistance is available. A recently developed *in vitro* model for the assessment of drug sensitivity should aid in defining the extent, if any, of resistance (Cedeño and Krogstad, 1983).

1.3. Giardia lamblia

Drug resistance in clinical cases has not been reported. Treatment failures occur but are often cured with a second course of therapy. Optimal dosage schedules still need to be defined that, along with reinfection, may account for the observed failures. An *in vitro* model for routine susceptibility testing was recently developed (Jokipii and Jokipii, 1980). An isolate from a patient clinically resistant to quinacrine or metronidazole (alone) was shown to be sensitive to these drugs *in vitro* (Smith *et al.*, 1982), indicating that resistance cannot yet be invoked as an explanation of treatment failures.

1.4. Trichomonas vaginalis

As recently as 1976, no confirmed *in vitro* resistance to metronidazole had been reported, although treatment failures and apparent *in vivo* resistance were known (Coombs, 1976). Strains could be made metronidazole resistant in the laboratory (Coombs, 1976; Meingassner and Mieth, 1976). Honigberg (1977) reviewed the extensive literature on experimental resistance, on *in vitro–in vivo* correlations, on strain differences in sensitivity, and on possible explanations of treatment failures.

However, recently an isolate of *T. vaginalis* from a clinically resistant case was shown to be insensitive to metronidazole *in vitro* (Thurner and Meingassner, 1978; Meingassner and Thurner, 1979) and to be cross-resistant to similar drugs. Other reports have since appeared, including isolates cross-resistant to ornidazole and tinidazole (Forsgren and Forssman, 1979; Heyworth *et al.*, 1980; Müller *et al.*, 1980; Kulda *et al.*, 1982). One report confirmed *in vitro* resistance in a mouse model and ruled out reinfection on clinical grounds; adequate serum metronidazole concentrations were also demonstrated (Kulda *et al.*, 1982). Although treatment failures may have other causes, including suboptimal dosing, reinfection, noncompliance, or drug inactivation by other flora (Meingassner and Heyworth, 1981), drug resistance must now be considered a contributing factor. As of 1982, such cases had been described from America, Sweden, Austria, and Britain.

Doubts have been raised about the clinical significance of these observations (Edwards, 1980), particularly since *in vitro* resistance can only be seen in cultures grown aerobically; in anaerobic conditions (the "natural" state for *T. vaginalis*), all strains are equally sensitive. However, in the *in vivo* state it is possible that a small proportion of organisms populate areas that are relatively aerobic and that, after metronidazole treatment, resistant types repopulate the depleted anaerobic site. This idea fits in with the observation that relapses, not continuous growth, typify clinical metronidazole resistance. Clearly more information is needed on the use of *in vitro* tests for drug resistance, on the implications of drug resistance for therapy, and on the extent of the problem (Edwards, 1980; Meingassner and Heyworth, 1981).

Little is known about the mechanism of resistance. *Tritichomonas foetus* resistant to metronidazole lacks the enzymes required for pyruvate oxidation and fails to reduce the drug to the active species (Čerkasovová *et al.*, 1980), but *T. vaginalis* does not appear to share this trait (Kulda *et al.*, 1982).

1.5. Leishmania spp.

Treatment failures have long been observed in the chemotherapy of leishmaniasis (cf. Beveridge, 1963; Bray, 1972; Steck, 1974; Peters, 1974a, 1976, 1980a; Marsden, 1979; Jha, 1983; Chulay *et al.*, 1983b). Reasons postulated for failure include derangements in the typical host–parasite interaction, poor host immune response, improper dosing and lack of understanding of pharmacokinetics, poor drug penetration into sites of infection, insensitivity of promastigotes, and, perhaps most important, species and strain differences in drug sensitivity (see above citations and Ercoli, 1966, Neal, 1972;

Rees *et al.*, 1980, 1984). Questions about the existence of selected drug-resistant mutants were difficult to resolve because most available *in vitro* and *in vivo* models were inadequate for this purpose (cf. Peters, 1976). However, several animal models were used to confirm the marked differences in drug sensitivity that exist among strains and species (Mattock and Peters, 1975*a,b;* Bjorvatn and Neva, 1979; Trotter *et al.*, 1980; Peters *et al.*, 1980). Using such a model, a Kenyan isolate of *L. donovani* was shown to be truly insensitive to pentavalent antimonials (Hanson *et al.*, 1983). After 15 hamster passages, however, the isolate had regained normal sensitivity. Whether this finding was attributable to unstable resistance or to overgrowth of drug-sensitive organisms present in the isolate is not clear.

Recently, a significant advance was achieved by Berman and colleagues on the development of a reliable *in vitro* model for the assay of drug sensitivity of these parasites (Berman and Wyler, 1980; Berman *et al.*, 1982; Berman, 1982). The organisms are grown in human macrophages. Sensitivity to antileishmanial drugs is well correlated with *in vivo* susceptibility at appropriate drug concentrations. Isolates from antimony-sensitive infections are killed *in vitro* by therapeutically relevant concentrations of these drugs. Of seven isolates obtained from cases of apparent antimony resistance, five proved fully sensitive *in vitro;* one of the truly resistant isolates was extremely insensitive to antimonials *in vitro* and probably represents the first irrefutable evidence of drug resistance in human infections of this type (Berman *et al.*, 1982). Cross-resistance between trivalent and pentavalent antimonials has also been observed in this model (Berman, 1982).

The implications of these findings for human infections are not clear. In most apparently drug-resistant cases, truly drug-resistant parasites are probably not present. Strain and subspecies differences undoubtedly account for some of the problem, but great improvements could be made by optimizing treatment regimens and increasing understanding of the clinical pharmacology of available drugs, areas in which much work needs to be done (Chulay *et al.*, 1983*a,b*). The use of the Berman *in vitro* system will be of great help in defining the type and extent of drug resistance.

1.6. Trypanosoma cruzi

Recent reviews of the chemotherapy of Chagas' disease (Brener, 1975; Kierszen-baum, 1984) indicate that no proven cases of true drug resistance in human infections have been reported. Isolates resistant to primaquine and nitrofurazone have been produced *in vitro* (Amrein, 1965). Also, strain differences in drug sensitivity are well known (Brener and Chiari, 1967; Haberkorn and Gönnert, 1972; Freeman *et al.*, 1975; Brener *et al.*, 1976; Andrade and Figueira, 1977; Cover and Gutteridge, 1981). Some treatment failures have been ascribed to the presence of drug-resistant strains (Schenone *et al.*, 1972; Andrade *et al.*, 1975, 1977), although this remains to be proved *in vitro*. The fact that nifurtimox, used at maximally tolerated doses for long periods of time, is differentially effective in different areas (cf. Kierszenbaum, 1984) may be explained by strain differences in sensitivity.

It is also interesting to note that *T. cruzi* possesses a competent, inducible cytochrome P-450 drug monooxygenase system that metabolizes standard substrates (Agosin et al., 1976, 1984). Although not every drug is a substrate for this system, and all metabolites are not inactive, this reaction, by virtue of the increased hydrophobicity of the products, may help reduce intracellular drug concentrations below the therapeutic level. More work must be done on the ability of these parasites to detoxify chemotherapeutic agents.

1.7. Trypanosoma brucei rhodiesense and T. b. gambiense

Information on the extent and characteristics of drug resistance in the human African trypanosomes has been thoroughly reviewed (Bishop, 1959; Williamson and Rollo, 1959; Williamson, 1959a, 1962, 1970; Schneider, 1963; Hawking, 1963, 1965; deRaadt and Seed, 1977; Apted, 1980; WHO, 1982). The phenomenon of drug resistance was first noted in trypanosomes, immediately after the development of arsenicals as the first antiprotozoal drugs (cf. Bishop, 1959; Williamson, 1970). It has since been noted for every available agent, one of which, tryparsamide, was eventually discarded because of the magnitude of the resistance problem. Laboratory experiments have demonstrated that resistance arises quite readily to arsenicals and dye derivatives, but less easily to suramin. Resistance is apparently related to reduced drug uptake (Williamson, 1959b). The stability of resistance is highly variable. Cross-resistance is very common but is unpredictable and may not be reciprocal; it appears to be generally based on the ionic characteristics of the drugs. In addition, strains that are resistant to one set of drugs may be hypersensitive to other unrelated compounds (Williamson et al., 1982).

These laboratory observations are of uncertain clinical relevance. Relapses occur in therapy with every available drug. Jennings and colleagues pioneered studies suggesting that at least some of these cases may be caused by behavioral changes in the parasite (Jennings et al., 1977, 1979, 1980; Gray et al., 1982; Williamson, 1983). Except for melarsoprol, none of the available drugs penetrates the blood-brain barrier and thus cannot eliminate CNS parasites. These studies convincingly demonstrated that in vivo strain differences resulting in relapsing infections and apparent drug resistance can be traced to different rates of initial CNS invasion, thus providing an escape from the drug; after clearance of blood parasites, the CNS colony could return and generate the relapse. Poltera and colleagues showed that a similar situation can occur with melarsoprol, which does cross the blood-brain barrier (Poltera, 1980; Poltera et al., 1981). These workers showed that the parasite can occupy areas such as the cerebral interstitium, where even melarsoprol penetrates poorly; thus, the parasite escapes the drug and generates relapses. Indeed, although melarsoprol relapse rates of about 5% for T. b. rhodiesense and of 10–30% for T. b. gambiense have been reported (cf. Poltera et al., 1981), these investigators were able to demonstrate that an apparently melarsoprol-resistant strain was in fact sensitive when examined in a mouse model.

Other factors can also cause treatment failures, including the innate differences in sensitivity known to characterize T. b. rhodiesense and T. b. gambiense (Apted, 1980); differences in sensitivity of amastigotes, procyclic trypomastigotes, and trypomastigotes (cf. Jennings *et al.*, 1980; Hill, 1980); suboptimal pharmacokinetics in animal models (Gilbert and Newton, 1980); and suboptimal blood levels achieved during chemotherapy (cf. Apted, 1980).

Despite the voluminous literature on experimental drug resistance, Apted noted as recently as 1980 that remarkably little hard evidence has accrued to show that clinical resistance has developed to suramin, pentamidine, or melarsoprol. The recent development of *in vitro* assay systems for determining trypanosomal drug sensitivity should greatly improve research in this area (Hill, 1980; Desjardins *et al.*, 1980).

1.8. *Plasmodium spp.*

A truly remarkable literature has accumulated on this topic, particularly the masterful tome by Peters (1970), but including many other contributions as well, e.g., Bishop (1959), Powell and Tigertt (1968), Thompson and Werbel (1972), WHO (1973, 1982), Elslager (1974), Peters (1974*b*, 1980*b*, 1982, 1984*a,b*), Tigertt and Clyde (1976), Wernsdorfer and Kouznetzov (1980), Wernsdorfer (1980), Bruce-Chwatt (1980, 1981), Ross Institute (1981), Harinasuta *et al.* (1982), Rieckmann (1983), Wyler (1983, 1984), Centers for Disease Control (1984), Doberstyn (1984). This discussion focuses primarily on areas of recent interest and those that have not, in our opinion, been adequately addressed.

1.8.1. *P. malariae*

This organism is known to respond slowly to treatment with a variety of antimalarials (cf. Dixon *et al.*, 1983). True drug resistance to proguanil and pyrimethamine has been reported (Peters, 1970), but this is of little clinical significance, since chloroquine (CQ) is fully effective. *p*-Aminobenzoic acid (PABA) antagonists are known to be relatively ineffective (Tigertt and Clyde, 1976).

1.8.2. *P. vivax*

This species is relatively insensitive to dihydrofolate reductase (DHFR) inhibitors (cf. Doberstyn *et al.*, 1979; Darlow *et al.*, 1982) and is unaffected by PABA antagonists (Tigertt and Clyde, 1976). True proguanil and pyrimethamine resistance has been observed (Peters, 1970). Despite occasional reports (Gupta, 1978), CQ resistance has not been demonstrated in *P. vivax;* a recently developed *in vitro* system can monitor the situation (Gajanana and Raichowdhuri, 1984). Strain differences in primaquine sensitivity are well known (Tigertt and Clyde, 1976; Grewal, 1981), but this is not true drug resistance; laboratory experiments have selected such mutants, but they have no clinical relevance thus far (Grewal, 1981).

1.8.3. *P. falciparum*

Drug resistance is of tremendous and depressing clinical significance. The current efficacy of chemotherapy is declining, a fact that has potentially devastating implications, and seriousness of the situation is difficult to overestimate (Peters, 1982, 1984*a;* Bruce-Chwatt, 1982; Doberstyn, 1984).

1.8.3a. Antibiotics. True drug resistance has not been reported for these compounds. Although they act slowly and may not be curative in cases involving high, threatening parasitemias, no conclusive evidence has been presented on decreased parasite sensitivity to them. One report of semiresistance to clindamycin (Hall *et al.*, 1975*a*) was based solely on treatment failures using what has proved a suboptimal dosing schedule (R. Westerman, personal communication). Attempts to generate clindamycin resistance in *P. falciparum in vitro* have not been successful (D. Krogstad, personal communication).

1.8.3b. Primaquine. Although clinically resistant strains of *P. falciparum* have not been described, it appears that exoerythrocytic schizonts of CQ-resistant strains are somewhat cross-resistant to primaquine (cf. Grewal, 1981), although gametocytes do not share the resistance (cf. Tigertt and Clyde, 1976). Since most investigators do not consider the mechanism of action of these drugs to be similar, these observations are intriguing. It would be very interesting to characterize the actions of primaquine on these strains in an *in vitro* system capable of analyzing drug effects on exoerythrocytic schizonts.

1.8.3c. PABA Antagonists. These drugs have met with widespread resistance when used alone (cf. Bruce-Chwatt, 1981), and this is considered to be true resistance. Pharmacokinetic variations due to the pharmacogenetics of N-acetyltransferase also contribute to treatment failures (cf. Tigertt and Clyde, 1976). Further work on the characterization of sulfa resistance will be advanced by the *in vitro* assay system developed by Brockelman and Tan-Ariya (1982; Tan-Ariya and Brockelman, 1983*a*). These workers report that a sulfa-sensitive strain requires PABA, whereas a sulfa-resistant strain does not (Tan-Ariya and Brockelman, 1983*b*); we have not found this to be true (Divo *et al.*, 1984). However, since these drugs are not routinely used alone in malaria chemotherapy, the problems of resistance to them are not the most important we face.

1.8.3d. DHFR Inhibitors. Clinical resistance to pyrimethamine and proguanil is geographically widespread but patchy (Bruce-Chwatt, 1981; Reacker *et al.*, 1981). Once resistance develops, it appears to be marked, and the drugs no longer have any effect (Peters, 1970). Cross-resistance is common but not absolute (cf. Schapira, 1984; Peters, 1970, 1980*b;* McLarty *et al.*, 1984). In rodent parasites, resistance to pyrimethamine can be caused by production of an altered DHFR with decreased affinity for the drug (Ferone *et al.*, 1969; Sirwaraporn and Yuthavong, 1984). These parasites appear to be at a biological disadvantage *in vivo* compared with sensitive strains (Rosario *et al.*, 1978). Recently, several explanations have been advanced to explain resistance to DHFR inhibitors in *P. falciparum.* Several possibilities are obvious, including an altered DHFR, DHFR gene amplification (cf. Pratt and Ruddon, 1979), decreased drug uptake, or enhanced uptake of folic acid or the products of folate metabolism (cf. Pratt, 1977). Lanners and Trager (1984) have presented ultrastructural evidence they consider suggestive of gene amplification; this hypothesis remains to be confirmed bio-chemically. McCutchen *et al.* (1984) have clearly shown in several *P. falciparum* clones that changes in K_m of pyrimethamine for DHFR and not gene amplification can account for pyrimethamine resistance. Finally, Milhous *et al.* (1985) find that resistant isolates of *P. falciparum* may obtain folate cofactors exogenously or synthesize them in unusual de novo pathways. It is of course possible that pyrimethamine pressure has selected mutants of each type in various areas. Clinically, the high degree of pyrimethamine resistance observed (1000–10,000 fold) argues against DHFR gene amplification, which in other systems is generally associated with a more modest degree of resistance (cf. Pratt and Ruddon, 1979). The fact that new DHFR inhibitors have been developed which are effective in drug-resistant strains (Peters, 1974b; Rozman and Canfield, 1979; Richards, 1979; Howells, 1982; Mamalis and Werbel, 1984) is only consistent with an altered DHFR mechanism of resistance, since the others predict essentially complete cross-resistance. Nonetheless, that such compounds exist argues that the potential of DHFR inhibitors as antimalarials has not been exhausted and that folate metabolism in *P. falciparum* is clearly more complex that previously thought (Ferone, 1977; Sherman, 1979; Tan-Ariya and Brockelman, 1983a; Chulav *et al.*, 1984; Milhaus *et al.*, 1985; Geary *et al.*, 1985b).

An altered DHFR active site may also lead to decreased affinity for the natural substrate, resulting in a less fit strain that would eventually be overgrown by sensitive parasites in the absence of drug pressure; this has indeed been observed. However, pyrimethamine-resistant strains can also spread and have been observed in areas in which the drug has rarely been used (cf. Clyde, 1967; Peters, 1970), suggesting that more than one mechanism of resistance can occur. Recent developments in *in vitro* systems for determining pyrimethamine sensitivity should enhance our understanding of this phenomenon (Nguyen-Dinh and Payne, 1980; Chen *et al.*, 1980; Nguyen-Dinh *et al.*, 1982; Lamont and Darlow, 1982; Thaithong and Beale, 1981; Eastham and Rieckmann, 1983; Schapira, 1984; Spencer *et al.*, 1984).

1.8.3e. Combinations of PABA Antagonists and DHFR Inhibitors. Resistance to combinations such as Fansider (sulfadoxine + pyrimethamine) has been fully documented recently and seems to be found throughout the regions in which such drugs are commonly used. A number of cases have been described; the reader is referred to some of the more recent for a survey (Hurwitz *et al.*, 1981; Chongsupphajaisiddhi and Sabchareon, 1981; Dixon *et al.*, 1982; Pinichpongse *et al.*, 1982; Johnson *et al.*, 1982; Oostburg and Jozefzoon, 1983; Ferraroni *et al.*, 1983; Hess *et al.*, 1983; Mazier *et al.*, 1984). Recently, Brockelman and colleagues (1982) showed the usefulness of Way-mouth's medium, which lacks PABA and folic acid, in measuring sensitivity to these compounds. Their results have been confirmed (Chulay *et al.*, 1984) using another medium. Interestingly, the combinations are generally effective against all but the most pyrimethamine-resistant strains (Bruce-Chwatt, 1981), and it will be important to define the additional mutation(s) necessary to create resistance to them.

1.8.3f. Quinoline-Containing Antimalarials. Strain variations in sensitivity to quinine have long been recognized (cf. Bishop, 1959), and recently decreased *in vitro* and *in vivo* sensitivity to this drug has been observed in areas in which it has been heavily used due to CQ resistance (Glew *et al.*, 1974; Chongsupphajaisiddhi *et al.*, 1981; Smrkovski *et al.*, 1982*b*; Webster *et al.*, 1985). It is relatively difficult to produce experimental quinine resistance (Peters, 1970), but this has been accomplished in *P. falciparum* (Clyde *et al.*, 1970; Glew *et al.*, 1978). Clinically, quinine is becoming extremely important again (see Chapter 3), and the problems of resistance are indeed threatening. In many areas, quinine is routinely combined with other drugs to ensure efficacy (Bruce-Chwatt, 1981) and, if extensive quinine resistance develops, chemotherapy will be severely compromised.

Mefloquine, a structural analogue of quinine with significant advantages (see Chapter 3) is now becoming available. It is indeed depressing to note that cases of mefloquine resistance have already been documented (Brockelman *et al.*, 1981; Boudreau *et al.*, 1982; Smrkovski *et al.*, 1982*a*; Bygbjerg *et al.*, 1983). It appears that areas in which quinine has been heavily used may show mefloquine resistance (S. Hoffman, personal communication). Quinine-resistant strains may develop mefloquine resistance as well, although the cross-resistance is certainly not absolute (Geary and Jensen, 1983; Webster *et al.*, 1985).

By far the most serious and intensely investigated area of drug resistance in *P. falciparum* is that relating to CQ. As noted, this subject has been thoroughly reviewed, but several interesting aspects should be discussed. First, the classification of various levels of resistance as described by WHO (1973) separates drug responsiveness into four general categories: S (sensitive to normal chemotherapeutic regimens), R-I (disappearance of parasitemia followed by a variably delayed recrudesence), R-II (reduction but not elimination of parasitemia), and R-III (little or no effect on parasitemia). In terms of classic antibiotic resistance, the last two categories are easily understood. However, it is difficult to explain the phenomenon of R-I resistance in biological terms. The initial clinical observations on this type of response showed that normal CQ dosing caused resolution of symptoms and apparent elimination of parasitemia, followed 1–2 weeks later by a return of both, while ruling out reinfection (Moore and Lanier, 1961). The patient described had three classic recrudescence episodes of this type. Thus, R-I resistance is a stable phenotype that can be reproduced in experimental hosts (Peters, 1970, 1974*b*; Campbell *et al.*, 1979) and characterized *in vitro* (Rieckmann *et al.*, 1978; Campbell *et al.*, 1979).

The mechanism of resistance is obscure. These strains show a moderately reduced CQ sensitivity *in vitro* (WHO, 1973) that may be sufficient to break through CQ concentrations achieved during prophylaxis but insufficient to survive concentrations achieved during therapy (see Chapter 3). If the delayed recrudescence was caused by the selection of a small number of drug-resistant parasites that would eventually reproduce to create symptoms, one would expect the recrudescent parasites to display an R-II or R-III response, but this is not the case. Rather, a response exactly like that seen initially is observed. Furthermore, adequate blood levels are maintained following therapy to ensure killing of the parasites (Yayon *et al.*, 1983) (see Chapter 3), so that it is not a case of small numbers of parasites struggling along until the blood concentration of CQ decreases sufficiently to permit full growth. Even if this were true, it is difficult to account for recrudescences that occur as long as 30 days or more after initial clearance (WHO, 1973; Campbell *et al.*, 1979).

It could also be that R-I resistance is a combination of traits, one of which (reduced CQ sensitivity) permits prophylaxis breakthrough and another that enables the parasite to evade and survive the immune response, reemerging when immunity wanes. It is clear that the host immune response has an important role in drug efficacy; much less CQ is needed to cure *falciparum* malaria in semi-immune individuals as compared with those who are nonimmune (cf. Peters, 1970). It could thus be that R-I parasites can survive both the drug and the immune response slightly better than sensitive strains, causing recrudescences when protection decreases. However, R-I responses can be duplicated in strains transferred to other human or primate hosts (with presumably different immune status), and R-I resistance is observed in such cases during the initial attack, at a time when the immune response has not developed.

One highly speculative possibility is based on an observation by Yayon *et al.* (1983), who found *in vitro* that a particular CQ concentration at a specific parasite age resulted in the "freezing" of parasites in the relatively CQ-insensitive ring stage, persisting in a morphologically normal state for at least 48 hr. Interestingly, the parasites used were obtained from an infected individual with an R-I response (Jensen *et al.*, 1981). The application of therapeutic CQ concentrations might result in a small number of inert ring stages (blood stage hypnozoites, as it were) that would not be destroyed by the spleen and that would resume growth and replication after CQ levels dropped. The ability of parasites to enter such a state could cause stable R-I resistance. Of course, this idea is unsubstantiated and difficult to test. No other alternative appears to be available, and it is certainly difficult to relate moderate drug resistance to delayed recrudescences. It would be interesting to attempt to infect other hosts with blood taken from an R-I case at various periods following initial parasite clearance and to attempt to culture organisms from such cases in CQ-free medium. If such experiments have been done, we are not aware of them. Such research is clinically important, since currently most CQ resistance in Africa is R-I. Can such infections be completely cured if a therapeutic schedule of CQ is administered 1 or 2 weeks after the initial parasite clearance? Such studies have important implications for individuals acquiring *falciparum* malaria in Africa.

Finally, it is interesting that in the initial case of R-I resistance, the infection eventually became R-II (Moore and Lanier, 1961). It would be important to know whether R-II and R-III mutants arise from further mutations in existing R-I strains or by unique selection from sensitive populations and to determine the mechanistic relationship of the mutations resulting in the three phenotypes.

Another area of the analysis of CQ resistance that needs some improvement is in optimizing *in vitro* assay systems for drug sensitivity, several of which have been described (Rieckmann *et al.*, 1968, 1978; Wernsdorfer, 1980; Nguyen-Dinh and Trager, 1980; Desjardins *et al.*, 1979; Deloron *et al.*, 1982; Geary *et al.*, 1983; Gajanana *et al.*, 1982; LeBras and Deloron, 1983; Nguyen-Dinh *et al.*, 1983). Some tests show a cutoff between sensitive and resistance strains at about 1 μM CQ, whereas for others this value is about 3×10^{-8} M. Although the latter value is in better agreement with clinical data, resistant strains in these systems are killed by $\leq 5 \times 10^{-7}\ M$; *in vivo*, blood levels up to 10 times this value are seen with no apparent effect on the parasite. Thus, an *in vitro* model system accurately representing the situation experienced by parasites *in vivo* is lacking. Although it is clear that reasonably good correlations between *in vitro* and *in vivo* sensitivity are obtained with any of the tests, absolute differences in sensitivity among R-I, R-II, and R-III isolates are not always found. Improvement can no doubt be made.

It has been suggested that cultivation tends to increase CQ resistance in *P. falciparum* strains (LeBras *et al.*, 1983) and that resistant strains grow better *in vitro* than do CQ-sensitive isolates (Thaithong, 1983). In our experience, this is certainly not always the case, but it is possible that such strains have some advantage *in vitro*. The relevance to the *in vivo* situation is not clear. It has been shown that resistant *P. chabaudi* lines overgrow sensitive isolates *in vivo* (Rosario *et al.*, 1978). However, if the mutation generating CQ resistance were to have given rise to parasites that grow better in humans (and thus were more fit and better adapted for survival), it seems odd that such mutations would not have been established by natural selection, resulting in an original predominance of CQ-resistant organisms. Nonetheless, it appears that CQ-resistant strains are transmitted better by *Anopheles* mosquitos in the presence of the drug (cf. Tigertt and Clyde, 1976).

There is a marked geographic variation in the distribution of CQ-resistant strains. Proven cases of resistance predominate in many areas of Southeast Asia (Harinasuta *et al.*, 1982) and South America (Ferraroni *et al.*, 1983) but are relatively uncommon in Africa. Indeed, until very recently, CQ resistance in Africa was restricted to nonimmune individuals (Peters, 1982). The reasons have not been fully defined, but several investigators have suggested that the immune response may play a role (Peters, 1970; Tigertt and Clyde, 1976; Targett, 1984). We recently showed that immunity in Africa includes an apparently cell-mediated component that acts intracellularly (Jensen *et al.*, 1982, 1983, 1984) and postulated that this factor may retard the development of drug resistance (Carlin *et al.*, 1984). Reports of *P. falciparum* infections in Africans that are sensitive *in vivo* but resistant *in vitro* are available (Spencer *et al.*, 1983a), suggesting that these are the source for the clinically resistant infections observed in nonimmune individuals. It remains to be shown how rapidly CQ resistance will spread in Africa. So far, no confirmed reports of this type from West Africa have been published. We recently cultured an R-II resistant parasite from a Sudanese (where no such cases have been reported) who acquired the infection in Tanzania, indicating the possibility of inter-African transfer of resistance (A. Farouk, M. Homeida, T. G. Geary, and J. B. Jensen, unpublished observations).

Another interesting feature of CQ-resistant *P. falciparum* is the lack of absolute cross-resistance to other QCA. This is not the case for many CQ-resistant rodent parasites (Peters, 1970, 1984b) but has been seen for amodiaquine, amopyroquine, and similar drugs in *Aotus* infections (cf. Elslager, 1974; Schmidt *et al.*, 1977) as well as *in vitro* (Smrkovski *et al.*, 1982; Geary and Jensen, 1983; Thaithong, 1983; Spencer *et al.*, 1983b). The continued sensitivity to amodiaquine of some CQ-resistant infections has been exploited therapeutically in some areas (Spencer *et al.*, 1983b; Noeypatimanond *et al.*, 1983; Watkins *et al.*, 1984) but is less successful elsewhere (Hall *et al.*, 1975*b*; Campbell *et al.*, 1983). Although cross-resistance has been noted in *P. falciparum* (cf. Peters, 1970; Elslager, 1974; Tigertt and Clyde, 1976), it is important to stress that this is not an absolute finding. Fairley (1946) reported that *P. falciparum* infections in Australian soldiers in Aitapie-Wewak were naturally resistant to quinacrine. The isolates were sensitive to quinine and CQ, but cross-resistance to 3-methylchloroquine (SN-6911; Sontochin) was found. *In vitro*, CQ-resistant strains are still sensitive to 3-methylchloroquine (Geary and Jensen, 1983). Such results suggest that the therapeutic potential of the 4-aminoquinolines has not been fully exhausted.

The lack of cross-resistance in CQ-resistant strains of *P. falciparum* to closely related drugs poses some difficulties for the currently favored hypothesis of the mechanisms of action of QCA (Fitch, 1983). It has been postulated that resistance is attributable to a decrease in receptors, which would result in absolute cross-resistance, or to a selective sequestration of the putative receptor from one ligand only (CQ). This latter possibility has not been found in other pharmacological systems and is not well documented.

The mechanism of CQ resistance has been thought to be a reduction in drug accumulation (Fitch, 1983). Thus, a CQ-resistant strain of *P. falciparum* accumulated less drug than did a CQ-sensitive isolate, but it accumulated normal amounts of amodiaquine, to which cross-resistance was not present (Fitch, 1973; Fitch *et al.*, 1974). However, good quantitative analyses of the relationships between accumulation and toxicity have not been published. The extent of CQ resistance in *P. falciparum* is typically about 30-fold (maximally) (cf. Geary and Jensen, 1983; Wernsdorfer, 1980), and the concentration–response curves of resistant and sensitive strains are generally parallel (Geary and Jensen, 1983), suggesting that the mechanism of action has not changed. From these results, we should expect a decrease in accumulation proportional to the decrease in sensitivity in resistant isolates. In recent studies (Geary *et al.*, 1985*a*), we have been able to show that the maximum difference in accumulation of high specific activity [^{3}H]chloroquine in *P. falciparum* is only about two- to threefold, and comparison of intracellular concentrations achieved 2 hr after exposure, at which time lethality is observed (Yayon *et al.*, 1983) with IC_{50} values, shows that killing occurs at different intracellular concentrations in different strains. This result is not compatible with the hypothesis that reduced uptake is the mechanism of resistance. It appears that our understanding of this phenomenon and of the mechanism of action of the QCA is far from complete (Ginsburg *et al.*, 1984).

Clonal analysis may be important in future work. Thaithong and colleagues showed that most clones from a multiply-resistant isolate of *P. falciparum* resembled the parental isolate in sensitivity but that one clone was much less resistant to chloroquine, pyrimethamine, and sulfadoxine + pyrimethamine (Thaithong, 1983; Thaithong *et al.*, 1984). Interestingly, the clones were sensitive to amodiaquine, quinine, and mefloquine. Graves *et al.* (1984) found that clones obtained from a CQ-resistant strain all possessed the moderate CQ resistance observed in the original isolate, while variations in pyrimethamine sensitivity of 1000-fold were seen. These results indicate that populations of *P. falciparum* are composed of individual organisms with a variety of drug sensitivity (as expected), and similar studies should be very profitable in the analysis of drug resistance.

2. DRUG RESISTANCE IN PROTOZOAL INFECTIONS OF ANIMALS

Protozoal infections in veterinary medicine constitute an enormous biological and economic problem, and considerable effort has been expended in the development of effective chemotherapy for such diseases. Primarily, these diseases are caused by trypanosomes and coccidia, and this discussion focuses heavily on them.

2.1. Trypanosoma spp.

A recent review by Leach and Roberts (1981) clearly summarized problems of drug resistance encountered in African countries in the treatment of animal infections caused by a variety of species of *Trypanosoma*. Many of the points discussed earlier for human trypanosomiasis (and cf. Williamson, 1962, 1970) hold true for trypanosomiasis of animals. Treatment failures can be result from underdosing (by underestimating total body weight of the treated animal) or from poor compliance to schedules of treatment. These conditions are also optimal for the selection of truly drug-resistant parasites, which clearly exist. The stability of resistance, the types and degree of cross-resistance, and the case-by-case implications of apparent drug resistance are areas in which considerable work remains to be done. Species variations in sensitivity and variations in sensitivity in different host species often make experimental data difficult to interpret. Nonetheless, problems in drug resistance have had serious implications for herd management of horses, cattle, camels, and other economically important species in Africa.

2.2. Coccidian Parasites

2.2.1. General

Although there are many protozoa of veterinary importance in domestic animals throughout the world, little has been published on drug resistance other than for the coccidia of poultry, particularly *Eimeria* species that infect chickens. During the late 1940s and early 1950s, when continuous administration of anticoccidial drugs in poultry feeds became a popular means of controlling coccidiosis in the United States, concern arose about the development of drug resistance (Waletzky *et al.*, 1954). There was the question of whether refractory strains of the various *Eimeria* species already existed (lack of sensitivity to drugs) or of whether resistance had begun to develop in response to drug use. There has since been ample evidence that significant resistance has developed to some drugs, which are no longer marketed, while other drugs have been widely and successfully used for many years. Failure of some newly introduced drugs to control certain species or isolates was often interpreted as lack of intrinsic activity. This appeared to have been the case for nitrophenide when first introduced. It had been proved effective against *E. tenella* and *E. necatrix* but was quite ineffective against *E. brunetti* (S. A. Edgar, unpublished data).

The earliest anticoccidial drugs for poultry had been screened most often against *E. tenella* alone, and most early drug-resistance studies in laboratories dealt with that species. Among the earliest papers published in the United States on drug resistance were those by Harwood and Stunz (1953), Waletzky *et al.* (1954), and Cuckler and Malanga (1955). In studying 40 field isolates from 14 American states, these last investigators found 43% resistant to nitrophenide, 45% to sulfaquinoxaline, and 57% to nitrofurazone. Some work has been done with *E. acervulina* (Fouré and Bennejean, 1973; Jeffers and Challey, 1973), *E. maxima* (Norton and Joyner, 1975), and others. Also, drug resistance by *E. meleagrimitis* and *E. adenoeides* of the turkey had been reported (Joyner and Norton, 1970, 1973). There have been several good reviews on this subject (Cuckler *et al.*, 1969; McLoughlin, 1970; Joyner and Norton, 1970; Ryley and Betts, 1973) as well as an excellent fairly recent review by Chapman (1978*b*). Thus, a detailed review is not given here. Notable among the many investigators of drug resistance are Chapman, Jeffers, and McLoughlin. There have apparently been no studies on the drug resistance of mammalian coccidia, even though some species are very important to the health of animals bred for human consumption.

2.2.2. Mechanisms of Resistance

Chapman (1978*b*) reported that nothing was known about the mechanisms of resistance in the coccidia and that this could possibly be attributed to lack of knowledge concerning the physiology of the parasites and the mode of action of anticoccidial drugs. Mechanisms proposed to explain how organisms become resistant to drugs included (1) alterations of cell permeability, (2) modification of the drug target sites, (3) reduction in the physiological importance of the target, and (4) synthesis of enzymes capable of inactivating inhibitors. Very little evidence is available to support these proposals, and none satisfactorily explains the development of resistance by *Eimeria* spp. to some drugs and not to others.

Smith and Galloway (1983) held that the effect of monesin does not depend on inhibition of one enzyme or on impairment of a metabolic pathway; it was their contention that coccidial resistance was less likely to develop against this drug than to some other anticoccidials because the mode of action is directed against the extracellular sporozoites and involves nonspecific interference with transmembrane sodium transport. They considered that this may be the reason why development of resistance by coccidia to monensin has been slow to occur.

2.2.3. Models for the Study of Resistance

Once a promising drug has been discovered, it is important to know what the chances are of its controlling most of the field isolates of the most important species of poultry coccidia and to estimate how long it may continue to control them. This is important because of the high cost of developing and obtaining approval to market a new drug.

Initially, two types of tests were conducted by different investigators to determine how quickly drug resistance might develop. One test involved propagating strains of *Eimeria*, usually *E. tenella*, in a series of passages in clean chickens in the presence of a drug in the ration. Such isolates were tested for drug sensitivity at the outset, then tested for sensitivity or resistance after a certain number of passages. The results of the later tests were compared with the original tests of the isolates; it was thus determined whether the parasites had developed a significant degree of resistance. Resistance was measured on the basis of mortality, growth, oocyst production, and sometimes other characters. Such procedures were tedious, and usually not more than one or two isolates or species were tested at the same time.

A variety of dosages of oocysts and levels of drugs have been used in attempting to develop resistance. Norton and Joyner (1975) believed it was best to employ large populations of oocysts against suboptimal levels of a drug to obtain rapid development of resistance. Drug levels were gradually increased until those parasites that passed through chickens either were or were not resistant. Other investigators thought it more important to expose parasites to use levels of drugs but used large populations of chickens and/or inoculated chickens with large numbers of oocysts (Chapman, 1978a).

Some tests were thus designed to speed up the development of drug resistance by inoculating chicks with large doses of oocysts or by using large numbers of birds. This technique was believed to increase the chances of a few resistant or mutant organisms completing their parasitic cycle in the presence of a drug. It was assumed that what happened in such laboratory studies would probably occur in the field. Deliberate administration of large doses of oocysts to large numbers of birds in the laboratory to speed up the development of drug resistance probably mimics what occurs in commercial poultry. Large doses of infective sporulated oocysts in the infected feces in the litter could be eaten by susceptible birds, and there are large populations of chickens or turkeys in most commerical flocks.

That many isolates of different species are partially or almost completely resistant to some commercially available anticoccidial drugs is well known. A large number of isolates from the major broiler-producing American states were tested in our laboratory as part of a 5-year study. Most isolates came from farms in which monensin had been fed for several years and where mild outbreaks had been diagnosed. Some isolates were partially resistant and a few were almost totally resistant to some drugs being marketed in this country, as measured by mortality, weight gain, feed efficiency and/or oocyst production, and some were not well controlled even by drugs to which they had never been exposed. No single drug was found most effective against all species or all isolates as measured by the aforementioned criteria. However, drugs that were effective against the most isolates were, in descending order, halofuginone, lasalocid, monensin, salinomycin, robenidine, decoquinate, and nicarbazin. Furazolidone, amprolium + ethopabate, zoalene, unistat, novostat, and roxarsone were least effective. Each drug was tested at the maximum approved level (Edgar and Flanagan, 1976).

A second method of testing for the development of drug resistance, one that we have used at our station since the demise of glycarbylamide, has been that of seeding the litter of certain floor pens with laboratory or field isolates of six or more of the most important species of *Eimeria*. The same drug is fed to birds in the same pens throughout a trial lasting a year or more. Each isolate is tested at the outset against the drug in question and possibly other drugs, then the same species of coccidia are isolated from the litter of respective drug pens. Each species is propagated, titrated for potency, and then tested again against the same drug(s). If there is no change in drug sensitivity after six or more broods, one can expect the drug to have a reasonable life span. In such a test there are usually at least 25–200 birds per drug with a series of broods on the same litter. Litters are checked during each grow-out of birds to make sure that some viable coccidia are present. Advantages of this method over some laboratory techniques are that (1) five or six or more species can be tested at once, (2) isolates are exposed to fairly large populations of chickens, (3) some chickens may be exposed to large doses of oocysts, and (4) five or six cycles of infection by a species can occur during the life of a 49-day-old broiler without handling birds or artificially harvesting and sporulating oocysts. Disadvantages of this method include (1) the necessity of avoiding tracking oocysts from other pens, and (2) the labor involved in isolating, identifying, propagating, titrating, and then testing each species recovered from the litter in susceptible chickens.

Among many who have demonstrated drug resistance to *E. tenella* in the laboratory were McLoughlin and Gardiner (1961) for glycarbylamide and McLoughlin and Chute (1971, 1973*a,b*), who found that resistance developed more readily to quinolines than to clopidol. Results with robenidine were variable and not easily compared with those for other drugs. In spite of widespread occurrence of isolates of chicken coccidia resistant to zoalene, the drug is still widely used in this country. We recently tested amprolium and zoalene against the eight species of *Eimeria* in a commercial vaccine (CocciVac) and found that amprolium was as effective against each species as it had been more than 25 years ago when first tested unpublished observation. By contrast, dinitolmide was not very efficacious against some of the species, and it never had been. None of the isolates had ever been exposed to either drug.

Norton and Joyner (1975) and Chapman (1978*b*) pointed out that if valid comparisons are to be made among drugs, experimental procedures should be standardized. Chapman's experience (1976*a*) with robenidine and *E. tenella* was that emergence of drug resistance was dose related. He also found that coccidia made partially resistant increased their resistance only when exposed to higher concentrations of the drug. He believed that this is how resistance may develop in the field.

Ryley and Betts (1973) stated that species and strains within species may differ in sensitivity to drugs regardless of whether they had ever been exposed to a drug. Chapman (1976*b*), Jeffers (1978), and others were unable to demonstrate coccidial resistance to monensin; however, Wood (1982), in comparing arprinocid, salinomycin, lasalocid, and monensin against nine predominantly *E. tenella* isolates from North Alabama farms, found five with considerable resistance to monensin as measured by mortality and weight gain. These five isolates were more resistant than any Alabama *E. tenella* isolates tested earlier (Edgar and Flanagan, 1976). The latter did not find any of the isolates of several species totally resistant to monensin, as was the case for some isolates tested against amprolium + ethopabate, roxarsone, furazolidone, dinitolmide, Unistat, clopidol, decoquinate, and robenidine.

The reason why coccidia have developed resistance to some drugs and not others is not fully understood. Nicarbazin has been widely used in broilers in this country for many years and, in our experience, has suppressed signs and symptoms of the disease about as well as any drug fed to floor-reared broilers.

Initially, the moderately high incidence of E. *tenella* infections found in monensin-medicated broiler flocks had been attributed by some (e.g., Chapman, 1978*b*) to represent incomplete drug efficacy rather than the development of drug resistance. Chapman and others were unable to demonstrate parasite resistance to monensin (1976*b*). Our own experience with many recent field isolates to which monensin had been fed for several years leads us to conclude that some resistance has developed. None of the earlier isolates of E. *tenella* tested earlier in our laboratory exhibited such resistance.

In his review on drug resistance in coccidia, Chapman (1978*b*) concluded that progress in the understanding of drug resistance can only come from greater knowledge of the mode of action of anticoccidial drugs. Those drugs to which the parasites became resistant rather quickly blocked intracellular multiplication of coccidia almost completely. By contrast, the ionophores were shown by Long and Jeffers (1982) to exert their primary action against the invasive, extracellular stages (sporozoites and merozoites) of *Eimeria*. This may be why they have proved so effective for so long.

There have been very few studies in which isolates from poultry farms were tested upon the introduction of a drug and in which new isolates from the same farms were tested later. One such study investigated the drug-resistant trends of coccidia in an integrated poultry company by Mathis et al. (1984). In comparing the results of recent tests of isolates with those of a previous study from the same farms in Georgia, these workers found that resistance patterns had changed over a 10-year period because of change in drugs used. Some older drugs were more effective in the contemporary tests than in the previous study. These investigators concluded that the ionophores appeared to be less effective today than when first introduced. Perhaps more studies of this type should be undertaken and could provide justification for shuttle programs.

·   A variety of criteria have been applied in measuring development of drug resistance. These include oocyst production, host weight gain, and mortality. In measuring drug resistance should one measure the effect of a drug on the parasites or the drug's effectiveness in preventing the effect of infection on the host? The poultry industry is concerned with whether a drug suppresses the effect of infection on the host, rather than with whether it suppresses multiplication of the parasites. Partial or complete failure of a drug should then be measured by mortality and morbid signs (listlessness, anorexia, dehydration, growth suppression, feed efficiency, and possibly pigmentation). Fecal scores, lesion scores, and oocyst production may not measure drug resistance in the practical sense.

Rapid development of drug resistance in laboratory testing (series of passages) was indicative of what happened during the brief commercial use of drugs such as glycarbylamide, quinolines, clopidol, and robenidine. These drugs almost completely blocked the multiplication in chickens of many field isolates. By contrast, ionophores such as monensin, lasalocid, and salinomycin allowed some completion of the life cycle of most isolates. It is possible that the former group of drugs caused severe genetic selection pressure in contrast to very little pressure exerted by the ionophores. One exception has been nicarbazin, which blocks multiplication of some isolates of most species almost completely, yet drug resistance has been very slow to develop in commercial broiler flocks.

2.2.4. Suggested Research Directions

There are several routes of investigation for the study of resistance to anticoccidial agents.

1. Determine whether shuttle programs reduce, prevent, or delay development of drug resistance. This would involve testing coccidial isolates from selected poultry houses, to determine their sensitivity to selected drugs before a shuttle program was introduced, and then testing drugs against isolates after several broods of chickens have been raised on shuttle programs.

2. Search for new effective anticoccidial drugs to replace those to which the most important species of coccidia are resistant. Seek drugs that have activity similar to ionophores or other characters important in delaying development of drug resistance. Test as soon as possible in the development of new drugs to determine how quickly resistance might develop.

3. Replace drug-resistant coccidia on premises with drug-susceptible ones of the most important species. This has been attempted with some success (S. A. Edgar, unpublished data).

4. Develop methods at least as effective as prophylactic medication for control of the disease, e.g., methods based on management, housing, immunization, or genetics. Some progress has been made with each of these methods, but all have shortcomings, and none is thoroughly adequate.

5. As a method of avoiding drug resistance, some advocate only the therapeutic use of drugs. Historically, treatment of outbreaks has been far less effective in preventing effects of coccidial infections in chickens and turkeys than has continuous prophylactic medication. Once a bird exhibits signs and symptoms of coccidiosis, no drug is effective.

6. Search for new drugs that do not inhibit multiplication of the parasites too greatly, thus avoiding quick and severe genetic selection of resistant populations, yet at the same time not allowing coccidial infections to interfere with peak performance of the host. Up to this point, there has not been a totally satisfactory explanation of the mode of action of anticoccidial drugs, but such knowledge may not be essential to the development of new effective drugs.

REFERENCES

Agosin, M., Naquira, C., Paulin, J., and Capdevila, J., 1976, Cytochrome P-450 and drug metabolism in *Trypanosoma cruzi:* Effects of phenobarbital, *Science* 194:195–197.
Agosin, M., Cherry, A., Pedemonte, J., and White, R., 1984, Cytochrome P-450 in culture forms of *Trypanosoma cruzi, Comp. Biochem. Physiol.* 78C:127–132.

Amrein, Y. U., 1965, Genetic transfer in trypanosomes. I. Syngamy in *Trypanosoma cruzi*, *Exp. Parasitol.* 17:261–267.

Andrade, S. G., and Figueira, R. M., 1977, Estudo experimental sobre a acão terapêutica da droga RO-7-1051 na infecção por differentes cepas do *Trypanosoma cruzi*, *Rev. Inst. Trop. Med. Sao Paulo* 19:335–341.

Andrade, S. G., Figueira, R. M., and Carvalho, M. L., 1975, Influência da cepa do *Trypanosoma cruzi* na reposta terapêutica experimental pelo Bayer 2502 (resultados do tratamento a longo prazo), *Rev. Inst. Med. Trop. Sao Paulo* 17:380–389.

Andrade, S. G., Andrade, Z. A., and Figueira, R. M., 1977, Estudo experimental sôbre resistência de uma cepa do *Trypanosoma cruzi* do Bay 2502, *Rev. Inst. Med. Trop. Sao Paulo* 19:124–129.

Apted, F. I. C., 1980, Present status of chemotherapy and chemoprophylaxis of human trypanosomiasis in the Eastern hemisphere, *Pharmacol. Ther.* 11:391–413.

Bakshi, J. S., Ghiara, J. M., and Nanivadekar, A. S., 1978, How does tinidazole compare with metronodazole? A summary report of Indian trials in amoebiosis and giardiasis, *Drugs* (Suppl. 1) 15:33–42.

Berman, J. D., 1982, *In vitro* susceptibility of antimony-resistant *Leishmania* to alternate drugs, *J. Infect. Dis.* 145:279.

Berman, J. D., and Wyler, J. D., 1980, An *in vitro* model for investigation of chemotherapeutic agents in Leishmaniasis, *J. Infect. Dis.* 142:83–86.

Berman, J. D., Chulay, J. D., Hendricks, L. D., and Oster, C. N., 1982, Susceptibility of clinically sensitive and resistant *Leishmania* to pentavalent antimony *in vitro*, *Am. J. Trop. Med. Hyg.* 31:459–465.

Beveridge, E., 1963, Chemotherapy of leishmaniasis, in: *Experimental Chemotherapy* (R. J. Schnitzer and F. Hawking, eds.), Vol. 1, pp. 257–287, Academic Press, London and New York.

Biagi, F., 1981, Amebiasis, *Antibiot. Chemother.* 30:20–27.

Bishop, A., 1959, Drug resistance in protozoa, *Biol. Rev.* 34:445–500.

Bjorvatn, B., and Neva, F. A., 1979, Experimental therapy of mice infected with *Leishmania tropica*, *Am. J. Trop. Med. Hyg.* 28:480–485.

Boudreau, E. F., Webster, H. K., Pavanand, K., and Thosingha, L., 1982, Type II mefloquine resistance in Thailand, *Lancet* 2:1335.

Bray, P. S., 1972, Leishmaniasis in the Old World, *Br. Med. Bull.* 28:39–43.

Brener, Z., 1975, Chemotherapy of *Trypanosoma cruzi* infections, *Adv. Pharmacol. Ther.* 13:1–44.

Brener, Z., and Chiari, E., 1967, Susceptibilitade de differentes amostras de *Trypanosoma cruzi* a vários agentes quimoterápicos, *Rev. Inst. Med. Trop. Sao Paulo* 9:197–207.

Brener, Z., Costa, C. A. G., and Chiari, C., 1976, Differences in the susceptibility of *Trypanosoma cruzi* to active chemotherapeutic agents, *Rev. Inst. Med. Trop. Sao Paulo* 18:450–455.

Brockelman, C. R., and Tan-Ariya, P., 1982, *Plasmodium falciparum* in continuous culture: a new medium for the *in vitro* test of sulfadoxine sensitivity, *Bull. WHO* 60:423–426.

Brockelman, C. R., Monkoleha, S., and Tan-Ariya, P., 1981, Decrease in susceptibility of *Plasmodium falciparum* to mefloquine in continuous cultures, *Bull. WHO* 59:249–252.

Bruce-Chwatt, L. J., 1980, *Essential Malariology*, Heinemann, London.

Bruce-Chwatt, L. J. (ed.), 1981, *Chemotherapy of Malaria*, World Health Organization, Geneva.

Bruce-Chwatt, L. J., 1982, Chemoprophylaxis of malaria in Africa: The spent "magic bullet," *B. Med. J.* 285:674–676.

Bygbjerg, A., Schapira, A., Flachs, H., Gomme, G., and Jepsen, S., 1983, Mefloquine resistance of falciparum malaria from Tanzania enhanced by treatment, *Lancet* 1:774–775.

Campbell, C. C., Chin, W., Collins, W. E., Teutsch, S. M., and Moss, D. M., 1979, Chloroquine-resistant *Plasmodium falciparum* from East Africa, *Lancet* 2:1151–1154.

Campbell, C. C., Payne, D., Schwartz, I. K., and Khatib, O. J., 1983, Evaluation of amodiaquine treatment of chloroquine-resistant *Plasmodium falciparum* malaria on Zanzibar, *Am. J. Trop. Med. Hyg.* 32:1216–1220.

Carlin, J. M., VandeWaa, J. B., Jensen, J. B., and Akood, M. A. S., 1984, African serum interference in the determinations of chloroquine sensitivity in *Plasmodium falciparum*, *Z. Parasitenk.* 70:589–597.

Cedeño, J. R., and Krogstad, D. J., 1983, Susceptibility testing of *Entamoeba histolytica*, *J. Infect. Dis.* 148:1090–1095.

Centers for Disease Control, 1984, Imported malaria among travelers—United States, *M.M.W.R.* 33:388–390.

Čerkasovová, A., Cerkasov, J., Kulda, J., and Demes, P., 1980, Metronidazole action on *Tritrichomonas foetus:* enzyme activities in the strains of a different resistance to the drug, in: *The Host-Invader Interplay* (H. van den Bossche, ed.), pp. 669–672, Elsevier/North-Holland Biomedical Press, Amsterdam.

Chacin-Bonilla, L., 1980, Successful treatment of human *Entamoeba policki* infections with metronidazole, *Am. Trop. Med. Hyg.* 29:521–523.

Chapman, H. D., 1975, *Eimeria tenella* in chickens: Development of resistance to quinoline anticoccidial drugs, *Parasitology* 71:41–49.

Chapman, H. D., 1976*a, Eimeria tenella:* Experimental studies in the development of resistance to robenidine, *Parasitology* 73:65–73.

Chapman, H. D., 1976*b, Eimeria tenella* in chickens: Studies on resistance to the anticoccidial drugs Monensin and Lasalocid, *Vet. Parasitol.* 2:187–196.

Chapman, H. D., 1978*a, Eimeria tenella:* Experimental studies on the development of resistance to amprolium, clopidol and methyl benzoquate, *Parasitology* 76:177–183.

Chapman, H. D., 1978*b,* Drug resistance in coccidia, in: *Avian Coccidiosis* (P. L. Long, K. N. Boorman, and R. M. Freeman, eds.), pp. 387–412, British Poultry Science, Edinburgh.

Chapman, H. D., 1979, Studies on the sensitivity of recent field isolates of *Eimeria maxima* to monensin, *Avian Pathol.* 8:181–186.

Chen, P., Lamont, G., Elliott, T., Kidson, C., Brown, G., Mitchell, G., Stace, J., and Alpers, M., 1980, *Plasmodium falciparum* strains from Papua New Guinea: Culture characteristics and drug sensitivity, *Southeast Asian J. Trop. Med. Publ. Health* 11:425–440.

Chongsupphajaisiddhi, T., and Sabchaeron, A., 1981, Sulfadoxine-pyrimethiamine resistant falciparum malaria in Thai children, *Southeast Asian J. Trop. Med. Publ. Health* 12:418–421.

Chongsupphajaisiddhi, T., Sabchaeron, A., and Attanath, P., 1981, *In vivo* and *in vitro* sensitivity of falciparum malaria to quinine in Thai children, *Ann. Trop. Paediatr.* 1:21–26.

Chulay, J. D., Anzeze, E. M., Koech, D. K., and Bryceson, A. D. M., 1983*a,* High dose sodium stibogluconate treatment of cutaneous leishmaniasis in Kenya, *Trans. R. Soc. Trop. Med. Hyg.* 77:717–721.

Chulay, J. D., Bhatt, S. M., Muigai, R., Ho, M., Gachihi, G., Were, J. B. O., Chunge, C., and Bryceson, A. D. M., 1983*b,* A comparison of three dosage regimens of sodium stibogluconate in the treatment of visceral leishmaniasis in Kenya, *J. Infect. Dis.* 148:148–155.

Chulay, J. D., Watkins, W. M., and Sixsmith, D. G., 1984, Synergistic antimalarial activity of pyrimethamine and sulfadoxine against *Plasmodium falciparum in vitro, Am. J. Trop. Med. Hyg.* 33:325–330.

Clyde, D. K., 1967, *Malaria in Tanzania, Oxford University Press, London.*

Clyde, D. F., Miller, R. M., DuPont, H. L., and Hornick, R., 1970, Treatment of falciparum malaria caused by strain resistant to quinine, *J.A.M.A.* 213:2041–2045.

Coombs, G. H., 1976, Studies on the activity of nitroimidazoles, in: *Biochemistry of Parasites and Host–Parasite Relationships* (H. van den Bossche, ed.), pp. 545–552, Elsevier/North-Holland Biomedical Press, Amsterdam.

Cover, B., and Gutteridge, W. E., 1981, Comparison of drug sensitivities of three strains of *Trypanosoma cruzi* in inbred A/Jax Mice, *Trans. R. Soc. Trop. Med. Hyg.* 75:274–281.

Cuckler, A., and Malanga, C. M., 1955, Studies on drug resistance to coccidia, *J. Parasitol.* 41:302–311.

Cuckler, A. C., McManus, E. C., and Campbell, W. C., 1969, Development of resistance to coccidia, *Acad. Vet. (Brno)* 38:87–99.

Darlow, B., Vrbova, H., Gibney, S., Jolley, D., Stace, J., and Alpers, M., 1982, Sulfadoxine-pyrimethamine for the treatment of acute malaria in children in Papua New Guinea. II. *Plasmodium vivax, Am. J. Trop. Med. Hyg.* 31:10–16.

Deloron, P., LeBras, J., Andrieu, B., and Hartman, J. F., 1982, Standardisation de l'épreuve de chémosensibilité *in vitro* de *Plasmodium falciparum, Path. Biol.* 30:585–588.

deRaadt, P., and Seed, J. R., 1977, African trypanosomes in man, in: *Parasitic Protozoa* (J. P. Kreier, ed.), Vol. 1, pp. 175–237, Academic Press, New York.

Desjardins, R. E., Canfield, C. J., Haynes, J. D., and Chulay, J. D., 1979, Quantitative assessment of antimalarial activity *in vitro* by a semiautomated microdilution technique, *Antimicrob. Agents Chemother.* 16:710–718.

Desjardins, R. E., Casero, R. A., Jr., Willet, G. P., Childs, G. E., and Canfield, C. J., 1980, *Trypanosoma rhodiesense:* Semiautomated microtesting for quantitation of antitrypanosomal activity *in vitro, Exp. Parasitol.* 50:260–271.

Divo, A. A., Geary, T. G., and Jensen, J. B., 1984, Nutritional requirements of *Plasmodium falciparum* in culture. I. Exogenously supplied dialyzable components necessary for continuous growth, *J. Protozool.* 32:59–64.

Dixon, K. E., Williams, R. G., Pongsupat, T., Pitaktong, U., and Phintuyothin, P., 1982, A comparative trial of mefloquine and Fansidar in the treatment of falciparum malaria: Failure of Fansider, *Trans. R. Soc. Trop. Med. Hyg.* 76:664–667.

Dixon, K. E., Pitaktong, U., Bamnetpandh, S., Teopipithaporn, S., and Na-Nakorn, A., 1983, Treatment of an acute case of *Plasmodium malariae* malaria with mefloquine, *Am. J. Trop. Med. Hyg.* 31:631–632.

Doberstyn, E. B., Teerakiartham, C., Andre, R. G., Phintayothin, P., and Noeypatimanondh, S., 1979, Treatment of vivax malaria with sulfadoxine-pyrimethamine and pyrimethamine alone, *Trans. R. Soc. Trop. Med. Hyg.* 73:15–17.

Doberstyn, E. B., 1984, Resistance of *Plasmodium falciparum, Experentia* 40:1311–1317.

Eastham, G. M., and Rieckmann, K. H., 1983, The activity of pyrimethamine and sulphadoxine against *Plasmodium falciparum* determined by the *in vitro* microtechnique, *Trans. R. Soc. Trop. Med. Hyg.* 77:91–93.

Edgar, S. A., and Flanagan, C., 1976, Susceptibility to recent field isolates of chicken *Eimeria* species to modern anticoccidial drugs, *Poultry Sci.* 55(5):2032.

Edwards, D. I., 1980, Mechanisms of selective toxicity of metronidazole and other nitroimidazole drugs, *Br. J. Vener. Dis.* 56:285–290.

Elslager, E. F., 1974, Recent advances in the chemotherapy of malaria, filariasis, and leprosy, in: *Progress in Drug Research* (E. Jucker, ed.), Vol. 18, pp. 99–172, Birkhäuser Verlag, Basel and Stuttgart.

Ercoli, N., 1966, Drug responsiveness in experimental cutaneous leishmaniasis, *Exp. Parasitol.* 19:320–326.

Fairley, N. H., 1946, Atebrin sensitivity of the Aitaipe-Wewak strains of *P. falciparum* and *P. vivax*—A field and experimental investigation by L. H. R. Medical Research Unit, Cairns, *Trans. R. Soc. Trop. Med. Hyg.* 40:229–273.

Ferone, R., Burchall, J. J., and Hitchings, G. H., 1969, *Plasmodium berghei* dihydrofolate reductase. Isolation, properties, and inhibition by antifols, *Mol. Pharmacol.* 5:49–59.

Ferone, R., 1977, Folate metabolism in malaria, *Bull WHO* 55:291–298.

Ferraroni, J. J., Alencar, F. H., and Shrimpton, R., 1983, Multiple drug resistance in falciparum malaria from Brazil, *Trans. R. Soc. Trop. Med. Hyg.* 77:138–139.

Ferraroni, J. J., Speer, C. A., Hayes, J., and Suzuki, M., 1981, Prevalence of chloroquine-resistant falciparum malaria in the Brazilian Amazon, *Am. J. Trop. Med. Hyg.* 30:526–530.

Fitch, C. D., 1973, Chloroquine-resistant *Plasmodium falciparum:* differences in the handling of ^{14}C-amodiaquine and ^{14}C-chloroquine, *Antimicrob. Agents Chemother.* 3:545–548.

Fitch, C. D., Chevli, R., and Gonzalez, Y., 1974, Chloroquine-resistant *Plasmodium falciparum:* effect of substrate on chloroquine and amodiaquine accumulation, *Antimicrob. Agents Chemother.* 6:757–762.

Fitch, C. D., 1983, Mode of action of antimalarial drugs, in: *Malaria and the Red Cell,* CIBA Foundation Symposium 94, pp. 222–232, Pitman, London.

Forsgren, A., and Forssman, L., 1979, Metronidazole-resistant *Trichomonas vaginalis, Br. J. Vener. Dis.* 55:351–353.

Fouré, N., and Bennejean, G., 1973, Les chimio-résistances acquises vis à vis des dérivés des quinoléines et de la pyridine, *Symp. Int. Coccidioses Tours* III:6.

Freeman, F., Wilson, P. L., and Kazam, B. H., 1975, *Trypanosoma cruzi:* Antimicrobial activity and strain differentiating properties of some five- and six-membered heterocyclic compounds on trypomastigotes, *Exp. Parasitol.* 38:181–190.

Gajanna, A., and Raichowdhuri, A. N., 1984, *Plasmodium vivax:* Micro *in vitro* test for assaying chloroquine sensitivity, *Trans. R. Soc. Med. Hyg.* 78:416–417.

Gajanana, A., Sivaraman, C. A., Sinha, S., Sivaraman, A., and Chowdhuri, A. N., 1982, An *in vitro* microtechnique for testing antimalarials—Use of cultured *Plasmodium falciparum* parasites, *Indian J. Med. Res.* 75:802–807.

Geary, T. G., and Jensen, J. B., 1983, Lack of cross-resistance to 4-aminoquinolines in chloroquine-resistant *Plasmodium falciparum in vitro*, *J. Parasitol.* 69:97–105.

Geary, T. G., Divo, A. A., and Jensen, J. B., 1983, An *in vitro* assay system for the identification of potential antimalarial drugs, *J. Parasitol.* 69:577–583.

Geary, T. G., Jensen, J. B., and Ginsburg, H., 1985a, Uptake of [^{3}H]-chloroquine by drug-sensitive and -resistant strains on the human malaria parasite *Plasmodium falciparum*, *Biochem. Pharmacol.* in press.

Geary, T. G., Divo, A. A., Bonnani, L. C., and Jensen, J. B., 1985b, Nutritional requirements of *Plasmodium falciparum* in culture. III. Further observations on essential nutrients and antimetabolites, *J. Protozool.* in press.

Gilbert, R. J., and Newton, B. A., 1980, Ethidium bromide: Host–trypanosome–drug interactions, in: *The Host–Invader Interplay* (H. van den Bossche, ed.), pp. 647–650, Elsevier/North-Holland Biomedical Press, Amsterdam.

Ginsburg, H., Geary, T. G., and Yayon, A., 1985, Current concepts and new ideas on the mechanism of action of chloroquine: A review, *Biochem. Pharmacol.* in press.

Glew, R. H., Briesch, P. E., Krotoski, W. A., Contacos, P. G., and Neva, F. A., 1974, Multidrug-resistant strain of *Plasmodium falciparum* from Eastern Colombia, *J. Infect. Dis.* 129:385–390.

Glew, R. H., Collins, W. E., and Miller, L. H., 1978, Selection of increased quinine resistance in *Plasmodium falciparum* in *Aotus* monkeys, *Am. J. Trop. Med. Hyg.* 27:9–13.

Graves, P. M., Carter, R., Keystone, J. S., and Seeley, D. C., Jr., 1984, Drug sensitivity and isoenzyme type in cloned lines of *Plasmodium falciparum*, *Am. J. Trop. Med. Hyg.* 33:212–219.

Gray, G. D., Jennings, F. W., and Hajduc, S. L., 1982, Relapse of monomorphic and pleomorphic *Trypanosoma brucei* infections in the mouse after chemotherapy, *Z. Parasitenk.* 67:137–145.

Grewal, R. S., 1981, Pharmacology of 8-aminoquinolines, *Bull. WHO* 59:397–406.

Gupta, V. K., 1978, The chloroquine-resistant chronic vivax malaria presenting as malarial cachexia and secondary hypersplenism (a case report), *Indian Peditra.* 15:171–173.

Haberkorn, A., and Gönnert, R., 1972, Animal experimental investigations on the activity of nifurtimox against *Trypanosoma cruzi*, *Arzneim. Forsch.* 22:1510–1581.

Hall, A. P., Doberstyn, E. B., Na-Nakorn, A., and Sonkom, P., 1975a, Falciparum malaria semi-resistant to clindamycin. *Br. Med. J.* 2:12–14.

Hall, A. P., Segal, H. E., Pearlman, E. J., Phintuyothin, P., and Kosakal, S., 1975b, Amodiaquine-resistant falciparum malaria in Thailand, *Am. J. Trop. Med. Hyg.* 24:595–580.

Hanson, W. L., Waits, V. B., Hendricks, L. D., Hockmeyer, W. T., Davidson, D. E., Jr., and Chapman, W. L., Jr., 1983, Relative insensitivity of a Kenyan strain of *Leishmania donovani* to pentavalent antimony therapy in hamsters, *J. Parasitol.* 69:446–447.

Harinasuta, T., Dixon, K. E., Warrell, D. A., and Doberstyn, E. B., 1982, Recent advances in malaria with special reference to Southeast Asia, *Southeast Asian J. Trop. Med. Publ. Health* 13:1–34.

Harwood, P. D., and Stunz, D. I., 1953, A search for drug-fast strains of *Eimeria tenella*, *J. Parasitol.* 39:268.

Hawking, F., 1963, Chemotherapy of trypanosomiasis, in: *Experimental Chemotherapy* (R. J. Schnitzer and F. Hawking, eds.), Vol. 1, pp. 129–256, Academic Press, New York and London.

Hawking, F., 1965, Chemotherapy of trypanosomiasis, in: *Experimental Chemotherapy* (R. J. Schnitzer and F. Hawking, eds.), Vol. 4, pp. 398–419, Academic Press, New York and London.

Hess, U., Timmermans, P. M., and Jones, M., 1983, Combined chloroquine/Fansidar-resistant malaria appears in East Africa, *Am. J. Trop. Med. Hyg.* 32:217–220.

Heyworth, R., Simpson, D., McNeillage, G. J. C., Robertson, D. H. H., and Young, H., 1980, Isolation of *Trichomonas vaginalis* resistant to metronidazole, *Lancet* 2:476–478.

Hill, G. C., 1980, Biochemical studies using *Trypanosoma rhodiesense* cultured infective trypomastigotes, in: *The Host–Invader Interplay* (H. van den Bossche, ed.), pp. 555–556, Elsevier/North-Holland Biomedical Press, Amsterdam.

Honigberg, B. M., 1977, Trichomonads of importance in human medicine, in: *Parasitic Protozoa* (J. P. Kreier, ed.), Vol. 1, pp. 332–454, Academic Press, New York.

Howells, R. E., 1982, Advances in chemotherapy, *Br. Med. Bull.* 38:193–199.

Hurwitz, E. S., Johnson, D., and Campbell, C. C., 1981, Resistance of *Plasmodium falciparum* to sulfadoxine-pyrimethamine (Fansidar) in a refugee camp in Thailand, *Lancet* 1:1068–1070.

Jeffers, T. K., 1978, *Eimeria tenella:* Sensitivity of recent field isolates to monensin, *Avian Dis.* 22:157–161.

Jeffers, T. K., and Challey, J. R., 1973, Collaterial sensitivity to 4-hydroxyquinolines in *Eimeria acervulina* strains resistant to metichlorpindol, *J. Parasitol.* 59:624–630.

Jennings, F. W., Whitelaw, D. D., and Urquhart, G. M., 1977, The relationship between duration of infection with *Trypanosoma brucei* in mice and the efficacy of chemotherapy, *Parasitology* 75:143–153.

Jennings, F. W., Whitelaw, D. D., Holmes, Ph. H., Chizyuka, H. G. B., and Urquhart, G. M., 1979, The brain as a source of relapsing *Trypanosoma brucei* infection in mice after chemotherapy, *Int. J. Parasitol.* 9:381–384.

Jennings, F. W., Urquhart, G. M., Murray, P. K., and Miller, B. M., 1980, "Berenil" and nitromidazole combinations in the treatment of *Trypanosoma brucei* infection with central nervous system involvement, *Int. J. Parasitol.* 10:27–32.

Jensen, J. B. (ed.), 1983, *In Vitro Cultivation of Protozoan Parasites,* CRC Press, Boca Raton.

Jensen, J. B., Capps, T. C., and Carlin, J. M., 1981, Clinical drug-resistant falciparum malaria acquired from cultured parasites, *Am. J. Trop. Med. Hyg.* 30:523–525.

Jensen, J. B., Boland, M. T., and Akood, M., 1982, Induction of crisis forms in cultured *Plasmodium falciparum* with human immune serum from Sudan, *Science* 216:1230–1233.

Jensen, J. B., Boland, M. T., Allan, J. S., Carlin, J. M., VandeWaa, J. A., Divo, A. A., and Akood, M. A. S., 1983, Association between human serum induced crisis forms in cultured *Plasmodium falciparum* and clinical immunity to malaria in Sudan, *Infect. Immun.* 41:1302–1311.

Jensen, J. B., Hoffman, S. L., Boland, M. T., Akood, M. A. S., Laughlin, L. W., Kurniawan, L., and Marwoto, H. A., 1984, Comparison of immunity to malaria in Sudan and Indonesia: Crisis-form versus merozoite-invasion inhibition, *Proc. Natl. Acad. Sci. U.S.A.* 81:922–925.

Jha, T. K., 1983, Evaluation of diamidine compound (pentamidine isethionate) in the treatment of resistant cases of kala-azar occurring in North Bihar, India, *Trans R. Soc. Trop. Med. Hyg.* 77:167–170.

Johnson, D. E., Roendej, P., and Williams, R. G., 1982, Falciparum malaria acquired in the area of Thai-Khmer border resistant to treatment with Fansidar, *Am. J. Trop. Med. Hyg.* 31:907–912.

Jokipii, A. M. M., and Jokipii, L., 1980, *In vitro* susceptibility of *Giardia lamblia* trophozoites to metronidazole and tinidazole, *J. Infect. Dis.* 141:317–325.

Joyner, L. P., and Norton, C. C., 1970, The response of recently isolated strains of *Eimeria meleagrimitis* to chemotherapy, *Res. Vet. Sci.* 11:349–353.

Joyner, L. P., and Norton, C. C., 1973, The drug-sensitivity of recently isolates strains of *Eimeria meleagrimitis* and a laboratory strain of *Eimeria adenoeides* in turkeys to ethopabate, *Res. Vet. Sci.* 14:279–284.

Joyner, L. P., and Norton, C. C., 1975, Robenidine dependence in a strain of *Eimeria maxima, Parasitology* 70:47–51.

Kierszenbaum, F., 1984, The chemotherapy of *Trypanosoma cruzi* infections (Chagas' disease), in: *Parasitic Disease* (J. Mansfield, ed.), Vol. 2, pp. 133–163, Marcel Dekker, New York.

Kulda, J., Vojtechovska, M., Tachezy, J., Demes, P., and Kunzova, E., 1982, Metronidazole resistance of *Trichomonas vaginalis* as a cause of treatment failures in trichomoniasis, *Br. J. Vener. Dis.* 58:394–399.

Lai, C. H., Tizard, I. R., and Ingram, D. G., 1974, Development of sulphonamide-resistant strains of *Toxoplasma gondii, Trans. R. Soc. Med. Hyg.* 68:257–258.

Lamont, G., and Darlow, B., 1982, Comparison of *in vitro* pyrimethamine assays and *in vivo* response to sulphadoxine-pyrimethamine in *Plasmodium falciparum* from Papua New Guinea, *Trans. R. Soc. Trop. Med. Hyg.* 76:797–799.

Lanners, H. N., and Trager, W., 1984, Intranuclear structures in pyrimethamine-resistant isolates of the malaria parasite *Plasmodium falciparum, Cell Biol. Int. Rep.* 8:221–225.

Leach, T. M., and Roberts, C. J., 1981, Present status of chemotherapy and chemoprophylaxis of animal trypanosomiasis in the Eastern hemisphere, *Pharmacol. Ther.* 13:91–147.

LeBras, J., and Deloron, P., 1983, *In vitro* study of drug sensitivity of *Plasmodium falciparum:* Evaluation of a new semi-micro test, *Am. J. Trop. Med. Hyg.* 32:447–451.

LeBras, J., Deloron, P., Ricour, A., Andrieu, B., Sarel, J., and Couland, J. P., 1983, *Plasmodium falciparum:* Drug sensitivity *in vitro* of isolates before and after adaptation to continuous culture, *Exp. Parasitol.* 56:9–14.

Long, P. L., and Jeffers, T. K., 1982, Studies on stage of action of ionophorous antibiotics against *Eimeria, J. Parasitol.* 68:363–371.

Mamalis, P., and Wirbel, L. M., 1984, Triazines, quinazolines and related dihydrofolate inhibitors, in: *Antimalarial Drugs,* Vol. II (W. Peters and W. H. G. Richards, eds.), *Handbook of Experimental Pharmacology,* Vol. 68, pp. 387–442, Springer-Verlag, New York.

Marsden, P. D., 1979, Current concepts in parasitology: Leishmaniasis, *N. Engl. J. Med.* 300:350–352.

Mathis, G. F., McDougald, L. R., and McMurray, B., 1984, Drug resistance trends in broiler coccidia in an integrated poultry company over a 10-year period, *Poultry Sci.* (Suppl. 1) 63:145.

Mattock, N. M., and Peters, W., 1975*a,* The experimental chemotherapy of leishmaniasis. I. Techniques for the study of drug action in tissue culture, *Ann. Trop. Med. Parasitol.* 69:349–357.

Mattock, N. M., and Peters, W., 1975*b,* The experimental chemotherapy of leishmaniasis. II. The activity in tissue culture of some antiparasitic and antimicrobial compounds in clinical use, *Ann. Trop. Med. Parasitol.* 69:359–371.

Mazier, D., Danis, M., Druilhe, P., Karabinis, A., Brucker, G., Félix, H., and Gentilini, M., 1984, Paludisme à *Plasmodium falciparum* multi-résistant contracté en Tanzanie, *Bull. Soc. Pathol. Exp.* 77:44–51.

McCutchen, T. F., Welsh, J. A., Dame, J. B., Quakyi, I. A., Graves, P. M., Drake, J. C., and Allegra, C. J., 1984, Mechanism of pyrimethamine resistance in recent isolates of *Plasmodium falciparum, Antimicrob. Agents Chemother.* 26:656–659.

McLoughlin, D. K., 1970, Coccidiosis: Experimental analysis of drug resistance, *Exp. Parasitol.* 28:129–136.

McLoughlin, D. K., and Gardiner, L., 1961, Drug resistance in *Eimeria tenella.* 1. The experimental development of a glycarbylamide-resistant strain, *J. Parasitol.* 47:1001.

McLoughlin, D. K., and Chute, M. B., 1971, Efficacy of decoquinate against 11 strains of *Eimeria tenella* and development of a decoquinate-resistant strain, *Avian Dis.* 15:342–345.

McLoughlin, D. K., and Chute, M. B., 1973*a,* The efficacy of nequinate against 13 strains of *Eimeria tenella* and the development of a nequinate-resistant strain. *Avian Dis.* 17:717–721.

McLoughlin, D. K., and Chute, M. B., 1973*b,* Efficacy of clopidol against 12 strains of *Eimeria tenella* and the development of a clopidol-resistant strain, *Avian Dis.* 17:425–429.

Meingassner, J. G., and Heyworth, P. G., 1981, Intestinal and urogenital flagellates, *Antibiot. Chemother.* 30:163–202.

Meingassner, J. G., and Meith, H., 1976, Cross-resistance of trichomonads to 5-nitroimidazole derivatives, *Experientia* 32:183–184.

Meingassner, J. G., and Thurner, J., 1979, Strain of *Trichomonas vaginalis* resistant to metronidazole and other 5-nitroimidazoles, *Antimicrob. Agents Chemother.* 15:254–247.

Milhous, W. K., Weatherly, N. F., Bowdre, J. H., and Desjardins, R. E., 1985, *In vitro* activities of and mechanisms of resistance to antifol antimalarial drugs, *Antimicrob. Agents Chemother.* 27 in press.

Moore, D. V., and Lanier, J. E., 1961, Observations on two *Plasmodium falciparum* infections with an abnormal response to chloroquine, *Am. J. Trop. Med. Hyg.* 10:5–9.

Müller, M., Meingassner, J. G., Miller, W. A., and Ledger, W. J., 1980, Three metronidazole-resistant strains of *Trichomonas vaginalis* from the USA, *Am. J. Obstet. Gynecol.* 138:808–812.

Neal, R. A., 1972, Effect of dihydrofolate reductase inhibitors on experimental cutaneous leishmaniasis with special emphasis on *Leishmania* isolates from Latin America, *Rev. Inst. Trop. Med. Sao Paulo* 14:341–351.

Neal, R. A., 1983, Experimental amoebiasis and the development of antiamoebic compounds, *Parasitology* 86:175–191.

Nguyen-Dinh, P., and Payne, O., 1980, Pyrimethamine sensitivity in *Plasmodium falciparum:* Determination *in vitro* by a modified 48-hour test, *Bull. WHO* 58:909–912.

Nguyen-Dinh, P., and Trager, W., 1980, *Plasmodium falciparum in vitro:* Determination of chloroquine sensitivity of three new strains by a modified 48-hour test, *Am. J. Trop. Med. Hyg.* 29:339–342.

Nguyen-Dinh, P., Spencer, H. C., Masaba, S. C., and Churchill, F. C., 1982, Susceptibility of *Plasmodium falciparum* to pyrimethamine and sulfadoxine/pyrimethamine in Kisumu, Kenya, *Lancet* 1:823–825.

Nguyen-Dinh, P., Magloire, R., and Chin, W., 1983, A simple field kit for the determination of drug susceptibility in *Plasmodium falciparum*, *Am. J. Trop. Med. Hyg.* 32:452–455.

Noeypatimanond, S., Malikul, S., Benjapong, W., Duriyananda, D., and Ungkasrithongkul, M., 1983, Treatment of *Plasmodium falciparum* malaria with a combination of amodiaquine and tetracycline in Central Thailand, *Trans. R. Soc. Trop. Med. Hyg.* 77:338–340.

Norton, C. C., and Joyner, L. P., 1975, The development of drug-resistant strains of *Eimeria maxima* in the laboratory, *Parasitology* 71:153–165.

Oostburg, B. F. J., and Jozefzoon, L. M. E., 1983, Fansidar-resistant *Plasmodium falciparum* infections in Surinam, *Trop. Georgr. Med.* 35:243–247.

Oshima, S., and Hoshino, M., 1977, Different susceptibilities of *Toxoplasma* strains to antitoxoplasmic drugs, *Jpn. J. Parasitol.* 26:127–131.

Pehrson, P., and Bengtsson, E., 1983, Treatment of non-invasive amoebiasis. A comparison between tinidazole alone and in combination with diloxanide furoate, *Trans. R. Soc. Trop. Med. Hyg.* 77:845–846.

Peters, W., 1970, *Chemotherapy and Drug Resistance in Malaria*, Academic Press, London.

Peters, W., 1974a, Drug resistance in trypanosomiasis and leishmaniasis, in: *Trypanosomiasis and Leishmaniasis*, CIBA Foundation Symposium 20, pp. 309–334, Elsevier, Amsterdam.

Peters, W., 1974b, Recent advances in antimalarial chemotherapy and drug resistance, in: *Advances in Parasitology* (B. Dawes, ed.), Vol. 12, pp. 69–114, Academic Press, London and New York.

Peters, W., 1976, The search for antileishmanial agents, in: *Biochemistry of Parasites and Host–Parasite Relationships* (H. Vanden Bossche, ed.), pp. 523–535, Elsevier/North-Holland Biomedical Press, Amsterdam.

Peters, W., 1980a, Therapy of intracellular parasitic infections with lysosomotropic drugs, in: *The Host–Invader Interplay* (H. Vanden Bossche, ed.), pp. 567–573, Elsevier/North-Holland Biomedical Press, Amsterdam.

Peters, W., 1980b, Chemotherapy of malaria, in: *Malaria* (J. P. Kreier, ed.), Vol. 1, pp. 145–283, Academic Press, New York and London.

Peters, W., 1982, Antimalarial drug resistance: An increasing problem, *Br. Med. Bull.* 38:187–192.

Peters, W., 1984a, History and current status of drug resistance, in: *Antimalarial Drugs* (W. Peters and W. H. G. Richards, eds.), Vol. 1, pp. 423–446, Springer-Verlag, New York.

Peters, W., 1984b, Experimental production of drug resistance, in: *Antimalarial Drugs*, Vol. I (W. Peters and W. H. G. Richards, eds.), *Handbook of Experimental Pharmacology*, Vol. 68, pp. 461–473, Springer-Verlag, New York.

Peters, W., Trotter, E. R., and Robinson, B. L., 1980, The experimental chemotherapy of leishmaniasis, VII. Drug responses of *L. major* and *L. mexicana amazonensis*, with an analysis of promising chemical leads to new antileishmanial agents, *Ann. Trop. Med. Parasitol.* 74:321–335.

Pfefferkorn, E. R., and Pfefferkorn, L. C., 1978, The biochemical basis for resistance to adenine arabinoside in a mutant of *Toxoplasma gondii, J. Parasitol.* 64:486–492.

Pinichpongse, S., Doberstyn, E. B., Cullen, J. R., Yisunsri, L., Thongsomban, Y., and Thimasarn, K., 1982, An evaluation of five regimens for the outpatient therapy of falciparum malaria in Thailand, 1980–81, *Bull. WHO* 60:907–912.

Poltera, A. A., 1980, Immunopathological and chemotherapeutic studies in experimental trypanosomiasis with special reference to the heart and brain, *Trans. R. Soc. Trop. Med. Hyg.* 74:706–715.

Poltera, A. A., Hochman, A., and Lamport, P. H., 1981, *Trypanosoma brucei:* The response to melarsoprol in mice with cerebral trypanosomiasis. An immunopathological study, *Clin. Exp. Immunol.* 46:81–102.

Powell, R. D., and Tigertt, W. D., 1968, Drug resistance of parasites causing human malaria, *Annu. Rev. Med.* 19:81–102.

Pratt, W. B., 1977, *Chemotherapy of Infection*, Oxford University Press, New York.

Pratt, W. B., and Ruddon, R. W., 1979, *The Anticancer Drugs*, Oxford University Press, New York.

Ralph, E. D., and Clark, D. A., 1978, Inactivation of metronidazole by anaerobic and aerobic bacteria, *Antimicrob. Agents Chemother.* 14:377–383.

Reacher, M., Campbell, C. C., Freeman, J., Doberstyn, E. B., and Brandling-Bennett, A. D., 1981, Drug therapy of *Plasmodium falciparum* malaria resistant to pyrimethamine-sulfadoxine (Fansidar), *Lancet* 2:1066–1068.

Rees, P. H., Kager, P. A., Keating, M. I., and Hockmeyer, W. T., 1980, Renal clearance of pentavalent antimony (sodium stibogluconate), *Lancet* 2:226–229.

Rees, P. H., Kager, P. A., Wellde, B. T., and Hockmeyer, W. T., 1984, The response of Kenyan kala-azar to treatment with sodium stibogluconate, *Am. J. Trop. Med. Hyg.* 33:357–361.

Richards, W. H. G., 1979, Some promising leads in experimental antimalarial drugs, in: *Advances in Pharmacology and Therapeutics* (M. Adolphe, ed.), Vol. 10, pp. 71–112, Pergamon Press, Oxford and New York.

Rieckmann, K. H., 1983, Falciparum malaria: The urgent need for safe and effective drugs, *Annu. Rev. Med.* 34:321–335.

Rieckmann, K. H., McNamara, J. V., Frischer, H., Stockert, T. A., Carson, P. E., and Powell, R. D., 1968, Effects of chloroquine, quinine, and cycloguanil upon the maturation of asexual erythrocytic forms of two strains of *Plasmodium falciparum in vitro*, *Am. J. Trop. Med. Hyg.* 17:661–671.

Rieckmann, H. H., Campbell, G. H., Sax, C. J., and Mrema, J. E., 1978, Drug sensitivity of *Plasmodium falciparum*. An *in vitro* microtechnique, *Lancet* 1:22–23.

Rosario, V. E., Hall, R., Walliker, D., and Beale, G. H., 1978, Persistence of drug-resistant malaria parasites, *Lancet* 1:185–187.

Ross Institute, 1981, Malaria prevention in travelers from the United Kingdom, *Br. Med. J.* 283:214–218.

Rozman, R. S., and Canfield, C. J., 1979, New experimental antimalarial drugs, *Adv. Pharmacol. Chemother.* 16:1–43.

Ryley, J. F., and Betts, M. J., 1973, Chemotherapy of chicken coccidiosis, *Adv. Pharmacol. Chemother.* 11:221–293.

Sanders, J., and Midved, T., 1971, Development of sulphonamide resistance in *Toxoplasma gondii*, *Acta Pathol. Microbiol. Scand. Sect. B* 79:531–533.

Sargeaunt, P. G., and Williams, J. E., 1978, The differentiation of invasive and non-invasive *Entamoeba histolytica* by isoenzyme electrophoresis, *Trans. R. Soc. Trop. Med. Hyg.* 72:519–521.

Sargeaunt, P. G., Jackson, T. F. H. G., and Simjee, A., 1982, Biochemical heterogeneity of *Entamoeba histolytica* isolates, especially those from liver abscesses, *Lancet* 1:1386–1388.

Schapira, A., 1984, Concomitant resistance to pyrimethamine and cycloguanil of chloroquine-resistant falciparum malaria from East Africa: An *in vitro* study of 12 isolates, *Trans. R. Soc. Trop. Med. Hyg.* 78:359–362.

Schenone, H., Concha, L., Aranda, R., Rojas, A., Knierim, F., and Rujo, M., 1972, Tratamiento de la infection chagasica cronica con "Lampit," *Biol. Chileno Parasitol.* 27:11–14.

Schmidt, L. H., Vaughn, D., Mueller, D., Crosby, R., and Hamilton, R., 1977, Activities of various 4-aminoquinolines against infections with chloroquine-resistant strains of *Plasmodium falciparum*, *Antimicrob. Agents Chemother.* 11:826–843.

Schneider, J., 1963, Traitement de la trypanosomiase africaine humaine, *Bull. WHO* 28:763–786.

Sherman, I. W., 1979, Biochemistry of *Plasmodium* (malarial parasites), *Microbiol. Rev.* 43:453–495.

Sirwaraporn, W., and Yuthavong, Y., 1984, Kinetic and molecular properties of dihydrofolate reductase from pyrimethamine-sensitive and pyrimethamine-resistant *Plasmodium chabaudi*, *Mol. Biochem. Parasitol.* 10:355–367.

Smith, C. K., and Galloway, R. B., 1983, Influence of monensin on cation inflex and glycolysis of *Eimeria tenella* sporozoites *in vitro*, *J. Parasitol.* 69:666–670.

Smith, P. D., Gillin, F. D., Spira, W. M., and Nash, T. E., 1982, Chronic giardiasis: Studies on drug sensitivity, toxin production, and host immune response, *Gastroenterology* 83:797–803.

Smrkovski, L. L., Buck, R. L., Alcantara, A. K., Rodriquez, C. A., and Uylanco, C. V., 1982a, In vitro mefloquine resistant *Plasmodium falciparum* from the Philippines, *Lancet* 2:322.

Smrkovski, L. L., Buck, R. L., Rodriquez, C. S., Wooster, M. T., Mayuga, J. L., and Rivera, D., 1982b, Chloroquine and quinine resistant *Plasmodium falciparum* on the island of Mindora, Philippines, 1982, *Southeast Asian J. Trop. Med. Publ. Health* 13:551–555.

Spencer, H. C., Kariuki, D. M., and Koech, D. K., 1983a, Chloroquine resistance in *Plasmodium falciparum* from Kenyan infants, *Am. J. Trop. Med. Hyg.* 32:922–925.

Spencer, H. C., Kipingor, T., Agure, R., Koech, D. K., and Chulay, J. D., 1983b, *Plasmodium falciparum* in Kisumu, Kenya: Differences in sensitivity to amodiaquine and chloroquine *in vitro*, *J. Infect. Dis.* 148:732–736.

Spencer, H. C., Watkins, W. M., Sixsmith, D. G., Koech, D. K., and Chulay, J. D., 1984, Correlation of a new *in vitro* test for pyrimethamine/sulfadoxine susceptibility with *in vivo* resistance in Kenyan *Plasmodium falciparum*, *Bull. WHO* 62:615–621.

Steck, E. A., 1974, The leishmaniases, in: *Progress in Drug Research* (E. Jucker, ed.), Vol. 18, pp. 289–351, Birkhäuser Verlag, Basel and Stuttgart.

Tan-Ariya, P., and Brockelman, C. R., 1983a, *Plasmodium falciparum:* Variations in *p*-aminobenzoic acid requirements as related to sulfadoxine sensitivity, *Exp. Parasitol.* 55:364–371.

Tan-Ariya, P., and Brockelman, C. R., 1983b, Continuous cultivation and improved drug responsiveness of *Plasmodium falciparum* in *p*-aminobenzoic acid deficient medium, *J. Parasitol.* 69:353–359.

Targett, G. A. T., 1984, Interactions between chemotherapy and immunity, in: *Antimalarial Drugs*, Vol. I (W. Peters and W. H. G. Richards, eds.), *Handbook of Experimental Pharmacology*, Vol. 68, pp. 331–348, Springer-Verlag, New York.

Thaithong, S., 1983, Drug resistant isolates of *Plasmodium falciparum* contain clones of different sensitivities, *Bull. WHO* 61:709–712.

Thaithong, S., and Beale, G. H., 1981, Resistance of ten Thai isolates of *Plasmodium falciparum* to chloroquine and pyrimethamine by *in vitro* tests, *Trans. R. Soc. Trop. Med. Hyg.* 75:271–273.

Thaithong, S., Beale, G. H., Fenton, B., McBride, J., Rosario, V., Walker, A., and Walliker, D., 1984, Clonal diversity in a single isolate of the malaria parasite *Plasmodium falciparum*, *Trans. R. Soc. Trop. Med. Hyg.* 78:242–245.

Thompson, P. E., and Werbel, L. M., 1972, *Antimalarial Agents, Chemistry and Pharmacology*, Academic Press, New York.

Thurner, J., and Meingassner, J. G., 1978, Isolation of *Trichonomas vaginalis* resistant to metronidazole, *Lancet* 2:738.

Tigertt, W. D., and Clyde, D. F., 1976, Drug resistance in the human malarias, *Antibiot. Chemother.* 20:246–272.

Trotter, E. R., Peters, W., and Robinson, B. L., 1980, The experimental chemotherapy of leshmaniasis, II. The development of rodent models for cutaneous infections with *L. major* and *L. mexicana amazonensis*, *Ann. Trop. Med. Parasitol.* 74:299–319.

Waletzky, E., Neal, R., and Hable, I., 1954, A strain of *Eimeria tenella* resistant to sulfonamides, *J. Parasitol.* 40:24.

Watkins, W. M., Spencer, H. C., Kariuki, D. M., Sixsmith, D. G., Boriga, D. A., Kipingor, T., and Koech, D. K., 1984, Effectiveness of amodiaquine as treatment for chloroquine-resistant *Plasmodium falciparum* infections in Kenya, *Lancet* 1:357–359.

Webster, H. K., Boudreau, E. F., Pavanand, K., Yongvanitchit, K., and Pang, L. W., 1985, Antimalarial drug susceptibility testing of *Plasmodium falciparum* in Thailand using a microdilution radioisotope method, *Am. J. Trop. Hyg.* 34:228–235.

Wernsdorfer, W. H., 1980, Field evaluation of drug resistance in malaria. *In vitro* micro test, *Acta Trop.* 37:222–227.

Wernsdorfer, W. H., and Kouznetzov, R. L., 1980, Drug resistant malaria: occurrence, control, and surveillance, *Bull. WHO* 58:341–352.

WHO, 1973, *Chemotherapy of Malaria and Resistance to Antimalarials*, WHO Tech. Rep. Ser. No. 529, WHO, Geneva.

WHO, 1982, Control of sleeping sickness due to *Trypanosoma brucei gambiense*, *Bull. WHO* 60:821–825.

Williamson, J., 1959a, Drug resistance in trypanosomes; selective interference with trypanocidal action, *Br. J. Pharmacol.* 14:431–442.

Williamson, J., 1959b, Drug resistance in trypanosomes; effects of metabolic inhibitors, pH and oxidation-reduction potential on normal and resistant *Trypanosoma rhodiesense*, *Br. J. Pharmacol.* 14:443–455.

Williamson, J., 1962, Chemotherapy and chemoprophylaxis of African trypanosomiasis, *Exp. Parasitol.* 12:274–322.

Williamson, J., 1970, Review of chemotherapeutic and chemoprophylactic agents, in: *The African Trypanosomiases* (H. W. Mulligan, ed.), pp. 125–221, Wiley–Interscience, New York.

Williamson, J., 1983, Drug sensitivity of pleomorphic *Trypanosoma rhodiesense, Trans. R. Soc. Trop. Med. Hyg.* 77:192–193.

Williamson, J., and Rollo, I. M., 1959, Drug resistance in trypanosomes; cross-resistance analyses, *Br. J. Pharmacol.* 14:423–430.

Williamson, J., March, J. C., and Scott-Finnigan, T. J., 1982, Drug synergy in experimental African trypanosomiasis, *Tropenmed. Parasitol.* 33:76–82.

Wood, L. D., 1982, The efficacy of four anticoccidial drugs (arprinocid, salinomycin, monensin, and lasalocid) against ten field isolates of chicken coccidia, M.S. thesis, Auburn University, 95 pp.

Wyler, D. J., 1983, Malaria-resurgence, resistance, and research, *N. Engl. J. Med.* 308:875–878.

Wyler, D. J., 1984, The ascent and decline of chloroquine, *J.A.M.A.* 251:2420–2422.

Yayon, A., VandeWaa, J., Yayon, M., Geary, T. G., and Jensen, J. B., 1983, Stage-dependent effects of chloroquine on *Plasmodium falciparum in vitro, J. Protozool.* 30:642–649.

III

Nematodes

11

Chemistry of Antinematodal Agents

MICHAEL H. FISHER

1. INTRODUCTION

Before 1938, no broadly useful drugs for the treatment of nematode infections existed. Limited activity was found in arsenicals and in various natural products such as nicotine and oil of chenopodium. The discovery of the anthelmintic activity of phenothiazine made available a moderately broadly active compound that, although not very potent, was virtually nontoxic. The benzimidazoles, reported in 1961, followed by the commercial success of thiabendazole, signaled a new era of truly broad-spectrum, safe, orally effective, antinematodal drugs. Considerable structure–activity studies in many research centers later produced a host of more potent benzimidazoles with activity expanded to lungworms, tapeworms, and liver flukes. The advent of tetramisole in 1965 followed by the L-isomer levamisole afforded a relatively safe oral or parenteral anthelmintic that has achieved widespread use, especially in cattle. Pyrantel and morantel were developed in the same period and have found their own special place, morantel as a ruminal bolus. The discovery of the avermectins in 1976 followed by the introduction of ivermectin as a broad-spectrum antiparasitic agent carried the search one stage further. Ivermectin is not only very potent and equally effective by the oral or parenteral routes but is also effective against ectoparasites. The search for better drugs continues in many research institutes, guided by mechanism of action studies and comparative biochemistry.

2. BENZIMIDAZOLES

The announcement of thiabendazole in 1961 marked the beginning of the modern era of broad-spectrum anthelmintic agents (Brown *et al.*, 1961). The original lead in the series was 2-phenyl benzimidazole, which was itself marketed for a brief period.

MICHAEL H. FISHER • Merck Sharp & Dohme Research Laboratories, Rahway, New Jersey 07065

Structure–activity studies indicated that the most potent compounds had an aromatic group at the 2-position. Substitution at the 4-position caused a decrease in activity. However, activity could be maintained with certain 5-substituents and even increased with 5-carbamates. Thiabendazole is metabolized to inactive 5-hydroxythiabendazole with a half-life ($t\frac{1}{2}$) of 11 min in the rat and is excreted as a mixture of the phenol and glucuronide.

THIABENDAZOLE

$C_{10}H_7N_3S$ mol. wt. 201.26

Synonyms: MK-360; Omnizole; Thiaben; Thibenzole; Bovizole; Eprofil; Equizole; Mintezol; Top Form Wormer; Mertect; Lombristop; Minzolum; Nemapan; Polival; TBZ; Tecto.

2-(4-thiazolyl-1H-benzimidazole; 4-(2-benzimidazolyl)thiazole

Crystals, m.p. 304–305°C; uv max (methanol): 298 nm (ε 23,330). Fluorescence max in acid solution: 370 nm (310-nm excitation).

Solubility: maximum solubility in water at pH 2.2: 3.84%; sol. in DMF; sl. sol. in alcohols, esters, chlorinated hydrocarbons.

Toxicity: LD_{50} orally in mice, rats, rabbits: 3.6, 3.1, >3.8 g/kg.

CAMBENDAZOLE

$C_{14}H_{14}N_4O_2S$;   mol. wt. 302.35

Synonyms: MK-905; Bonlam; Bovicam; Cambenzole; Cambet; Equiben; Novazole; Noviben.

[2-(4-Thiazolyl)-1H-benzimidazol-5-yl]carbamic acid 1-methylethyl ester; 2-(4-thiazolyl)-5-benzimidazolecarbamate isopropyl ester; 5-isopropoxycarbonylamino-2-(4-thiazolyl)benzimidazole; 5-isopropoxycarbonylaminothiabendazole isopropyl 2-(4-thiazolyl)-5-benzimidazolecarbamate

Odorless, white crystalline solid, m.p. 238–240°C (dec).

Solubility: sol. in alcohol, dimethylformamide; sp. sol. in acetone; sl. sol. in benzene; v. sl. sol. in 0.1 M HCl; practically insol. in isooctane and water (0.02 mg/ml);

stable in acid and base in range of pH 1–12; uv max (0.1 N HCl): 319, 232 nm ($A_{1\,cm}^{1\%}$ 740, 670).

Notes: Cambendasole is more potent than thiabendazole presumably because of its 10-fold extension of half-life (Hoff *et al.*, 1970). However, the price paid for this increase in duration of action was teratogenicity in some species. A considerable breakthrough in the medicinal chemistry of anthelmintic benzimidazoles came with the discovery that the aromatic substituent at the 2-position could be replaced by a carbamate group with an increase in activity (Actor *et al.*, 1967). Methyl carbamates proved the most potent, but a further increase in activity was achieved by 5-substitution, resulting in the development of a new series of highly potent benzimidazole anthelmintic drugs, unfortunately, in several instances at the expense of teratogenicity and increased residues.

PARBENDAZOLE

$C_{13}H_{17}N_3O_2$ mol. wt. 247.29

Synonyms: SKF 29044; Helmatac; Verminum; Worm Guard.

(5-Butyl-$1H$-benzimidazol-2-yl)carbamic acid methyl ester; methyl 5-butyl-2-benzimidazolecarbamate; 5-butyl-2-(carbomethoxyamino)benzimidazole

Crystals from aqueous ethanol, mp 225–227° (dec); uv max (95% ethanol/liter N HCl): 282, 288 nm (ϵ 16,200, 20,000).

Solubility: pract. insol. in water.

Toxicity: LD_{50} orally in mice and rats: >4 g/kg.

OXIBENDAZOLE

$C_{12}H_{15}N_3O_3$ mol. wt. 249.27

Synonyms: SKF 30310; Anthelcide EQ; Equitac.

(5-Propoxy-$1H$-benzimidazol-2-yl)carbamic acid methyl ester; 5-propoxy-2-benzimidazolecarbamic acid methyl ester; 5-propoxy-2-(carbomethoxyamino)benzimidazole

Crystals, m.p. 230–230.5°C.

Preparation: Theodorides *et al.* (1973).

MEBENDAZOLE

$C_{16}H_{13}N_3O_3$ mol. wt. 295.35

Synonyms: R 17635; Ovitelmin; Pantelmin; Telmin; Vermirax; Vermox.

(5-Benzoyl-1*H*-benzimidazol-2-yl)carbamic acid methyl ester; 5-benzoyl-2-ben-
zimidazolecarbamic acid methyl ester; methyl 5-benzoyl-2-benzimidazole-
carbamate

Crystals from acetic acid and methanol, m.p. 288.5°C.

Toxicity: LD_{50} orally: >80 mg/kg in sheep; >40 mg/kg in mice, rats, and chickens.

Preparation: Brugmans *et al.* (1971), Walker and Knight (1972).

FLUBENDAZOLE

$C_{16}H_{12}FN_3O_3$ mol. wt. 313.30

Synonyms: R 17889; Flumoxal; Flumoxane; Flubenol; Flutelmin.

[5-(4-Fluorobenzoyl)-1*H*-benzimidazol-2-yl]carbamic acid methyl ester; 5-(*p*-fluo-
robenzoyl)-2-benzimidazolecarbamic acid methyl ester

Crystals, m.p. 260°C

Toxicity: LD_{50} in mice, rats, guinea pigs (mg/kg): >2560 orally.

Preparation: Raeymaekers *et al.* (1978).

FENBENDAZOLE

$C_{15}H_{13}N_3O_2S$ mol. wt. 299.35

Synonyms: HOE 881v; Panacur.

[5-(Phenylthio)-1*H*-benzimidazol-2-yl]carbamic acid methyl ester; 5-(phenylthio)-2-
benzimidazolecarbamic acid methyl ester; methyl 5-(phenylthio)-2-
benzimidazolecarbamate

Light brownish-gray, odorless, tasteless crystalline powder, m.p. 233°C (dec).
Solubility: insol. in water; insol. or only v. sl. sol. in the usual solvents; freely soluble in DMSO.
Preparation: Baeder *et al.* (1974).

OXFENDAZOLE

$C_{15}H_{13}N_3O_3S$ mol. wt. 315.35
Synonyms: RS 8858; Synanthic; Systamex.
[5-(Phenylsulfinyl)-1*H*-benzimidazol-2-yl]carbamic acid methyl ester; methyl-5-(phenylsulfinyl)-2-benzimidazolecarbamate; 5-phenylsulfinyl-2-carbomethoxyaminobenzimidazole

Crystals from chloroform-methanol, m.p. 253°C (dec).
Toxicity: LD_{50} in dogs, rats, and mice: >1600, >6400, >6400 mg/kg.
Preparation: Averkin et al. (1975).

ALBENDAZOLE

$C_{12}H_{15}N_3O_2S$ mol. wt. 265.33
Synonyms: SKF 62979; Valbazen; Zental.
[5-(Propylthio)-1*H*-benzimidazol-2-yl]carbamic acid methyl ester; methyl 5-(propylthio)-2-benzimidazolecarbamate; 5-(propylthio)-2-carbomethoxyaminobenzimidazole

Colorless crystals, m.p. 208–210°C.
Preparation: Theodorides *et al.* (1976).

CYCLOBENDAZOLE

$C_{13}H_{13}N_3O_3$ mol. wt. 259.25
Synonyms: CC-2481; R-17147; Haptocil.
[5-(Cyclopropylcarbonyl)-1*H*-benzimidazol-2-yl]carbamic acid methyl ester; ciclobendazole

Crystals from acetic acid, m.p. 250.5°C.

Preparation: Raeymaekers *et al.* (1978).

Note: Febantel and thiophanate are included with benzimidazoles because they have been shown to metabolize to benzimidazoles *in vivo*, although it has not been conclusively demonstrated whether they are simply prodrugs or whether they also have intrinsic benzimidazolelike activity by mimicking the spatial arrangement of atoms.

FEBANTEL

$C_{20}H_{22}N_4O_6S$ mol. wt. 446.49

Synonyms: Bay Vh 5757; Bay h 5757; Rinital.

[[2-(Methoxyacetylamino)-4-(phenylthio)phenyl]carbonimidoyl]biscarbamic acid dimethyl ester; dimethyl[[2-(2-methoxyacetamido)-4-(phenylthio)phenyl]imidocarbonyl]dicarbamate

Crystals, m.p. 129–130°C.

Preparation: Wollweber *et al.* (1978).

THIOPHANATE

$C_{14}H_{18}N_4O_4S_2$ mol. wt. 370.44

Synonyms: Cercobin; Topsin; Nemafax.

[1,2-Phenylenebis(iminocarbonothioyl)]biscarbamic acid diethyl ester; 4,4′-*o*-phenylenebis[3-thioallophanic acid]diethyl ester; 1,2-bis(3-ethoxycarbonyl-2-thioureido)benzene

O,O-DIMETHYL ANALOGUE

$C_{12}H_{14}N_4O_4S_2$ mol. wt. 342.26

Colorless prisms, m.p. 181.5–182.5°C.

Solubility: sol. in acetone, methanol, chloroform, acetonitrile; sl. sol. in other organics; insol. in water.

Toxicity: LD_{50} orally in rats, mice, guinea pigs, rabbits: 3.40, 6.64, 3.64, 2.27 g/kg.

Preparation: Eichler (1973).

3. IMIDAZOTHIAZOLES

In 1966, workers at Janssen Pharmaceutica reported a remarkably active series of broad-spectrum anthelmintic compounds: the 6-arylimidazo[2,1-b]thiazoles. Interestingly, the lead compound in the series was a prodrug that cyclized to an imidazothiazole in chickens, the species used in the screening program. A considerable number of the 6-aryl compounds synthesized exhibited a high order of anthelmintic activity, but the compound selected for commercial development was the racemic 6-phenyl derivative tetramisole. After resolution, all the anthelmintic activity was found to reside in the L-isomer, which was developed as levamisole, thereby increasing the margin of safety.

TETRAMISOLE-LEVAMISOLE

$C_{11}H_{12}N_2S$ mol. wt. 204.1

Synonyms: Hydrochloride, $C_{11}H_{13}ClN_2S$, Bayer 9051, McN-JR-8299, R 8299, Anthelvet, Citarin, Nilverm, Orovermol, Ripercol, Levasole, Spartakon.

2,3,5,6-Tetrahydro-6-phenylimidazo-[2,1-b]thiazole;   DL-6-phenyl-2,3,5,6-tetrahydroimidazol[2,1-b]thiazole; tetramizole

Crystals, m.p. 87–89°C.

Preparation: Raeymaekers *et al.* (1966).

Solubility: sol. in water (21 g/100 ml at 20°C), methanol, propylene glycol; sp. sol. in ethanol; sl. sol. in chloroform, hexane, acetone.

Toxicity: LD_{50} in mice, rats: 22, 24 mg/kg iv; 84, 130 mg/kg sc; 210, 480 mg/kg orally.

D-(+)-form, dexamisole, m.p. 60–61.5°C; $[\alpha]_D^{25}$ +85.1° (c = 10 in chloroform);

D-(+)-form hydrochloride, R 12563, m.p. 227–227.5°; $[\alpha]_D^{20}$ +125° (c = 0.7 in water);

L-(−)-form, levamisole, m.p. 60–61.5°; $[\alpha]_D^{25}$ −85.1° (c = 10 in chloroform);

L-(−)-form hydrochloride, R 12564, Ergamisol, Levasole, Nemicide, Solaskil, Stimamizol, Tramisol, Worm-Chek, m.p. 227–229°C; $[\alpha]_D^{20}$ −124° ± 2° (c = 0.9 in water).

Notes: The only other imidazothiazole anthelmintic agent that has been developed commercially is butamisole, which emerged from studies on levamisole derivatives (Spicer and Hand, 1975).

BUTAMISOLE

$C_{15}H_{19}N_3OS$ mol. wt. 289.40

2-Methyl-*N*[3-(2,3,5,6-tetrahydroimidazo[2.1-*b*]thiazol-6-yl)phenyl]propanamide;
     (−)-2-methyl-3′-(2,3,5,6-tetrahydroimidazo[2,1-*b*]thiazol-6-yl)propionanilide

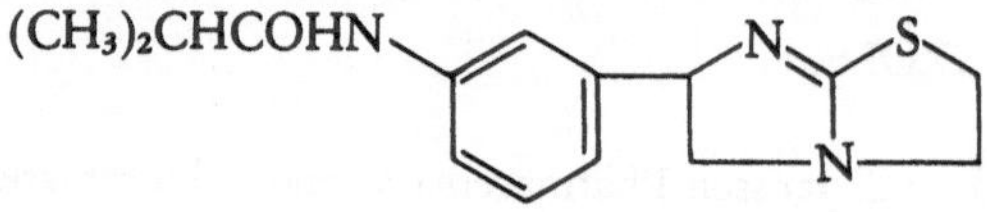

$(CH_3)_2CHCOHN$

Hydrochloride

$C_{15}H_{20}ClN_3OS$
Synonyms: CL 206214, Styquin.

4. TETRAHYDROPYRIMIDINES

In 1959, 2-thenylmercapto-2-imidazoline (I) was reported from Pfizer Laboratories to have broad-spectrum anthelmintic activity in rodents. Its lack of activity in sheep was ascribed to rapid metabolism to 2-imidazolidinone and 2-thenylthiol (Lynch and Nelson, 1959).

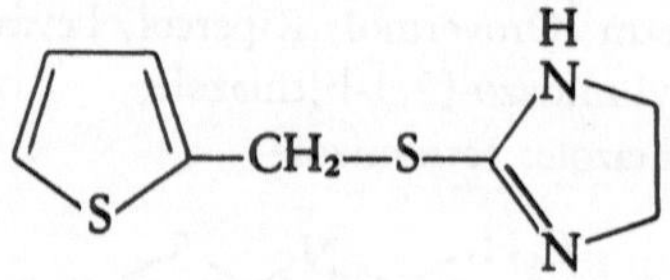

CH_2—S

An extensive search for compounds designed to overcome this liability resulted in the discovery that the cyclic amidine could be five or six membered and that the link between the two rings could be —CH_2CH_2— or —CH=CH—. Three commercial anthelmintic agents—pyrantel, oxantel, and morantel—grew out of this research.

PYRANTEL

$C_{11}H_{14}N_2S$ mol. wt. 206.32

1,4,5,6-Tetrahydro-1-methyl-2-[2-thienyl)ethenyl]pyrimidine

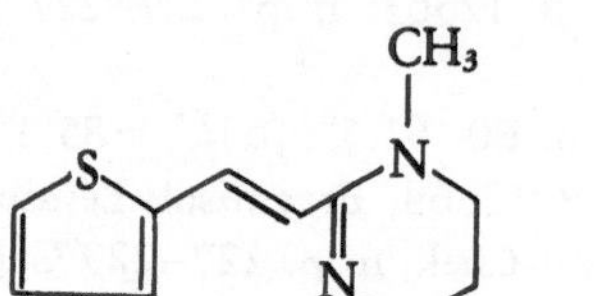

CH_3

Crystals from methanol, m.p. 178–179°C.
Preparation: Austin *et al.* (1966).

Tartrate
$C_{15}H_{20}N_2O_6S$
Synonyms: CP-10423-18, Strongid, Banminth.
White crystals from hot methanol, m.p. 148–150°C; uv max (water): 312nm (ε 3.27).

PAMOATE

$C_{34}H_{30}N_2O_6S$ mol. wt. 594.6
Synonyms: CP-10423-16, pyrantel embonate; Antiminth; Cobantel; Combantrin; Helmex; Piranver.
Solubility: Mixture with oxanted pamoate (1 : 1), Quantrel.

OXANTEL

$C_{13}H_{16}N_2O$ mol. wt. 216.28
3-[2-(1,4,5,6-Tetrahydro-1-methyl-2-pyrimidinyl)ethyl]phenol; (E)-*m*-[2-(1,4,5,6-tetrahydro-1-methyl-2-pyrimidinyl)vinyl]phenol;   1-methyl-1,4,5,6-tetrahydro--2-[2-(3-hydroxyphenyl)vinyl]pyrimidine; CP 14445

HYDROCHLORIDE

$C_{13}H_{17}ClN_2O$ mol. wt. 252.77
Crystals from ethanol, m.p. 207–208°C; uv max (water): 231, 274 nm (ε 12,700; 20,100).

PAMOATE

$C_{49}H_{48}N_4O_8$ mol. wt. 820.29
Synonyms: CP 14445-16; oxantel embonate; Telopar.
Note: Mixture with pyrantel pamoate (1 : 1), Quantel.
Preparation: McFarland and Howes (1972).

MORANTEL

$C_{12}H_{16}N_2S$ mol. wt. 220.33
1,4,5,6-Tetrahydro-1-methyl-2-[2-(3-methyl-2-thienyl)ethenyl]pyrimidine

$$CH_3 \quad H$$

Crystals from chloroform + benzene, m.p. 239–241°C.
Preparation: McFarland *et al.* (1969).

Tartrate

$C_{16}H_{22}N_2O_6S$, CP 12009-18, Suiminth.

5. ORGANOPHOSPHATES

Organophosphate anthelmintic agents were generally selected from the huge number of compounds synthesized as agricultural pesticides. Since they are all AChE inhibitors, those that have commercial value in animals or man depend for their safety on tissue or enzyme specificity. In the case of dichlorvos, which has a high vapor pressure, the compound is incorporated into a resin from which the active ingredient is slowly released.

COUMAPHOS

Phosphorothioic acid 0-(3-chloro-4-methyl-2-oxo-^2H-1-benzopyran-7-yl)0,0-diethyl
    ester; 3-chloro-7-hydroxy-4-methylcoumarin 0-ester with 0,0-diethyl phos-
    phorothioate; 3-chloro-4-methylumbelliferone, 0-ester with 0,0-diethyl phos-
    phorothioate; 0,0-diethyl 0-(3-chloro-4-methyl-7-coumarinyl)phosphorothioate;
    0,0-diethyl 0-(3-chloro-4-methylumbelliferone)thiophosphate
$C_{14}H_{16}ClO_5PS$ mol. wt. 362.78
Synonyms: Coumafos; Bayer 21/199; Asuntol; Baymix; Co-Ral; Meldane; Muscatox;
    Resitox.

Crystals, m.p. 91°C. The commercial product may be slightly brownish.
Solubility: practically insol. in water; somewhat sol. in acetone, chloroform, corn oil.
    Stable in water.
Toxicity: LD_{50} in female, male rats: 16, 41 mg/kg orally.
Note: Minor ingredient of Neguvon A, see under Trichlorfon.
Preparation: Krueger *et al.* (1959).

TRICHLORFON

$C_4H_8Cl_3O_4P$ mol. wt. 257.45

Synonyms: Chlorofos; metrifonate; trichlorphene; Bayer L 13/59; Vermicide Bayer 2349; Combot Equine; Danex; Dipterex; Neguvon; Dyrex; Anthon; Dylox; Bilarcil; Tugon; Proxol; Foschlor.

(2,2,2-Trichloro-1-hydroxyethyl)phosphonic acid dimethyl ester; 0,0-dimethyl-1-hydroxy-2,2,2-trichloroethylphosphonate; 0,0-dimethyl-2,2,2-trichloro-1-hydroxyethylphosphonate

$$\begin{array}{c} \quad\quad\quad O\quad OH \\ CH_3O \quad \| \quad | \\ \qquad\quad P-CHCCl_3 \\ CH_3O \end{array}$$

White crystals, m.p. 83–84°C. d_{40}^2 1.73. n_D^{20} 1.3439. Vapor pressure at 20°C: 7.8 × 10^{-6} nm Hg.

Solubility: sol. at 25°C; water 15.4 g/100 ml; chloroform 75 g/100 ml; ether 17 g/100 ml; benzene 15.2 g/100 ml; v. sl. sol. in pentane and hexane; dec. by alkali.

Toxicity: LD_{50} orally in male, female rats: 630, 560 mg/kg.

Note: Neguvon A contains trichlorfon and, as a minor ingredient, coumaphos, q.v.

HALOXON

$C_{14}H_{14}Cl_3O_6P$ mol. wt. 415.61

7[[Bis(2-chloroethoxy)phosphinyl]oxy]-3-chloro-4-methyl-2H-1-benzopyran-2-one; 3-chloro-7-hydroxy-4-methylcoumarin-bis(2-chloroethyl)phosphate; 0,0-bis(β-chloroethyl)-0-(3-chloro-4-methyl-7-coumarinyl)phosphate; 3-chloro-7-hydroxy--4-methyl-2H-1-benzopyran-2-one-bis(chloroethyl)phosphate; 3-chloro-4-methyl-umbelliferone bis (2-chloroethyl)phosphate; 3-chloro-4-methylumbelliferone-di(2-chloroethyl)phosphate; 0,0-di(2-chloroethyl)-0-(3-chloro-4-methylcoumarin-7-yl)phosphate; galoxone; helmirone; No. 96H60; Galloxon; Loxon; Luxon.

$$\begin{array}{c} \qquad\qquad O \\ ClCH_2CH_2O \quad \| \\ \qquad\qquad P-O-\text{(coumarin ring)} \\ ClCH_2CH_2O \\ \qquad\qquad\qquad\qquad Cl \\ \qquad\qquad\qquad\qquad CH_3 \end{array}$$

Crystals from ethanol, m.p. 91°C.

Toxicity: LD_{50} orally in rats: 900 mg/kg.

Preparation: Brown *et al.* (1962).

NAFTALOFOS

$C_{16}H_{16}NO_6P$ mol. wt. 349.29

Synonyms: BAY 9002; Bayer 25820; ENT-25567; S-940; Maretin; Rametin.

2-[(Diethoxyphosphinyl)oxy]-1*H*-benz[de]isoquinoline-1,3(2*H*)-dione;   *N*-hydroxynaphthalimide diethyl phosphate; *0,0*-diethyl-*0*-naphthaloximide phosphate; naphthalophos; phthalophos

Minute crystals; the commercial product has a brown to tan color, m.p. 174–179°C.
Solubility: pract. insol. in water; sp. sol. in the usual organic solvents; fairly sol. in
   methylene chloride.
Preparation: Lorenz and Wegler (1957).

DICHLORVOS

$C_4H_7Cl_2O_4P$ mol. wt. 220.98
Phosphoric acid 2,2-dichloroethenyl dimethyl ester; phosphoric acid 2,2-dichlorovinyl
   dimethyl ester; *0,0*-dimethyl-*0*-(2,2-dichlorovinyl)phosphate
Synonyms: Dichlorophos; dichlorovos; DDVP; SD 1750; Astrobot; Atgard; Canogard;
   Dedevap; Dichlorman; Divipan; Equigard; Equigel; Estrosol; Herkol; Nogos;
   Nuvan; Task; Vapona.

Liquid; pract. nonflammable; d_4^{25} 1.415. b.p. 20 140°C; b.p. 1.0 84°C; b.p. 0.5 72°C;
   b.p. 0.01 30°C; n_D^{25} 1.451. Vapor pressure at 20°: 1.2×10^{-2} mm Hg.
Solubility: misc. with alcohol and most nonpolar solvents; sol. in water: $\sim$1 g/100 ml;
   in glycerol: $\sim$0.5 g/100 ml.
Toxicity: LD_{50} orally in male and female rats: 80, 56 mg/kg.
Preparation: Whetstone and Harman (1960).

6. AVERMECTINS AND MILBEMYCINS

The avermectins and milbemycins are two groups of closely related natural products, both of which are 16-membered cyclic lactones with a spiroketal system comprising two six-membered rings. The principal difference is that the avermectins have an α-L-oleandrosyl-α-L-oleandrosyloxy substituent at the 13-position, whereas the milbemycins have no substituent (Albers-Schonberg *et al.*, 1981; Takiguchi *et al.*, 1980).

components A: R_5 – CH_3 components 1: X = – CH = CH –

components B: R_5 = H

components a: R_{26} = C_2H_5 components 2: X = – CH_2 $\overset{OH}{\underset{\equiv}{CH}}$ –
components b: R_{26} = CH_3

The only compounds that have been commercialized so far are avermectin B_1 (abamectin) and its 22,23-dihydro derivative (ivermectin) (Chabala *et al.*, 1980), although there is some interest in 13-deoxy-22,23-dihydroavermectin B_{1b} aglycone, also known as Milbemycin B41-D (Mrozik *et al.*, 1983; Mishima *et al.*, 1983).

ABAMECTIN

Synonyms: AVM; C-076; MK-936.
Note: Contains at least 80% of avermectin B_{1a} and not more than 20% of avermectin B_{1b}.

Avermectin B_{1a}

$C_{48}H_{72}O_{14}$; mol wt: 872. $[\alpha]_D^{27}$ + 55.7 ± 2° (c = 1.06 in chloroform); uv max (methanol): 237, 243, 252 nm (ϵ 29,120; 31,850; 20,510).

Avermectin B_{1b}

$C_{47}H_{70}O_{14}$ mol. wt. 858.

IVERMECTIN

Synonyms: 22,23-Dihydroavermectin B_1; 22,23-dihydro C-076B_1; MK-933; Heartguard 30; Cardomec; Eqvalen; Ivomec.

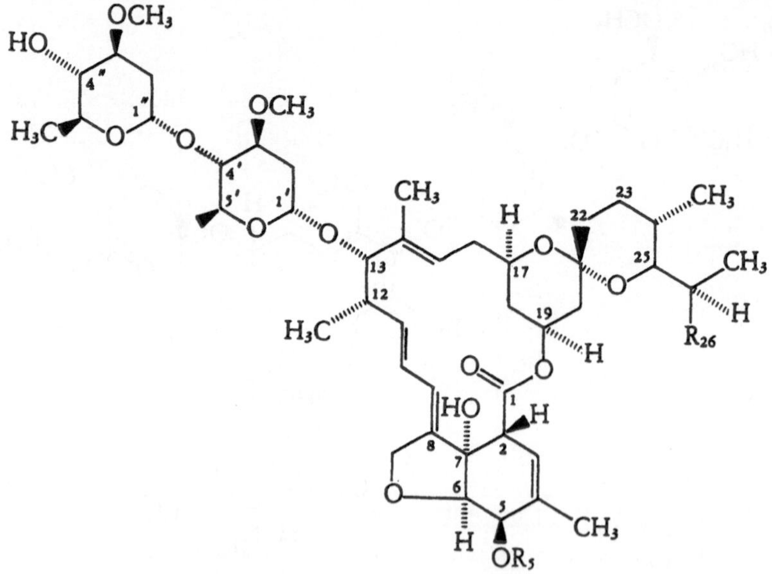

Semisynthetic derivative of the avermectins, q.v. Ivermectin contains at least 80% of 22,23-dihydroavermectin B_{1a} and less than 20% of 22,23-dihydroavermectin B_{1b}. Off-white powder; $[\alpha]_D + 71.5 \pm 3°$ ($c = 0.755$ in chloroform); uv max (methanol): 238, 245 nm (ϵ 27,100; 30,100).

Component B_{1a}

$C_{48}H_{74}O_{14}$ mol. wt. 874

5-0-Demethyl-22,23-dihydroavermectin A_{1a}; 22,23-dihydroavermectin B_{1a}; 22,23-di-hydro C-076B_{1a}

$R = C_2H_3$

Crystals from ethanol/water, m.p. 155–157°C.

Component B_{1b}

$C_{47}H_{72}O_{14}$ mol. wt. 860

5-0-Demethyl-25-de(1-methylpropyl)-22,23-dihydro-25-(1-methylethyl)avermectin A_{1a}; 22,23-dihydroavermectin B_{1b}

$R = CH_3$

7. MISCELLANEOUS ANTINEMATODAL COMPOUNDS

Phenothiazine was the first broad-spectrum anthelmintic agent brought into general use (Bernthsen, 1883). Structure–activity studies demonstrated no useful analogues.

PHENOTHIAZINE

$C_{12}H_9NS$ mol. wt. 199.26

10H-Phenothiazine

Synonyms: Thiodiphenylamine; dibenzothiazine; Phenoxur; Contaverm; Fenoverm; Padophene; Phenegic; Lethelmin; AFI-Tiazin; Antiverm; Biverm; Fentiazin; Helmetina; Nemazine; Orimon; Phenoverm; Reconox; Souframine; Vermitin; Phenovis.

Yellow, rhombic leaflets or diamond-shaped plates from toluene or butanol, m.p. 185.1°C. Sublimes at 130°C at 1 mm. b.p. 760 371°C.; b.p. 40 290°C.

Solubility: freely sol. in benzene; sol. in ether, in hot acetic acid; sl. sol. in alcohol and in mineral oils; pract. insol. in petroleum ether, chloroform, water.

7.1. Piperazines

Piperazine has long been used for the treatment of ascarid infections (Martin and Martell, 1948). The only derivative to be widely used commercially is diethylcarbamazine, which has antifilarial activity.

PIPERAZINE

$C_4H_{10}N_2$ mol. wt. 86.14

Synonyms: Hexahydropyrazine; piperazidine; diethylenediamine; Lumbrical; Worm-Away; Wurmirazin.

Leaflets from alcohol, m.p. 106°C; salty taste; b.p. 760 146°; strong base: K at 25°C = 6.4×10^{-5}, absorbs water and CO_2 from air.

Solubility: freely sol. in water, glycerol, glycols; 1 g dissolves in 2 ml of 95% alcohol; insol. in ether; pH of a 10% aq. sol: 10.8–11.6.

HEXAHYDRATE

$C_4H_{10}N_2 6H_2O$ mol. wt. 198.12

Synonyms: Anthalazine; Arpezine; Arthriticine; Ascaril; Dispermin; Eraverm (syrup); Helmifren; Parid; Piavetrin; Tasnon (elixir); Upixon; Vermicompren (syrup); Vermisol.

Crystals from water (containing 44.34% anhydrous piperazine) m.p. 44°C; b.p. 125–
   130°.

Solubility: freely sol. in water; sol. in alcohol (about 1 : 2); pract. insol. in ether; pH of a
   10% aq. soln.: 10.8–11.8.

Note: The piperazine commercially available is usually this hydrate.

PHOSPHATE

$C_4H_{13}N_2O_4P$ mol. wt. 183.97

Synonyms: Eraverm (tablets); Pincets; Pinisirup; Piperaverm (tablets); Piperazate; Pri-
   psen; Tasnon (tablets). Uvilon (tablets).

Minute crystals.

Solubility: v. sl. sol. in water; pH of sat. aq. soln.: 6.5

PIPERAZINE ADIPATE

$C_{10}H_{20}N_2O_4$ mol. wt. 232.28

*Synonyms:*Hexanedioic acid compound with piperazine (1 : 1); Dietelmin; Entacyl; Oxyzin (tablets); Vermicompren (tablets); Nometan; Vermilass; Oxypaat; Pipadox;
   Oxurasin; Adiprazine.

Prisms, m.p. 256–257°C; stable to heat and air; pleasant, sl. acidic taste.

Solubility: dissolves slowly; sol. in 100 ml water at 20°C: 5.53 g, at 30°C; 6.61 g, at
   56.3°C: 10.14 g; in 100 g methanol at 25°C: 0.02 g; pract. insol. in absolute
   ethanol, isopropanol, dioxane; aq. solns. of 0.02–0.01 M have pH 5.45; this pH
   is only sl. affected by increases in ionic strength caused by the addition of simple
   neutral salts.

Toxicity: LD_{50} orally in mice: 11.4 g/kg.

PIPERAZINE CITRATE

$C_{24}H_{46}N_6O_{14}$ mol. wt. 642.68

Synonyms: Tripiperazine dicitrate; Antepar; Multifuge; Oxucide; 3P-2C; Piperaverm
   (syrup); Pipizan Citrate; Pinrou; Piptelate; Ta-Verm; Exelmin; Rhomex;
   Nemadital; Pinozan; Pipracid syrup); Exopin; Uvilon (syrup); Oxyzin (syrup);
   Parazine; Helmezine; Arpezine.

Crystals, dec. 182–187°C.

Solubility: freely sol. in water; pract. insol. in alcohol, ether, chloroform; pH of a 10%
   aq. soln: 5.0–6.0.

PIPERAZINE EDETATE CALCIUM

$C_{14}H_{24}CaN_4O_8$ mol. wt. 416.45

(Ethylenedinitrilo)-tetraacetic acid piperazine calcium salt

Synonyms: Piperazine calcium edetate; piperazine calcium edathamil; Justelmin; Perin.

Dihydrate crystals; sl. salty taste.

Solubility: freely sol. in water; v. sl. sol. in alcohol, chloroform; pract. insol. in ether;
   pH of aq. soln.: 4.3–5.4.

PIPERAZINE TARTRATE

$C_8H_{16}N_2O_6$ mol. wt. 236.23

Synonyms: Piperate; Veroxil; Noxiurotan; Papavermin; 1P-1T.

Crystals, dec. 258–263°C; formed from 1 mole piperazine and 1 mole tartaric acid.

Solubility: sol. in g/100 ml at 25°C: water 26; alcohol 0.01; chloroform 0.01; pH of 1% soln.: 4.8.

DIETHYLCARBAMAZINE

$C_{10}H_{21}N_3O$ mol. wt. 199.29

N,N-Diethyl-4-methyl-1-piperazinecarboxamide

Synonyms: 1-Diethylcarbamoyl-4-methylpiperazine; carbamazine; 1-diethylcarbamyl-4-methylpiperazine; 84L; RP 3799; Carbilazine; Caricide; Cypip; Ethodryl; Notezine; Spatonin.

$$CON(C_2H_5)_2$$

$$CH_3$$

Crystals, m.p. 47–49°C; b.p. 3 108.5–111°C.

Preparation: Kushner *et al.* (1948).

Hydrochloride

$C_{10}H_{22}ClN_3O$

Crystals from acetone, m.p. 156.5–157°C.

Solubility: v. sol. in water; sol. in chloroform, dioxane.

Citrate (hydrogen citrate)

$C_{16}H_{29}N_3O_8$ mol. wt. 235.79

Synonyms: Franocide; Filazine; Loxuran; Longicid; Dirocide; Filarabits; Hetrazan.

Crystals m.p. 141–143°C.

Solubility: freely soluble in water (>20% at 20°C); sp. sol. in cold alcohol; freely sol. in hot alcohol; pract. insol. in benzene, acetone; ether, chloroform.

Toxicity: LD_{50} orally in rats: 1.38 g/kg.

Phosphate

$C_{10}H_{24}N_3O_5P$ mol. wt. 306.26

Synonym: Ditrazin.

Crystals.

Solubility: freely sol. in water.

7.2. *Chlorinated Hydrocarbons*

Chlorinated hydrocarbons such as *n*-butyl chloride and tetrachloroethylene have been largely replaced by other, safer, more useful drugs. However, both compounds are still used in small animals such as cats and dogs.

n-BUTYL CHLORIDE

C_4H_9Cl mol. wt. 92.57

Synonyms: 1-Chlorobutane; *n*-propylcarbinyl chloride; butyl chloride.

Liquid. Highly flammable; d_4^{15} 0.89197; d_4^{20} 0.88648; d_4^{25} 0.88098; m.p. $-123.1°C$; b.p. 760 78.5°C; n_D^{20} 1.40223; flash pt.: $-6.7°C$ ($+20°F$).

Solubility: pract. insol. in water (0.066% at 12°C); misc. with alcohol, ether.

Toxicity: LD_{50} orally in rats: 2.67 g/kg.

Preparation: Whaley and Copenhaver (1938).

TETRACHLOROETHYLENE

C_2Cl_4 mol. wt. 165.85

$Cl_2C = CCl_2$

Synonyms: Perchloroethylene; ethylene tetrachloride; Tetrachlorethylene; Nema; Tetracap; Tetropil; Perclene; Ankilostin; Didakene.

Colorless, nonflammable liquid; ethereal odor; d_4^{15} 1.6311; d_4^{20} 1.6230; b.p. 121°C; solidifies at about $-22°C$; n_D^{20} 1.5055.

Solubility: sol. in $\sim$10,000 vol water; misc. with alcohol, ether, chloroform, benzene.

Toxicity: LD_{50} orally in mice: 8.85 g/kg; lethal concn. for mice in air: 5925 ppm; human toxicity: narcotic in high concns.; defatting action on skin can lead to dermatitis.

Review: Peters and Neumann (1932).

7.3. *Phenols*

Many phenols have been reported to have some degree of anthelmintic activity. However, the only compound used routinely against nematodes is disophenol.

DISOPHENOL

$C_6H_3I_2NO_3$ mol. wt. 390.93

2,6-Diiodo-4-nitrophenol

Synonyms: DNP; Ancylol.

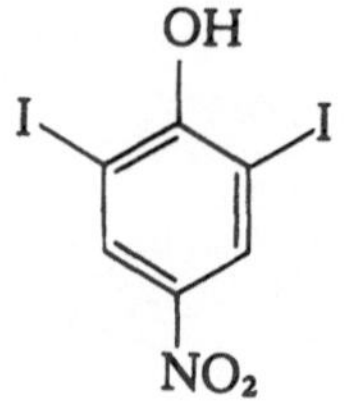

Light yellow, feathery crystals from glacial acetic acid, m.p. 157°C.

Solubility: freely sol. in alcohol, v. sp. sol. in water.

Toxicity: LD_{50} in rats, mice: 170, 212 mg/kg orally; 105, 88 mg/kg iv; 105, 107 mg/kg ip; 122, 110 mg/kg sc.

Preparation: Datta and Prosad (1917).

7.4. Arsenicals

Organic arsenic compounds have wide biological activity, including toxicity, presumably related to the known ability of arsenic to bind sulfhydryl groups. One compound is worthy of mention, as it is widely used in dog heartworm disease.

ARSENAMIDE

$C_{11}H_{12}AsNO_5S$ mol. wt. 377.26

[[[4-(Aminocarbonyl)phenyl]arsenidene]bis(thio)bisacetic   acid;   [[(p-carbamoylphe-
nyl)arsylene]dithio]diacetic   acid;   bis[carboxymethylmercapto](p-carbamylphe-
nyl)arsine;   p-[bis(carboxymethylmercapto)arsino]benzamide;   diothioglycolyl-p-
arsenobenzamide; 4-carbamylphenyl-bis[carboxymethylthio]arsenite

Synonyms: Thioarsenite; thiacetarsamide; Caparsolate; Caparside.

$$As(SCH_2COOH)_2$$

$$CONH_2$$

White crystalline powder.

Solubility: sp. sol. in cold water; appreciably sol. in water above 90°C; sp. sol. in cold methanol, ethanol; v. sol. in these solvents when they are warm; insol. in warm isopropyl ether; $pK_a = 4$; the disodium salt is stoichiometrically formed in aq. soln. at pH 7–8.

Preparation: Gough and King (1930).

7.5. Ethanolamines

Anthelmintic activity is often found among compounds with the general structure

$$-O-CH_2-CH_2-\overset{|}{\underset{|}{N}}{}^+-$$

The nitrogen atom may be either quaternary or protonated at physiological pH.

BEPHENIUM

N,N-Dimethyl-N-(2-phenoxyethyl)benzenemethanaminium

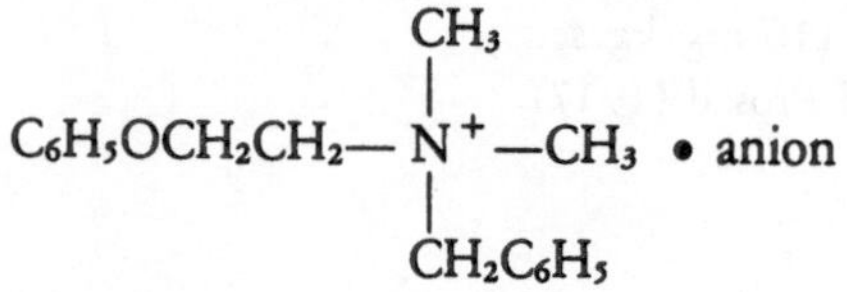

$$C_6H_5OCH_2CH_2-\overset{\overset{\displaystyle CH_3}{|}}{\underset{\underset{\displaystyle CH_2C_6H_5}{|}}{N^+}}-CH_3 \quad \bullet \quad \text{anion}$$

Preparation: Copp *et al.* (1958).

Hydroxynaphthoate

$C_{28}H_{29}NO_4$

Benzyldimethyl(2-phenoxyethyl)ammonium 3-hydroxy-2-naphthoate
Synonyms: Alcopar(a), Benfeniol, Lecibis, Nemex.
Crystals, m.p. 170–171°C.

Pamoate

$C_{57}H_{60}N_2O_8$

Benzyldimethyl(2-phenoxyethyl)ammonium-4,4'-methylenebis[3-hydroxy-2-
      haphthoate]
Synonyms: Bephenium embonate, Frantin.
Dihydrate, pale yellow solid from water, m.p. 144–160°C.

Chloride

$C_{17}H_{22}ClNO$

Crystals from acetone, m.p. 135–136°C

Bromide

$C_{17}H_{22}BrNO$

Crystals from isopropanol + ethyl acetate, m.p. 144.5–146°C

Iodide

$C_{17}H_{22}INO$

Crystals from methanol + ether, m.p. 146–147°C.

THENIUM CLOSYLATE

$C_{21}H_{24}ClNO_4S$ mol. wt. 454.02

N,N-Dimethyl-N-(2-phenoxyethyl)-2-thiophenemethanaminium salt with 4-chlo-
      robenzenesulfonic   acid;   dimethyl(2-phenoxyethyl)-2-thenylammonium p-
      chlorobenzenesulfate
Synonyms: 611C55; Bancaris; Canopar.

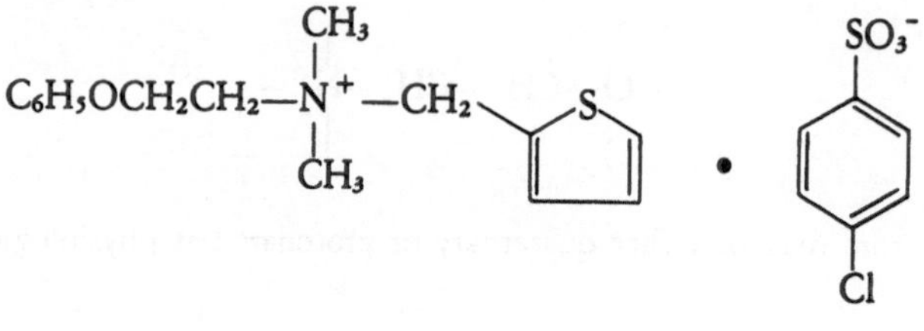

Crystals from isopropanol + ether, m.p. 159–160°C.
Solubility: sol. in water at 20°C: 0.6% w/v.
Preparation: Burrows and Lillis (1962).

METHYRIDINE

$C_8H_{11}NO$ mol. wt. 137.18
2-(β-methoxyethyl)pyridine
Synonyms: Dekelmin; Promintic.

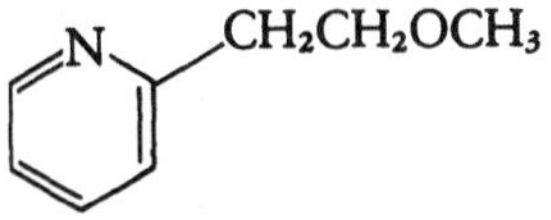

Sweet-smelling liquid, b.p. 17 94–96°C; d^{20} 0.988; n_D^{20} 1.4975; $pK_a = 5.5$.
Solubility: v. sol. in water and common solvents.
Preparation: Broome and Greenhalgh (1961).

Sulfate

Mintic.

Hydrochloride

m.p. 104–105°C.

Note: Although methyridine is structurally not an ethanolamine, it is included along with bephenium and thenium because it is presumably a part of the same broad class.

7.6. *Cyanine Dyes*

Many of the early leads in medicinal chemistry of nematode diseases came from work on compounds originally prepared as dyes. It was reasoned that because dyes bind well to natural fibers, they might bind to receptors as well. Two dyes remain in general use:

PYRVINIUM CHLORIDE

$C_{26}H_{28}ClN_3$ mol. wt. 417.99
6-Dimethylamino-2-[2-(2,5-dimethyl-1-phenyl-3-pyrrolyl)vinyl]-1-methylquinolinium chloride
Synonyms: Viprynium chloride; SN 4395.

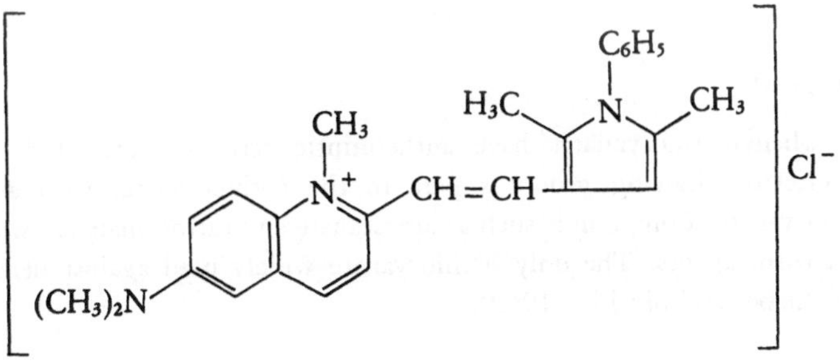

Dihydrate, deep red powder, dec. 249–251°C.
Solubility: sp. sol. in water.
Preparation: Van Lare and Brooker (1950).

PYRVINIUM PAMOATE

$C_{75}H_{70}N_6O_6$ mol. wt. 1151.44

6-(Dimethylamino)-2-[2-(2,5-dimethyl-1-phenyl-1H-pyrrol-3-yl)ethenyl]-1-methyl-
   quinolinium, salt with 4,4'-methylenebis[3-hydroxy-2-naphthalene-carboxylic
   acid] (2 : 1); bis(6-dimethylamino)-2-[2-(2,5-dimethyl-1-phenylpyrrol-3-yl)vin-
   yl]-1-methylquinolinium]-4.4'-methylenebis(3-hydroxy-2-naphthoate);   6-(dimethylamino)-2-[2-(2,5-dimethyl-1-phenyl]-3-pyrryl)vinyl]-1-methylquinoli-
   nium salt of 2,2'-dihydroxy-1,1'-dinaphthylmethane-3,3'-dicarboxylic acid
Synonyms: Pyrvinium embonate; viprynium embonate; Alnoxin; Molevac; Neo-Oxy-
   paat; Pamovin; Poquil; Povan; Povanyl; Pyrcon; Altolat; Tolapin; Tru; Vanquil;
   Vanquin; Vermitiber.
Bright orange or orange-red to almost black precipitate, m.p. 210–215°C (softens at
   190°C). Stable to heat, light, and sir.
Solubility: sl. sol. in chloroform, methoxyethanol; v. sl. sol. in alcohol; pract. insol. in
   water, ether.

DITHIAZANINE IODIDE

$C_{23}H_{23}IN_2S_2$ mol. wt. 518.47

3-Ethyl-2-[5-(3-ethyl-2-(^{3}H)-benzothiazolylidene)-1,3-pentadienyl]benzothiazolium
   iodide; 3,3'-diethylthiadicarbocyanine iodide
Synonyms: Abminthic; Anelmid; Anguifugan; Delvex; Dejo; Deselmine; Dilombrin;
   Dizan; Nectocyd; Partel; Telmicid; Telmid.

Green needles from methanol, dec. 248°C.
Solubility: Pract. insol. in water; can be solubilized with polyvinylpyrrolidone.
Preparation: Kendall and Edwards (1946).

7.7. *Isothiocyanates*

Many phenyl*iso*thiocyanates have anthelmintic activity, particularly those in
which an electron drawing group is para to the *iso*thiocyanate, such as *p*-nitro-
phenyl*iso*thiocyanate. Compounds such as amoscanate and nitroscanate are widely used
as anti-tapeworm agents. The only *iso*thiocyanate widely used against nematodes is
bitoscanate (Lieber and Slutkin, 1962).

BITOSCANATE

$C_8H_4N_2S_2$ mol. wt. 192.24

1,4-Diisothiocyanatobenzene;   phenylene-1,4-diisothiocyanate; isothiocyanic acid *p*-phenylene ester

Synonym: Jonit.

SCN—⬡—NCS

Tasteless, odorless, colorless needles, from acetic acid or acetone, m.p. 132°C.

7.8. Other Compounds

Suramin was originally introduced into human medicine for the treatment of trypanosomiasis and later became widely used for onchocerciasis. It is also a product that emerged from the dye industry.

SURAMIN SODIUM

$C_{51}H_{34}N6O_{-23}S_6$ mol. wt. 1429.21

8,8'-[Carbonylbis[imino-3,1-phenylenecarbonylimino(4-methyl-3,1-phe-nylene)carbonylimino]]bis-1,3,5-naphthalenetrisulfonic acid hexasodium salt; hexasodium-*sym*-bis(*m*-aminobenzoyl-*m*-amino-*p*-methylbenzoyl-1-naphthylamino-4,6,8-trisulfonate)carbamide

Synonyms: Bayer 205; 309F; Antrypol; Germanin; Moranyl; Naganol; Naganin; Naphuride Sodium.

White, slightly pink, or cream-colored powder; sl. bitter taste; hygroscopic,

Solubility: freely sol. in water, in physiological salt solution; sp. sol. in 95% alcohol; insol. in benzene, ether, petroleum ether, chloroform; aq. solns. are neutral to litmus.

Toxicity: LD_{40} iv in mice: 50 mg/kg.

Preparation: Dressel and Kothe (1961).

Phthalofyne

$C_{14}H_{14}O_4$ mol. wt. 246.25

1,2-Benzenedicarboxylic acid mono(1-ethyl-1-methyl-2-propynyl) ester; phthalic acid
    1-ethyl-1-methyl-2-propynyl ester; 1-ethyl-1-methyl-2-propynyl acid phthalate;
    3-methyl-1-pentyn-3-yl acid phthalate
Synonyms: Ftalofyne; NSC-25614; Whipcide.

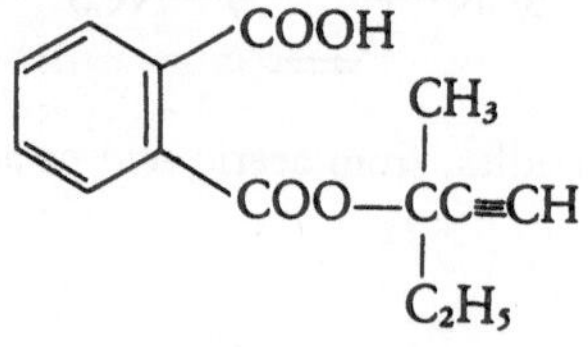

Crystals from benzene or hexane, m.p. 96–98°C; weak acid.
Solubility: sl. sol. in water; unstable in strong alkali.
Preparation: Sugimoto and Okumura (1954).

7.9. *Miscellaneous Natural Products*

Many natural products have been reported to display some degree of anthelmintic
activity. Other than the avermectins and milbemycins, three compounds are worthy of
mention:

HYGROMYCIN B

$C_{20}H_{37}N_3O_{13}$ mol. wt. 527.54

0-6-Amino-6-deoxy-L-glycero-D-galactoheptopyranosylidene-(1→2–3)-O-β-D-tal-
    opyranosyl-(1→5)-2-deoxy-N^3-methyl-D-streptamine
Synonym: Hygromix.

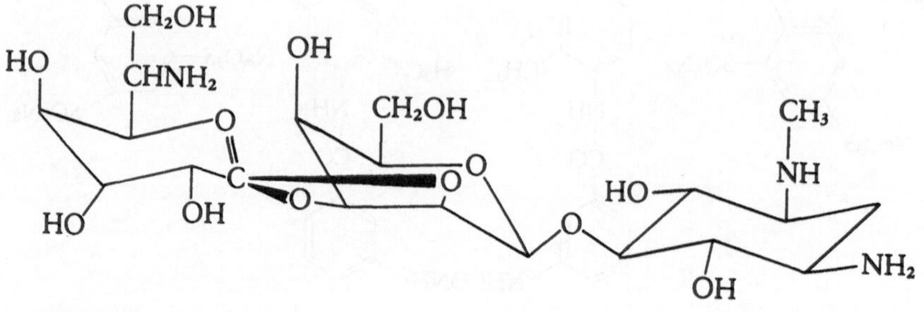

Amorphous powder, dec. 160–180°C; weakly basic; pK_a 7.1–8.8; $[\alpha]_D^{20}$ + 20.2° ($c =$
    1 in water).
Solubility: freely sol. in water, methanol, and ethanol; pract. insol. in less polar
    solvents.
Preparation: Mann and Bromer (1958).

α-SANTONIN

$C_{15}H_{18}O_3$ mol. wt. 246.19

3a,5,5a,9b-Tetrahydro-3,5a-9-trimethylnaphtho[1,2-b]furan-2,8-(3H,4H)-dione;
   1,2,3,4,4a,7-hexahydro-1-hydroxy-α,4a,8-trimethyl-7-oxo-2-naphthaleneacetic
   acid γ-lactone; l-santonin

(−)-Form

Tabular crystals, orthorhombic sphenoidal, m.p. 170–173°C; almost tasteless with
   bitter aftertaste; $[\alpha]_D^{25}$ −170 to −175° (c = 2 in alcohol); becomes yellow on
   exposure to light; irritating to mucous membranes; d 1.187.

Solubility: one part dissolves in 5000 parts of cold water, in 250 parts of boiling water,
   in 280 parts of 50% alcohol at 17°C, in 10 parts of boiling 50% alcohol, in 44
   parts of cold 90% alcohol, in 3 parts of boiling 90% alcohol, in 125 parts of cold
   ether, in 72 parts of boiling ether, in 4.3 parts of cold chloroform.

(±)-Form

Colorless plates from methanol, m.p. 181°C; uv max (ethanol): 241 nm (log ε 4.10).

(+)-Form

Colorless plates from methanol, m.p. 172°C: $[\alpha]_D^{20}$ + 165.9° (c = 1.92 in ethanol).
Preparation: Corey (1955).

KAINIC ACID

$C_{10}H_{15}NO_4$ mol. wt. 213.23

2-Carboxy-4-(1-methylethyl)-3-pyrrolidineacetic   acid;   2-carboxy-3-carboxy-
   methyl-4-isopropenylpyrrolidine; digenic acid; α-kainic acid; L_5-xylokainic acid
Synonyms: Digenin; Helminal.

Needles, dec. 251°C; $[\alpha]_D^{24}$ − 14.8° (c = 1.01); intense absorption at 6.05 and 11.2
   μm.

Solubility: sol. in water; insol. in ethanol; stable in boiling aq. solns.
Preparation: Nitta *et al.* (1958).

ACKNOWLEDGMENTS. Most of the structures and physical data cited in this chapter were abstracted from the *Merck Index,* Tenth Edition (1983), Martha Windholz, Editor, published by Merck and Co., Inc., Rahway, New Jersey.

REFERENCES

Actor, P., Anderson, E. L., DiCuollo, C. J., Ferlauto, R. J., Hoover, J. R. E., Pagano, J. F., Ravin, L. R., Scheidy, S. F., Stedman, R. J., and Theodorides, V. J., 1967, New broad spectrum anthelmintic, methyl 5(6)-Butyl-2-benzimidazole-carbamate, *Nature (Lond.)* 215:321–322.

Albers-Schonberg, G., Arison, B. H., Chabala, J. C., Douglas, A. W., Eskola, P., Fisher, M. H., Lusi, A., Mrozik, H., Smith, J. L., and Tolman, R. L., 1981, Avermectins. Structure determination, *J. Am. Chem. Soc.* 103:4216–4221.

Austin, W. C., Courtney, W., Danilewicz, J. C., Morgan, D. H., Conover, L. H., Howes, H. L., Jr., Lynch, J. E., McFarland, J. W., Cornwell, R. L., and Theodorides, V. J., 1966, Pyrantel tartrate, a new anthelmintic effective against infections of domestic animals, *Nature (Lond.)* 212:1273–1274.

Averkin, E. A., Beard, C. C., Dvorak, C. A., Edwards, J. A., Fried, J. H., Kilian, J. G., Schiltz, R. A., Kistner, T. P., Drudge, J. H., Lyons, E. T., Sharp, M. L., and Corwin, R. M., 1975, Methyl 5(6)-phenylsulfinyl-2-benzimidazolecarbamate, A new, potent anthelmintic, *J. Med. Chem.* 18:1164–1166.

Baeder, C., Bahr, H., Christ, O., Duwel, D., Kellner, H. J,, Kirsch, R., Loewe, H., Schultes, E., Schutz, E., and Westen, H., 1974, Fenbendazole: A new, highly effective anthelmintic, *Experientia* 30:753–754.

Barthel, W. F., Giang, P. A., and Hall, S. A., 1954, Dialkyl α-hydroxyphosphonates derived from chloral, *J. Am. Chem. Soc.* 76:4186–4187.

Bernthsen, A., 1883, Zur Kenntniss des Methylenblau und verwandter Farbstoffe, *Ber.* 16:2896–2904.

Broome, A. W. J., and Greenhalgh, N., 1961, A new anthelmintic with unusual properties, *Nature (Lond.)* 189:59–60.

Brown, H. D., Matzuk, A. R., Ilves, I. R., Peterson, L. H., Harris, S. A., Sarett, L. H., Egerton, J. R., Yakstis, J. J., Campbell, W. C., and Cuckler, A. C., 1961, Antiparasitic drugs. IV. 2-(4′-thiazolyl)-benzimidazole, A new anthelmintic, *J. Am. Chem. Soc.* 83:1764–1765.

Brown, N. C., Hollinshead, D. T., Kingsbury, P. A., and Malone, J. C., 1962, A new class of compounds showing anthelmintic properties, *Nature (Lond.)* 194:379.

Brugmans, J. P., Thienpont, D. C., van Wijngaarden, I., Vanparijs, O. F., Schuermans, V. L., and Lauwers, H. L., 1971, Mebendazole in enterobiasis: Radiochemical and pilot clinical study in 1,278 subjects, *J. A. M. A.* 217:313–316.

Burrows, R. B., and Lillis, W. G., 1962, Thenium, a new anthelmintic for dog and cat hookworms, *Am. J. Vet. Res.* 23:77–80.

Chabala, J. C., Mrozik, H., Tolman, R. L., Eskola, P., Lusi, A., Peterson, L. H., Woods, M. F., Fisher, M. H., Campbell, W. C., Egerton, J. R., and Ostlind, D. A., 1980, Ivermectin, a new broad-spectrum antiparasitic agent, *J. Med. Chem.* 23:134–1136.

Copp, F. C., Standen, O. D., Scarnell, J., Rawes, D. A., and Burrows, R. B., 1958, A new series of anthelmintics, *Nature (Lond.)* 181:183.

Corey, J., 1955, The stereochemistry of santonin, β-santonin and artemisin, *J. Am. Chem. Soc.* 77:1044–1045.

Datta, R. L., and Prosad, N., 1917, Halogenation. XVI. Iodination by means of nitrogen iodide or by means of iodine in the presence of ammonia, *J. Am. Chem. Soc.* 39:441–457.

Dressel, O., and Kothe, R., 1961, The discovery of germanin, *J. Chem. Ed.* 38:620–621.

Eichler, D. A., 1973, The anthelmintic activity of thiophanate in sheep and cattle, *Br. Vet. J.* 129:533–543.

Gough, G. A. C., and King, H., 1930, Trypanocidal action and chemical constitution. Part IX. Aromatic acids containing an amide group, *J. Chem. Soc.* 669–694.

Hoff, D. R., Fisher, M. H., Bochis, R. J., Lusi, A., Waksmunski, F., Egerton, J. R., Yakstis, J. J., Cuckler, A. C., and Campbell, W. C., 1970, A new broad spectrum anthelmintic: 2-(4-thiazolyl)-5-isopropoxycarbonylaminobenzimidazole, *Experientia* 26:550–551.

Kendall, J. D., and Edwards, H. D., 1946, Dicarbocyanine dyes, U.S. Pat. 2,412,815.

Krueger, H. R., Casida, J. E., and Niedermeier, R. P., 1959, Bovine metabolism of organophosphorus insecticides. Metabolism and residues associated with dermal application of Co-ral to rats, a goat, and a cow, *J. Agr. Food Chem.* 7:182–188.

Kushner, S., Brancone, L. M., Hewitt, R. I., McEwen, W. L., and Subbarow, Y., Stewart, H. W., Turner, R. J., and Denton, J. J., 1948, Experimental chemotherapy of filariasis. V. The preparation of derivatives of piperazine, *J. Org. Chem.* 13:144–153.

Lieber, E., and Slutkin, R., 1962, Diisothiocyanates and derivatives, *J. Org. Chem.* 27:2214–2217.

Lorenz, W., and Wegler, R., 1957, Verfahren zur Herstellung von Phosphorsaure-bzw. Thiophosphor-saureestern, Ger. Pat. 962,608.

Lynch, J. E., and Nelson, B., 1959, Preliminary Anthelmintic Studies with *Nematospiroides dubius* in Mice, *J. Parasitol.* 45:659–662.

Mann, R. L., and Bromer, W. W., 1958, The isolation of a second antibiotic from *Streptomyces hygroscopicus*, *J. Am. Chem. Soc.* 80:2714–2716.

Martin, W. B., and Martell, A. E., 1948, Preparation of piperazine, *J. Am. Chem. Soc.* 70:1817–1818.

McFarland, J. W., and Howes, H. L., Jr., 1972, Novel anthelmintic agents. 6. Pyrantel analogs with activity against whipworm, *J. Med. Chem.* 15:365–368.

McFarland, J. W., Conover, L. H., Howes, H. L., Jr., Lynch, J. E., Chisholm, D. R., Austin, W. C., Cornwell, R. L., Danilewicz, J. C., Courtney, W., and Morgan, D. H., 1969, Novel anthelmintic agents. II. Pyrantel and other cyclic amidines, *J. Med. Chem.* 12:1066–1079.

Mishima, H., Ide, J., Muramatsu, S., and Ono, M., 1983, Milbemycins D, E, F, G, H, J and K, *J. Antibiot.* **XXXVI**(8):980–989.

Mrozik, H., Chabala, J. C., Eskola, P., Matzuk, A., Waksmunski, F., Woods, M., and Fisher, M. H., 1983, Synthesis of milbemycins from avermectins, *Tetrahedron Lett.* 24:5333–5336.

Nitta, I., Watase, H., and Tomiie, Y., 1958, Structure of kainic acid and its isomer, allokainic acid, *Nature (Lond.)* 181:761–762.

Peters, V. K., and Neumann, L., 1932, Über die Photochemische Acetylenchlorierung, *Angew. Chem.* 45:261–266.

Raeymaekers, A. H. M., Allewijn, F. T. N., Vandenberk, J., Demoen, P. J. A., Van Offenwert, T. T. T., and Janssen, P. A. J., 1966, Novel broad-spectrum anthelmintics. Tetramisole and related derivatives of 6-arylimidazo[2,1-b]-thiazole, *J. Med. Chem.* 9:545–551.

Raeymaekers, A. H. M., Van Gelder, J. L. H., Roevens, L. F. C., and Janssen, P. A. J., 1978, Synthesis and anthelmintic activity of alkyl-(5-acyl-1-H-benzimidazol-2-yl) carbamates, *Arzneimittelforsch.* 28:586–594.

Spicer, L. D., and Hand, J. J., 1975, Method of using 6-substituted amino phenyl-2,3,5,6-tetrahydro-[2,1-b]-thiazoles, U.S. Pat. 3,899,583.

Sugimoto, N., and Okumura, K., 1954, 3-Methyl-1-pentyn-3-ol acid phthalate, Jpn. Pat. 1833 ('54).

Takiguchi, Y., Mishima, H., Okuda, M., Terao, M., Aoki, A., and Fukuda, R., 1980, Milbemycins, a new family of macrolide antibiotics: Fermentation, isolation and physico-chemical properties, *J. Antibiot.* 33:1120–1127.

Theodorides, V. J., Chang, J., DiCuollo, C. J., Grass, G. M., Parish, R. C., and Scott, G. C., 1973, Oxibendazole, a new broad spectrum anthelmintic effective against gastrointestinal nematodes of domestic animals, *Br. Vet. J.* 129:xcvii–xcviii.

Theodorides, V. J., Gyurik, R. J., Kingsbury, W. D., and Parish, R. C., 1976, Anthelmintic activity of albendazole against liver flukes, tapeworms, lung and gastrointestinal roundworms, *Experientia* 32:702–703.

Van Lare, E., and Brooker, L. G. S., 1950, Pyrrole dimethinecyanine dyes, U.S. Pat. 2,515,912.

Walker, D., and Knight, D., 1972, The anthelmintic activity of "mebendazole": A field trial in horses, *Vet. Rec.* 90:58–65.

Whaley, A. M., and Copenhaver, J. E., 1938, Preparation of some lower alkyl chlorides from the corresponding alcohols using zinc chloride and concentrated hydrochloric acid, *J. Am. Chem. Soc.* 60:2497–2498.

Whetstone, R. R., and Harman, D., 1960, Insecticidally active esters of phosphorus acids and preparation of the same, U.S. Pat. 2,956,073.

Wollweber, H., Kolling, H., Widdig, A., Thomas, H., Schulz, H.-P., and Murmann, P., 1978, Febantel, a new broad-spectrum anthelmintic, *Arzneimittelforsch.* 28:2193–2195.

12

Nematode Infections of Man

Intestinal Infections

DAVID BOTERO

1. INTRODUCTION

In most underdeveloped regions of the world, especially the tropical areas, intestinal helminthiases present high prevalence rates, similar to those found a half-century ago (Botero, 1981). The varied and sometimes important symptomatology caused by these worms, the lowering of work efficiency, and the deterioration of nutritional status are deleterious consequences requiring efficient confrontation not only by traditional measures such as installation of latrines, potable water, wearing of shoes, instruction, and personal hygiene, but also by medical treatment to individuals or to affected populations.

This chapter briefly notes some principles and methods. Mention is made, in alphabetical order, of the major intestinal nematode infections of man, specifying the drugs of choice and the alternative drugs, briefly explaining the indications of treatment. Other less common infections and their treatments are briefly mentioned as well. Finally the anthelmintic drugs are considered, in alphabetical order, in relationship to efficacy, dosages, indications, contraindications, and side effects. A recently published comprehensive review of the treatment of intestinal helminthiases in man may be found in Sturchler (1982).

2. GENERAL PRINCIPLES AND METHODS

Antiparasitic chemotherapy for intestinal human nematode infections is one of the fields that has shown important advances in recent years, as reviewed by Vanden

DAVID BOTERO • Section of Parasitology, School of Medicine, University of Antioquia, Medellin, Colombia.

Bossche (1981). The newer anthelmintics are much safer than the old ones, and most of them have the desirable characteristic of being effective in short treatments or even in a single dose. This facilitates community-based treatments, an important control measure used to reduce the prevalence rates of these parasites in endemic areas (Botero, 1979). Absence of toxicity, good tolerance, single dose, and low cost are the characteristics that an effective anthelmintic should have for being the ideal drug for deworming campaigns. A drug that has satisfactory activity against all human intestinal nematodes has not yet been discovered, but in few other medical fields has chemotherapy reached the level of ample efficacy and low toxicity presented by the anthelmintics.

Intestinal nematode infections are easily established in laboratory animals, and many animal models have been used to discover and evaluate anthelmintic drugs. For references to sources of information on such methods, see Chapter 14. A recent report (World Health Organization, 1981) recommended continuance of attempts to develop better anthelmintic drugs; for this purpose, proper clinical trial methods must be used. In another WHO report, reference was made to the factors in the helminth life cycles affecting the evaluation of drug efficacy, and pitfalls in experimental design were noted (Davis, 1973). Botero (1976) discussed important hints and precautions necessary for good clinical trials in intestinal helminthiases and considered such points as who should do the trials and where, when a new anthelmintic should be studied, the tolerance and dose range to be studied, the assessment of efficacy, and the parasitological methods. In this matter, emphasis was placed on the need for repeated and replicated egg counts for a period of 4 weeks after treatment for ascariasis, trichuriasis, and hookworm infections. In hookworm infection, it is necessary to differentiate the species of parasite by examining the cultured larvae or by identifying the adult worms. For enterobiasis, egg counts are not feasible, and reliance should be placed on the Scotch-tape technique for determining the presence or absence of eggs. To establish complete cure, the method should be applied for 7 consecutive days beginning 1 week and 3 weeks after treatment. For strongyloidiasis, drug efficacy is also judged in an all-or-none fashion, and repeated fecal examinations (using direct and concentration methods) are necessary as well as culture and isolation of larvae. For the other less common intestinal nematode infections, specific methods and precautions are necessary for proper clinical trials.

3. MAJOR INFECTIONS AND THE DRUGS OF CHOICE

3.1. Ascariasis

Ascaris lumbricoides lives in the lumen of the small intestine and is easily reached by anthelmintics through direct contact. All infections should be treated—even the light ones—since even a single parasite may migrate to an abnormal place and produce significant pathology. Community-based treatments are highly recommended in this parasitic infection, which is associated with protein-energy malnutrition in children (Stephenson *et al.*, 1983).

Drugs of choice: pyrantel pamoate, albendazole, and mebendazole.
Alternative drugs: piperazine and levamisole.

3.2. Enterobiasis

Enterobius vermicularis is a parasite of the large intestine, where it lives in the lumen and migrates through the anus to deposit eggs on the perianal skin. It is easily transmitted directly from person to person, and treatment is necessary especially in children, who are frequently reinfected if the close contacts are not also cured.

Drugs of choice: pyrantel pamoate, albendazole, and mebendazole.
Alternative drug: piperazine, pyrvinium pamoate.

3.3. Hookworm Infections

Necator americanus and *Ancylostoma duodenale* are important causes of iron deficiency anemia; infections caused by these parasites should always be treated because both live many years, and even light infections may lower the hemoglobin levels in undernourished patients. Iron therapy is also required in anemic patients. *Ancylostoma ceylanicum* in Asia presents similar characteristics, although on a smaller scale.

Drugs of choice: pyrantel pamoate, albendazole, and mebendazole.
Alternative drug: bephenium hydroxynaphthoate.

3.4. Strongyloidiasis

Strongyloides stercoralis lives in the interior of the small intestinal wall but may spread to the large intestine and viscera in cases of immunosuppression, when it may be fatal (Carvalho Filho, 1978). Anthelmintics for intestinal or disseminated strongyloidiasis should act in the tissues and for this reason need to be absorbed. All cases should be treated because of the danger of dissemination and long-lasting infection resulting from the autoinfection cycle.

Drug of choice: thiabendazole.
Alternative drug: cambendazole, if approved for human use. For disseminated infections, no treatment is known to be reliable, but cambendazole or high-dose mebendazole therapy may prove effective. Ivermectin is highly active against extraintestinal larvae of *S. stercoralis* in mice, so this compound offers promise of efficacy against the disseminated infection in man (Grove, 1983).

3.5. Trichuriasis

Trichuris trichiura inserts the anterior part of its body into the colonic mucosa, producing small lesions that may be responsible for colitis and even a dysenteric syndrome in heavily infected children. Only light infections in well nourished patients do not produce symptoms, and treatment in these cases is not as crucial as in heavy infections.

Drugs of choice: mebendazole, oxantel pamoate.
Alternative drug: albendazole.

4. LESS COMMON INTESTINAL NEMATODE INFECTIONS

4.1. Trichinosis

Trichinella spiralis reaches maturity in the small intestine. The adult worms are believed to live only for a few weeks and to produce light symptoms; for this reason, anthelmintic treatment is often not recommended. However, since the adults are the source of the more pathogenic muscle-dwelling larvae, some authorities believe that anthelmintic treatment should always be directed against the adults, as well as the larvae (Pawlowski, 1983). In cases of presumptive infection (ingestion of infected meat within the previous few days) or in heavy infections that have been diagnosed in the early phase, attempts should be made to sterilize or remove the worms residing in the intestine. For this purpose, patients may be given mebendazole at 200 mg/day for 4 days or pyrantel at 10 mg/kg per day for 4 days (Pawlowski, 1983). For treatment of the muscle phase, see Chapter 13.

4.2. Trichostrongyliasis

Trichostrongylus orientalis is the main etiological agent, predominating in Asia, although other species of the same genus are also occasional human parasites. Enteritis and other pathological changes have been found in this parasitic infection, but it is usually asymptomatic. Pyrantel and bephenium have been used successfully for treatment.

4.3. Intestinal Capillariasis

Capillaria philippinensis, recently found in the Philippines and Thailand, is acquired by eating raw fish and produces enteritis, malabsorption, and diarrhea. Thiabendazole is effective with prolonged therapy, but mebendazole is.the drug of choice.

4.4. Intestinal Angiostrongyliasis

Angiostrongylus costaricensis, a newly discovered parasite in Latin America, produces a tumorlike lesion in the colon. Some cases require surgical intervention; the anthelmintics that have been tried have shown very little benefit.

4.5. Anisakiasis, Oesophagostomiasis, and Gnathostomiasis

These uncommon intestinal parasitic infections of man, found mainly in Asia, are produced by different species of *Anisakis*, *Oesophagostomum*, and *Gnathostoma*, which are animal parasites. Most cases of these infections are treated by surgery, since the granulomatous lesions are not susceptible to anthelmintic therapy.

5. ANTHELMINTICS AND THEIR USAGE

5.1. Albendazole

Albendazole, a benzimidazole carbamate, is the most recent broad-spectrum anthelmintic for use in man. It has been used for several years in veterinary medicine. The use of albendazole in human helminthiasis has been reported in the proceedings of a recent symposium (Firth, 1983). It offers the advantage of single-dose treatment for several infections. A single oral dose of 100 mg (approximately 1.5 mg/kg) is highly effective against *Enterobius vermicularis*, while 400 mg is highly effective against *Ascaris lumbricoides* and *Ancylostoma duodenale*. The 400 mg dosage is also effective against *Necator americanus* but less so than against the other hookworm. The difference in susceptibility may, to some extent, be related to intensity of infection and geographical strain of parasite as well as to interspecific difference. In trials against *N. americanus* in Thailand dosages of 400, 600 or 800 mg gave cure rates of only 35, 44 and 69%, respectively (Chitchang *et al.*, 1983). In contrast, other studies have shown a cure rate of 100% against *A. duodenale*, and 91% against light infections of *N. americanus* (Pene *et al.*, 1982; Rossignol and Coulaud, 1983). In *Strongyloides* infection a 3-day treatment, using 400 mg daily, has shown unsatisfactory results and even a dosage of 800 mg, given once daily for 3 days, resulted in a cure rate of only 77% (Coulaud *et al.*, 1982). More studies are necessary to determine the efficacy in this parasitic infection (Rossignol and Maisonneuve, 1983; Pene *et al.*, 1982). The efficacy of albendazole against *T. trichiura* seems to be inferior to that of mebendazole (Amato Neto *et al.*, 1983). Albendazole is rapidly, though slightly, absorbed after oral administration. The absorbed portion is fully metabolized, the chief metabolite being the sulphoxide derivative. This anthelmintically active metabolite reaches peak concentration in plasma after 2.5 hr, has a half-life of 8.5 hr, and is eliminated in the urine. Although the proportion of albendazole that is absorbed is low, it is considerably higher than in the case of mebendazole. While albendazole has only recently been introduced into human medicine, it appears to be very well tolerated. A review of multinational trials involving almost 1500 patients indicated that side effects had occurred in only 6% (Rossignol and Coulaud, 1983). They were mild and transient, the most common being epigastric pain (2.2%) and diarrhea (2.0%). Since albendazole, like mebendazole, is known to produce embryotoxicity and teratogenicity in laboratory animals, the use of either drug in pregnant women is not recommended, especially during the first trimester of pregnancy.

5.2. Bephenium Hydroxynaphthoate

This drug is poorly absorbed from the intestine and has been used mainly in the treatment of *A. duodenale* at a dosage of 5 g (containing 2.5 g of the base) for adults, and one-half this dose for children. The results in the treatment of *N. americanus* are unsatisfactory (Botero and Castaño, 1973). Although the drug acts against *A. lumbricoides*, it is not recommended in this parasite because there are more effective drugs and because of poor tolerance of bephenium. The side effects are mainly gastrointestinal (GI) symptoms such as nausea, vomiting, abdominal pain, diarrhea, and anorexia. Other general symptoms are dizziness and headache. These side effects occurred in 60% of cases. Bephenium hydroxynaphthoate should not be used in hypertensive patients because, if absorbed in considerable amount, it may cause a marked drop in blood pressure. For the same reason, caution is necessary in using this drug during pregnancy. Such disadvantages are likely to result in the decline in the use of this product, especially considering that there are other more effective and better-tolerated drugs for the treatment of hookworm infections.

5.3. Cambendazole

This is another benzimidazole derivative that has been used in veterinary medicine. It has been used very little in human patients, as the necessary safety studies have not been completed. Nevertheless, studies in Brazil in cases of human strongyloidiasis have demonstrated excellent results and no side effects; Amato Neto *et al.* (1978) and Baransky *et al.* (1978) used a single dose of 5 mg/kg, which resulted in cure rates of better than 90%—even higher than those found with thiabendazole. The marked efficacy of cambendazole has also been demonstrated in experimentally infected mice (Grove, 1982). It is hoped that more clinical trials are done with this drug and that the toxicological studies show no undesirable effects, since there is great need for a good and well-tolerated treatment for strongyloidiasis.

5.4. Levamisole

Levamisole, an isomer of tetramisole, has been effectively used in human patients harboring *A. lumbricoides* at a single dose of 150 mg for adults and 40–80 mg for children (Thienpont *et al.*, 1969; Moens *et al.*, 1978). It also has an effect on hookworms and *S. stercoralis*. Soluble in water, this substance is readily absorbed. It is well tolerated. A few cases of intestinal symptoms and dizziness have been reported as the only side effects. Levamisole has been undergoing clinical trials for diseases resulting from immunodeficiencies and for some malignancies (Renoux *et al.*, 1976), based on findings that it enhances the immunological defense of the patients, probably by stimulating the production of T lymphocytes. In such cases, levamisole has been administered at a dosage of 300 mg/day for 3 days weekly, continued for several months, with good tolerance.

5.5. Mebendazole and Flubendazole

Mebendazole (reviewed by Vanden Bossche *et al.*, 1982) is the most commonly used benzimidazole derivative. It is very slightly absorbed from the intestinal tract. This anthelmintic shows a broad spectrum of activity, being effective against *T. trichiura*, hookworms, *A. lumbricoides*, and *E. vermicularis*. The usual dose is 100 mg twice per day, for 3 days, both in children and adults (Pena-Chavarria *et al.*, 1973; Sargent *et al.*, 1974). A single dose of 100–200 mg is sufficient for enterobiasis (Brugmans *et al.*, 1971). It is not considered satisfactory in the treatment of *Strongyloides*, but a very high dosage of 1500 mg/day for 14 days was highly effective in a patient with an infected blind intestinal loop who had failed to respond to thiabendazole therapy (Wilson and Kauffman, 1983). There is general agreement on the lack of toxic effects and on the absence of side effects. In a small number of cases, *Ascaris* has been seen to migrate to the mouth in children who were heavily infected by this parasite and who were under treatment with mebendazole. In regard to teratogenicity, it was found that mebendazole, when given during the period of organogenesis in rodents, induces fetal abnormalities, consisting mainly of skeletal defects in the ribs and tail. Neither teratogenic nor embryotoxic effects were observed in dogs, sheep, or horses. As a precaution, this drug should not be used during the first months of pregnancy.

Flubendazole, a fluorine analogue of mebendazole, has produced results similar to those of mebendazole (Schenone *et al.*, 1977; Kan, 1983). It apparently differs from mebendazole in that tests have failed to demonstrate teratogenicity in rodents. As in the case of mebendazole, a single oral dose of 100 mg is sufficient for enterobiasis, while broad-spectrum use requires 100 mg b.i.d. for 3 days. The properties of flubendazole have been reviewed by Vanden Bossche (1982).

5.6. Oxantel

This compound is an analogue of pyrantel and shows particularly good efficacy against *T. trichiura*. A single dose of 10 mg/kg is effective in light infections, while the same dosage given daily for 3 days cures most severe infections (Lee *et al.*, 1976). According to unofficial reports from the Chinese literature of 1983, workers in China gave oxantel to approximately 400 patients (1 g over a period of 2–3 days) and obtained 70% cure of *Trichuris*, with mild and transient side effects in 17% of cases; in approximately 50 patients given mebendazole (200 mg/kg b.i.d. × 2–3 days), the cure rate was only 22%. The combination of oxantel and pyrantel widens the spectrum of activity to cover the three major soil-transmitted nematodes—*Ascaris*, hookworms, and *Trichuris*—as well as *Enterobius*. Its use as a single dose in communities with endemic intestinal helminthiases has shown beneficial effects, maintaining low prevalence rates of these parasites when administered periodically (Botero *et al.*, 1984). Oxantel is well tolerated.

5.7. Piperazine

Piperazine has been in use for almost 30 years and still is widely used in many countries as an inexpensive popular anthelmintic. Initial studies in group treatments in

Africa in 1954 showed it to be well accepted by patients who observed the elimination of roundworms. This interesting episode in the introduction of piperazine was very nicely described by Goodwin (1980). Efficacy of the drug is limited to *A. lumbricoides* and *E. vermicularis* at a dosage of 50 mg/kg, divided into three to five doses and given daily for 5 days (Davis, 1973). Several salts are used, such as hexahydrate, citrate, phosphate, adipate, and tartrate, all of which are soluble in water and readily absorbable from the intestine. Because there is a wide range between the therapeutic and the toxic dosages, drug reactions are uncommon. In a few cases, piperazine produces nausea, vomiting, and diarrhea. When a large amount of the drug is swallowed or when the drug accumulates in the body, as occurs mainly in cases of renal insufficiency, dramatic toxic effects are seen, but fortunately they are transient and do not leave sequelae. These symptoms are caused by the action of piperazine on the myoneural mammalian junctions, which produces a blocking effect. The symptomatology is muscular incoordination, ataxia, vertigo, difficulty in speech, confused mental state, muscular weakness, and myoclonic contractions. It may produce or exacerbate epileptic seizures in predisposed patients. Piperazine is contraindicated in patients with renal or hepatic insufficiency and in epileptic patients.

5.8. Pyrantel Pamoate

This compound is insoluble in water and is very slightly absorbed from the intestine. Pyrantel is effective against ascariasis and enterobiasis in a single dose of 10 mg/kg and against hookworms in a 3-day treatment at the same daily dose (Botero and Castaño, 1973; Sanati and Ghadirian, 1971). The drug is well tolerated, and no toxic effects have been reported. In clinical trials (Botero and Castaño, 1973) only 20% of treated patients described side effects; these were light and consisted of dizziness, drowsiness, and intestinal symptoms, such as nausea, vomiting, diarrhea, and abdominal pain. There are no known contraindications for this anthelmintic. In combination with oxantel it is used as an polyvalent drug, effective in population-based treatments as mentioned above.

5.9. Pyrvinium Pamoate

This red cyanine dye is not appreciably absorbed from the intestinal tract. Its only use is in the treatment of *E. vermicularis* infection, as a single oral dose of 5 mg/kg (Beck *et al.*, 1959). The drug is well tolerated, but GI symptoms and dizziness have been reported. It stains clothes and stools red. Pyrvinium has been displaced by the newer anthelmintics in the treatment of pinworms.

5.10. Thiabendazole

Used for many years in the treatment of strongyloidiasis, thiabendazole is still considered the drug of choice for this disease, at a dosage of 25 mg/kg per day, divided in three doses with meals (Campbell and Cuckler, 1969). In disseminated strongyloidiasis, the daily dosage can be increased to 50 mg/kg for 5–8 days. An absorbable drug effective against larval forms of nematodes, thiabendazole has also been used in the treatment of cutaneous larva migrans. Experimentally, it has been useful in trichinosis and visceral larva migrans. Thiabendazole is rapidly absorbed and excreted *via* the urine. It is also absorbed from the skin. Side effects are common, with 50% of cases showing symptoms of intolerance, the most frequent being dizziness. Other side effects observed are GI symptoms, such as nausea, vomiting, abdominal pain, diarrhea, and anorexia. Headache, drowsiness, and lethargy have also been reported. Side effects are lowered when the daily dose is fractionated and administered after meals. A few cases of erythema multiforme and Stevens-Johnson syndrome, with two fatalities, have been reported as significant toxic effects.

REFERENCES

Amato Neto, V., Sinto, T., Pedro, R. de J., Levi, G. C., Tsukumo, M. K. K., de Moraes, V. M. C., and Correa, L. de L., 1978, Nossas observacoes iniciais sobre a eficacia do cambendazole no tratamento da estrongiloidiase, *Rev. Inst. Med. Trop.* 20:161–163.

Amato-Neto, V., Moreira, A. A. B., Campos, R., Lazzaro, E. S. M., Chiaramelli, M. C. G., Pinto, P. L. S., Da Silva, G. R., Nishioka, S., and de A. e Leite, R. M., 1983, Tratamento da ancilostomiase, ascaridiase e tricocefaliase por mejo do albendazol ou do mebendazol, *Rev. Inst. Med. Trop.* 25:294–299.

Baransky, M. C., Silva, A. F. da, Kotaka, P. I., Gomez, N. R., Giovannoni, M., and Telles, J. E. Q., 1978, Tratamento da estrongiloidiase humana com novo antihelmintico, o cambendazole. Estudo duplo cego, *Rev. Inst. Med. Trop. Sao Paulo* 20:213–218.

Beck, J. W., Saavedra, D., Antell, G. J., and Tejeiros, B., 1959, The treatment of pinworm infections in humans (enterobiasis) with pyrvinium chloride and pyrvinium pamoate, *Am. J. Trop. Med. Hyg.* 8:349–352.

Botero, C. A., Calad, G. A., Cardona, E. A., Correa, D. H., and Gonzalez, C. M., 1984, Epidemiologia de las helmintiasis intestinales en una zona rural de Antioquia, Colombia (Control por tratamiento comunitario), *Medicina Universidad Pontificia Bolivariana* 3:65–76.

Botero, D., 1976, Clinical trial methodology in intestinal parasitic disease, *Clin. Pharmacol. Ther.* 19:630–637.

Botero, D., 1979, Posibilidades de control de las geohelmintiasis mediante tratamientos en masa, *Bol. Chile. Parasitol.* 34:39–43.

Botero, D., 1981, Persistence of the endemic intestinal parasitoses in Latin America, *Bull. Pan. Am. Health Org.* 15:241–248.

Botero, D., and Castaño, A., 1973, Comparative study of pyrantel pamoate, bephenium hydroxinaphthoate and tetrachloroethylene in the treatment of *Necator americanus* infections, *Am. J. Trop. Med. Hyg.* 22:45–52.

Brugmans, J. P., Thienpont, D. C., Van Wijngaarden, I., Vanparijs, O. F., Schermans, V. L., and Lauwers, H. L., 1971, Mebendazole in enterobiasis. Radio-chemical and pilot clinical study in 1,278 subjects, *J.A.M.A.* 217:313–316.

Campbell, W. C., and Cuckler, A. C., 1969, Thiabendazole in the treatment and control in parasitic infections in man, *Tex. Rep. Biol. Med.* (Suppl. 2) 27:665–692.

Calvalho Filho, E., 1978, Strongyloidiasis. *Clin. Gastroenterol.* 7:179–200.

Chitchang, S., Leelayoova, S., and Piamjinda, T., 1983, Albendazole in the treatment of hookworm infestation in Thailand, *J. Med. Assoc. Thailand* 66:45–48.

Coulaud, J. P., Deluol, A. M., Cenac, J., and Rossignol, J. F., 1982, L'albendazole dans le traitement de la strongyloidose: à propos de 66 observations, *Bull. Soc. Pathol. Exot. Fil.* 75:530–533.

Davis, A., 1973, *Drug Treatment of Intestinal Helminthiases*, 125 pp., World Health Organization, Geneva.

Firth, M. (ed.), 1983, Albendazole in helminthiasis, in: *International Congress Symposium Series*, No. 57, Royal Society of Medicine, London.

Goodwin, L. G., 1980, New drugs for old diseases, *Trans. R. Soc. Trop. Med. Hyg.* 74:1–7.

Grove, D. I., 1982, *Strongyloides ratti* and *S. stercoralis:* The effects of thiabendazole, mebendazole and cambendazole in infected mice, *Am. J. Trop. Med. Hyg.* 31:469–476.

Grove, D. I., 1983, The effects of 22,23-dihydroavermectin B$_1$ on *Strongyloides ratti* and *S. stercoralis* infections in mice, *Ann. Trop. Med. Parasitol.* 77:405–410.

Kan, S. P., 1983, The anthelmintic effects of flubendazole on *Trichuris trichiura* and *Ascaris lumbricoides*, *Trans. R. Soc. Trop. Med. Hyg.* 77:668–670.

Lee, E. L., Kyngkaran, N., Grieve, A. W., Robinson, M. J., and Dissanaike, A. S., 1976, Therapeutic evaluation of oxantel pamoate (1,4,5,6-tetrahydro-1-methyl-2-(trans-3-hydroxystyryl)pyrimidine pamoate) in severe *Trichuris trichiura* infection, *Am. J. Trop. Med. Hyg.* 25:563–567.

Moens, M., Dom, J., Burke, W. E., Schlossberg, S., and Schermans, V., 1978, Levamisole in ascariasis. A multicenter controlled evaluation, *Am. J. Trop. Med. Hyg.* 27:897–904.

Pawlowski, Z. S., 1983, Clinical aspects in man, in: *Trichinella and Trichinosis* (W. C. Campbell, ed.), pp. 367–401, Plenum Press, New York.

Peña-Chavarria, A., Swatzwelder, J. C., Villarejos, V. M., and Zeledon, R., 1973, Mebendazole an effective broad spectrum anthelmintic, *Am. J. Trop. Med. Hyg.* 22:592–595.

Pene, P., Mojon, M., Garin, J. P., Coulaud, J. P., and Rossignol, J. F., 1982, Albendazole: a new broad spectrum anthelmintic. Double blind multicenter clinical trial, *Am. J. Trop. Med. Hyg.* 31:263–266.

Renoux, G., Renoux, M., Teller, M. N., McMahon, S., and Gyillaumin, J. M., 1976, Potentiation of T-cell mediated immunity by levamisole, *Clin. Exp. Immunol.* 25:288–296.

Rossignol, J. F., and Coulaud, J. P., 1983, Summary of clinical trials worldwide (evaluation of albendazole in Europe, West Africa and Asia as a single-dose anthelmintic: report on 1455 patients), in: *Albendazole in Helminthiasis* (M. Firth, ed.), *International Congress Symposium Series*, No. 57, Royal Society of Medicine, London, pp. 19–27.

Rossignol, J. F., and Maisonneuve, H., 1983, Albendazole: Placebo-controlled study in 870 patients with intestinal helminthiasis, *Trans. R. Soc. Trop. Med. Hyg.* 17:707–711.

Sanati, A., and Ghadirian, E. G., 1971, Treatment of enterobiasis with pyrantel pamoate in Iran, *J. Trop. Med. Hyg.* 74:160–161.

Sargent, R. G., Savory, A. M., Mina, A., and Lee, P. R., 1974, A clinical evaluation of mebendazole in the treatment of trichuriasis, *Am. J. Trop. Med. Hyg.* 23:375–377.

Schenone, H., Galdames, M., Insunza, E., Jimenez, M., Romero, E., and Bloomfield, R., 1977, Flubendazol en el tratamiento de infecciones por nematodes intestinales en niños, *Bol. Chil. Parasitol.* 32:85–86.

Stephenson, L. S., Cromptom, E. W. T., Latham, M. C., Arnold, S. E., and Jansen, A. A. J., 1983, Evaluation of a four year project to control *Ascaris* infection in children in two Kenyan villages, *J. Trop. Pediatr.* 29:175–184.

Sturchler, D., 1982, Chemotherapy of human intestinal helminthiases: A review, with particular reference to community treatment, *Adv. Pharmacol. Chemother.* 19:129–154.

Thienpont, D., Brugmans, J., Abadi, K., and Tanamal, S., 1969, Tetramisole in the treatment of nematode infections of man, *Am. J. Trop. Med. Hyg.* 18:520–525.

Vanden Bossche, H., 1981, Peculiar targets in anthelmintic chemotherapy, *Biochem. Pharmacol.* 29:1981–1990.

Vanden Bossche, H., Rochette, F., and Horig, C., 1982, Mebendazole and related anthelmintics, *Adv. Pharmacol. and Chemother.* 19:67–128.

Wilson, K. H., and Kauffman, C. A., 1983, Persistent *Strongyloides stercoralis* in a blind loop of the bowel: successful treatment with mebendazole, *Arch. Intern. Med.* 143:357–358.

World Health Organization, 1981, *Intestinal Protozoan and Helminthic Infections*, Technical Report Series 666, World Health Organization, Geneva.

13

Nematode Infections of Man

Extraintestinal Infections

DAVID A. DENHAM

1. INTRODUCTION

Despite a plethora of anthelmintics active against the nematodes parasitizing the human gut, as illustrated in Chapter 12, far fewer drugs have been or can be used in the treatment of those nematodes that parasitize other organs. This chapter deals with the chemotherapy of diseases caused by such nematodes.

2. INTRALYMPHATIC FILARIAE

2.1. Methods of Detecting Activity against Wuchereria and Brugia

Most of the original screening for filaricides active against the lymphatic dwelling filariae used *Litomosoides carinii*. It was with this parasite in naturally infected cotton rats, captured from the wild, that Hewitt *et al.* (1947) detected the filaricidal activity of diethylcarbamazine (DEC). The original paper on DEC and *Litomosoides carinii* and the dog heartworm, *Dirofilaria immitis*, suggested that DEC killed adult worms, but all subsequent experimentation has failed to confirm macrofilaricidal activity against these parasites. It is possible that in these naturally infected cotton rats the worms were adversely affected by an immune response that potentiated the action of DEC.

There are very considerable differences between the biochemistry of *L. carinii* and all the other filariae that have been studied, as *L. carinii* is a obligate aerobe, whereas the other filariae are facultative anaerobes (Rew and Saz, 1977; Barrett, 1983). Fortunately, *Brugia* spp. infect jirds (*Meriones unguiculatus*) (Ash and Riley, 1970), so that a much more relevant screen can be used. However, a mathematical analysis of both

DAVID A. DENHAM • London School of Hygiene & Tropical Medicine, London WC1E 7HT, England.

subcutaneously and intraperitoneally induced infections shows that groups of up to 10 jirds are needed to obtain statistically valid results if an observed decrease in worm burden of 50% is to be accepted as reliable (Denham *et al.*, 1984). Suswillo and Denham (1977) developed a technique for transplanting adult *Brugia* into the peritoneal cavities of jirds as part of some experiments on hybridization of the different *Brugia* spp. These workers noted that when adult *Brugia* were recovered from the peritoneal cavities of jirds and implanted into peritoneal cavities of naive jirds there was a remarkably consistent recovery of adult worms from the recipients and the adult worms lived for several months. This system is now used in several laboratories sponsored by the special program of the World Bank/UNDP/WHO. Full methodology for this screen has been published elsewhere (Denham, 1982*b*).

Secondary screening can be carried out either in jirds infected by inoculation of infective larvae or in cats similarly infected. Infections with *B. pahangi* in cats are very reliable, and the worms are in the same intralymphatic anatomical site as they are in man. If infective larvae are injected subcutaneously into the foot, virtually all adults are found in the lymphatics below the popliteal lymph node, making the post mortem examination very simple and rapid.

In experimental animals with *Brugia* infections, many compounds have been shown to be macrofilaricidal. Several benzimidazole carbamates, such as mebendazole, flubendazole, albendazole, fenbendazole, and oxibendazole, kill adult *Brugia*, but only if injected (Denham *et al.*, 1978, 1979, 1981). So far none has been active when given *per os*. It will be interesting to see whether albendazole, which is now being used orally in man against intestinal nematodes and which was not active orally in cats (Denham *et al.*, 1980), has any activity against the filariae in man by the enteral route. Ivermectin has very little effect on experimental *Brugia* infections (Denham, 1982*a*), but it would still be worth testing to see its effects in man because it has such varied effects on filarial worms (Campbell, 1982).

2.2. *Wuchereria bancrofti and Brugia spp. in Man*

Only one anthelmintic has been widely used against these widespread and pathogenic filarial worms. This anthelmintic, diethylcarbamazine (DEC), was first described by Hewitt *et al.* (1947), the result of a research program initiated because of the large number of American marines and soldiers who suffered various clinical forms of filariasis contracted in the South Pacific during World War II. Its use against *W. bancrofti* was first described by Santiago-Stevenson *et al.* (1947).

In man, as in many experimental models, there can be no doubt that DEC is microfilaricidal. In *W. bancrofti* infections relatively few side effects are reported, but in people with either *B. malayi* or *B. timori* the side effects are severe. Partono *et al.* (1979) described in graphic terms the side effects of DEC in patients with *B. timori* infections.

DEC has also been used in a successful program for the control of a human helminthic disease with chemotherapy. Starting in French Oceania, and now through virtually the whole of the South Pacific, DEC has been used to prevent the development of bancroftian filariasis. These programs were summarized by Hawking and Denham

(1976). With a few variations, DEC was given to all the inhabitants of the target islands once monthly at 6 mg/kg for 1 year, for a total dose of 72 mg/kg. After 1 year, any microfilaremic patients were treated for another year. While this regimen does not eliminate the infection, it does prevent the development of any new clinical signs.

A dose rate of 50–72 mg/kg is most commonly used for the treatment of lymphatic filariasis, but the ways in which this overall level is achieved are manifold. In most hospitals the DEC will be given over a few days, whereas Partono used very low starting levels to avoid some of the side effects in *B. timori* patients (Partono, 1984; Partono *et al.*, 1984).

There has been controversy about whether DEC kills adult *W. bancrofti* or *B. malayi* in man. Ch'en (1964) produced the only direct evidence by biopsying lymphatics and finding dead worms. The results from the South Pacific strongly suggest that DEC either kills or sexually sterilizes *W. bancrofti* as most treated patients remain amicrofilaremic. Ottesen (1984) recently reviewed this subject and concludes that if a full course of treatment is given DEC is definitely macrofilaricidal. Partono showed that DEC treatment can reverse some of the more dramatic consequences of filarial infection (Partono, 1984; Partono *et al.*, 1979).

Few other drugs have been used against the lymphatic filariae. Suramin was shown to be macrofilaricidal (Thooris, 1956), but its use cannot be justified. Mebendazole has also been used and appears to be active, especially if used in conjunction with levamisole (Narasimhan *et al.*, 1978), but has to be used at very high levels and for long periods. Although DEC is a very useful chemotherapeutic for the lymphatic filariases, a one-shot macrofilaricide would have very great advantages, especially in control programs.

3. *ONCHOCERCA VOLVULUS* INFECTIONS

3.1. Screening Methods for Onchocercicidal Drugs

No rodent species has been successfully infected with *O. volvulus* or any of the other species of *Onchocerca*. The only filaria of rodents with a skin-dwelling microfilaria is *Monanema globulosa*. This filaria is a natural parasite of striped mice and other rodents in East Africa and is transmitted by the ard tick *Haemophysalis leachi* (Muller and Nelson, 1975). Bianco and Denham (1984) showed that DEC is microfilaricidal in infected jirds and that a Mazzoti-type reaction occurs in these animals. However, a new microfilaricide is not really needed, so this model has little applicability. The current "official" attitude to primary screening is to use either *B. pahangi* or *Dipetalonema viteae*, or both, as a primary screen (Goodwin, 1984). The only infection currently available for secondary screening is *Onchocerca* spp. infection of cattle. Denham and Mellor (1976) were the first to test an anthelmintic against a species of *Onchocerca* in cattle. They used cattle naturally infected with *O. lienalis* to test the arsenical compound E synthesized by Dr. E. A. H. Friedheim. Copeman (1979) showed that *O. gibsoni* infections give much more reliable results. His system involves treating naturally infected cattle and at autopsy removing nodules and processing these for histopathological investigation.

Copeman has successfully used this system as a routine screen for several potentially onchocercicidal drugs. He has shown that several benzimidazole carbamates are embryotoxic but not adulticidal. He also found that ivermectin was microfilaricidal but that subsequent to the cessation of treatment, skin microfilarial levels soon reached levels higher than they were before treatment. Duke (1962) experimentally infected chimpanzees (*Pan troglodytes*) with *O. volvulus* and carried out a series of experiments with different drugs (Duke, 1977).

3.2. Chemotherapy in Man

Onchocerciasis is probably the most debilitating of all the nematode infections afflicting man, causing appalling skin disease and blindness, and yet the chemotherapy of this disease is very unsatisfactory. DEC is highly microfilaricidal, and yet the very destruction of the microfilariae greatly increases the skin pathology. Mazzoti (1948) was the first to describe this reaction, which now bears Mazzoti's name. So intense and specific is the Mazzoti reaction that it has been used as a diagnostic procedure in patients in whom the disease is suspected but in whom microfilariae cannot be demonstrated. The use of DEC also exacerbates eye lesions, at least temporarily (Anderson and Fuglsang, 1976, 1978). Metrifonate also kills microfilariae of *O. volvulus* but, as it kills many fewer microfilariae, it also produces lower levels of Mazzoti reactions than does DEC (Salazar-Mallen *et al.*, 1971; Awadzi and Gillies, 1980).

Ivermectin has been shown to be microfilaricidal and to produce minimal reaction, but it has not yet been used in patients with high mirofilarial levels (Aziz *et al.*, 1982; Coulaud *et al.*, 1983, 1984). Ivermectin is also reported to prevent embryogenesis in adult female *O. volvulus*. Follow-up studies with ivermectin are being conducted.

Suramin has been used extensively as an adulticide in *O. volvulus* infected patients (Duke, 1968). It is administered by intravenous injection, which has both advantages and disadvantages. The major problem with suramin is that it is unpredictably toxic in some patients and deaths associated with treatment are by no means uncommon. The arsenical compound Mel W has also been used in the treatment of onchocerciasis and like suramin kills both adult *O. volvulus* and some patients (Duke, 1968). There is a very clear need for a nontoxic adulticide for the chemotherapy of onchocerciasis.

Rivas-Alcala *et al.* (1984) examined the effects of mebendazole and levamisole on human onchocerciasis. Mebendazole had good embryostatic effects on female *O. volvulus* and levamisole rather less effect. A combination of mebendazole and levamisole had an even greater effect on embryogenesis than either drug given separately.

4. LOA LOA

DEC is the drug of choice for *Loa loa* infections, being both micro- and macrofilaricidal (Bonnin and Moretti, 1950). The dosage is 5 mg/kg per day for 3 weeks. However, care should be taken with the treatment of patients with very high microfilarial counts, as meningoencephalitis may occur. Plasmaphoresis has been used to reduce the microfilarial levels before treatment with DEC (Saeed *et al.*, 1984). There are no known rodent hosts of *L. loa* (Suswillo *et al.*, 1976), although it will mature in various monkeys (Duke, 1964).

5. OTHER TISSUE-DWELLING NEMATODES

5.1. Angiostrongylus cantonensis and A. malaysiensis

These zoonotic infections mature in rats. In man larvae become arrested in the brain and cause eosinophilic encephalomeningitis. This disease is comparatively rare but is serious and occasionally fatal.

Cuckler *et al.* (1965) treated infected rats for 3 weeks with 0.1% thiabendazole in the diet. These workers found that the young worms, which are clinically significant in man, were completely susceptible to this regimen. Kliks *et al.* (1982) treated human patients with 50 mg thiabendazole per day for 3 days but reported no change in the clinical status of their patients. Ambu *et al.* (1982) had extremely encouraging results with mebendazole and levamisole in rats infected with *A. malaysiensis*. With mebendazole, they obtained 97% cures with 5 × 1 mg/kg and 100% cures with 5 × 5 mg/kg. With levamisole, they obtained 90% cures with 5 × 1 mg/kg and 100% cures with 5 × 5 mg/kg. Ishii *et al.* (1983) obtained a 60% reduction in *A. cantonensis* in rats treated with 1 mg/kg ivermectin; this suggests that further experimentation using multiple doses of ivermectin is called for.

There is clearly room for a great deal more work on the experimental and clinical chemotherapy of *Angiostrongylus* spp. infections. However, there is doubt as to whether the death of larvae in the brain will worsen or improve the human patient's condition.

5.2. Toxocara canis

This ascarid parasite of dogs causes visceral larva migrans and neurological complications in man (usually in young children), but there have been very few attempts to use chemotherapy to kill larvae in human patients. As with so many other tissue-dwelling nematodes, there has been doubt about whether the death of larvae would exacerbate or improve the human condition. However, Bekhti (1984) treated a patient with visceral larvae migrans for 21 days with 1 g of mebendazole three times a day and obtained a clinical cure.

Toxocara canis will develop to the inhibited larval stage in mice, and there have been numerous experiments with established anthelmintics in this model. Burren (1968) described a screening method using this model. Nicholas and Stewart (1979) fed fenbendazole and oxfendazole in the diet and found both compounds to be highly effective in killing *T. canis* larvae. This system was also used by Holt *et al.* (1981) and Abdel Hameed (1984).

Dubey (1979) showed that fenbendazole will kill inhibited larvae of *T. canis* in dogs. Similar results with this and other benzimidazole carbamates, including albendazole, have been obtained by S. Lloyds and E. J. L. Soulsby (personal communication). As albendazole can be used in man, it must have potential for the treatment of visceral larva migrans especially in the light of the encouraging results of Bekhti (1984).

5.3. Hookworm Infections

During their migration through the lungs, hookworms, especially *Necator americanus,* produce a pneumonitis (called Löffler's syndrome). Albendazole has been used successfully to treat the lung stages in humans experimentally infected with *N. americanus* (J. F. Rossignol, 1984, unpublished data).

Necatur americanus and various animal *Ancylostoma* spp. cause cutaneous larva migrans. The inflammatory lesion is caused by the immune response to the excretory products of the migrating larvae. Oral thiabendazole has been used to treat larva migrans (Stone and Mullins, 1963), but this type of treatment has been replaced by topical application of thiabendazole in either DMSO or petroleum jelly. Battistini (1969) published a superb paper on this form of treatment and, as Stone says in the article following Battistini's, it is difficult to imagine a more effective, less expensive, and less toxic treatment for this condition. Coulaud *et al.* (1982) reported that 5-day treatment with albendazole *per os* at 400 mg/day was effective in killing the larvae and stopping the pruritis. The cost of the latter treatment must be manyfold higher.

5.4. Dracunculus medinensis Infection

This is a very debilating disease, for which no satisfactory chemotherapy exists. Muller (1979) reviewed the attempts made to affect the course of this disease, which is complicated by the fact that the life cycle of the parasite in man takes one year. Although several established anthelmintics have been used to treat patients with dracontiasis, Muller (1971) believes that any beneficial effect of treatment with thiabendazole, niridazole or metronidazole is due to the anti-inflammatory effect of these drugs, which allows the worms to be withdrawn from the ulcer more easily. This is well illustrated by the results of Sastry *et al.* (1978). These workers treated patients with 50–75 mg thiabendazole per kg and found that in 79% of patients there was a rapid loss of the female *D. medinensis.* Mebendazole also produces an alleviation of clinical signs and allows the worms to be more easily withdrawn. However, it does not appear to have any adverse effect on worms that have not emerged through the skin, as new ulcers with viable worms develop after treatment of patients with patent ulcers.

5.5. Trichinella spiralis Infections

The chemotherapy of *Trichinella* infections has been recently reviewed in detail by Campbell and Denham (1983).

5.5.1. Screening of Anti-Trichinella Compounds

Jenkins and Carrington (1981) described an *in vitro* screen for detecting anti-*Trichinella* activity. Excysted muscle larvae are incubated at 37°C in culture medium, with the test compound added, in plastic culture trays for 4 days. Any abnormality in the larvae as compared with the control cultures indicates some kind of efficacy by the test compound.

Probably the best *in vivo* screen is to infect mice and feed them a diet containing the test compound for the ensuing 28–35 days and to harvest larvae by digestion of the mice 1 week later. This method will detect all known active compounds but is very prodigal of compound. Alternatively compounds could be administered daily by gavage beginning 2 hr after infection and continuing for 5 days. This regimen would select virtually every compound shown to be active (the exception is methyridine, which must be given parenterally and which, although useful in experimental work, has no clinical application).

5.5.2. Clinical Trichinellosis

Trichinella infections are normally acquired on a single, often identified, occasion. It is possible to reduce the intensity of muscle infection by using anthelmintics such as pyrantel (10 mg/kg for 4 days), which affect the adult worms. There is no positive proof that any drug will either sexually sterilize or kill adult *Trichinella* in man, but evidence from experimental infections of rodents suggests that frequent long-term use of several benzimidazole carbamates will sexually sterilize and possibly kill adult worms. Such a compound will also kill developing larvae and encysted larvae. Mebendazole is currently the drug of choice for this purpose (Pawlowski, 1983) and has been widely used for the treatment of human trichinellosis, being more effective and less toxic than the previous drug of choice, thiabendazole. Guidelines now being prepared by the World Health Organization are expected to suggest that mebendazole should be used at dosages higher than the 5.0 mg/kg per day now recommended. Now that albendazole is being used for other infections, it will be interesting to see its effects on human trichinellosis, especially since it is better absorbed than mebendazole and is highly effective against *Trichinella* in mice (McCracken, 1978).

There is little likelihood that a drug would be especially developed for the treatment of trichinellosis. The only hope for improved chemotherapy lies with the exploitation of drugs developed for more general use.

ACKNOWLEDGMENTS. The author is on the External Scientific Staff of the Medical Research Council and wishes to thank Cherie Wright for patiently typing this manuscript several times.

REFERENCES

Abdel-Hamfeed, A. A., 1984, Effect of thiabendazole on the migration of *Toxocara canis* larvae in the mouse, *Parasitol.* 70:226–231.

Abo-Shehada, M. N., and Herbert, I. V., 1984, Anthelmintic effect of levamisole, ivermectin, albendazole and fenbendazole on larval *Toxocara canis* infection in mice, *Res. Vet. Sci.* 36:87–91.

Ambu, S., Kwa, B. H., and Mak, J. W., 1982, Studies on the experimental chemotherapy of *Angiostrongylus malaysiensis* infection in rats with mebendazole and levamisole, *Trans. R. Soc. Trop. Med. Hyg.* 76:458–462.

Anderson, J., and Fuglsang, H., 1976, Ocular onchocerciasis: "At risk" patients and their treatment, *Tropenmed. Parasitol.* 26:13.

Anderson, J., and Fuglsang, H., 1978, Further studies on the treatment of ocular onchocerciasis with diethylcarbamazine and suramin, *Br. J. Ophthalmol.* 62:450–457.

Ash, L. R., and Riley, J. M., 1970, Development of *Brugia pahangi* in the jird, *Meriones unguiculatus*, with notes on infections in other rodents, *J. Parasitol.* 56:962–968.

Awadzi, K., and Gilles, H. M., 1980, The chemotherapy of onchocerciasis. III. Comparative study of diethylcarbamazine (DEC) and metrifonate, *Ann. Trop. Med. Hyg.* 74:199–210.

Aziz, M. A., Diallo, S., Diop, I. M., Larivere, M., and Porta, M., 1982, Efficacy of ivermectin in human onchocerciasis, *Lancet* 2:171–173.

Barrett, J., 1983, Biochemistry of filarial worms, *Helm. Abst. A.* 52:1–18.

Battistini, F., 1969, Treatment of creeping eruption with topical thiabendazole, *Tex. Rep. Biol. Med.* 27:645.

Bekhti, A., 1984, Mebendazole in toxocariasis, (letter), *Ann. Int. Med.* 100:463.

Bianco, A. E., and Denham, D. A., 1984, The action of diethylcarbamazine on the skin-dwelling microfilariae of *Monanema globulosa* (Nematoda: Filarioidae) in rodents, *Tropenmed. Parasitol.* 35:55–57.

Bonnin, H., and Moretti, G. F., 1950, Preuves cliniques et biopsiques de l'action léthale d'un dérivé de la piperazine sur la filaire *Loa loa* adulte, *Bull. Soc. Pathol. Exot.* 43:279–282.

Burren, C. H., 1968, Experimental toxocariasis. II. *Toxocara canis* in the mouse as a system for testing compounds of potential anthelmintic activity, *Z. Parasitaikd.* 30:162–170.

Campbell, W. C., 1982, Efficacy of the avermectins against filarial parasites: A short review, *Vet. Res. Commun.* 5:251–262.

Campbell, W. C., and Denham, D. A., 1983, Chemotherapy, in: *Trichinella and Trichinosis* (W. C. Campbell, ed.), pp. 335–366, Plenum Press, New York.

Ch'en, T. T., 1964, Demonstration of macrofilaricidal action of hetrazan, antimony and arsenic preparations in man, *Chinese Med. J.* 83:625–640.

Copeman, D. B., 1979, An evaluation of the bovine—*Onchocerca gibsoni, Onchocerca gutturosa* model as a tertiary screen for drugs against *Onchocerca volvulus* in man, *Tropenmed. Parasitol.* 30:469–474.

Coulaud, J. P., Binet, D., Voyer, C., Samson, C., Moreau, G., Rossignol, J. F., 1982, Traitement du syndrome de *larva migrans* cutane "Larbish" par l'albendazole, *Bull. Soc. Pathol. Exot.* 75:534–537.

Coulaud, J. P., Larivière, M., Gervais, M. C., Gaxotte, P., Aziz, A., Deluol, A. M., and Cenac, J., 1983, Traitement de l'onchocercose humaine par l'ivermectine, *Bull. Soc. Pathol. Exot.* 76:681–688.

Coulaud, J. P., Larivière, M., Aziz, M. A., Gervais, M. C., Gaxotte, P., Deluol, A. M., and Cenas, J., 1984, Invermectin in onchocerciasis, *Lancet* 1:526–527.

Cuckler, A. C., Egerton, J. R., and Alicata, J. E., 1965, Therapeutic effect of thiabendazole on *Angiostrongylus cantonensis* infection in rats, *J. Parasitol.* 51:392–396.

Denham, D. A., 1979, A review of methods for testing compounds for filaricidal activity, *J. Helminthol.* 53:175–187.

Denham, D. A., 1980, Anthelmintic properties of flubendazole against *Dipetalonema viteae* in jirds, *Trans. R. Soc. Trop. Med. Hyg.* 74:829.

Denham, D. A., 1982a, The effects of some avermectins on the growth of *Brugia pahangi*, *Methods Findings Exp. Clin. Pharmacol.* 4:347–350.

Denham, D. A., 1982b, The methodology of screening for filarial activity using *Brugia pahangi*, in: *Animal Models in Parasitology* (D. Owen, ed.), pp. 93–104, Macmillan, London.

Denham, D. A., and Mellor, P., 1976, The anthelmintic effects of a new compound "E" (Freidheim) on *Onchocerca gutturosa* in the cow—A possible tertiary screening system for drug action against *O. volvulus* in man, *J. Helminthol.* 50:49–52.

Denham, D. A., Suswillo, R. R., and Rogers, R., 1978, Studies with *Brugia pahangi*. 19. Anthelmintic effects of mebendazole, *Trans. R. Soc. Trop. Med. Hyg.* 72:546–647.

Denham, D. A., Samad, R., Cho, S-Y., Suswillo, R. R., and Skippins, S. C., 1979, The anthelmintic effects of flubendazole on *Brugia pahangi, Trans. R. Soc. Trop. Med. Hyg.* 73:673–676.

Denham, D. A., Liron, D. A., and Brandt, E., 1980, The anthelmintic effects of albendazole on *Brugia pahangi, J. Helminthol.* 54:199–200.

Denham, D. A., Brandt, E., and Liron, D. A. 1981, Anthelmintic effects of oxibendazole on *Brugia pahangi*, *J. Parasitol.* 67:123.

Denham, D. A., Suswillo, R, R., and Chusattayanond, W., 1984, Parasitological observations on *Meriones unguiculatus* singly or multiply infected *Brugia pahangi*, *Parasitology* 88:295–301.

Dubey, J. P., 1979, Effect of fenbendazole on *Toxocara canis* larvae in tissues of infected dogs, *Am. J. Vet. Res.* 40:698–699.

Duke, B. O. L., 1962, Experimental transmission of *Onchocerca volvulus* from man to a chimpanzee, *Trans. R. Soc. Trop. Med. Hyg.* 56:271.

Duke, B. O. L., 1964, Studies on loiasis in monkey. IV. Experimental hybridization of the human and simian strains of *Loa*, *Ann. Trop. Med. Parasitol.* 58:390–408.

Duke, B. O. L., 1968, The effect of drugs on *Onchocerca volvulus*. 3. Trials of suramin at different dosages and a comparison of the brands Antrypol, Moramyl and Naganol, *Bull. WHO* 39:157–167.

Duke, B. O. L., 1970, The effects of drugs on *Onchocerca volvulus*. A trial of Malarsonyl potassium. *Bulletin of the World Health Organization* 42:115–117.

Duke, B. O. L., 1977, The effects of some drugs—Pentamidine, Stibocaptate, Hoechst 33258, F151, Compound "E" and Nifurtimox—on *Onchocerca volvulus* in chimpanzees, *Tropenmed. Parasitol.* 28:447–455.

Goodwin, L. G., 1984, Chemotherapy, *Trans. R. Soc. Trop. Med. Hyg. (Suppl.)* 78:1–8.

Hawking, F., and Denham, D. A., 1976, The distribution of human filariasis throughout the world. Part 1. The pacific region; including New Guinea, *Trop. Dis. Bull.* 73:348–373.

Hewitt, R. I., Kushner, S., Stewart, H. W., White, E., Wallace, W. S., and Subbarow, Y., 1947, Experimental chemotherapy of filariasis. III. Effect of 1-diethyl-carbamyl-4-methylpiperazine hydrochloride against naturally acquired filarial infections in cotton rats and dogs, *J. Lab. Clin. Med.* 32:1314–1329.

Holt, P. E., Clarkson, M. J., and Kerslake, M., 1981, Anthelmintic tests on *Toxocaris canis* infection in mice, *Vet. Rec.* 108:308–309.

Ishii, A. I., Terada, M., Kino, H., Hayashi, M., and Sano, M., 1983, Studies on chemotherapy of parasitic helminths: Effects of avermectin Bla on *Angiostrongylus cantonensis* in rats, *Int. J. Parasitol.* 13:491–498.

Jenkins, D. C., and Carrington, T. S., 1981, An *in vitro* screening test for compounds active against the parenteral stages of *Trichinella spiralis*, *Tropenmed. Parasitol.* 32:31–34.

Kliks, M. M., Kroenke, K., and Hardman, J. M., 1982, Eosinophilic radiculomyeloencephalitis: An angiostrongyliasis outbreak in American Samoa related to ingestion of *Achatina fulica* snails, *Am. J. Trop. Med. Hyg.* 31:1114–1122.

McCracken, R. O., 1978, Efficacy of mebendazole and albendazole against *Trichinella spiralis* in mice, *J. Parasitol.* 64:214–219.

Mazzoti, L., 1948, Posibilidad de utilizar como medio diagnostico auxiliar en la oncocercosis, las reacciones allergicas consecutivas a la administracion del "Hetrazan," *Rev. Inst. Sal. Enferm. Trop.* 9:235–237.

Muller, R., 1971, The possible mode of action of some chemotherapeutic agents in guinea worm disease, *Trans. R. Soc. Trop. Med. Hyg.* 65:843–844.

Muller, R., 1979, Guinea worm disease: Epidemiology, control, and treatment, *Bull. WHO* 57:683–689.

Muller, R. L., and Nelson, G. S., 1975, *Ackertia globulosa* sp.n. (Nematoda: Filarioidea) from rodents in Kenya, *J. Parasitol.* 61:606–609.

Narasimham, M. V. V. L., Roychowdhury, S. P., Das, M., and Rao, C. K., 1978, Levamisole and mebendazole in the treatment of Bancroftian infection, *Southeast Asian J. Trop. Med. Publ. Health* 9:571–575.

Nicholas, W. L., and Stewart, A. C., 1979, The action of benzimidazoles on the larval stages of *Toxocara canis* in the mouse, *Ann. Trop. Med. Parasitol.* 73:57–62.

Ottesen, E. A., 1984, The action of diethylcarbamazine on adult worms of the lymphatic-dwelling filariae *Wuchereria bancrofti*, *Brugia malayi* and *Brugia timori* in man, WHO/FIL/84.174 pp. 1–24. (WHO document described as "not formal publication" but can be obtained from Geneva on request.)

Partono, F., 1984, Filariasis in Indonesia: Clinical manifestations and basic concepts of treatment and control. *Trans. R. Soc. Trop. Med. Hygi.* 78:9–12.

Partono, F., Purnomo, and Soewarta, A., 1979, A simple method to control *Brugia timori* by diethylcarbamazine administration, *Trans. R. Soc. Trop. Med. Hyg.* 73:536–542.

Partono, F., Purnomo, Soewarta, A., and Sri Oemijati, 1984, Low dosage diethylcarbamazine administered by villagers for the control of timorian filariasis, *Trans. R. Soc. Trop. Med. Hyg.* 78:370–372.

Pawlowski, Z. S., 1983, Clinical aspects in man, in: *Trichinella and Trichinosis* (W. C. Campbell, ed.), pp. 367–401, Plenum Press, New York.

Rew, R. S., and Saz, J. F., 1977, The carbohydrate metabolism of *Brugia pahangi* micorilariae, *J. Parasitol.* 63:123–129.

Rivas-Alcala, R., Mackenzie, C. D., Gomez-Rojo, E., Greene, B. M., and Taylor, H. R., 1984, The effects of diethylcarbamazine, mebendazole and levamisole on *Onchocerca volvulus in vivo* and *in vitro*, *Tropenmed. Parasitol.* 35:71–77.

Saeed, A. A., Green, P. J., Naoroz, M., Lee, H. A., and Venkat Ramon, G., 1984, *Loa loa*: the use of a blood cell separator to reduce microfilaraemia before specific chemotherapy, *J. Infection* 9:161–166.

Salazar-Mallen, M., Gonzalez-Barranco, D., and Del Carmen Moutes, H., 1971, Quinaoterapia de la oncocercosis con metrifonate, *Rev. Inst. Med. Trop. Sao Paulo* 13:363–368.

Santiago-Stevenson, D., Oliver-Gonzalez, J., and Hewitt, R. I., 1947, Treatment of filariasis *bancrofti* with 1-diethylcarbamazine-4-methylpiperazine hydrochloride ("hetrazan"), *J.A.M.A.* 135:708–712.

Sastry, S. C., Kumar, J. K., and Lakshminarayana, V., 1978, The treatment of drancontiasis with thiabendazole, *J. Trop. Med. Hyg.* 81:32–35.

Shafei, A. Z., 1976, Preliminary report on the therapeutic effect of mebendazole in guinea worm infection, *J. Trop. Med. Hyg.* 79:197–200.

Stone, O. J., and Mullins, J. F., 1963, First use of thiabendazole in creeping eruption, *Tex. Rep. Biol. Med.* 21:422–424.

Suswillo, R. R., and Denham, D. A., 1977, A new system of testing for filaricidal activity using transplanted adult *Brugia* in the jird, *J. Parasitol.* 63:591–592.

Suswillo, R. R., Nelson, G. S., Muller, R., McGreevy, P. B., Duke, B. O. L., and Denham, D. A., 1976, Attempts to infect jirds (*Meriones unguiculatus*) with *Wuchereria bancrofti*, *Onchocerca volvulus*, *Loa loa* and *Mansonella ozzardi*, *J. Helminthol.* 50:132–133.

Thooris, G. C., 1956, Le traitement expérimental de la filariose a *Wuchereria bancrofti* en Oceanie Française par la suramine, *Bull. Soc. Pathol. Exot.* 49:1138–1157.

Wilson, T., 1950, Hetrazan in the treatment of filariasis due to *Wuchereria malayi*, *Trans. R. Soc. Trop. Med. Hyg.* 44:49–66.

14

Nematode Infections of Domestic Animals

Gastrointestinal Infections

SUSAN MARRINER and JAMES ARMOUR

1. PRINCIPLES OF CONTROL

Anthelmintics have been used for many years to treat clinical outbreaks of gastrointestinal (GI) helminthiasis. With the advent of modern drugs that are both broader in spectrum and much less toxic than many of the early compounds, large-scale prophylactic use of anthelmintics has increased enormously. At its simplest, prophylactic use of drugs involves treatment of susceptible animals at intervals frequent enough to prevent accumulation of heavy parasite burdens. This can be expensive and is not ideal, since generally the greater the use of a drug, the more likely it is that resistance to it will arise. In many situations, knowledge of the epidemiology of the disease permits strategic timing of drug treatments which, in combination with certain management practices, makes for a reduction in the number of treatments required. Efficient control programs for grazing cattle and sheep are based on knowledge of seasonal fluctuations of infective (L_3) larval stages on pasture. In temperate countries in the northern hemisphere, sufficient L_3 overwinter on pasture to infect susceptible animals grazing the following spring, culminating in fresh infections and in eggs being deposited in the feces; however, these burdens are seldom sufficient to cause a clinical effect. Most noningested overwintered L_3 die off by late June, and the buildup of pasture L_3 that occurs in midsummer is primarily attributable to hatching of eggs deposited the same year. Thus, the treatment of young cattle with anthelmintics 3 and 6 weeks after commencing spring grazing in April or May will markedly reduce subsequent pasture contamination. If treatment is delayed until July and is combined with removal to pasture not grazed by cattle that year, there will be no need for further treatments until the end of the grazing season.

SUSAN MARRINER • Department of Veterinary Pharmacology, University of Glasgow Veterinary School, Glasgow G61 1QH, Scotland.   JAMES ARMOUR • Department of Veterinary Parasitology, University of Glasgow Veterinary School, Glasgow G61 1QH, Scotland.

Since a high proportion of L_3 stages of certain nematodes, notably *Ostertagia* spp. ingested during autumn become arrested at the fourth larval stage, treatment of susceptible cattle at housing with an agent effective against these stages will prevent type II ostertagiasis, which occurs when the larvae resume their development the following spring.

A refinement of the early-season treatment described above is the incorporation of anthelmintic into a slow-release preparation administered to cattle at the beginning of the grazing system. Continuous release of the drug prevents development of ingested larvae over a prolonged period. One drug, morantel, is available in this form as a slow-release bolus that lodges in the reticulorumen and protects against ingested gut larvae for a period of approximately 90 days. At the end of this time, most remaining overwintered larvae on pasture will have succumbed, leaving the pasture effectively clean for the rest of the grazing season. Success of this system is dependent on all animals being treated at turnout or, if outwintered, before infections acquired early in the year become patent, so that pasture levels of larvae remain low. Treated animals must not be moved onto pasture grazed by untreated animals the same year, as once drug release has ceased they become fully susceptible. Control programs using the same principles but timed to suit the local epidemiology are employed in the temperate southern hemisphere and in many parts of the subtropics. To date there have been very few reports of similar measures being adopted in the tropics.

In sheep the major source of contamination of pasture for the lambs is the enormous rise in fecal egg output by the ewes during the periparturient period. Effective control by anthelmintic treatment of the ewes from 4 weeks before lambing to 8 weeks afterward, followed by a move to safe pastures, greatly reduces the larval challenge to the lambs. Where safe pastures are not available, most farmers resort to regular anthelmintic therapy of the lambs.

A similar relaxation of immunity to nematode infections occurs in sows during the periparturient period; treatment of sows at the time of entry to the farrowing house will do much to reduce the number of infective stages available to the sucking pigs. Treatment of young pigs at the time of removal to the fattening house and again 8 weeks later with 6-monthly treatment of boars provides an effective control program for intensive pig systems. Where pigs are kept at pasture, similar principles of control are adopted as for ruminants, although some species such as *Ascaris suum* are difficult to control because of the longevity of the eggs.

Most control programs in horses consist simply of regular repeated treatments of all grazing animals at 4–6-week intervals with broad-spectrum drugs. Specific treatment of young foals for *Parascaris equorum* and *Strongyloides westeri* may be carried out as well. Where arterial larval stages of *Strongylus vulgaris* are a problem, specific therapy is also indicated, but regular treatment should reduce the requirement for this.

In cats and dogs, control of gastrointestinal nematodes is carried out for esthetic reasons as well as for control of clinical disease. In the case of *Toxocara canis*, prevention of contamination of the environment is an important public health consideration, and young puppies should be treated frequently from the age of 2 weeks to 6 months to prevent ascarid infections from becoming patent.

The advent of drugs such as avermectins, which are highly effective against early larval stages as well as adults and are also extremely persistent, should markedly reduce the frequency of treatment required in many control programs. This high efficacy of the newer compounds together with the potential for limiting pasture contamination by the use of systems such as the morantel bolus over several grazing seasons would appear to offer the potential for almost total control of parasitic gastroenteritis in grazing animals. However, such rigorous control carries inherent risks in that it may seriously impair the development of immunity to the parasite by the host, resulting in a totally susceptible population of animals, with the potential for economic disaster should the control program break down for any reason.

2. ROUTES OF ADMINISTRATION

Anthelmintics for treatment of gastrointestinal nematode infections may be given parenterally, topically, orally, or by intraruminal injection. A wide variety of oral formulations are in use for many drugs, including tablets, drenches, gels, pastes, granules, and powders for inclusion in feed or water. There has been considerable interest in prolonged-release formulations of anthelmintics to provide continuous long-term prophylactic control, but only morantel is commercially available in this form as an intraruminal bolus.

Parenteral administration by injection, or oral administration by tablet, drench, or paste is an accurate way of ensuring adequate dosage of drug for each individual in all species. In companion animals fed individually, in-feed administration is also satisfactory.

In intensive pig and poultry systems, in-feed or in-water medication is the most practical means of administration; it is usually satisfactory, as treatment under modern systems of management is aimed at the removal of subclinical infections in order to enhance productivity, rather than at controlling frank disease. In cattle and sheep, however, it is impossible to ensure adequate intake of drug by all members of a group on in-feed or in-water medication; although this method is convenient from the point of view of reduced handling requirements, it cannot be regarded as satisfactory, especially in the face of clinical disease, where appetite is commonly depressed. Incorporation of anthelmintics into feedblocks for treatment of grazing animals being given supplementary feeding is also practiced. The benzimidazole and probenzimidazole drugs particularly lend themselves to this form of administration, since they are known to have increased efficacy, especially against inhibited larval stages and other problem parasites when given in divided-dose regimens (Prichard et al., 1978). However, there remains the problem of individual variation in uptake, with some animals taking excessive amounts of drug and others a subtherapeutic dose (Bogan and Marriner, 1983). This is wasteful of anthelmintic on the one hand and likely to lead to the emergence of resistant strains of nematodes on the other.

One consideration regarding the oral drenching of ruminants that has received considerable attention is the possibility of closure of the reticular (esophageal) groove, leading to a varying proportion of the drench bypassing the rumen and being delivered directly to the omasum/abomasum. Ruminal bypass with drenches such as levamisole is unimportant in terms of efficacy, as this drug acts rapidly on the nematode, and it is the maximum concentration to which the worms are exposed rather than the period of exposure that is important. With the benzimidazoles, however, it would appear that activity increases with duration of exposure of the parasites to a threshold concentration of drug. Delivery of the modern highly insoluble compounds directly to the abomasum results in reduced dissolution and uptake of the drugs into the systemic compartment and a reduced period of exposure of lumen-dwelling parasites to dissolved drug in the GI fluid, the reservoir effect of the rumen being lost. Closure of the groove and ruminal bypass has been widely regarded as a possible explanation for the occasionally variable activity of fenbendazole against inhibited larval stages of *Ostertagia ostertagi* in cattle (Duncan *et al.*, 1977). To circumvent the possibility of ruminal bypass, one of the modern benzimidazole drugs, oxfendazole, has recently been marketed as an intra-ruminal preparation for delivery by a special gun.

Levamisole is currently the only anthelmintic available as a topical preparation for pour-on application along the back of cattle only. The efficacy of levamisole against gastrointestinal nematodes when given by the pour-on route is good but is not as good as when given by the oral or subcutaneous route. This probably reflects the much lower blood concentrations measured after topical treatment (Forsyth *et al.*, 1983; S. E. Marriner and J. A. Bogan, unpublished observations). Forsyth *et al.* (1983) further suggest that anthelmintic uptake and efficacy vary considerably according to the climatic conditions at the time of application, making the pour-on route less reliable than conventional routes.

3. TESTING OF ANTHELMINTIC DRUGS

Initial screening of compounds for anthelmintic activity is usually carried out in laboratory species, principally rats and mice, for reasons of cost and convenience and also because usually only very small quantities of such compounds are synthesized. *Nippostrongylus* spp. infections in the rat, *Nematospiroides dubius* and *Syphacia obvelata* in the mouse, and *Ascaridia* spp. in chickens are common screens for efficacy against gastrointestinal parasites. *In vitro* screening tests have been developed. Early attempts used free-living stages of trichostrongylids (Tiner, 1958) and, more recently and more usefully, *in vitro* culture systems of parasitic stages of trichostrongyloids, have been utilized (Jenkins *et al.*, 1980). Systems using entirely free-living nematodes have also been described (Simpkin and Coles, 1981). Many compounds showing activity against free-living nematodes, however, have little effect on parasitic species, and some active compounds are only detected by such a screen at extremely high concentrations (Jenkins, 1982). One further problem with *in vitro* screens is that prodrugs, which are themselves inactive but which are metabolized to active metabolites in the host, may possibly be missed. Unless the metabolic pathway is similar in rodents and in the target species, prodrugs may also be missed in the rodent screens. Drugs warranting further investigation after preliminary screening are then evaluated in the target species using a number of tests. For further information on assay methods, see Coles (1984).

3.1. Critical Tests

Critical testing involves collection and counting of all worms passed in the feces of infected animals for a period of days after treatment with the anthelmintic. The animal is then either slaughtered and all remaining worms counted or, less commonly, may be treated with an anthelmintic drug of proven efficacy and further worm expulsion noted.

Efficacy in terms of percentage of total worms expelled can then be calculated. It is advisable to collect feces from untreated control animals at the same time, as worm expulsion can occur for reasons other than anthelmintic treatment. Critical tests are extremely time consuming and are really only applicable for parsites of the small and large intestine, since parasites passing the whole length of the intestinal tract tend to be digested and therefore missed.

3.2. Controlled Tests

In controlled testing, two groups of animals are similarly infected. One group is then treated with the test drug, while the other group is left untreated. After a suitable interval, both are killed, the worms are counted, and the percentage efficacy is calculated from the difference in burdens of treated and control animals. If single inoculations of infective larvae are used rather than trickle infections or naturally acquired infections, the time of treatment can be varied in order to assess anthelmintic activity against different larval stages. Killing is carried out after sufficient time has elapsed for surviving larvae to become adult. Controlled tests are preferred to other tests.

3.3. Fecal Egg Counts

Fecal egg counts of infected animals both before and after treatment have been widely used as an indicator of anthelmintic efficacy. Their value in the testing of new drugs is limited for the following reasons: (1) drugs may suppress egg production by the worms without killing them, (2) they give no information about the effect of the drug on immature stages, and (3) fecal egg counts are not a reliable indicator of the size of worm burden. They are of greater value in assessing the value of the drug in field outbreaks of parasitic disease.

3.4. Tests for Arrested Larvae

For anthelmintics to be evaluated against arrested larval stages, testing must be carried out under conditions that favor the arrest of a high percentage of ingested larvae. This may be done using naturally acquired infections at a specific time of year or using experimental infections where the infective stage has been exposed artificially to conditions likely to cause arrested larval development in the host.

3.5. Tests for Ovicidal Activity

Ovicidal activity may be evaluated *in vitro* by the egg-hatch test as described by Coles and Simpkin (1977). Nematode eggs from fresh (within 4 hours of leaving the host) fecal samples are incubated *in vitro* in contact with the drug. The percentage of eggs embryonating in the presence of the drug is compared with that of controls (no drug). Final demonstration, however, must be made by assessing the potential infectivity of eggs passed by treated animals, as some drugs (e.g., oxfendazole) are ovicidal in animal studies but not in the *in vitro* test. Once a drug has been evaluated by controlled studies in both artificial and naturally acquired infections, the optimum dosage regimen decided, and basic toxicological testing done, it is then evaluated in the field in outbreaks of disease and in control programs.

4. DRUGS IN CURRENT USE

The drugs in current use can be classified as either broad spectrum or narrow spectrum. Broad-spectrum drugs include the benzimidazoles, imidothiazoles, tetrahydropyrimidines, organophosphorus compounds, avermectins, and nitroscanate. Narrow-spectrum anthelmintics include piperazine and compounds such as disophenol and closantel, which are occasionally used to treat specific gastrointestinal nematodes. These drugs are considered for use in each species according to their chemical groupings and their efficiency summarized in tabular form. Anthelmintic efficacy has been graded (Tables I–VI) in a manner similar to that proposed by Armour (1982).

4.1. Broad-Spectrum Drugs

4.1.1. Benzimidazoles

A number of different benzimidazoles are currently marketed: thiabendazole, cambendazole, oxibendazole, mebendazole, flubendazole, fenbendazole, albendazole, and oxfendazole. In addition, the anthelmintic activity of febantel and thiophanate results from the formation of benzimidazoles (in the case of febantel, these are fenbendazole and oxfendazole) by *in vivo* hepatic metabolism; they are commonly referred to as probenzimidazoles. The benzimidazole group of drugs has wide application in all species. They are probably the least toxic of all the anthelmintics; it has been impossible to find an LD_{50} for thiabendazole and fenbendazole. Five members of the group have been found to be teratogenic—cambendazole, mebendazole, parbendazole, oxfendazole, and albendazole—limiting their use in pregnant animals. Withdrawal periods for the benzimidazoles vary considerably from zero for both meat and milk in the case of thiabendazole up to 5 days for milk and up to 28 days for meat in the case of some of the other derivatives, with parbendazole and cambendazole not recommended for use in lactating cattle.

Table 1. Benzimidazoles Used in Cattle[a]

| Drug (formulation) | Efficiency | | | Dose rate (mg/kg) |
| | Adults | Larvae | | |
		Developing	Arrested	
Thiabendazole (in feed, drench, paste)	A	B	O	66–110
Parbendazole (drench)	A	B	O	20–30
Oxibendazole (drench)	A	B	O	10
Cambendazole (paste)	A	B	O	25
Fenbendazole (drench, in feed)	A	A	A/B	7.5
Oxfendazole (drench, intraruminal injection)	A	A	A/B	4.5
Albendazole (drench)	A	A	A/B	7.5
Febantel (drench)	A	A	A/B	7.5 (increase for arrested larvae)
Thiophanate (drench, in feed)	A	A	B	66–132 (divided doses for arrested larvae)

[a] A, >90% efficacy; B, 75–90% efficacy; C, 50–75% efficacy; D, less than 50% efficacy; O, no activity.

4.1.1a. Cattle. The activity of the benzimidazoles currently used against the common gastrointestinal nematodes of cattle is shown in Table I. Thiabendazole displays good activity against adult worms, is less effective against immature stages, and in conventional usage has no activity against arrested larval stages. Subsequently developed members of the group, such as parbendazole, cambendazole, and oxibendazole, have similar activity to that of thiabendazole but require lower dose rates. They also have better activity against ascarids and, in the case of mebendazole and cambendazole, against lungworms and cestodes. The most recently developed members of the group—fenbendazole, oxfendazole, and albendazole—have an extended spectrum of activity that is highly effective against adult, immature, and arrested larval stages of important nematodes and also show activity against cestodes and trematodes. Febantel and thiophanate also have good activity against adult and developing larval stages but must be given at a higher dose rate (febantel) or be divided dose over 5 days (thiophanate) to ensure good activity against arrested larvae. All the benzimidazoles and probenzimidazoles are ovicidal.

It has been suggested that the greater potency and spectrum of activity of the most recently developed compounds is a function of their pharmacokinetic behavior rather than of intrinsic differences in activity. Because they are much less soluble than earlier members of the group, their dissolution rate, passage along the GI tract, and absorption into the systemic circulation are markedly slowed compared with that of thiabendazole. Maximum plasma concentrations of fenbendazole and oxfendazole occur between 24 and 36 hr after oral dosing in sheep (Marriner and Bogan, 1981a,b) and cattle (Prichard *et al.*, 1978; Ngomuo *et al.*, 1984), and measurable concentrations in plasma and in abomasal fluid persist for up to 5 days after a single dose. By contrast, thiabendazole reaches maximum plasma concentrations by 5 hr and is rapidly excreted over 48–72 hr (Tocco *et al.*, 1964). There is some evidence that if concentrations of thiabendazole in the gut and in the plasma are maintained by continuous infusion or repeated administration, albeit at very high dose rates, this drug will remove arrested larvae of *Ostertagia ostertagi* in cattle (Prichard *et al.*, 1978). It is as yet uncertain whether it is plasma concentrations or concentrations of drug in the GI fluid that are most important for efficacy against gastrointestinal nematodes. During the first month of pregnancy, care should be taken not to exceed the manufacturer's recommended dose rate of albendazole or oxfendazole; otherwise, the benzimidazoles are of very low topicity.

4.1.1b. Sheep. The activity of the benzimidazoles against common gastrointestinal helminths of sheep is shown in Table II. Activity of the different compounds is similar to that found in cattle, except that arrested larvae in sheep are more susceptible than those in cattle to thiabendazole, and a doubling of the dose rate gives good efficacy against these stages. *Nematodirus battus* infection in lambs also requires an increase in dose rate for thiabendazole, thiophanate, and parbendazole. Sheep are more sensitive than cattle to the teratogenicity of the benzimidazoles; parbendazole and cambendazole are not recommended for use during the first month of pregnancy, and recommended dose rates for oxfendazole and albendazole should not be exceeded.

Table II. Benzimidazoles Used in Sheep[a]

Drug (formulation)	Adults	Efficiency Larvae Developing	Arrested	Dose rate (mg/kg)
Thiabendazole (drench, in feed)	A	A/C	A/C	44 (88 for *N. battus* and arrested larvae)
Mebendazole (drench)	A	A/C	?[b]	15
Parbendazole (drench, in feed)	A	A/C	?	20
Oxibendazole (drench)	A	A/C	?	10
Cambendazole (paste)	A	A/B	?	20
Fenbendazole (drench, in feed)	A	A	A	5
Oxfendazole (drench, paste)	A	A	A	5
Albendazole (drench, in feed)	A	A	A	5
Febantel (drench)	A	A/B	A/B	5
Thiophanate (drench, in feed, feed blocks)	A	A/B	A/B	50

[a] See Table I for abbreviations.
[b] ?, Very few data available.

Table III. Anthelmintics Used for Pigs[a]

Drug	Ascaris suum adults/larvae	Hyostrongylus rubidus adults/larvae	Trichuris suis adults/larvae	Oesophagostomum spp. adults/larvae	Dose rate (mg/kg) (in feed unless stated)
Thiabendazole	D/D	A/C	D/D	A/C	50
Parbendazole	A/D	A/D	B/?	A/D	32
Cambendazole	A/B	A/C	D/D	A/C	20
Fenbendazole	A/B	A/A	A/D	A/B	5 (single feed or over 5–16 days)
Flubendazole	A/B	A/A	A/D	A/B	4 (single feed or over 10 days)
Febantel	A/C	A/C	A/D	A/C	32 (ppm in feed over 5 days)
Thiophanate	A/C	A/B	A/B	A/B	67 (single feed or over 14 days)
Dichlorvos	A/D	A/D	A/A	A/D	10–40
Tetramisole	A/B	A/C	B/B	B/B	15
Levamisole	A/A	A/B	B/B	B/B	7.5 (sc)
Ivermectin	A/A	A/A	?[b]	B/B	0.3 (sc)

[a]See Table I for abbreviations.
[b]?, very few data available.

4.1.1c. Pigs. Table III shows the activity of the drugs used in pigs, as well as their activity against the common gut nematodes. As in ruminants, the more recent benzimidazoles have a broader spectrum of activity than the earlier ones but, unlike the situation in ruminants, none is uniformly effective against adult and larval stages of all the common parasites in the pig. Flubendazole and fenbendazole are probably the most widely effective. Most of the compounds may be administered as a single dose in feed or as divided doses in feed over 5–14 days. Divided-dose regimens are generally more effective than single doses. None of the drugs is particularly active against *Strongyloides ransomi*. Several of the benzimidazoles have good activity against early stages of *Trichinella spiralis*. Flubendazole has recently been shown to eliminate intestinal or migratory stages in experimental infections in pigs when given at 32 ppm in feed for 14 days. Higher doses, at 125 ppm, are effective against encysted larvae (Thienpont and Vanparijs, 1980), and several other modern derivatives have shown activity against tissue stages of experimental infections in rats and mice.

4.1.1d. Horses. Benzimidazoles used in the horse, with details of their activity, are shown in Table IV. Derivatives for use in this species are formulated as pastes or as granules for in-feed administration. Most are active against adult and intestinal larval stages of large and small strongyles and mature *Oxyuris* spp. in the large intestine. Activity against nematodes of the small intestine, *Parascaris equorum* and *Strongyloides*

Table IV. Anthelmintics Used in Horses[a]

Drug (formulation)	P. equorum	Efficiency/Strongyles				Oxyuris equi	Dose rate
		S. vulgaris	S. edentatus	Small			
Thiabendazole (powder, in feed, paste)	C/D	A	A	A		A	44–50 × 2 for ascarids
Mebendazole (paste, granules)	A	A	B	B		A	8.8
Oxibendazole (paste)	A	A	A	A		A	10
Cambendazole (paste)	A	A	A	A		A	20
Fenbendazole (granules, suspension)	A	A	A	A		A	5 × 2 for ascarids
Oxfendazole (paste, granules)	A	A	A	A		A	10
Febantel (paste)	A	A	A	A		A	6
Pyrantel embonate (paste, granules)	A	A	B/C	A		C	19 (equivalent to 6.6 free base)
Dichlorvos (resin, pellets)	A	A	B	A/B		A	35
Metriphonate (paste)	A	O	O	O		A	35
Ivermectin (paste)	A	A	A	A		A	0.2
Piperazine (powder)	A	C/D	D	A		D	88 (free base)

[a]See Table I for abbreviations.

westeri, is more variable. Thiabendazole must be given at least twice the strongyle dose rate for activity against *P. equorum,* and fenbendazole must be given at seven times the dose rate for good activity against *S. westeri.* Mebendazole, oxfendazole, and febantel are poorly effective against this parasite. Cambendazole is effective against both *S. westeri* and *P. equorum,* although not licensed for use in horses in many countries. Only cambendazole and oxfendazole appear to be particularly effective against *Trichostrongylus axei* in the horse.

Migratory stages of large and small strongyles (cyathostomes) are much less susceptible to the older benzimidazoles than are adults; only oxfendazole, used as a single treatment at the recommended dose, has good efficacy (Kingsbury and Reid, 1981). Fenbendazole, at increased dose rates or alternatively at recommended dose rates daily for 5 days, also gives good control over tissue stages, and experimentally albendazole has been shown effective against *S. vulgaris* larvae in the cranial mesenteric artery (Georgi *et al.,* 1980). Toxicity of these drugs is low, with the exception of albendazole at very high doses, 25 mg/kg three times daily for 5 days, has been reported as being fatal (Georgi *et al.*, 1980). Cambendazole should be avoided during the first trimester of pregnancy. Palatability of the benzimidazoles is generally good.

4.1.1e. Dogs and Cats. Single-dose administration of benzimidazoles is poorly effective against the common gut nematodes of these species. This is probably related to the lower water content of digesta compared with that of herbivores, resulting in very limited dissolution and therefore bioavailability. By contrast, divided-dose administration is highly effective. Mebendazole and fenbendazole are both licenced for use in dogs and cats and are effective against the intestinal stages of *Toxocara* spp., *Toxascaris* spp., *Trichuris vulpis, Uncinaria stenocephala,* and *Ancylostoma caninum.* Mebendazole is administered as tablets at a dose rate of 6–50 mg/kg (2 days for ascarids only), and fenbendazole is given at 20 mg/kg per day for 5 days.

Prenatal infection of pups with *T. canis* can be prevented by treating pregnant bitches with fenbendazole at a dose rate of 50 mg/kg per day for the last 22–27 days of pregnancy. Infection *via* the milk can also be reduced by continuation of treatment for 12–18 days postwhelping. Such a regimen is highly expensive and, since *T. canis* eggs in the environment are widespread and extremely resistant to desiccation, it is questionable whether this is preferable to control of the intestinal stages in the pup. More recently, it has been shown that extremely high doses—150 mg/kg per day for 3 days—of fenbendazole or albendazole before mating can almost eliminate *T. canis* larvae from all tissues except the brain (Lloyd and Soulsby, 1983). Caution should be exercised, however, in using albendazole at this high dose rate.

4.1.1f. Poultry. Thiabendazole, mebendazole, and cambendazole have been used for the treatment of *Ascaridia, Heterakis,* and *Capillaria* infections of turkeys and chickens. Thiabendazole at 0.1% in feed for 3 days is effective against adult and immature *Ascaridia,* as is cambendazole at a single dose of 30 mg/kg and mebendazole in feed at 60 ppm for 7 days. Mebendazole and cambendazole are also effective against adult *Heterakis* infections. Higher doses (70–100 mg/kg) of cambendazole are effective against *Capillaria* spp.; thiabendazole is much less effective against this parasite. A temporary fall in host egg production may follow treatment with benzimidazoles.

4.1.2. Imidothiazoles

The two compounds in this chemical grouping that are used as anthelmintics are tetramisole and levamisole. Tetramisole is a racemic mixture of D and L forms, and levamisole is the L form. Since anthelmintic potency resides in the L form and toxicity resides equally in both, levamisole is used at one-half the dose rate of tetramisole and is therefore safer. The therapeutic index of these compounds is relatively low, especially in horses (Clarkson and Beg, 1971) and in dogs and cats, and their use for gastrointestinal nematode infections is restricted to ruminants, pigs, and poultry. Many levamisole preparations have a contraindication to concurrent use with organophosphorus compounds, as levamisole has some anticholinesterase activity. Recently, it has been recog-

Table V. Nonbenzimidazole Anthelmintics Used in Cattle[a]

Drug (formulation)	Adults	Efficiency Larvae Developing	Arrested	Dose rate (mg/kg)
Levamisole (subcutaneous injection drench, in feed, in water, pour-on)	A	A	D	7.5
Morantel (drench, slow-release bolus)	A	B	D	13.5 g free base to release 90 mg/day for at least 60 days
Ivermectin (subcutaneous injection)	A	A	A	0.2
Crufomate (in feed)	A/B	C	O	40 or 17/day for 3 days
Coumaphos (in feed, drench)	A/B	C	O	15 or 2/day for 6 days
Metriphonate (drench, subcutaneous injection)	A/B	C	O	60–80

[a]See Table I for abbreviations.

nized that levamisole does not lower the therapeutic index of organophosphates (Hsu, 1980). The withdrawal period for levamisole is 24 hr for milk and 3 (cattle and sheep) to 5 days for meat (pigs).

4.1.2a. Cattle. The activity of levamisole is shown in Table V. The drug has good activity against adult and developing larval stages but not against arrested larvae. Incontrast to the benzimidazoles, it is not ovicidal. Levamisole is nonteratogenic and is safe for use in pregnant animals. Although the therapeutic index is lower than that of many other anthelmintics, toxicity is rarely seen. When it does occur, it is caused by a stimulant effect on ganglia and is manifested by salivation, bradycardia, muscular tremors, and, in the extreme case, death from respiratory failure. In-feed, drench, subcutaneous injection, and pour-on formulations are available.

4.1.2b. Sheep. The anthelmintic activity of levamisole in sheep is similar to that in cattle, although the drug has activity against many arrested fourth-stage larvae in this species. Toxicity has been seen in lambs, and dosages should be calculated carefully, especially with subcutaneous injection, which gives higher blood concentrations than does drenching. Details of levamisole and other nonbenzimidazoles are given in Table VI.

4.1.2c. Pigs. Injectable formulations of levamisole may be used in pigs and are probably the drug of choice in clinical parasitism, where appetite may be depressed. In-feed preparations are available for administration in a single feed. Levamisole has good activity against *Ascaris suum, Hyostrongylus rubidus, Oesophagostomum* spp. and *Strong-*

Table VI. Nonbenzimidazoles Used in Sheep

| | | Efficiency | | |
| | | | Larvae | |
Drug (formulation)	Adults	Developing	Arrested	Dose rate (mg/kg)
Levamisole (subcutaneous injection, drench, in feed)	A	A/B	A/B	7.5
Morantel tartrate (drench)	A	B	?[b]	10
Ivermectin (drench)	A	A	A	0.2

[a]See Table I for abbreviations.
[b]?, few data are available.

yloides ransomi. Activity against *Trichuris suis* is variable (Table IV). It is also effective against the acanthocephalan, *Macrocanthorynchus hirudinaceus.*

4.1.2d. Poultry. Levamisole is effective in poultry against mature and immature *Ascaridia, Capillaria,* and *Heterakis* spp. at a dose rate of 25 mg/kg. The drug is given in the drinking water. In contrast to other species, levamisole appears to be very safe in poultry, although a minor drop in egg production may occur in laying birds. The withdrawal period is 3 days for eggs and meat.

4.1.3. Tetrahydropyrimidines

Pyrantel and its methyl analogue, morantel, are the two members of this group that are currently available. A further derivative, oxantel, has been investigated experimentally. The drugs are administered by the oral route to cattle, sheep, pigs, and horses as the tartrate or embonate (pamoate) salts. Morantel is more potent than pyrantel, requiring a lower dose rate; it also has a higher LD_{50}. Neither drug is particularly toxic, however, and can be used in pregnant as well as young animals. Toxicity results from nicotinic effects on ganglia.

4.1.3a. Cattle. Pyrantel and morantel have high efficacy against adult stages of gut nematodes but are less active against larval stages and have minimal activity against arrested larvae. They are not ovicidal. In many countries, the only available preparation is the slow-release morantel tartrate bolus. A single bolus, delivered by special balling gun, is designed to remain in the rumen and to release the drug at the rate of 90 mg/kg (base) daily for at least 60 days.

4.1.3b. Sheep. Activity in sheep is similar to that in cattle, although greater efficacy has been found against some immatures, and efficacy against all stages of *Nematodirus* is high. Table VI gives details.

4.1.3c. Pigs. Pyrantel and morantel are highly effective against adult *Ascaris* and *Oesophagostomum* and *Hyostrongylus* when given as a single dose in feed. Activity against *Trichuris* and *Strongyloides* is lacking. Pyrantel has been used as continuous low-level prophylaxis for ascarid infection in young pigs. Experimentally, oxantel has been shown to have good activity against *Trichuris* but little activity against other gut nematodes (Robinson, 1979).

4.1.3d. Horses. The activity of pyrantel against common gut nematodes in the horse is shown in Table IV. Activity against adult *S. vulgaris, S. equinus,* the small strongyles or cyathostomes and ascarids is very high; against *S. edentatus* slightly lower; and against *Oxyuris* variable. As in cattle, larval mucosal stages are relatively unsusceptible to pyrantel. In horses, the embonate (pamoate) salt is used: because it has lower solubility than the tartrate, it remains in higher concentration in the more distal regions of the gut, thereby providing activity against worms in the large intestine. Pyrantel is formulated as a paste and as granules for in-feed administration; it is a safe, effective drug for use in most equine parasite-control programs, especially where benzimidazole-resistant strains have been reported.

4.1.4. Organophosphates

A wide variety of organophosphorus compounds have been examined for anthelmintic activity, and several have been marketed for use. They are only available, however, in a limited number of countries. In general, they are not as widely effective as other broad-spectrum drugs, especially in ruminants, and they have largely been superseded. Organophosphorus compounds also tend to have a lower therapeutic index than that of other broad-spectrum drugs, toxicity being attributable to inhibition of cholinesterase with typical cholinergic signs—salivation, myosis, diarrhea, muscle fasciculations, and respiratory embarrassment. Severe toxic signs should be treated by atropine administration.

4.1.4a. Cattle. Haloxon, trichlorphon, coumaphos, and crufomate are the common organophosphorus compounds used in cattle. They have good activity against adult *Haemonchus* and *Cooperia* spp. but tend to be less effective against *Ostertagia, Trichostrongylus,* and *Oesophagostomum* spp. Activity against immatures is much lower. Rapidly metabolized organophosphates such as coumaphos have a zero milk withdrawal period and may be used for the treatment of lactating cattle.

4.1.4b. Sheep. Activity of the organophosphorus compounds in sheep is similar to that in cattle, but the therapeutic index is low in sheep. Haloxon is probably the safest of the compounds mentioned.

4.1.4c. Pigs. Dichlorvos is the only organophosphorus compound widely used in pigs. The active compound is incorporated into a polyvinyl chloride (PVC) resin pellet, which acts as a slow-release carrier. Drug diffuses out of the carrier during its passage through the GI tract, markedly increasing the safety of the compound. Efficacy against adult worms is high but is less good against larvae. Dichlorvos is one of the most useful drugs for the treatment of *Trichuris suis* infection.

4.1.4d. Horses. Dichlorvos and metriphonate (trichlorphon) are the two organophosphorus compounds used in horses. Dichlorvos resin pellets are used in feed for broad-spectrum activity against adult stages of strongyles ascarids and oxyurids. Palatability is low, limiting its use. Metriphonate is used against bots in the stomach and, although it has good activity against ascarids and oxyurids, is not used for specific treatment of these parasites. A paste formulation is used that can cause local irritation of the oral mucosa. This drug is not recommended for use during the first 4 months or the last month of gestation.

4.1.4e. Poultry. Organophosphorus compounds are occasionally used in poultry for treatment of *Capillaria* infections. In-feed coumaphos, 0.004% for 10–14 days or haloxon, 25 mg/kg, in 1 day's food is effective. Poultry are occasinally poisoned by ingestion of dichlorvos resin pellets passed in the feces of horses. The pellets accumulate in the gizzard, resulting in high blood concentrations and toxicity.

4.1.5. Avermectins

Ivermectin is the only avermectin derivative so far available. It has a very broad spectrum of activity against nematodes and is a highly potent compound, being active at dose rates measured in micrograms. Ivermectin appears to be highly effective against adult and larval stages of most of the gastrointestinal nematodes so far tested against, although it is not ovicidal. Formulations for cattle, sheep, pigs, and horses are available as paste, drench, or injection. The efficacy and safety of ivermectin have been reviewed by Campbell and Benz (1984). The withdrawal period of ivermectin is lengthy, at 21–28 days for meat, and it is not used in lactating dairy cattle.

4.1.5a. Cattle. The activity of ivermectin against gastrointestinal nematodes of cattle is shown in Table V. In this species, the route of administration is subcutaneous injection. The compound is extremely persistent in tissues. Limited studies so far suggest that it protects against the development of at least some genera of infective larvae for a period of approximately 2 weeks (Barth, 1983; Bremner *et al.*, 1983), as well as being highly effective against adults, immatures, and arrested larvae at the time of administration. The toxicity of ivermectin *per se* is low, although a few adverse reactions have been seen in animals treated when large numbers of larvae of *Hypoderma* spp. have been present in the esophageal wall or spinal canal. It is safe for use in pregnant animals.

4.1.5b. Sheep. A drench formulation of ivermectin is available for sheep, the efficacy of which is similar to that seen in cattle (Table V). Transient coughing has been seen after drenching, but otherwise toxicity is low.

4.1.5c. Pigs. Subcutaneous injection of ivermectin at a slightly higher dose rate than is used for other species is recommended in pigs. Although few studies have been published, it would appear that ivermectin is highly effective against *Ascaris suum* and *Strongyloides ransomi* including somatic third stage larvae in the pregnant animal (Barth and Preston, 1985) but that activity against *Oesophagostomum* spp. and *Trichuris suis* is more variable (Stewart *et al.*, 1981; Schillhorn van Veen and Gibson, 1983). Stewart *et al.* (1981) suggest that an interval longer than the 14-day treatment-slaughter used by them may have resulted in increased efficacy against these parasites. Campbell and Benz (1984) report that the drug is highly effective against the intestinal stages of *T. spiralis.*

4.1.5d. Horses. Ivermectin was marketed for horses as an intramuscular injection or paste formulation. However, some injection site reactions have occurred with the parenteral formulation, a few of which have become infected with clostridial bacteria and have been fatal, and a small number of sudden deaths have been reported immediately after injection. As a result, the injectable formulation has been withdrawn in most countries and the well-tolerated oral preparation is recommended.

Efficacy against all common gastrointestinal nematodes is high with both formulations (Torbert *et al.*, 1982), although fecal egg counts would appear to be depressed for slightly longer periods with the parenteral treatment (French *et al.*, 1983). Ivermectin is highly effective against 7-day migratory stages of fourth-stage larvae of *S. vulgaris* (Slocombe and McCraw, 1980). High efficacy against later larval stages has also been shown in some studies (Slocombe *et al.*, 1982) and lower efficacy in others (Klei and Torbert, 1980; DiPietro *et al.*, 1982). It is also reported effective against tissue larval stages of the small strongyles, but whether this includes larval stages, arrested at the third stage, is uncertain because of the limitations of the techniques used to evaluate efficacy against this stage (J. L. Duncan, personal communication). It would appear that the time of necropsy after treatment may be important in obtaining true efficacy figures with ivermectin, since the drug requires periods of greater than 2 weeks to exert its killing effect on these larvae.

4.1.5e. Dogs and Cats. Commercial preparations are not available for these species, although experimental work suggests that efficacy in dogs is high (Yazwinski *et al.*, 1982).

4.1.6. Nitroscanate

This compound is used exclusively in dogs for the treatment of gastrointestinal nematodes and cestodes. Boray *et al.* (1979) showed it to be highly effective against hookworms but ineffective against *Trichuris vulpis.* Activity against ascarids is also high at the recommended dose rate of 50 mg/kg. The drug consists of micronized particles in tablet form.

4.2. Narrow-Spectrum Drugs

4.2.1. Piperazine

Piperazine is used almost exclusively for the treatment of ascarid infections in young pigs, horses, dogs, cats, and poultry. It is frequently combined with other drugs such as thiabendazole to improve their activity against ascarids. It is not active against migratory stages. In all species, salts such as citrate or adipate are formulated as tablets or powders and administered in feed or by stomach tube. The drug is well tolerated even by very young animals.

4.2.1a. Pigs. In addition to activity against adult ascarids, piperazine has activity against adult *Oesophagostomum* spp. in pigs. It is usually given as the citrate in 1 day's feed.

4.2.1b. Horses. Piperazine has good activity against adult small strongyles and some activity against large strongyles (Table IV). It is usually given by stomach tube, as the dose is large.

4.2.1c. Cats and Dogs. All the common ascarids are susceptible to piperazine, which is usually given in tablet form to cats and dogs.

4.2.1d. Poultry. Ascaridia spp. in poultry may be controlled by 0.2–0.4% piperazine in feed or 0.1–0.2% in water consumed over a period of a few hours. Alternatively, 50–100 mg per bird is effective. *Heterakis* spp. are not susceptible to piperazine.

4.2.2. Closantel

This salicylanilide is an effective flukicide, with activity also against certain blood-sucking nematodes, including *Haemonchus contortus* in sheep (Hall *et al.*, 1980), and against large strongyles, including migrating *S. vulgaris* larvae in horses (Guerrero *et al.*, 1983). The reason for its lack of activity against non-blood-sucking nematodes is attributed to the fact that closantel binds very strongly to plasma proteins and that only blood feeders apparently take up sufficient drug for activity. Not only is it very effective against adult and immature species of *H. contortus* at the time of administration but, because of its long persistence in the body bound to plasma proteins, it protects against development of ingested larvae for at least 30 days after treatment at a dose rate of 10 mg/kg intraruminally (Hall *et al.*, 1981).

4.2.3. Disophenol

This compound is effective against mature *H. contortus*. Prevention of the establishment of mature worm burdens can be achieved by subcutaneous injection at a dose rate of 10 mg/kg. Recent reports of 30–60 days protection (Hall *et al.*, 1981) are somewhat shorter than earlier claims of 6 months (Gordon, 1974). Disophenol has also been used in dogs and cats for the treatment of hookworm infections at dose rates similar to those in sheep.

REFERENCES

Armour, J., 1983, Modern anthelmintics for farm animals, in: *Pharmacological Basis of Large Animal Medicine* (J. A. Bogan, P. Lees, and A. T. Yoxall, eds.), pp. 174–200, Blackwell Scientific Publications, London.

Barth, D., 1983, Persistent anthelmintic effect of ivermectin in cattle, *Vet. Rec.* 113:300.

Barth, D., and Preston, J. M., 1985, Efficacy of ivermectin against somatic *Strongyloides ransomi* larvae, *Vet. Rec.* 116:366–367.

Bogan, J. A., and Marriner, S. E., 1983, Uptake of fenbendazole by grazing sheep with access to feed blocks containing fenbendazole, *Br. Vet. J.* 139:223–237.

Boray, J. C., Strong, M. B., Allison, J. R., von Orelli, M., Sarasin, G., and Gfeller, W., 1979, Nitroscanate a new broad spectrum anthelmintic against nematodes and cestodes of dogs and cats, *Aust. Vet. J.* 55:45–53.

Bremner, K. C., Berrie, D. A., and Hotson, I. K., 1983, Persistence of the anthelmintic activity of ivermectin in calves, *Vet. Rec.* 113:569.

Campbell, W. C., and Benz, G. W., 1984, Ivermectin: A review of efficacy and safety, *J. Vet. Pharmacol. Ther.* 7:1–16.

Clarkson, M. J., and Beg, M. K., 1971, Critical tests of levamisole as an anthelmintic in the horse, *Ann. Trop. Med. Parasitol.* 65:87–91.

Coles, G. C., 1984, Models of infections due to intestinal worms, in: *Animal Models in the Evaluation of Chemotherapy of Infectious Disease* (O. Zak and M. A. Sande, eds.), Academic Press, New York (in press).

Coles, G. C., and Simpkin, K. G., 1977, Resistance of nematode eggs to the ovicidal activity of benzimidazoles, *Res. Vet. Sci.* 22:386–387.

DiPietro, J. A., Todd, K. S., Lock, T. F., and McPherron, T. A., 1982, Anthelmintic activity of ivermectin given intramuscularly in horses, *Am. J. Vet. Res.* 43:145–148.

Duncan, J. L., Armour, J., Bairden, K., Jennings, F. W., and Urquhart, G. M., 1977, The activity of fenbendazole against inhibited fourth stage larvae of *Ostertagia ostertagi*, *Vet. Rec.* 101:249.

Forsyth, B. A., Gibbon, A. J., and Pryor, D. E., 1983, Seasonal variation in anthelmintic response by cattle to dermally applied levamisole, *Aust. Vet. J.* 60:141–146.

French, D. D., Torbert, B. J., Chapman, M. R., Klei, T. R., and Pierce, R. J., 1983, Comparison of the antistrongyle activity of a micellar formulation of ivermectin given parenterally and per os, *Vet. Med.* 78:1778–1781.

Georgi, J. R., Rendano, V. T., Kind, J. M., Bianchi, D. G., and Theodorides, V. J., 1980, Equine verminous arteritis: Efficiency and speed of larvicidal activity as influenced by dosage of albendazole, *Cornell Vet.* 70:147–152.

Gordon, M. McL., 1974, Disophenol(2,6-diiodo-4-nitrophenol)—A remarkable anthelmintic, Proc. Third Int. Cong. Parasit. 3:1392–1393.

Guerrero, J., Michael, B. F., Rohovsky, M. W., and Campbell, B. P., 1983, The activity of closantel as an equine antiparasitic agent, *Vet. Parasitol.* 12:71–77.

Hall, C. A., McDonell, P. A., and Graham, J. M., 1980, Anthelmintic activity of closantel against benzimidazole resistant strains of *Haemonchus contortus* and *Trichostrongylus colubriformis* in sheep, *Aust. Vet. J.* 56:461–462.

Hall, C. A., Kelly, J. D., Whitlock, H. V., and Ritchie, L., 1981, Prolonged anthelmintic effect of closantel and disophenol against a thiabendazole selected resistant strain of *Haemonchus contortus* in sheep, *Res. Vet. Sci.* 31:104–106.

Hsu, W. H., 1980, Toxicity and drug interactions of levamisole, *J. Am. Vet. Med. Assoc.* 176:1166–1169.

Jenkins, D. C., 1982, *In Vitro Screening Tests for Anthelmintics in Animal Models in Parasitology* (D. G. Owen, ed.), pp. 173–186, Macmillan, London and Basingstoke.

Jenkins, D. C., Armitage, R., and Carrington, T. S., 1980, A new primary screening test for anthelmintics utilising the parasitic stages of *Nippostrongylus brasiliensis* in the rat, *S. Parasitkd.* 63:261–264.

Kingsbury, P. A., and Reid, J. F. S., 1981, Anthelmintic activity of paste and drench formulations of oxfendazole in horses, *Vet. Rec.* 109:404–407.

Klei, T. R., and Torbert, B. J., 1980, Efficacy of ivermectin (22,23-dihydroavermectin B_1) against gastrointestinal parasites in ponies, *Am. J. Vet. Res.* 41:1747–1750.

Lloyd, S., and Soulsby, E. J. L., 1983, Prenatal and transmammary infections of *Toxocara canis* in dogs: Effect of benzimidazole-carbamate anthelmintics on various developmental stages of the parasite, *J. Small Anim. Pract.* 24:763–768.

Marriner, S. E., and Bogan, J. A., 1981a, Pharmacokinetics of fenbendazolein sheep, *Am. J. Vet. Res.* 42:1146–1148.

Marriner, S. E., and Bogan, J. A., 1981b, Pharmacokinetics of oxfendazole in sheep, *Am. J. Vet. Res.* 42:1143–1145.

Ngomuo, A. J., Marriner, S. E., and Bogan, J. A., 1984, The pharmacokinetics of fenbendazole and oxfendazole in cattle, *Vet. Res. Commun.* 8:187–193.

Prichard, R. K., Hennessy, D. R., and Steel, J. W., 1978, Prolonged administration: A new concept for increasing the spectrum and effectiveness of anthelmintics, *Vet. Parasitol.* 4:309–315.

Robinson, M., 1979, Efficacy of oxantel tartrate against *Trichuris suis* in swine, *Vet. Parasit.* 5:223–235.

Schillhorn van Veen, T. W., and Gibson, C. D., 1983, Anthelmintic activity of ivermectin in pigs naturally infected with *Ascaris* and *Trichuris*, *Am. J. Vet. Res.* 44:1732–1733.

Simpkin, K. G., and Coles, G. C., 1981, The use of *Caenorhabditis elegans* for anthelmintic screening, *J. Chem. Tech. Biotech.* 31:66–69.

Slocombe, J. O. D., and McCraw, B. M., 1980, Evaluation of pyrantel pamoate nitramisole and avermectin B1a against migrating *Strongylus vulgaris* larvae, *Can. J. Comp. Med.* 44:93–100.

Slocombe, J. O. D., McCraw, B. M., Pennock, P. W., and Vasey, J., 1982, Effectiveness of ivermectin against later 4th stage *Strongylus vulgaris* in ponies, *Am. J. Vet. Res.* 43:1525–1529.

Stewart, T. B., Marti, O. G., and Hale, O. M., 1981, Efficacy of ivermectin against five genera of swine nematodes and the hog louse *Haematopinus suis*, *Am. J. Vet. Res.* 42:1425.

Thienpont, D., and Vanpariys, O., 1980, Prophylactic and curative action of flubendazole against experimental Trichinellosis in pigs, in: *Proceedings of the Fifth International Conference on Trichinellosis, Noordwijk aan Zee. The Netherlands, September 1980*, pp. 343–346.

Tiner, J. D., 1958, A preliminary *in vitro* test for anthelmintic activity. *Exp. Parasitol.* 7:292–305.

Tocco, D. J., Buhs, R. P., Brown, H. P., Matzuk, A. R., Mertel, H. E., Harman, R. E., and Trenner, N. R., 1964, The metabolic fate of thiabendazole in sheep, *J. Med. Chem.* 7:399–405.

Torbert, B. J., Kramer, B. S., and Klei, T. R., 1982, Efficacy of injectable and oral paste formulations of ivermectin against gastrointestinal parasites in ponies, *Am. J. Vet. Res.* 43:1451–1453.

Yazwinski, T. A., Tilley, W., and Greenway, T., 1982, Efficacy of ivermectin in the treatment of artificially induced canine mixed gastrointestinal helminthiasis, *Vet. Med.* 77:225–226.

15

Nematode Infections of Domestic Animals

Extraintestinal Infections

LYNDIA SLAYTON BLAIR and THOMAS R. KLEI

1. INTRODUCTION

This chapter considers those nematodes of domestic animals that live as adults outside the gastrointestinal (GI) tract. Migrating stages of intestinal worms such as *Ancyclostoma, Ascaris, Strongylus,* or *Trichinella* are not discussed, nor are worms found accidentally at such sites. The diversity of parasites in this group is clearly demonstrated by the number of superfamilies represented; these include the Filaroidea, Metastrongyloidea, Spiruroidea, Strongyloidea, and Trichuroidea. The variety and number of species prohibit presentation of complete details, and coverage is necessarily selective.

2. GENERAL PRINCIPLES AND METHODS

Although their life cycles are distinct, extraintestinal nematodes share some characteristics that are important to the host–parasite interactions and pose similar difficulties in regard to treatment and development of new anthelmintics. All dwell as third-stage larvae (L3), fourth-stage larvae (L4), adults, and embryos or first-stage larvae (L1) in a variety of host tissues. Many have prolonged migratory phases during their life cycles that result in long prepatent periods. Most of these nematodes have indirect life cycles and utilize specific invertebrate intermediate hosts. In addition, the quantitation of parasite numbers in tissue is often difficult, and the methods for assessment of these

LYNDIA SLAYTON BLAIR • Merck Institute for Therapeutic Research, Rahway, New Jersey 07065. THOMAS R. KLEI • Department of Veterinary Science, Louisiana Agricultural Experimental Station, Louisiana State University and Agricultural and Mechanical College, Baton Rouge, Louisiana 70803.

infections in living animals or at necropsy vary greatly between investigators. These factors add substantially to the difficulty of producing experimental infections for controlled laboratory investigations. Because of these biological factors, few of these life cycles have been well defined and laboratory models and *in vitro* culture methods are of limited availability.

For tissue nematodes, particularly the filariae, the cuticle may have a more active role in the uptake of nutrients and drugs than the gut (Howells, 1980). Biochemical pathways may also differ (Barrett, 1983). Two main trends for catabolic pathways are found in parasitic helminths, homolactic fermentation, and carbon dioxide fixation involving a partial reverse tricarboxylic acid (TCA) cycle (Barrett, 1984). In general, homolactic fermentation is found in blood and tissue parasites and carbon dioxide fixation in gut parasites (Barrett, 1984).

In order for a drug to be effective, it (or the consequences of its action) must reach the parasite in sufficient strength for a period of time long enough to damage the worm. For the GI nematode, temporary paralysis or narcosis may be enough—i.e., when the worm awakens, its host will have gone. Such an effect is unlikely to be of equal benefit in an extraintestinal site. Development of continuous slow-release methods of anthelmintic treatment may assist in providing sufficient drug pressure to tissue dwelling worms.

Because most anthelmintics are relatively toxic and because concentrations of drug tend to decrease as one moves from the site of introduction, it is often a problem to deliver an appropriate amount of chemical to worms in an extraintestinal location. Drugs given *per os* (or at any site where the parasite is not found) must be absorbed and transported to the site of the parasite. The current emphasis in targeting drugs by packaging them in liposomes, combining them with monoclonal antibodies specific for the parasite or its location, and so forth, may help solve these problems.

Anthelmintic killing of parasites in extraintestinal tissues, vessels, and airways poses problems related to the host response not generally seen in the treatment of parasites of the GI tract. Remnants and intact dead parasites not flushed from the host are either destroyed or encapsulated by inflammatory responses. These inflammatory reactions may be extensive, occluding vessels or producing space-occupying lesions, resulting in serious systemic disease. In addition, the release of toxic or antigenic material from dead nematodes may elicit systemic reactions or lesions.

In general, less is known about the extraintestinal nematodes than about the GI worms. Not surprisingly, the available treatments and experimental methods for assessing efficacy are more apt to be unsatisfactory. For many extraintestinal nematode species, nothing at all has been shown to be effective, and there are many for which attempts at chemotherapy have not even been reported.

The most relevant screen for drug efficacy is a controlled trial in the target host against the target parasite. A full understanding and characterization of the activity profile would require a test against known numbers of organisms of known ages. For the extraintestinal worms of domestic animals, this approach represents an impractical ideal.

In practice, screening against extraintestinal nematodes is usually the secondary evaluation of compounds already known to possess biological activity. Most often, knowledge of tissue nematode activity follows an evaluation of GI nematode activity by one of the methods described in Chapter 12. Approaches to antifilarial screening are discussed in Chapter 13.

Campbell (1983) cautioned against thinking of parasites as intestinal or extraintestinal in the search for new drugs. All the above generalities run the risk of being oversimplified. Certainly the drug–parasite–host interactions are very complex and poorly understood.

The search for, and evaluation of, anthelmintics for tissue nematodes has been hampered in many cases by a lack of basic knowledge of the parasites and by limited ability to manipulate the host–parasite models under controlled laboratory conditions. Some of the problems (e.g., our ignorance of what preventive drugs actually do to preadult heartworm) can be readily solved with greater effort; others (e.g., the long life cycles) will continue to add to the frustrations of working with these worms for some time.

3. TREATMENT OF EXTRAINTESTINAL NEMATODES

For convenience, we have divided the species covered into filariae, lungworms, and other extraintestinal nematodes.

3.1. Filariae

Adult filarial nematodes inhabit the body cavities, blood vessels, lymphatics, and subcutaneous tissues of animals. Typically, the life cycles within the definitive hosts involve long prepatent periods during which the parasite molts twice and may migrate extensively through many tissues and organs. Microfilariae, the progeny of the adult parasites, may be found in the peripheral blood or in the skin. The microfilariae are ingested by an appropriate arthropod vector and after further development are passed to a new host as L3.

For the purpose of chemotherapy, the life cycle stages are traditionally viewed as preadult or developing larvae (L3, L4, and early L5 larvae), adults, and microfilariae (L1 larvae). Anthelmintic activity against the filariids is not only species and stage specific but site and host specific as well. For example, microfilariae of *Brugia pahangi* experimentally injected into mice are sensitive to ivermectin if they are within the bloodstream but are insensitive if they are located intraperitoneally (Devaney and Howells, 1984). Microfilariae of *B. pahangi* in the bloodstream of birds or cats are insensitive to ivermectin (Denham, quoted by Campbell, 1982). Similar contrasts can be drawn for diethylcarbamazine. More basic information is needed about these drug–host–parasite interactions before they will appear logical.

Pathological effects resulting from drug activity against filariae are dependent on the stage affected and on the location of the parasite. Pathological effects are not generally associated with the treating (and presumed killing) of the developing stages in the subcutaneous connective tissue. Nor does killing adult parasites (such as *Dipetalonema reconditum* or *Parafilaria bovicola*) within the subcutaneous muscle and connective tissue seem to harm the host.

Anthelmintic efficacy against microfilariae may induce a severe host reaction especially when large numbers of microfilariae are present. Killing of *Onchocerca* microfilariae in horses with diethylcarbamazine has been associated with pruritic dermatitis. The reactions in response to diethylcarbamazine treatment of filarial infections are generally more severe than those elicited by levamisole or ivermectin.

Several drugs, notably the organophosphates, are contraindicated in heartworm-infected animals because they cause death or migration of the adult worms to the pulmonary circulation and death of microfilariae, which then become microemboli throughout the vascular system, resulting in disseminated intravascular coagulation (DIC) (Barsanti and Greene, 1975). Death of adult heartworm from arsenical treatment may result in marked inflammation, pulmonary thromboemboli, thrombosis, and infarcts; it is recommended that activity of the host be restricted for several weeks after treatment. Steroid treatment is frequently recommended to reduce the postadulticide lesions, but there is evidence that prednisolone reduces efficacy of thiacetarsamide (Rawlings *et al.*, 1983*a*). Aspirin is also used to regulate platelet aggregation following adulticide therapy; its use reduces the radiological signs of pulmonary disease after arsenical treatment (Rawlings *et al.*, 1983*a*).

Selected common filarial parasites of domestic animals are listed in Table I, together with treatments reported to be effective against them. Of these, *D. immitis*, the canine heartworm, is the most studied and the one for which treatment and prevention are common. The recommended procedures for the management of canine heartworm disease are summarized in the Proceedings of the Heartworm Symposium '83 (American Heartworm Society, 1983).

The ability of existing drugs to kill adult heartworm is unsatisfactory. Although several arsenicals have been shown to exhibit adulticidal properties, thiacetarsamide is the only one readily available worldwide. Its efficacy in naturally infected dogs, necropsied to assess efficacy, varies from none at all to complete effect. In experimentally infected beagles, Blair and co-workers (1983) found the efficacy to vary as a function of age and sex. Male worms were more susceptible than females, and very young (2 months) and very old (2 years) were more susceptible than the rest (4 months, 6 months, 12 months, 18 months). Other investigators have suggested host-related variations in thiacetarsamide pharmacodynamics as a possible explanation for the extreme variation in efficacy (Rawlings *et al.*, 1983*b*). Heartworm infections involving the life-threatening condition known as vena cava syndrome are not amenable to chemotherapeutic treatment but can be treated by surgical removal of worms (Jackson, 1975).

Diethylcarbamazine is a very effective prophylactic treatment, but it must be given daily from the beginning of mosquito season until 2 months beyond. In many areas, this represents continuous treatment. It may not be given safely to dogs with circulating microfilariae (Powers *et al.*, 1981).

Treatment of microfilariae is unsatisfactory in that no approved drug is consistently marketed. Dithiazanine, the standard for many years, is available intermit-

Table I. Filarial Worms of Domestic Animals and Drugs Shown to Be Efficacious

Parasite	Stage[a]	Drug	Dosage (mg/kg)	Reference
Dirofilaria immitis	D	Diethylcarbamazine	5.5 daily, mosquito season + 2 months	American Heartworm Society (1983)
	D	Thiacetarsamide	2.2 b.i.d. × 2 at 2 months postinfection	Blair *et al.* (1983)
	D	Ivermectin	0.003 monthly	McCall *et al.* (1983)
	A	Thiacetarsamide	2.2 b.i.d. × 2	American Heartworm Society (1983); Blair *et al.* (1983)
	A	Melarsoprol	100	Blair and Campbell (1979)
	M	Dithiazanine	11 × 7–10	American Heartworm Society (1983)
	M	Levamisole	5 × 6–10	American Heartworm Society (1983)
	M	Ivermectin	0.05	American Heartworm Society (1983)
Dipetalonema reconditum	M	Levamisole	5 × 5	Scholtens *et al.* (1981)
	M	Ivermectin	0.25	Lindemann and McCall (1983)
Onchocerca cervicalis	M	Ivermectin	0.2 intramuscular	Klei *et al.* (1980)
			0.1 subcutaneous	Egerton *et al.* (1981)
	M		0.2 oral	French *et al.* (1984)
	M	Diethylcarbamazine	20 × 3	Chauve (1983)
Onchocerca gibsoni	D	Ivermectin		Copeman (1983)
	A	Suramin	9 × 6, 17 × 7	Copeman (1979)
	A	CGP6140	40 × 5	Striebel *et al.* (1982)
	M	Ivermectin	0.0125	Copeman, cited by Campbell (1982)
	M	Diethylcarbamazine	20 × 5	Copeman (1979)
	M	CGP6140	40 × 5	Striebel *et al.* (1982)
Onchocerca gutturosa	D	Ivermectin		Copeman (1983)
	A	Suramin	9 × 6, 17 × 7	Copeman (1979)
	M	Ivermectin	0.0125	Copeman, cited by Campbell (1982)
	M	Diethylcarbamazine	20 × 5	Copeman (1979)
Parafilaria bovicola	A	Nitroxynil	20	Wellington and Van Schalkwyk (1982)
	A	Ivermectin	0.2	Swan *et al.* (1983) Merker (1985)
	A	Levamisole	10 × 5, 15 × 2	Viljoen (1976)
	A	Fenbendazole	20–100 × 5	Viljoen (1976)
Setaria equina	A	Ivermectin	0.2–0.5	Klei *et al.* (1980)
Stephanofilaria okinowaensis		Trichlorphon + sulfanilamide	20% trichlorphon; 5% sulfanilamide	Dewan and Baki (1976)
		Levamisole	7.5 × 2	Ueno and Chibana (1980)

[a]D, preadult developing stages; A, adult; M, microfilariae.

tently. Consequently, ivermectin and levamisole, neither of which is approved for this purpose, are widely used (American Heartworm Society, 1983; Jackson, 1984).

Ivermectin is still in the developmental stages for use in dogs (Campbell *et al.*, 1983), and any use in dogs of the formulations marketed for large animals must be regarded as experimental. Broad-spectrum anthelmintic dosages may not have adequate safety margins for use in dogs. Certain dogs, particularly of the collie breed, have been reported to be uniquely susceptible to ivermectin toxicity (Seward *et al.*, 1985). Different formulations of ivermectin vary in potency against *D. immitis,* and recommended use levels will depend on the formulation made available. In experimental animals a single dose many times less than that required for broad-spectrum anthelmintic activity has been shown to prevent maturation of adult heartworm if given 1 or 2 months postinfection (Blair and Campbell, 1980). It is not active against the adults (Campbell, 1982).

Ivermectin is the most promising new component of the antifilarial arsenal. Activity against bovine and equine filariae is rapidly changing the way in which such infections are treated. Use of ivermectin to treat *O. cervicalis* in horses has helped determine that the microfilariae are involved in the cause and pathogenesis of dermatitis in horses (Herd and Donham, 1983). There is also evidence to suggest that ivermectin has prophylactic efficacy against *Onchocerca* in cattle (Copeman, 1983).

The number of focal cutaneous hemorrhages in cattle infected with *Parafilaria bovicola* was reduced by 100% within 14 days after a single subcutaneous treatment with ivermectin at 0.2 mg/kg. Comparison with untreated controls after 83 days showed that the number of subcutaneous lesions, total lesion area, and mass of tissue trimmed from carcases were reduced by 88.2, 98.7, and 98.8%, respectively. Curiously, oral treatment did not work. Swan *et al.* (1983) concluded that the effects of ivermectin on *Parafilaria* probably result from activity against the adults. Similar results with subcateneous treatment have been reported by Merker (1985).

3.2. Lungworms

This category is not meant to imply taxonomic status but rather location within the host. *Elaphostrongylus* is included because of its similarity to other metastrongyles, even though the adult worm inhabits tissues other than the lungs. The parasites and drugs used to treat them are listed in Table II. Parasites of the genera *Dictyocaulus* of ruminants and horses and *Metastrongylus* of pigs are the most common and the most extensively studied owing to their pathogenicity and occurrence in commercially important animals. Thus, numerous controlled studies report the efficacy of various anthelmintics against these parasites. Other genera listed in Table II are more sporadic in their occurrence and in the severity of the diseases they produce. Absence of specific drugs on the list for any given parasite is not necessarily indicative of lack of effect. This is particularly true for newer drugs such as ivermectin, which are likely to be highly effective against many of the minor genera inhabiting the lungs, even though the tests and/or reports have yet to surface.

Table II. Nematodes Parasitizing Lungs of Domestic Animals and Drugs Shown to Be Efficacious

Parasite	Host	Drug	Dosage (mg/kg)	Reference
Dictyocaulus viviparus	Cattle	Fenbendazole	7.5	Cawthorne (1984)
		Oxfendazole	4.5	Cawthorne (1984)
		Albendazole	7.5	Cawthorne (1984)
		Febantel	7.5	Cawthorne (1984)
		Levamisole	7.5	Cawthorne (1984)
		Ivermectin	0.2	Cawthorne (1984)
Dictyocaulus filaria	Sheep, goats	Fenbendazole	5.0	Cawthorne (1984)
		Oxfendazole	5.0	Cawthorne (1984)
		Albendazole	5.0	Cawthorne (1984)
		Mebendazole	15.0	Cawthorne (1984)
		Febantel	5.0	Cawthorne (1984)
		Levamisole	7.5	Cawthorne (1984)
		Ivermectin	0.2	Cawthorne (1984)
Dictyocaulus arnfieldi	Equine	Thiabendazole	440 × 2	Lyons *et al.* (1982)
		Mebendazole	15–30 × 5	Clayton and Trawford (1981)
		Ivermectin	0.2	Lyons *et al.* (1985)
Protostrongylus sp.	Sheep, goats	Febantel	10, 45	Acedo *et al.* (1980)
		Fenbendazole	10, 15	Dakkak *et al.* (1979)
Neostrongylus sp.	Sheep, goats	Febantel	10, 45	Acedo *et al.* (1980)
		Fenbendazole	10, 15	Ramisz *et al.* (1979)
Mullerius sp.	Sheep, goats	Fenbendazole	10	Himonas *et al.* (1980)
		Albendazole	10	Himonas *et al.* (1980)
		Mebendazole	40	Himonas *et al.* (1980)
		Febantel	5, 10, 45	Acedo *et al.* (1980)
		Ivermectin	0.2	Gregory *et al.* (1985)
Cystocaulus sp.	Sheep, goats	Fenbendazole	10, 15	Dakkak *et al.* (1979)
		Febantel	5, 10, 45	Acedo *et al.* (1980)
Elaphostrongylus rangiferi	Reindeer	Mebendazole	6 × 10	Rehbinder *et al.* (1982)
Elaphostrongylus cervi	Deer	Fenbendazole	7.5 or 3 × 5	Prosl and Kutzer (1980)
Metastrongylus sp.	Swine	Flubendazole	1.5 × 5	Bradley *et al.* (1983)
		Fenbendazole	3, 5 × 3	Stewart *et al.* (1981a)
		Oxfendazole	3	Corwin (1977)
		Levamisole	8	Cawthorne (1984)
		Tetramisole	15	Cawthorne (1984)
		Ivermectin	0.3	Cawthorne (1984)
Filaroides osleri	Dogs	Thiabendazole	70 × 2 + 140 × 21	Hill and McChesney (1976)
		Levamisole	7.5 × 30	Darke (1976)
Filaroides hirthi	Dogs	Levamisole	8 × 5	Georgi *et al.* (1976)
		Albendazole	50 b.i.d. × 5	Georgi *et al.* (1978)
Aelurostrongylus abstrusus	Cats	Fenbendazole	50 × 3	Roberson and Burke (1980)
		Levamisole	15–20 × 5–6	Scott (1973, 1975)

(continued)

Table II (Continued)

Parasite	Host	Drug	Dosage (mg/kg)	Reference
Crenosoma vulpis	Dogs	Levamisole	8	Stockdale and Smart (1975)
Capillaria aerophila	Dogs	Levamisole	5 × 5, 3× at 9-day intervals	Norsworthy (1975)
		Ivermectin	0.2	Evinger *et al.* (1985)
Syngamus sp.	Poultry	Thiabendazole	0.1% diet × 14–21	Cawthorne (1984)
		Mebendazole	120 ppm × 14	Cawthorne (1984)
		Fenbendazole	20 × 3–4	Ssenyonga (1982)
		Febantel	120 ppm × 6	Enigk and Dey-Hazra (1978)
		Levamisole	25	Cawthorne (1984)
		Nitroxynil	24	Cawthorne (1984)
Cyathosoma sp.	Waterfowl	Tetramisole	40 × 3	Denev and Vasilev (1973)
Mammomonogamus sp.	Cattle, other mammals	Tetramisole	15	Floser and Mitterpak (1982)

Reports of efficacy for drugs against lungworms are often based on resolution of clinical signs and failure to find first stage lungworm larvae in the feces after treatment. Results of these observations if only carried out for short periods may be questionable, as L1 larvae may reappear after prolonged periods suggesting efficacy of the drug against L1 or reproductive efficacy of female worms rather than adult worms. In this regard, it is interesting to note that ivermectin was apparently ineffective, at doses of 0.2 to 0.4 mg/kg, against adult *Parelaphostrongylus tenuis,* the protostrongylid meningeal worm of deer, but was effective against L1 and L3 stages of this parasite, which are not protected by the blood brain barrier (Kocan and Olsen, 1983).

The severity of adverse reactions to the killing of lungworms appears to be related to the location of the parasites within the respiratory tree. Only transient bouts of coughing are seen following treatment of nematodes inhabiting the trachea, bronchi, and larger bronchiole (*Metastrongylus* sp., *Capillaria areophia*). However, effective treatment of some nematodes inhabiting deeper airways or the lung parenchyma has been reported to produce severe reactions. Such reactions, many resulting in fatalities, have been described following treatment of *D. viviparus* infections of cattle (Jarrett *et al.,* 1980). Exacerbation of lesions and clinical signs has been reported following albendazole treatment of *Filaroides hirthi* in dogs (Georgi *et al.,* 1978). The death of one dog infected with *F. milksi* (Barsanti and Prestwood, 1983) and of several sheep infected with large numbers of *Mullerius capillaris* following levamisole treatment have been attributed to shock following release of antigens from the nematodes (Halhead, 1968).

Table III. *Extraintestinal Nematode Infections of Domestic Animals Other Than Those Due to Filariae and Lungworms and Drugs Reported Efficacious against Them*

Parasite	Host	Drug	Dosage (mg/kg)	Reference
Stephanurus dentatus	Swine	Levamisole	8	Stewart *et al.* (1977)
		Fenbendazole	3 × 3	Stewart *et al.* (1981c)
		Ivermectin	0.5	Stewart *et al.* (1981b)
		Flubendazole	1.5 × 5	Bradley *et al.* (1983)
Thelazia sp.	Mammals, birds	Levamisole (cattle) (bolus)	5.4–11.9	Lyons *et al.* (1981b)
		Levamisole (cattle)	12.5	Auro (1974)
		Febantel (horses)	10	Alvesten (1982)
		Ivermectin	0.2	Carmichael and Soll (1985)
Capillaria plica	Dogs	Fenbendazole	50 × 3	Gillespie (1983)
		Albendazole	50 × 10–14	Senior (1980)

3.3. Other Extraintestinal Nematodes of Domestic Animals

Few species of nematodes other than filariids and "lungworms" live as adults outside the GI tract. Those cited in this chapter are *Stephanurus dentatus,* the swine kidney worm, *Thelazia* spp., parasites of the conjunctival sac and lacrimal ducts of mammals and birds, and *Capillaria plica,* a trichurid nematode inhabiting the urinary tracts of canine and feline hosts. Drugs reported to be efficacious against these parasites are shown in Table III. The few reported efficacy studies involved naturally infected animals.

Efficacy of levamisole against *S. dentatus* appears to be limited to parasitism in the urinary tract as compared with other drugs (fenbendazole, febantel, ivermectin) efficacious against *S. dentatus* in other tissues as well.

Efficacy of drugs against *Thelazia* spp. appears to be variable, with some reports indicating tetramisole (15 mg/kg) or levamisole (5 mg/kg) to be efficacious when given orally or parenterally and others indicating injection of levamisole into the conjunctival sac (Soulsby, 1982) or bolus formulation (Lyons *et al.,* 1981b) to be more efficacious against bovine *Thelazia* spp. Observations on efficacies of 15 anthelmintics against *T. lacrymalis* in horses suggested that all were ineffective (Lyons *et al.,* 1981a). Carmichael and Soll (1985) found a single subcutaneous injection of ivermectin > 97% effective against natural infections of cattle. Variable results reported may be attributable to the numerous species of *Thelazia* and hosts involved as well as technical and drug formulation differences among these studies.

Efficacy of anthelmintics against *C. plica* are limited to improvement of clinical signs in cases of *C. plica*-induced cystitis treated with elevated doses of fenbendazole (Gillespie, 1983) or albendazole (Senior, 1980).

316 LYNDIA SLAYTON BLAIR and THOMAS R. KLEI

REFERENCES

Acedo, C., Hernandez, J. A. C., and Galindo, J. G., 1980, Effect of febantel on different species of lungworms in naturally infected sheep, *Vet. Med. Rev.* 1:27–34.

Alvesten, G., 1982, Treatment of *Thelazia lacrymalis* infection in horses (with febantel), *Svensk. Vet.* 34(6):255–257.

American Heartworm Society, 1983, Recommended procedures for the management of canine heartworm disease, in: *Proceedings of the Heartworm Symposium 1983, Orlando, Florida, February 11–13, 1983* (G. F. Otto, ed.), pp. 181–183, Veterinary Medicine Publishing Company, Edwardsville, Kansas.

Auro, S. K., 1974, The use of "Nilverm" (Tetramisole) in the control of clinical signs of *Thelazia rhodesi* (eyeworm) infection in cattle, *Bull. Epizoot. Dis. Afr.* 22(3):275–277.

Barrett, J., 1983, Biochemistry of filarial worms, *Helminth. Abst. A, Anim. Hum. Helminth.* 52(1):1–18.

Barrett, J., 1984, The anaerobic end-products of helminths, *Parasitology* 88(1):179–198.

Barsanti, J. A., and Greene, C. E., 1975, Disseminated intravascular coagulation in a heartworm infected dog treated with dichlorvos, *Small Anim. Clin.* 31(3):110–112.

Barsanti, J. A., and Prestwood, A. K., 1983, Parasitic disease of the respiratory tract, in: *Current Veterinary Therapy.* VIII. (R. W. Kirk, ed.), pp. 241–246, W. B. Saunders, Philadelphia.

Blair, L. S., and Campbell, W. C., 1980, Efficacy of ivermectin against *Dirofilaria immitis* larvae in dogs 31, 60, and 90 days after infection, *Am. J. Vet. Res.* 41(12):2108.

Blair, L. S., Malatesta, P. F., Gerckens, L. S., and Ewanciw, D. V., 1983, Efficacy of thiacetarsamide in experimentally infected dogs at 2,4,6,12 or 24 months post-infection with *Dirofilaria immitis*, in: *Proceedings of the Heartworm Symposium 1983, Orlando, Florida, February 11–13, 1983* (G. F. Otto, ed.), pp. 130–133, Veterinary Medicine Publishing Company, Edwardsville, Kansas.

Bradley, R. E., Guerrero, J., Becker, H. N., Michael, B. F., and Newcomb, K., 1983, Flubendazole: Dose range and efficacy studies against common internal parasites of swine, *Am. J. Vet. Res.* 44(7):1329–1333.

Campbell, W. C., 1982, Efficacy of the avermectins against filarial parasites: A short review, *Vet. Res. Commun.* 5:251–262.

Campbell, W. C., 1983, Progress and prospects in the chemotherapy of nematode infections of man and other animals, *J. Nematol.* 15(4):608–615.

Campbell, W. C., Blair, L. S., and Seward, R. L., 1983, Ivermectin vs. heartworm: The present status, in: *Proceedings of the Heartworm Symposium '83, Orlando, Florida, February 11–13, 1983* (G. F. Otto, ed.), pp. 146–150, Veterinary Medicine Publishing Company, Edwardsville, Kansas.

Carmichael, I. H., and Soll, M. D., 1985, Efficacy of ivermectin against *Thelazia*, World Association for Advancement in Veterinary Parasitology, Sao Paulo, Rio de Janeiro, Brazil, in press.

Cawthorne, R. J. G., 1984, *Anthelmintics for Cattle, Sheep, Goats, Pigs, Horses and Poultry*, Ministry of Agriculture, Fisheries and Food, Central Veterinary Laboratory, New Haw Weybridge, Surrey, England.

Chauve, C., 1983, Microfilariasis in a pony. *Sci. Vet. Med. Comp.* 85(1):45–46 (in French).

Clayton, H. M., and Trawford, A. F., 1981, Anthelmintic control of lungworm in donkeys, *Equine Vet. J.* 13(3):192–194.

Copeman, D. B., 1979, An evaluation of the bovine-*Onchocerca gibsoni, Onchocerca gutturosa* model as a tertiary screen against *Onchocerca volvulus* in man, *Tropenmed. Parasitol.* 30(4):469–474.

Copeman, D. B., 1983, The bovine *Onchocerca* model in selection of chemotherapeutic agents against human onchocerciasis, p. 6, *Abstracts of the World Association for the Advancement of Veterinary Parasitology, 10th International Conference, August 18–20, 1983*, Perth, Western Australia.

Corwin, R. M., 1977, Critical evaluation of oxfendazole as a swine anthelmintic, *Am. J. Vet. Res.* 38(4):465–467.

Dakkak, A., Cabaret, J., and Ouhelli, H., 1979, Comparative efficacy of fenbendazole and tetramisol against sheep helminths in Morocco. I. Protostrongyles and *Dictyocaulus* filariae, *Rec. Med. Vet.* 155(9):703–711.

Darke, P. G. G., 1976, Use of levamisol in the treatment of parasitic tracheobronchitis in the dog, *Vet. Rec.* 99:293–294.

Denev, I., and Vasilev, I., 1973, Therapeutic effect of tetramisole in *Cyathostoma bronchialis* infection in geese, *Vet. Nauk.* 10(7):3–8 (in Bulgarian).

Denham, D. A., 1982, (unpublished data), cited in: Campbell, W. C., 1982, Efficacy of the avermectins against filarial parasites: A short review, *Veterinary Research Communications* 5:251–262.

Devaney, E., and Howells, R. E., 1984, The microfilaricidal activity of ivermectin in vitro and in vivo, *Tropenmed. Parasitol.* 35(1):47–49.

Dewan, M. L., and Baki, M. A., 1976, Use of Neguvon (Bayer) for treatment and eradication of stephanofilariasis (humpsore) in zebu cattle, *Bangladesh Vet. J.* 10(1/4):47–50.

Egerton, J. R., Brokken, E. S., Suhayda, D., Eary, C. H., Wooden, J. W., and Kilgore, R. L., 1981, The antiparasitic activity of ivermectin in horses, *Vet. Parasitol.* 8(1):83–88.

Enigk, K., and Dey-Hazra, A., 1978, The treatment of roundworm infections in wild mammals and birds with Rintal (R), *Vet. Med. Rev.* 2:195–203.

Evinger, J. V., Kazacos, K. B., Cantwell, H. D., 1985, Ivermectin for treatment of nasal capillariasis, *J. Am. Vet. Med. Assoc.* 186(2):174–175.

Floser, R., and Mitterpak, J., 1982, Efficacy of tetramisol (Vermisol) against *Mammonogamas laryngeus* in cattle in Cuba, *Veterinarstvi* 32(5):210.

French, D. D., Klei, T. R., McClure, J. J., Miller, R. I., O'Neill, C. S., and Foil, L., 1984, Efficacy of ivermectin in injectable and paste formulations in the resolution of cutaneous lesions associated with *Onchocerca cervicalis* infections, *Proceedings of the 29th Annual Meeting of the American Association of Veterinary Parasitologists, New Orleans, Louisiana, July 15–17, 1984*, p. 10.

Georgi, J. R., Fleming, W. J., Hirth, R. S., and Cleveland, D. J., 1976, Preliminary investigation of the life history of *Filaroides hirthi* Georgi and Andersen 1975, *Cornell Vet.* 66(3):309–323.

Georgi, J. R., Slauson, D. O., and Theodorides, V. J., 1978, Anthelmintic activity of albendazole against *Filaroides hirthi* lungworms in dogs, *Am. J. Vet. Res.* 39(5):803–806.

Gillespie, D., 1983, Successful treatment of canine *Capillaria plica* cystitis, *Vet. Med. Small Anim. Clin.* 78(5):681–682.

Gregory, E., Foreyt, W. J., and Breeze, R., 1985, Efficacy of ivermectin and fenbendazole against lungworms, *Vet. Med.* 80:114–117.

Halhead, W. A., 1968, Tetramisol toxicity in sheep infected with *Mullerius capillaris*, *Vet. Rec.* 83:58.

Herd, R. P., and Donham, J. C., 1983, Efficacy of ivermectin against *Onchocerca cervicalis* microfilarial dermatitis in horses, *Am. J. Vet. Res.* 44(6):1102–1105.

Hill, B. L., and McChesney, A. E., 1976, Thiabendazole treatment of a dog with *Filaroides osleri*, *J. Am. Anim. Hosp. Assoc.* 12:487–489.

Himonas, C. A., Haralambidis, S. T., and Liakos, V. D., 1980, Treatment of *Mullerius capillaris* infection in goats, *Bull. Hell. Vet. Med. Soc.* 31(4):233–243.

Howells, R. E., 1980, *Filariae: Dynamics of the Surface. The Host Invader Interplay* (H. Van den Bossche, ed.), pp. 69–84, Elsevier/North-Holland Biomedical Press, Amsterdam.

Jackson, R. F., 1975, The venae cavae syndrome, in: *Proceedings of the Heartworm Symposium 1974, Auburn, Alabama, March 16–17, 1974* (G. Otto, R. F. Jackson, and W. F. Jackson, ed.), pp. 48–50. VM Publishing, Bonner Springs, Kansas.

Jackson, R., 1984, Ivermectin again, *Am. Heartworm Soc. Bull.* 10(3):9–10.

Jarrett, W. F. H., Urguhart, G. M., and Bairden, K., 1980, Treatment of parasitic bronchitis, *Vet. Rec.* 106(6):135.

Klei, T. R., Torbert, B. J., Ochoa, R., 1980, Efficacy of ivermectin (22,23-dihydroavermectin B1) against adult *Setaria equina* and microfilariae of *Onchocerca cervicalis* in ponies, *J. Parasitol.* 66(5):859–861.

Kocan, A. A., and Olsen, S. K., 1983, Ivermectin (MK-933) versus *Parelaphostrongylus tenuis*, *J. Wildl. Dis.* (Suppl. 3) 19:4.

Lindemann, B. A., and McCall, J. W., 1983, Microfilaricidal activity of ivermectin against *Dipetalonema reconditum*, *J. Vet. Pharmacol. Ther.* 6(1):75–76.

Lyons, E. T., Drudge, J. H., and Tolliver, S. C., 1981a, Apparent inactivity of several antiparasitic compounds against the eye worm *Thelazia lacrymalis* in equids, *Am. J. Vet. Res.* 42(6):1046–1047.

Lyons, E. T., Drudge, J. H., Tolliver, S. C., Hemken, R. W., and Button, F. S., 1981b, Preliminary tests for activity of levamisole against natural infections of eyeworms in dairy calves, *Vet. Med. Small Anim. Clin.* 76(8):1199–1201.

Lyons, E. T., Drudge, J. H., Zygmont, S. M., Twehues, J. L., Downing, R. G., and Sutton, H. H., 1982, Clinical history of lungworm disease in a foal, *Vet. Med. Small Anim. Clin.* 77(10):1533–1537.

Lyons, E. T., Drudge, J. H., and Tolliver, S. C., 1985, Ivermectin: Emphasis on controlled tests of activity against natural infections of *Dictyocaulus arnfieldi* and *Trichostrongylus axei* in donkeys, *Vet. Med.*, in press.

McCall, J. W., Cowgill, L. M., Plue, R. E., and Evans, T., 1983, Prevention of natural acquisition of heartworm infection in dogs by monthly treatment with ivermectin, in: *Proceedings or the Heartworm Symposium 1983, Orlando, Florida, February 11–13, 1983* (G. F. Otto, ed.), pp. 150–152, Veterinary Medicine Publishing Company, Edwardsville, Kansas.

Merker, M. K., 1985, Treatment with ivermectin of cattle naturally infested with *Parafilaria bovicola* in Burundi, *Trop. Anim. Health Prod.* 17(1):1–2.

Norsworthy, G. O., 1975, Feline lungworm treatment case report, *Feline Pract.* 5:14.

Powers, K. G., Parbuoni, E. L., and Furrow, R. D., 1981, *Dirofilaria immitis:* I. Adverse reactions associated with diethylcarbamazine therapy in microfilaremic dogs, in: *Proceedings of the Heartworm Symposium 1980, Dallas, Texas, February 23–24, 1980* (G. F. Otto, ed.), pp. 108–116, Veterinary Medicine Publishing Company, Edwardsville, Kansas.

Prosl, H., and Kutzer, E., 1980, Biology and control of *Elaphostrongylus cervi*, *Z. Jagdwiss.* 26(4):198–207.

Ramisz, A., Urban, E., and Balicka, A., 1979, Studies on the suitability of preparation fenbendazole (Panacure-Hoechst) for the control of nematodes of the family Protrostrongylidae in sheep, *Med. Wet.* 35(12):709–711.

Rawlings, C. A., Keith, J. C., Lewis, R. E., Losonsky, J. M., and McCall, J. W., 1983a, Aspirin and prednisolone modification of radiographic changes caused by adulticide treatment in dogs with heartworm infection, *J. Am. Vet. Med. Assoc.* 182(2):131–136.

Rawlings, C. A., Keith, J. C., and McCall, J. W., 1983b, Thiacetarsamide efficiency: One more study, using a different research model, in: *Proceedings of the Heartworm Symposium 1983, Orlando, Florida, February 11–13, 1983* (G. F. Otto, ed.), pp. 141–145, Veterinary Medicine Publishing Company, Edwardsville, Kansas.

Rehbinder, C., Forssell, I., Nordqvist, M., and von Szokolay, P., 1982, Efficacy of mebendazole on *Elaphostrongylus rangiferi* in reindeer, in: *Wildlife Diseases of the Pacific Basin and Other Countries, Proceedings of the Fourth International Conference of the Wildlife Disease Association, Sydney, Australia, August 25–28, 1981* (M. E. Fowler, ed.), pp. 208–212, Wildlife Disease Association, Ames, Iowa.

Roberson, E. L., and Burke, T. M., 1980, Evaluation of granulated fenbendazole (22.2%) against induced and naturally occurring helminth infections in cats, *Am. J. Vet. Res.* 41(9):1499–1502.

Scholtens, R. G., Legendre, A. M., and Weigel, J. P., 1981, Treatment of dogs with *Dipetalonema reconditum* microfilaremias, in: *Proceedings of the Heartworm Symposium 1980, Dallas, Texas, February 23–24, 1980* (G. F. Otto, ed.), pp. 106–107, Veterinary Medicine Publishing Company, Edwardsville, Kansas.

Scott, D. W., 1973, Current knowledge of aelurostrongylosis in the cat, *Cornell Vet.* 63(3):483–500.

Scott, D. W., 1975, Lungworm treatment, *Feline Pract.* 5(3):5.

Senior, D. F., 1980, *Capillaria plica* infections in dogs, *J. Am. Vet. Med. Assoc.* 176(9):901–905.

Seward, R. L., Blair, L. S., Plue, R. E., and Brokken, E. S., 1985, The efficacy and safety of ivermectin in dogs, in: *Proceedings of the World Veterinary Congress, Perth, Australia, August 25–26, 1983*, in press.

Soulsby, E. J. L., 1982, *Helminths, Arthropods and Protozoa of Domesticated Animals*, Lea & Febiger, Philadelphia, pp. 290–291.

Ssenyonga, G. S. Z., 1982, Efficacy of fenbendazole against helminth parasites of poultry in Uganda, *Trop. Anim. Health Prod.* 14(3):163–166.

Stewart, T. B., Fincher, G. T., Marti, O. G., and McCormick, W. C., 1977, Efficacy of levamisol against the swine kidney worm *Stephanurus dentatus*, *Am. J. Vet. Res.* 38(12):2081–2082.

Stewart, T. B., Marti, O. G., and Hale, O. M., 1981a, Efficacy of fenbendazole against five genera of swine parasites, *Am. J. Vet. Res.* 42(7):1160–1162.

Stewart, T. B., Marti, O. G., and McCormick, W. C., 1981b, Efficacy of ivermectin against the swine kidney worm *Stephanurus dentatus*, *Am. J. Vet. Res.* 42(8):1427–1428.

Stewart, T. B., Marti, O. G., and McCormick, W. C., 1981c, Efficacy of fenbendazole against the swine kidney worm *Stephanurus dentatus*, *Am. J. Vet. Res.* 42(9):1627–1629.

Stockdale, P. H. G., and Smart, M. E., 1975, Treatment of crenosomiasis in dogs, *Res. Vet. Sci.* 18(2):178–181.

Striebel, H. P., Sanger, I., Copeman, D. B., and Lammler, G., 1982, Antifilarial activities of amoscanate and CGP6140, in: *Proceedings of the Fifth International Congress of Parasitology, Toronto, Canada, August 7–14, 1982, Molecular Parasitology*, pp. 527–528.

Swan, G. E., Soll, M. D., Carmichael, I. H., Schroder, J., 1983, Efficacy of ivermectin against *Parafilaria bovicola*, *Vet. Rec.* 113(12):260.

Ueno, H., and Chibana, T., 1980, Clinical and parasitological evaluations of levamisole as a treatment for bovine stephanofilariasis, *Vet. Parasitol.* 7(1):59–68.

Viljoen, J. H., 1976, Studies on *Parafilaria bovicola* (Tubangui 1934). I. Clinical observations and chemotherapy, *J. South Afr. Vet. Assoc.* 47(3):161–169.

Wellington, A. C., and Van Schalwyk, L., 1982, The effect of a single injection of nitroxynil at 20 milligrams per kilogram live mass in the treatment of *Parafilaria bovicola* infestations in cattle, *J. South Afr. Vet. Assoc.* 53(2):91–94.

16

Mode of Action of Antinematodal Drugs

ROBERT S. REW and RAYMOND H. FETTERER

1. INTRODUCTION

The purpose of this chapter is to describe biochemical or physiological events observed in nematodes exposed to an anthelmintic. Whether these pharmacologically mediated events truly represent a mode of action is difficult to prove, and the action described may represent a secondary event unrelated to the mode of action or it may be part of a series of events involved in the killing process.

Mode-of-action investigations of anthelmintics known to be active *in vivo* are designed to tell us how the drug affects a biochemical or series of biochemical events; these studies also attempt to show that these events are required for nematode survival, but not for host survival, under the conditions of the measurements. If the function measured is the site of primary activity of the drug, these studies achieve their goal. If the event(s) can be monitored quantitatively, that event can be used for screening structure–activity relationships to identify the most active analogue in a series or identify new molecules that may serve as anthelmintics against that site.

Mode-of-action studies with known antinematodal compounds have tentatively identified two general and one specific area(s) as sites of anthelmintic activity, glucose metabolism, neuromuscular coordination and microtubular function, as potential sites unique in some way to the parasite and required for survival (Table I). Specific sites under glucose catabolism include glucose transport, glycogen metabolism, phosphofructokinase, fumarate reductase, oxygen uptake, and ATPase. Specific sites under neuromuscular coordination include acetylcholinesterase, cholinergic and GABAergic (γ-aminobutyric acid) neurons, and muscle membranes. These functions have been used for structure–activity studies but to date have not yielded a new class of antinematodal compounds. However, as we understand the biochemical and molecular details of these

---

ROBERT S. REW • Merck Sharp & Dohme Research Laboratories, Rahway, New Jersey 07065.   RAYMOND H. FETTERER • Animal Parasitology Institute, Agricultural Research Service, U.S. Department of Agriculture, Beltsville, Maryland 20705.

Table I. Proposed Mode of Action for Antinematodal Drugs

Drug class	Mode of action
Phenothiazine	Interruption of microtubular function (?)
Benzimidazoles	Interruption of microtubular function
Imidazoles, quaternary ammonium salts, pyrimidines, pyridines	Cholinergic ganglionic blockers
Avermectins	Chloride channel opener at GABA-mediated inter-neuron .
Organophosphates	Acetylcholinesterse inhibitors
Piperazine	Hyperpolarization of muscle membrane (chloride channel opener; GABA-agonist)
Piperazine derivative, diethylcarbamazine	Opsonization for immune destruction
Antimonials	Inhibition of phosphofructokinase
Arsenicals	Bind to sulfhydryl proteins
Naphthalene sulfonic acid	DHFR or protein kinase or pyridine nucleotide utilization inhibition
Isothiocyanate	Glucose transport, synthesis into glycogen and cata-bolism inhibition
Cyanine dyes	Glucose transport or oxidative metabolism inhibition
Substituted phenols and salicylanilides	Uncouple electron-transport-associated phosphoryla-tion

functions and others more completely, a more rational approach to drug design will become a reality.

2. IMPORTANT PHYSIOLOGICAL REQUIREMENTS OF NEMATODES

Physiological requirements for survival of adult parasitic nematodes are restricted mainly to maintaining energy levels *via* the catabolism of carbohydrates and to maintaining an appropriate feeding site *via* neuromuscular coordination. Little evidence of lipid metabolism (Barrett *et al.*, 1970; Meyer and Meyer, 1972; Frayha, 1974; Ward and Fairbairn, 1970), nucleic acid metabolism, or protein metabolism (other than egg laying) is available, at least such as would indicate that inhibition by a chemical compound threatens the viability of the parasite without affecting the host. This limitation also restricts the types of compounds for which one would expect an anti-nematodal effect; for example, antibacterials affecting prokaryotic DNA, RNA, protein, or cell wall metabolism would not be expected to be active against a eukaryotic nematode (reviewed by Rew, 1978; Prichard, 1978; Coles, 1977; Eckert and Kohler, 1982; Saz and Bueding, 1966). Exceptions would be the work of Jaffe and of Howells, respectively, on suramin effects on purine salvage pathways and nucleotide transport inhibition in filariid nematodes. Jaffe (1980) demonstrated a methyltetrahydrofolate (CH_3FH_4)-dependent killing mechanism for suramin (10^{-5} M) against filariids *in vitro* and a 50% inhibition of NADP-dependent 10-formyl-FH_4 dehydrogenase by 5 × 10^{-6} M suramin. Howells *et al.* (1981) demonstrated a chemosterilant effect of 5-

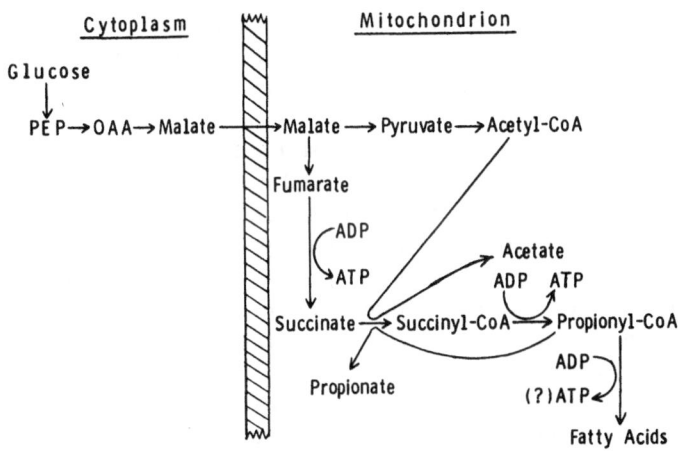

Figure 1. Ascaris pathway for glucose catabolism.

fluorouracil and 5-fluorodeoxyuridine against filariids *in vivo*. These reports may signal the need for a more careful examination of potential sites in nucleic acid metabolism.

2.1. Glucose Metabolism

Studies on metabolism of carbohydrates in parasitic nematodes have demonstrated three principles: (1) glucose is the primary substrate, (2) few species completely decarboxylate the glucose molecule, and (3) organic acids and alcohols are the major end products of metabolism. Oxygen requirements among the various genera, species, and life stages of the nematodes vary greatly. For example, adult *Litomosoides carinii* require oxygen for survival and motility (Bueding, 1949), whereas a closely related adult filariid, *Brugia pahangi*, has no oxygen requirement and catabolizes glucose to lactate alone (Wang and Saz, 1974). However, the microfilarial stage of *B. pahangi* excretes lactate, acetate, and CO_2, when given glucose, and requires oxygen for acetate production and motility, but not survival (Rew and Saz, 1977). If any generalization might be made in the majority of examples available, eggs and larval stages of parasitic nematodes have tricarboxylic acid (TCA) cycle enzymes and cytochromes up through L3; however, L4 and adult nematodes generally lose their oxygen requirement, certain of their TCA cycle enzymes, and cytochrome oxidase.

Most in-depth studies of glucose catabolism in adult parasitic nematodes have been done with *Ascaris suum*, since it is large and obtained easily from most local abattoirs. These studies have revealed that glucose is catabolized through the classic Embden-Meyerhof-Parnas pathway to phosphoenolpyruvate (PEP) (Fig. 1). Unlike mammalian systems, the *Ascaris* system contains an active cytoplasmic PEP carboxykinase (PEP–CK) and has essentially no pyruvate kinase (PK) to catabolize PEP further. PEP is carboxylated to OAA (Saz and Lescure, 1969) and a very active cytoplasmic malate dehydrogenase (MDH) converts oxalacetate to malate (Bueding and

Saz, 1968). Malate serves as the mitochondrial substrate (Saz, 1970), where it undergoes a dismutation to succinate and pyruvate, generating 1 mole of NADH through the malic enzyme (ME) (Saz and Hubbard, 1957; Saz and Lescure, 1969) and regenerating 1 mole of NAD through an electron-transport-associated fumarate reductase (FR) (Saz and Vidrine, 1959; Kmetec and Bueding, 1961; Bueding, 1962). One mole of ATP is generated through a site I phosphorylation coupled to the FR (Kmetec and Bueding, 1961; Seidman and Entner, 1961; Saz and Lescure, 1969), and a redox balance is achieved in the mitochondrion without the need for oxygen. Apparently, the NADH generated is formed in the intermembrane space of the mitochondrion (Rew and Saz, 1974) and the translocation of the hydride ion to the electron-transport-associated FR requires an NADH : NAD transhydrogenase (TH) located on the inner membrane (Kohler and Saz, 1976).

Further catabolism of pyruvate and succinate has recently been shown to involve a substrate level phosphorylation in which energy of the succinyl-CoA bond is conserved in the succinyl CoA decarboxylation to propionate (Saz and Pietrazak, 1980). Acetate, propionate, and their condensation products are the primary end products excreted by the worm (Bueding and Yale, 1951; Saz and Weil, 1960; Bueding, 1962; Mata, *et al.*, 1977). An additional site of ATP generation could involve the β-ketoreductase with conservation of energy from the CoA bond in formation of branched-chain volatile fatty acids (VFA), but supporting data are not available.

Type and percentage of end-product accumulation differ among the nematodes and depend partly on the ratio of cytoplasmic PEPCK/PK (Bueding and Saz, 1968). If the PK predominates, cytoplasmic products such as lactate or ethanol predominate; if the PEPCK predominates, mitochondrial products such as succinate, acetate, propionate, VFAs, and *n*-propanol are the major excreted end products.

Several of the enzymes demonstrated in these reactions are unique or have unique locations or directions from the host. PEPCK, ME, TH, FR, and β-oxidation enzymes are all among these unique reactions and may serve as potential targets for chemotherapeutic attack.

2.2. Neuromuscular Coordination

In addition to carbohydrate metabolism, the neuromuscular system of nematodes has been identified as the second general site of action of anthelmintic compounds. Proper neuromuscular control is critical in maintenance of proper parasite location within the host as well as in the more subtle, but equally important, movements such as copulation and feeding. The neuromuscular physiology of many economically and medically important nematodes has not been investigated because of both their small size and the difficulty in maintaining them *in vitro*.

The large size and relative abundance of adult female *A. suum* have made this parasite the primary model for the study of nematode neurophysiology. The free-living nematode *Caenorhabditis elegans*, because of its short generation time, ease of cultivation, and well-studied genetics, has emerged as another important model for the study of nematode neurobiology (Zuckerman, 1980).

The basic structure and function of nematode systems have been well reviewed elsewhere (Johnson and Stretton, 1980). There are, however, unique features in neuromuscular function of nematodes that may serve as a basis of selective action of nematocides.

The membrane potential of *Ascaris* somatic muscle is about −30 mV but, unlike classic vertebrate muscle cells, *Ascaris* muscle is relatively insensitive to changes in extracellular potassium (Del Castillo *et al.*, 1964a–c; DeBell *et al.*, 1963). Theoretical and experimental analyses indicate that an active transport system contributes significantly to resting membrane potential (Brading and Caldwell, 1971). This transport system apparently involves active transport of organic ions that may represent an adaptation to the high concentration of organic acids found in *Ascaris* pseudocoelomic fluid. Neither the biochemical mechanisms nor selective inhibitors of this system have been reported.

Considerable interest has centered on the putative neurotransmitters of nematodes. Convincing evidence has accumulated that acetylcholine (Ach) is the excitatory neurotransmitter at the neuromuscular junction. Acetylcholine causes muscle depolarization and contraction, which can be blocked by tubocurarine and potentiated by cholinesterase inhibitors (Del Castillo *et al.*, 1963). Biochemical studies have also shown that the enzyme choline acetyltransferase is also present in neural tissue and is selectively associated with excitatory motor neurons (Johnson and Stretton, 1980).

Evidence for an inhibitory transmitter in nematodes is less satisfactory, although studies on *Ascaris* muscle have shown that GABA depolarizes muscle cells (Del Castillo *et al.*, 1964b), causes a dose-dependent relaxation of muscle strips (Ash and Tucker, 1966), and activates a choloride conductance in isolated muscle cells (Martin, 1982). The localization of GABA and associated synthetic enzymes has not been reported.

2.3. Microtubular Integrity

Importance of microtubular integrity to the survival of nematode parasites may be defined by extrapolation from microtubular function in other systems or by inhibitions of functions as a result of benzimidazole exposure (see Section 3.2). Microtubular functions in other systems include cell division, axoplasmic transport, cell movement, and cell-to-cell communication. These functions in nematodes as demonstratd by benzimidazole action include egg laying, egg hatching, larval development, substrate transport, enzyme activity, and enzyme secretion.

3. CHEMICAL CLASSES OF ANTINEMATODAL COMPOUNDS AND THEIR EFFECTS

3.1. Phenothiazine

Mode-of-action studies of phenothiazine and its derivatives cover a wide range of disciplines. Phenothiazine has been used as an antipsychotic agent, an anthelmintic, and recently as an antiprotozoal compound. Numerous studies on the site of anti-psychotic mode of action of phenothiazine have demonstrated a number of molecular interactions, including dopamine receptors (Seeman, 1981), calmodulin (Levin and Weiss, 1979), and microtubules (Appurao and Cann, 1981; Poffenbarger and Fuller, 1977; Hinman and Cann, 1976). Anthelmintic mode-of-action studies have examined the motility and acetylcholinesterase (AchE) of adult ascarids, demonstrating an inhibition of motility *in vitro* and a partial inhibition of AchE [19% inhibition by $2 \times 10^{-3} M$ PTZ (Hutchinson and Probert, 1972) and 45% inhibition by $10^{-4} M$ PTZ (Knowles and Casida, 1966)] at high concentrations of PTZ. Recently, PTZ has been shown to block motility and cell growth of *Trypanosoma brucei in vitro* at $10^{-5} M$ (Seebeck and Gehr, 1983). Electron microscopic examination of the treated protozoan cells revealed a disruption in cytoskeletal microtubules.

The repeated correlation between microtubular integrity and phenothiazine action in nonhelminth systems, coupled with certain circumstantial observations in helminth systems would tend to support a microtubular inhibition hypothesis of action mechanism in nematodes. Kelly *et al.* (1981) reported that benzimidazole-resistant *Haemonchus contortus* developing eggs and larvae were also resistant to phenothiazine. Biochemical and resistance studies have indicated that benzimidazoles act as microtubule inhibitors in exerting their anthelmintic effect (Rew, 1978), together indicating the likely possibility of a common action for PTZ and benzimidazoles. (See the following section and refer to Chapter 17).

3.2. Benzimidazoles

Mode-of-action studies with benzimidazoles (BZs) can be separated into three categories: (1) fumarate reductase inhibition, (2) inhibition of glucose transport, (3) interruption of microtubular function. Most of the recent work suggests that category 3 represents the primary underlying mechanism.

1. *Fumarate Reductase*

Prichard (1970) demonstrated complete inhibition of NADH oxidation in the presence of fumarate by $10^{-3} M$ thiabendazole (TBZ) in *H. contortus* homogenates. Additional support for this information was demonstrated by Prichard (1973), who showed that although 85% of the NADH oxidation in the presence of fumarate was inhibited by $10^{-3} M$ TBZ in homogenates of a TBZ-susceptible strain of *H. contortus*, no inhibition was seen even at $2 \times 10^{-3} M$ TBZ in homogenates of a resistant strain. Studies by Malkin and Camacho (1972) and by Romanowski *et al.* (1975) further demonstrated a similar difference between BZ-sensitive and BZ-resistant *H. contortus*.

2. *Glucose Transport*

Vanden Bossche and de Nollin (1973) demonstrated an inhibition of glucose transport into *A. suum* and *Trichinella spiralis* larvae at $10^{-5} M$ or $10^{-6} M$ mebendazole (MBZ), resulting in a demonstrable reduction in glycogen reserves. However, other studies indicated that the glucose tranpsort inhibition was specific among BZs for MBZ alone.

3. Microtubules

Several types of evidence have implicated microtubules in the mechanism of BZ action. Electron microscopic studies following MBZ treatment of *A. suum* or *Syngamus trachea* by Borgers *et al.* (1975) demonstrated a disappearance of demonstrable microtubules in the gut cell. Subsequently, Friedman and Platzer (1980) demonstrated that BZs would prevent binding of [^{14}C]colchicine to crude *Ascaris* egg tubulin at 10^{-8} M and that 10^{-6} M BZs were required to prevent binding to purified mammalian brain tubulin. Recently, N. C. Sangster, R. K. Prichard, and E. Lacey (unpublished data) demonstrated that AchE secretion (possibly microtubule mediated), colchicine binding, and microtubular integrity are inhibited by TBZ and/or oxfendazole (OFZ) at lower concentrations in BZ-sensitive *Trichostrongylus colubriformis* than in a BZ-resistant strain.

The observation of cross-resistance among all tested benzimidazoles in controlled efficacy trials (Colglazier *et al.*, 1975) makes it likely that BZs have a common mode of action. Unpublished observations by E. Lacy, R. K. Prichard, and R. S. Rew, on egg hatch, fumarate reductase, and glucose transport, respectively, in BZ-sensitive and BZ-resistant strains of *Haemonchus contortus* would indicate that these functions are inhibited with all BZs tested (including TBZ and MBZ) at 5–10 times higher concentrations of BZs in the BZ-resistant strain. In addition, colchicine, its analogues, and podophyllotoxin, all known microtubular inhibitors, display comparable inhibitory effects, and colchicine and its analogues display differential effects between BZ-sensitive and BZ-resistant *H. contortus* comparable to those of the BZs. These data would indicate that all previously published BZ modes of action have a common basis—microtubular interruption. Apparently, inhibition of egg hatching, larval development, glucose transport, and fumarate reductase involves the tubulin molecule either directly or by conformational alternation of a protein (i.e., FR) that is spatially associated with the tubulin–drug interaction (see Chapter 17).

3.3. Imidazoles and Other Cholinergic Agonists

Bephenium and thenium are cholinergic agonists, that is, they bind to Ach binding sites, cause an Ach-like response and cannot be inactivated by acetylcholinesterase (Eyre, 1970). Consistent with their cholinergic properties, these compounds cause a contraction of *Ascaris* muscle (Broome, 1961). Pyrantel and its analogue morantel also appear to act as cholinergic agonists (Eyre, 1970; Forbes, 1972). Pyrantel, in common with nicotine and decamethonium, causes paralysis and contracture of vertebrate skeletal muscle. Pyrantel also causes a slowly developing contracture of *Ascaris* muscle strips and depolarization of muscle cells (Aubry *et al.*, 1970). The vertebrate ganglion stimulating agent, dimethylphenylpiperazium, also causes a contracture of *Ascaris* muscle, while the ganglionic blocking agents hexamethonium, mecamylamine, and pempidine block the action of levamisole on *Ascaris* muscle (Van Nueten, 1972; Coles *et al.*, 1974). Coles *et al.* (1974) observed that the small percentage of *Ascaris* that recovered from treatment with levamisole did not exhibit the expected contraction when injected with bephenium, methyridine, and pyrantel but did contract in presence of Ach, suggesting that all four compounds may be acting in the same manner but not directly at the neuromuscular junction.

The most convincing evidence that levamisole acts as a cholinergic agonist at the neuromuscular junction comes from an elegant study of the cholinergic receptor in *C. elegans* (Lewis *et al.*, 1980). These studies, using a cutworm assay to permit cuticle permeation by drugs, reveal that the pharmacological specificity of nematode neuromuscular cholinergic receptors is most like that of a vertebrate nicotinic ganglionic receptor. Levamisole appears to act as both an antagonist and an agonist on this receptor. Lending further support to a cholinergic mechanism for the paralyzing action of levamisole is the observation that mutants of *C. elegans* highly resistant to the paralyzing effects of levamisole respond very poorly to cholinergic agonists effective on the wild type, although the mutants respond to the noncholinergic muscle agonist, ouabain (Lewis *et al.*, 1980). Larval isolates of the levamisole-sensitive ruminant parasite *Ostertagia circumcincta* are paralyzed by levamisole in a dose-dependent manner. Larval isolates from parasite strains clinically resistant to levamisole show decreased dose–response paralysis to levamisole and morantel (Martin and LeJambre, 1979). The observation that parasites clinically resistant to levamisole exhibit an altered response to morantel supports the hypothesis that levamisole and morantel act via the same cholinergic mechanism.

In addition to a cholinergic action, other mechanisms for levamisole action have been proposed. Levamisole has been shown to affect nematode metabolism by inhibition of fumarate reductase (FR) (Vanden Bossche and Janssen, 1967). It seems unlikely that inhibition of FR is the primary effect of levamisole, since relatively high concentrations of levamisole are required to inhibit FR, administration of levamisole to infected host does not alter the adenylate energy charge in *Nematospiroides dubius* (Sharpe, 1980) and adult *B. pahangi* that contains no FR is paralyzed by levamisole (Wang and Saz, 1974). More recently, levamisole has been shown to increase the rate of incorporation of glucose into glycogen in *L. carinii* without altering glycolysis (Komuniecki and Saz, 1982). Although it is likely that the effects of levamisole on parasite metabolism are secondary to a paralytic effect, the possibility that these metabolic effects do contribute to overall anthelmintic efficacy of the compound cannot be ruled out.

In addition to its anthelmintic properties levamisole has also been shown to stimulate the mammalian immune system (Mikulikova and Trnavskg, 1980) and to improve cellular immunity in malnourished animals (Olusi *et al.*, 1979). The relationship between the immunomodulatory properties and nematocidal effects of levamisole is unknown.

3.4. Ivermectin

Ivermectin (IVM) is the newest class of nematocides available. Observations on some nematode species demonstrate a triphasic response to IVM comprising an initial loss of locomotor activity where parasites remain sensitive to touch, a recovery phase and a final complete loss of motor activity (Wright et al., 1984). Picrotoxin and bicuculline, GABA antagonists, block this effect of IVM on parasite motility.

Neurophysiological studies indicate that IVM may interfere with the function of the GABA system in nematodes. Using selective stimulation of either interneurons or excitatory motor neurons, Kass et al. (1980) demonstrated that IVM blocks motor neurons in the ventral nerve cord of Ascaris. Transmission between inhibitory neurons and muscle is also blocked by IVM. These observations suggest that IVM stimulates inhibitory neurons directly or causes release of GABA from presynaptic terminals. IVM has been shown to stimulate GABA release from mammalian synaptosomes (Pong et al., 1980). However, IVM and GABA do not act at the same receptor, since they do not compete for the same site in a dog brain preparation (Pong and Wang, 1980). Since IVM neither depolarizes nematode muscle cells nor mimics the lengthening effect of GABA when injected into an adult Ascaris (Kass et al., 1980), it appears that IVM does not act directly on the muscle but interferes with synaptic transmission in the nematode nerve cord.

Studies on invertebrate model systems support a hypothesis that IVM action is associated with GABA systems. IVM applied to the lobster stretcher muscle eliminates inhibitory postsynaptic potentials by increasing muscle membrane conductance to chloride ions, an effect blocked by the GABA antagonist picrotoxin (Fritz et al., 1979). Detailed analyses, however, suggest that effects of IVM on muscle chloride conductance may be due to an increase in tonic release of GABA from presynaptic terminals (Pong et al., 1980). An association of IVM with chloride channels has also been observed in studies on identified central snail neurons (A. J. Bokitch and R. J. Walker, unpublished data). When IVM is applied to snail neurons containing either inhibitory GABA or ACh receptors, a chloride conductance is activated. These observations suggest that IVM has the ability to activate chloride channels coupled with more than one specific neurotransmitter receptor.

The available evidence supports a hypothesis that IVM paralyzes nematodes by activating a membrane chloride conductance in neurons of the nerve cord, either directly or by stimulating a presynaptic release of GABA. Since GABA systems are widely distributed in the vertebrate CNS, the selectivity of IVM as a nematocide most likely results from the inability of IVM to reach its target in the host CNS, while sites in the nematode parasite are readily accessible to IVM.

Unlike a number of other nematocides, IVM appears to be without effect on pathways of nematode carbohydrate metabolism (Kass et al., 1980). A recent study contends, however, that IVM exerts its antiparasitic activity by inhibiting chitin synthesis (Calcott and Fatig, 1984). This mechanism for the action of IVM seems unlikely for two reasons: (1) the IVM used in this study was only partially purified leaving the possibility that antibiotic contaminants were present, and (2) chitin has only a very limited distribution in nematode species and is found only in eggshell (Lestan, 1969); therefore, inhibition of chitin synthesis would not account for the broad-spectrum efficacy of IVM on adult nematodes.

3.5. Organophosphates

Since excitatory neuromuscular transmission in nematodes is cholinergic, AchE is required for postsynaptic inactivation of Ach. Inhibition of AchE results in continued depolarization of postsynaptic junction with resultant paralysis (Lee and Hodsden, 1963; Hart and Lee, 1966). Organophosphates such as crufomate, dichlorovos, haloxon, and triclorophon inhibit nematode AchE at concentrations as low as 10^{-13} M (Knowles and Casida, 1966). Although organophosphates are potent inhibitors of nematode AchE these compounds are also inhibitors of mammalian AchE and may result in toxic responses (Jamnadas and Thomas, 1979).

3.6. Piperazine and Diethylcarbamazine

Piperazine causes a flaccid paralysis of Ascaris muscle with resultant paralysis. Application of piperazine to isolated Ascaris muscle causes a hyperpolarization of muscle membranes (Del Castillo et al., 1964a,b). A more recent study using voltage-clamp techniques to investigate the effects of piperazine on muscle membrane conductance demonstrated that the reversal potential of both GABA and piperazine were similar to each other and close to that of the predicted Nernst potential for chloride (Martin, 1982). It was concluded from these studies that piperazine acts as a GABA agonist of relatively low potency on extra synaptic GABA receptors located on muscle bellies of Ascaris muscle.

The antifilarial drug diethylcarbamazine (DEC), a piperazine derivative, has been in widespread use for more than 30 years, but its mode of action still remains poorly understood. Although DEC appears to lack in vitro activity against microfilariae, Hawking et al. (1950) reported that DEC affects the worm's surface and thus prepares the parasites for phagocytosis by host immune system. In vitro studies show that DEC enhances leukocyte adherence to microfilariae in the presence of immune serum (Chandrasekaran et al., 1980; MacKenzie, 1980; Piessens and Beldekas, 1979). A recent study demonstrates that DEC may act directly on phagocytic cells rather than on the nematode's surface (King et al., 1983).

Although studies on the mode of action of DEC have concentrated on its effects on the host immune system, studies on isolated Ascaris muscle indicate that DEC can activate cholinergic receptors on muscle membrane and thus depolarize muscle cells (Martin, 1982). The cholinergic effects of DEC are probably not related to the antifilarial action of DEC.

Although piperazine-like pharmacological effects can be demonstrated for DEC, lack of in vitro activity or in vivo activity in immunologically naive hosts against microfilariae (mf) indicates an immune system–drug interaction as the mode of action. Sasa (1976) summarized the work of Kobayashi and associates, who demonstrated five features of DEC action: (1) mf treated with DEC in vitro and injected into an uninfected cotton rat survived as well as untreated mf; (2) mf removed from a DEC-treated cotton rat survived in vitro as well as untreated mf; (3) mf transferred to a clean cotton rat, then treated with DEC 3–48 days later were not removed from circulation; (4) immune serum from a cotton rat with a patent filarial infection when transferred to a previously clean cotton rat with transferred mf allowed for a transient mf reduction with DEC treatment; and (5) full DEC activity was expressed against mf after adult worms were transplanted to an uninfected cotton rat, but only 15 or more days after transplantation.

3.7. Salicylanilides and Substituted Phenols

Rafoxanide, closantel and disophenol are active against blood-ingesting nematodes. Their mode of action appears to involve uncoupling of electron transport from ATP generation, (Vanden Bossche, 1972) (see Chapter 25). The combination of blood-ingesting lifestyle and long serum half-life seems to be required for nematode activity of these types of compounds.

3.8. Antimonials

Saz and Dunbar (1975) demonstrated an inhibition of filarial phosphofructokinase (PFK) by the antimonial, stibophen, similar to that shown by Bueding and Fisher (1966) against the enzyme from the blood fluke Schistosoma mansoni (see Chapter 21). PFK appears to be a rate-limiting enzyme in filariids and appears to be 80 times more sensitive than the host enzyme.

3.9. Arsenicals

Several mode of action studies have been done with arsenicals against adult filariids. As would be expected from an arsenical because of its ability to bind -SH groups on a protein, several inhibitory actions have been demonstrated.

3.10. Naphthalene Sulfonic Acid

Walter and co-workers (1980a,b, 1981) have demonstrated an inhibition of lactate dehydrogenase, malate dehydrogenase, malic enzyme, and protein kinase, while Jaffe (1980) showed inhibition of folate metabolism by suramin. Which of these, if any, is a primary mode of action is unknown, but each may have a role in the filaricidal activity of suramin.

3.11. Isothiocyanate

Glucose uptake and incorporation into glycogen were inhibited in L. carinii and B. pahangi after treatment of infected jirds with amoscanate (Nelson and Saz, 1984). In addition, end-product accumulation of glucose catabolism was similarly reduced.

3.12. Cyanine Dyes

Bueding (1949) demonstrated an irreversible inhibition of oxygen uptake for adult *L. carinii,* an oxygen-requiring nematode, with dithiazinine. However, *Trichuris vulpis,* an anaerobic adult nematode, was also sensitive to dithiazinine, as well as pyrivinium and styrylpyridinium, apparently due to the inhibition of glucose transport (Bueding *et al.,* 1960).

4. NEW AREAS FOR ANTINEMATODAL DRUGS

Unique physiological mechanisms of parasitic nematodes that lend themselves, at least theoretically, to attack by chemicals that would not affect the host are egg laying, egg hatching, larval development, and adult mating. Approaches for control of this nature are directed mainly at reduction in the reproductive potential of the parasite species, not cure of the infected individual. However, with new controlled-release formulations to interfere with larval functions at the time of initial infestation, such sites may serve for both types of control mechanism.

Phenothiazine salt blocks have been used for many years to "clean up" pastures by virtue of a depression in egg laying and larval development. Reversible egg laying inhibition, and inhibition of egg hatching and larval development can be demonstrated for BZs *in vitro* and/or *in vivo.* Hawkins *et al.* (1981) recently showed that a light-activated dye will inhibit egg hatch in fecal material when fed to nematode-infested sheep. If the potential to limit parasite development with these existing drugs or newly developed drugs can be realized in new formulations, a new avenue for parasite control may be expressed.

Indications of ecdysonelike and/or juvenile hormonelike molecules being involved in control of larval development are more and more frequent (see Sommerville, 1982; Davey, 1982). A more thorough understanding of the details of development may open a new area of chemotherapy aligned to the insect growth regulators; and such agents may represent a new class of inhibitors that could be enhanced by controlled-release formulations.

Sex pheromones may be important in the mating of adult parasitic nematodes (Bone *et al.,* 1978; Stringfellow, 1984). Interference with these chemical mating cues may provide another avenue for pasture sterilization.

A final area for consideration may be an alteration of the environment of the parasite within the host to make it untenable for survival. Recently, cimetidine, a H_2 blocker that stops gastric acid secretion, has been shown to decrease or eliminate gastrointestinal nematodes (Hall and Oddy, 1984). This approach may open a new direction for further development.

REFERENCES

Appurao, A. G., and Cann, J. R., 1981, A comparative study of the interaction of chlorpromazine, trifluoperazine and promethazine with mouse brain tubulin, *Mol. Pharmacol.* 19:295–301.

Ash, A., and Tucker, J., 1966, Inhibition of *Ascaris* muscles by gamma-aminobutyric acid: A possible new assay method, *Nature (Lond.)* 209:306–307.

Aubry, M., Cowell, P., Davey, M., and Shevde, S., 1970, Aspects of the pharmacology of a new anthelmintic: Pyrantel, *Br. J. Pharmacol.* 38:332–344.

Barrett, J., Cain, G. D., and Fairbairn, D., 1970, Sterols in *Ascaris lumbricoides* (Nematoda), *Macracanthorhynchus hirudinaceus* and *Moniliformis dubius* (Acanthocephala), and *Echinostoma revolutum* (Trematoda), *J. Parasitol.* 56:1004–1008.

Bone, L. W., Shorey, H. H., and Gaston, L. K., 1978, *Nippostrongylus brasiliensis:* factors influencing movements of males toward a female pheromone, *Exp. Parasitol.* 44:100–108.

Borgers, M., de Nollin, S., de Brabander, M., and Thienpoint, D., 1975, Influence of the anthelmintic mebendazole on microtubules and intracellular organelle movement in nematode intestinal cells, *Am. J. Vet. Res.* 36:1153–1166.

Brading, A., and Caldwell, P,, 1971, The resting membrane potential of the somatic muscle cells of *Ascaris lumbricoides, J. Physiol. (Lond.)* 217:624.

Broome, A. W. J., 1961, Studies on the mode of action of methyridine, *Br. J. Pharmacol. Chemother.* 17:327–338.

Bueding, E., 1949, Studies on the metabolism of the filarial worm, *Litomosoides carinii, J. Exp. Med.* 89:107–130.

Bueding, E., 1962, Comparative aspects of carbohydrate metabolism, *Fed. Proc.* 21:1039–1046.

Bueding, E., and Fisher, J., 1966, Factors affecting the inhibition of phosphofructokinase activity of *Schistosoma mansoni* by trivalent organic antimonials, *Biochem. Pharmacol.* 15:1197–1121.

Bueding, E., and Saz, H. J., 1968, Pyruvate kinase and phosphoenol pyruvate carboxylase activities of *Ascaris* muscle, *Hymenolepis diminuta*, and *Schistosoma mansoni, Comp. Biochem. Physiol.* 24:511–518.

Bueding, E., and Yale, H. W., 1951, Production of alpha-methylbutyric acid by bacteria-free *Ascaris lumbricoides, J. Biol. Chem.* 193:411–423.

Bueding, E., Kmetec, E., Swartzwelder, C., Abadie, S., and Saz, H. J., 1960, Biochemical effects of dithiazinine on the canine whipworm, *Trichuris vulpis, Biochem. Pharmacol.* 5:311–322.

Calcott, P., and Fatig, R., 1984, Inhibition of chitin metabolism by avermectin in susceptible organisms, *J. Antibiot.* 37(3):253–259.

Chandrasekaran, B., Ghirnikar, S., and Harinath, B., 1980, Effect of diethylcarbamazine and diethylcarbamazine-N-oxide on microfilariae *in vitro* in the presence of immune sera and leukocytes, *Indian J. Exp. Biol.* 18:1179–1180.

Coles, G. C., 1977, The biochemical mode of action of some modern anthelmintics, *Pestic. Sci.* 8:536–543.

Coles, G. C., East, J. M., and Jenkins, S. M., 1974, The mode of action of four anthelmintics, *Experientia* 30:1265.

Colglazier, M. L., Kates, K. C., and Enzie, F. D., 1975, Cross-resistance to other anthelmintics in an experimentally produced cambendazole-resistant strain of *Haemonchus contortus* in lambs, *J. Parasitol.* 61:778–779.

Davey, K. G., 1982, Growth and Moulting, in: *Aspects of Parasitology* (E. Merovitch, ed.), pp. 58–67, McGill University, Montreal.

DeBell, J., Del Castillo, J., and Sanchez, V., 1963, Electrophysiology of somatic muscle cells of *Ascaris lumbricoides, J. Cell Comp. Physiol.* 62:159–178.

Del Castillo, J., De Mello, W. C., and Morales, T., 1963, The physiological role of *Ascaris lumbricoides, Arch. Int. Physiol.* 71:741–757.

Del Castillo, J., De Mello, W. C., and Morales, T. A., 1964a, Mechanisms of paralyzing action of piperazine on *Ascaris* muscle, *Br. J. Pharmacol.* 22:463–477.

Del Castillo, J., De Mello, W. C., and Morales, T. A., 1964b, Inhibiting action of gamma-aminobutyric acid (GABA) on *Ascaris* muscle, *Experientia* 20:141–143.

Del Castillo, J., De Mello, W. C., and Morales, T. A., 1964c, Influence of some ions on the membrane potential *Ascaris* muscle, *J. Gen. Physiol.* 48:129–140.

Eckert, J., and Kohler, P., 1982, in: *Facts and Reflections. IV. Resistance of Parasites to Anthelmintics* (F. H. M.

Borgsteede, Sr., Aa. Henriksen, and H. J. Over, eds.), pp. 67–79, Central Veterinary Institute, Lelystad, Netherlands.

Eyre, P., 1970, Some pharmacodynamic effects of the nematocides: Methyridine, tetramisole and pyrantel, *J. Pharm. Pharmacol.* 22:26–36.

Forbes, L., 1972, Toxicological and pharmacological relations between levamisole, pyrantel and diethylcarbamazine and their significance in helminth chemotherapy, *Southeast Asian J. Trop. Med. Publ. Health* 3(2):235–241.

Frayha, G., 1974, Synthesis of certain cholesterol precursors by hydatid protoscoleces of *Echinococcus granulosus* and cysticerci of *Taenia hydatigena, Comp. Biochem. Physiol.* 49B:93–98.

Friedman, P., and Platzer, E., 1980, The molecular mechanism of action of benzimidazoles in embryos of *Ascaris suum,* in: *The Host Invader Interplay* (H. Vanden Bossche, ed.), pp. 595–604, Elsevier/North-Holland Biomedical Press, Amsterdam.

Fritz, L., Wang, C., and Gorio, A., 1979, Avermectin B_1a irreversibly blocks postsynaptic potentials at the lobster neuromuscular junction by reducing muscle membrane resistance, *Proc. Natl. Acad. Sci. U.S.A.* 76(4):2062–2066.

Hall, C. A., and Oddy, V. H., 1984, Effect of cimetidine on abomasal pH and *Haemonchus* and *Ostertagia* in sheep, *Res. Vet. Sci.* 36:316–319.

Hart, R. J., and Lee, R. M., 1966, Cholinesterase activities of various nematode parasites and their inhibition by the organophosphate anthelmintic haloxon, *Exp. Parasitol.* 60:227–231.

Hawking, F., Sewell, P., and Thurston, J. P., 1950, The mode of action of hetrazan on filarial worms, *Br. J. Pharmacol.* 3:285.

Hawkins, J. A., Healey, M. C., Heitz, J. R., and Johnson, M. H., 1981, Xanthene dyes: A new approach for control of bovine gastrointestinal nematodes, in: *Proceedings of the Twenty-Sixth American Association of Veterinary Parasitology, St. Louis, Mo.,* p. 5.

Hinman, N. D., and Cann, J. R., 1976, Reversible binding of chlorpromazine to brain tubulin, *Mol. Pharmacol.* 12:769–777.

Howells, R. E., Tinsley, J., Devaney, E., and Smith, G., 1981, The effect of 5-fluorouracil and 5-fluorocytosine on the development of the filarial nematodes *Brugia pahangi* and *Dirofilaria immitis, Acta Trop.* 38:289–304.

Hutchinson, G. W., and Probert, A. J., 1972, *Ascaris suum:* Kinetic properties, tissue specificity, and ultrastructural localization of cholinesterases, *Exp. Parasitol.* 32:109–116.

Jaffe, J. J., 1980, Filarial folate-related metabolism as a potential target for selective inhibitors, in: *The Host Invader Interplay* (H. Vanden Bossche, ed.), pp. 605–614, Elsevier/North-Holland Biomedical Press, Amsterdam.

Jamnadas, V., and Thomas, J., 1979, Metriphonate and organophosphate poisoning, *Centr. Afr. J. Med.* 25(6):130.

Johnson, C., and Stretton, A., 1980, Neural control of locomotion in *Ascaris:* Anatomy, Electrophysiology and Biochemistry, in: *Nematodes as Biological Models* (B. Zuckerman, ed.), pp. 159–196, Academic Press, New York.

Kass, J., Wang, C., Walround, J., and Stretton, A., 1980, Avermectin B_1a a paralyzing anthelmintic that affects interneurons and inhibitory motor neurons in *Ascaris, Proc. Natl. Acad. Sci. U.S.A.* 77(10):6211–6215.

Kelly, J. D., Whitlock, H. V., Gunawan, M., Griffin, D., Porter, C. J., and Martin, I. C. A., 1981, Anthelmintic efficacy of low-dose phenothiazine against strains of sheep nematodes susceptible or resistant to thiabendazole, levamisole, and morantel tartrate: Effect on patent infections, *Res. Vet. Sci.* 30:161–169.

King, C., Greene, B., and Spangnvolo, P., 1983, Diethylcarbamazine citrate, an antifilarial drug, stimulates human granulocyte adherence, *Antimicrob. Agents Chemother.* 24(3):453–456.

Kmetec, E., and Bueding, E., 1961, Succinic reduced diphosphopyridine nucleotide oxidase systems of *Ascaris* muscle, *J. Biol. Chem.* 236:584–591.

Knowles, C. O., and Casida, J. E., 1966, Mode of action of organophosphate anthelmintics. Cholinesterase inhibition in *Ascaris lumbricoides, J. Agric. Food Chem.* 14:566–572.

Kohler, P., and Saz, H. J., 1976, Demonstration and possible function NADH : NAD$^+$ transhydrogenase from *Ascaris* muscle mitochondria, *J. Biol. Chem.* 251:2217–2225.

Komuniecki, P., and Saz, H. J., 1982, The effect of levamisole on glycogen synthase and the metabolism of *Litomosoides carinii, J. Parasitol.* 68(2):221–227.

Lee, R. M., and Hodsden, M. R., 1963, Cholinesterase activity in *Haemonchus contortus* and its inhibition by organophosphorus anthelmintics, *Biochem. Pharmacol.* 12:1241–1252.

Lestan, P., 1969, The biochemistry of chitin and its occurrence in helminths, *Helminthologica* 10:29–37.

Levin, R. M., and Weiss, B. J., 1979, Selective binding of antipsychotics and other psychoactive agents to the calcium-dependent activity of cyclic nucleotide phosphodiesterase, *Pharmacol. Exp. Ther.* 208:454–459.

Lewis, J., Wu, C., Levine, J., and Berg, H., 1980, Levamisole-resistant mutants of the nematode *Caenorhabditis elegans* appear to lack pharmacological acetylcholine receptors, *Neuroscience* 5:967–989.

MacKenzie, C., 1980, Eosinophil leukocytes in filarial infections, *Trans. R. Soc. Trop. Med. Hyg. (Suppl.)* 74:51–58.

Malkin, M. F., and Camacho, R. M., 1972, The effect of thiabendazole on fumarate reductase from thiabendazole-sensitive and resistant *Haemonchus contortus, J. Parasitol.* 58:845–846.

Martin, P., and LeJambre, L., 1979, Larval paralysis as an *in vitro* assay of levamisole and morantel tartrate resistance in *Ostertagia, Vet. Sci. Commun.* 3(2):159–164.

Martin, R. J., 1982, Electrophysiological effects of piperazine and diethylcarbamazine on *Ascaris suum* somatic muscle, *Br. J. Pharmacol.* 77:255–265.

Mata, Z. S., Saz, H. J., and Pasto, D. J., 1977, 2-Methylacetoacetate reductase and possible propionyl coenzyme A condensing enzyme activity in branched chain volatile fatty acid synthesis by *Ascaris lumbricoides, J. Biol. Chem.* 252:4215–4224.

Meyer, F., and Meyer, H., 1972, Loss of fatty acid biosynthesis in flatworms, in: *Comparative Biochemistry of Parasites* (H. Vanden Bossche, ed.), pp. 383–389, Academic Press, New York.

Mikulikova, D., and Trnavskg, K., 1980, Effect of levamisole on lysosomal enzyme release from polymorphonuclear leukocytes and intracellular levels of cAMP and cGMP after phagocytosis of monosodium urate crystals, *Agents Actions* 10(4):374–377.

Nelson, N. F., and Saz, H. J., 1984, Effects of amoscanate on the utilization of glucose by *Brugia pahangi* and *Litomosoides carinii, J. Parasitol.* 70:194–196.

Olusi, S., Jessop, W., and Shoroye, A., 1979, Effects of levamisole on the immune responses of experimentally malnourished rats, *Pediatr. Res.* 13:1237–1239.

Piessens, W., and Beldekas, M., 1979, Diethylcarbamazine enhances antibody-mediated cellular adherence to *Brugia malayi* microfilariae, *Nature (Lond.)* 282:845–847.

Poffenbarger, M., and Fuller, G. M., 1977, Effects of psychotropic drugs of neurotubule assembly, *J. Neurochem.* 28:1167–1174.

Pong, S. S., and Wang, C. C., 1980, The specificity of high affinity binding of avermectin B_1a to mammalain brain, *Neuropharmacology* 19:311–317.

Pong, S. S., Wang, C. C., and Fritz, L., 1980, Studies on the mechanism of action of avermectin B_1a: Stimulation of release of gamma-aminobutyric acid from brain synaptosomes, *J. Neurochem.* 34(2):351–358.

Prichard, R. K., 1970, Mode of action of the anthelmintic thiabendazole in *Haemonchus contortus, Nature (Lond.)* 228:684–685.

Prichard, R. K., 1973, The fumarate reductase reaction of *Haemonchus contortus* and the mode of action of some anthelmintics, *Int. J. Parasitol.* 3:409–417.

Prichard, R. K., 1978, Anthelmintics, *Course Vet. Aust.* 39:421–463.

Rew, R. S., 1978, Mode of action of common anthelmintics, *J. Vet. Pharmacol. Ther.* 1:183–198.

Rew, R. S., and Saz, H. J., 1974, Enzyme localization in the anaerobic mitochondria of *Ascaris lumbricoides, J. Cell Biol.* 63:125–135.

Rew, R. S., and Saz, H. J., 1977, The carbohydrate metabolism of *Brugia pahangi* microfilariae, *J. Parasitol.* 63:123–129.

Romanowski, R. D., Rhoads, M. L., Colglazier, M. L., and Kates, K. C., 1975, Effect of cambendazole, thiabendazole, and levamisole on fumarate reductase in cambendazole-resistant and sensitive strains of *Haemonchus contortus, J. Parasitol.* 61:777–778.

Sasa, M., 1976, Experimental chemotherapy, in: *Human Filariasis,* pp. 747–753, University of Tokyo Press, Tokyo.

Saz, H. J., 1970, Comparative energy metabolisms of some parasitic helminths, *J. Parasitol.* 56:634–642.

Saz, H. J., and Hubbard, J. A., 1957, The oxidative decarboxylation of malate by *Ascaris lumbricoides, J. Biol. Chem.* 225:921–933.

Saz, H. J., and Dunbar, G., 1975, The effect of stibophen on phosphofructokinases and aldolases of adult filariids, *J. Parasitol.* 61:794–801.

Saz, H. J., and Bueding, E., 1966, Relationships between anthelmintic effects and biochemical and physiological mechanisms, *Pharmacol. Rev.* 18:871–894.

Saz, H. J., and Lescure, O. L., 1969, The functions of phosphoenol pyruvate carboxykinase and malic enzyme in the anaerobic formation of succinate by *Ascaris lumbricoides, Comp. Biochem. Physiol.* 30:49–60.

Saz, H. J., and Pietrzak, S. M., 1980, Phosphorylation associated with succinate decarboxylation to propionate in *Ascaris* mitochondria, *Arch. Biochem. Biophys.* 202:388–395.

Saz, H. J., and Vidrine, A., 1959, The mechanism of formation of succinate and propionate by *Ascaris lumbricoides* muscle, *J. Biol. Chem.* 234:2001–2005.

Saz, H. J., and Weil, A., 1960, The mechanism of the formation of alpha-methylbutyrate from carbohydrate by *Ascaris lumbricoides* muscle, *J. Biol. Chem.* 235:914–918.

Seebeck, T., and Gehr, P., 1983, Trypanocidal action of neuroleptic phenothiazines in *Trypanosoma brucei, Mol. Biochem. Parasitol.* 9:197–208.

Seeman, P., 1981, Brain dopamine receptors, *Pharmacol. Rev.* 32:229–313.

Seidman, I., and Entner, N., 1961, Oxidative enzymes and their role in phosphorylation in sarcosomes of adult *Ascaris lumbricoides, J. Biol. Chem.* 236:915–919.

Sharpe, M. J., 1980, Changes in adenylate energy charge of *Nematospiroides dubius* and *Trichostrongylus colubriformis* paralyzed by levamisole *in vivo, Parasitology* 81:593–601.

Sommerville, R. I., 1982, The mechanics of moulting in nematodes, in: *Aspects of Parasitology* (E. Meerovitch, ed.), pp. 407–433, McGill University, Montreal.

Stringfellow, F., 1984, A unique Bioassay: *Haemonchus contortus* adult spicule sheaths attract conspecific larvae, *Proc. Helminthol. Soc.* 51:163–165.

Vanden Bossche, H., 1972, Studies on the phosphorylation in *Ascaris* mitochondria, in: *Comparative Biochemistry of Parasites* (H. Vanden Bossche, ed.), pp. 455–469, Academic Press, New York.

Vanden Bossche, H., and de Nollin, S., 1973, Effects of mebendazole on the absorption of low molecular weight nutrients by *Ascaris suum, Int. J. Parasitol.* 3:401–407.

Vanden Bossche, H., and Janssen, P., 1967, The biochemical mechanism of action of the anthelmintic drug tetramisole, *Life Sci.* 6:1781–1792.

Van Nueten, J., 1972, Pharmacological Aspects of Tetramisole, in: *Comparative Biochemistry of Parasitology* (H. Vanden Bossche, ed.), pp. 101–116, Academic Press, New York.

Walter, R. D., and Schulz-Key, H., 1980a, Interaction of suramin with protein kinase I from *Onchocerca volvulus,* in: *The Host Invader Interplay* (H. Vanden Bossche, ed.), pp. 709–712, Elsevier/North-Holland Biomedical Press, Amsterdam.

Walter, R. D., and Schulz-Key, H., 1980b, *Onchocerca volvulus:* Effect of suramin on lactate dehydrogenase and malate dehydrogenase, *Tropenmed. Parasitol.* 31:55–58.

Walter, R. D., and Albiez, E. J., 1981, Inhibition of NADP-linked malic enzyme from *Onchocerca volvulus* and *Dirofilaria immitis* by suramin, *Mol. Biochem. Parasitol.* 4:53–60.

Wang, E. J., and Saz, H. J., 1974, Comparative biochemical studies of *Litomosoides carninii, Dipetalonema viteae, Brugia pahangi* adults, *J. Parasitol.* 60:316–321.

Ward, C. W., and Fairbairn, D., 1970, Enzymes of beta-oxidation and the tricarboxylic acid cycle in adult *Hymenolepis diminuta* and *Ascaris lumbricoides, J. Parasitol.* 56:1009–1012.

Wright, D., Birtle, A., and Roberts, I., 1984, Triphasic locomotor response of a Plant parasitic nematode to avermectin: Inhibition by the GABA antagonists bicuculline and picrotoxin, *Parasitology* **88**:375–382.

Zuckerman, B. (ed.), 1980, *Nematodes as Biological Models, Behavioral and Developmental Models,* Vol. 1. Academic Press, New York, 305 pp.

17

Drug Resistance in Nematodes

PETER J. WALLER and ROGER K. PRICHARD

1. INTRODUCTION

Drug resistance in nematodes is almost solely confined to the strongylid parasites of the alimentary tract of grazing livestock. Few reports have been made on the resistance in plant-parasitic nematodes (Foot, 1980), and none for nematode parasites of man. Unlike drug resistance in bacteria, protozoa, and arthropods, resistance in nematodes to anthelmintics has been slow to develop and is patchy in worldwide distribution. However, this does not constitute grounds for complacency. It is not necessary for anthelmintic resistance to have reached a high level to be a serious problem. Evidence that it has increased from negligibly small levels and that it exists in two of the three widely used broad-spectrum drug groups means it would be foolhardy to assume that its prevalence and thus importance will not escalate, unless effective countermeasures are undertaken.

One of the major limitations to increasing productivity following intensification of the grazing livestock industries during the past three decades has been the greater range and severity of animal health problems, of which diseases caused by nematode parasites were prominent. The pharmaceutical industry met this challenge with the development of new "wonder drugs" that included the modern broad-spectrum anthelmintics. They were cheap compared with other agricultural inputs, and their very wide range of high-level efficiency fostered the view that eradication of the effects of nematode infection on animal production, if not of the parasites themselves, could be achieved by frequent treatment. The timing of treatment was also often guided by considerations of convenience rather than based on epidemiological principles. This approach led to considerable inefficiency and overuse of anthelmintics; it is not surprising that resistant nematode populations have now been selected.

PETER J. WALLER • McMaster Laboratory, CSIRO, Division of Animal Health, Glebe, New South Wales 2037, Australia. ROGER K. PRICHARD • Institute of Parasitology, McGill University, Macdonald College, Ste. Anne-de-Bellevue, Quebec H9X 1CO, Canada.

Differences between countries, or regions, in the extent and magnitude of anthelmintic resistance are largely the result of accident rather than design. This may be attributed to (1) differences in the relative importance of nematode species and their impact on health and productivity, (2) differences in management and ways in which anthelmintics have been used, and (3) the extent to which resistance has been investigated. However, it is vital that anthelmintic resistance be recognized as a problem of increasing importance that poses a serious threat to profitable livestock production in the future. Only by understanding and counteracting the factors most likely to enhance its selection will resistance be prevented from increasing to the point of widespread control failure such as that which has occurred for certain arthropod pests.

2. DETECTION OF RESISTANCE

The failure of animals to respond to anthelmintic treatment should not be taken to indicate nematode resistance, without further investigation. Lack of response may be attributable to other causes, such as faulty administration, underdosing, incorrect choice of anthelmintic, or rapid reinfection or resumption of development of relatively drug-tolerant hypobiotic stages of the parasite. Malnutrition or concurrent disease conditions may also lead to reduced anthelmintic efficacy. In making a diagnosis of resistance, and before any testing is carried out, a complete clinical history should be obtained, in order to eliminate other causes of anthelmintic failure. Accurate diagnosis of resistance requires specific testing.

2.1. Indirect Methods

Two approaches commonly employed in the detection of resistance are the fecal egg-count depression test and *in vitro* assays. Both have their advantages and disadvantages, but neither provides totally unequivocal evidence of the presence or absence of resistance.

2.1.1. Fecal Egg-Count Depression Test

Nematode egg counts in the feces of groups of animals are assessed both before and 5–10 days after treatment. The fecal egg-count depression (FECD) test does not require highly trained personnel, expensive resources, or sophisticated equipment and facilities. It is therefore a suitable method for survey investigations when all available drugs can be readily compared, at different dose rates and using different routes of administration. Failure of an anthelmintic to reduce egg counts considerably indicates resistance, but in mixed infections only one species may be resistant. Therefore, in addition to this test, infective larvae derived from pre- and post-treatment fecal cultures must be differentiated. If egg counts are low, this method may fail to detect resistance. Also, for some species, particularly *Ostertagia* spp., there is not always a direct correlation between egg production and numbers of worms present. Egg counts will not detect the presence of immature worms that survive treatment, develop, and contribute to the post-treatment egg count. In addition, worm egg counts may only be temporarily suppressed with no reduction in worm numbers; egg counts should therefore be repeated 10–14 days after treatment.

Care should also be taken when interpreting resistance of *Ostertagia* spp. in sheep to levamisole on the basis of post-treatment fecal egg counts. Waller *et al.* (1983) obtained persistent positive *Ostertagia* spp. egg counts following repeated treatment with this drug but, when isolated and tested *in vivo*, the strain was found to be fully susceptible.

2.1.2. In Vitro Assays

Egg-hatch assays have been developed to discriminate between resistant and susceptible strains for both the benzimidazoles (Le Jambre, 1976; Coles and Simpkin, 1977) and levamisole (Dobson *et al.*, 1985), based on differences in the proportion of eggs that fail to hatch in solutions of increasing concentration of drug. The test for benzimidazoles exploits the ovicidal properties of these drugs; commonly used in research laboratories, it has been adapted for survey investigations (Whitlock *et al.*, 1980*b;* N. J. Campbell, personal communication). The levamisole test is based on the differences in the rate of return from paralysis of unhatched larvae in resistant and susceptible strains. Because the index of response is the occurrence of hatching, this test overcomes the problems of the reversible nature of paralysis, the subjectivity in judging whether or not a larva is paralyzed, and the parabolic response–dose relationship—all associated with the infective larval motility test described by Martin and Le Jambre (1979).

These methods are fast, inexpensive, and repeatable if only a single species is involved. They also have the advantage of greater sensitivity in detecting very low levels of resistance than is possible with the FECD test. Such differences between the two techniques need to be recognized, particularly when assessing results of field surveys for resistance. For example, in New Zealand, a survey by Kettle *et al.* (1981, 1982), involving 90 farms on both islands using the FECD method, detected only two genuine cases of benzimidazole resistance, whereas a survey based on egg-hatch (Kemp and Smith, 1982) of 52 farms on the North Island estimated benzimidazole resistance to be present on 20% of properties. These results indicate that benzimidazole resistance was not causing control failures at the time of investigation; however, resistance genes were present in a significant proportion of properties, and continued intensive use of benzimidazole anthelmintics would be likely to select rapidly for high level resistance.

However, *in vitro* tests require greater attention to technical detail and better facilities than do FECD tests; they are also susceptible to false-positive results. Variations in resistance parameters (e.g., EC_{50}, EC_{95}, regression parameters) have been reported between and even within laboratories following tests using the same parasite isolate (Martin *et al.*, 1981; Waller *et al.*, 1983). To overcome this problem, it is therefore important for laboratories carrying out these tests to maintain appropriate reference strains, particularly those known to be anthelmintic susceptible, so that comparisons can be made in parallel with the suspected resistant lines and resistance ratios (EC_{50} resistant strain/EC_{50} susceptible strain) can be calculated. Ideally, these susceptible strains should be derived from a common source and thus act as international reference strains.

2.2. Direct Methods

The most definite method of assessing anthelmintic efficacy, and thus resistance, is by a controlled test (Turton and Clark, 1974; Powers et al., 1982). Adult worm burdens are compared between untreated and treated groups of animals artificially infected with susceptible or resistant isolates of nematodes. A more informative test is obtained if serial dose rates are used enabling dose—response parameters to be calculated and then used for predictive purposes or to monitor changes in response with time. As these in vivo tests are very expensive in terms of labor and animals required, their applicability is restricted.

3. DEVELOPMENT OF ANTHELMINTIC RESISTANCE IN THE FIELD

Resistance has been detected most commonly among the trichostrongylid nematodes of sheep and goats (reviewed by Donald 1983a; Kelly and Hall, 1979; Prichard et al., 1980). Regions considered to have a serious problem are usually those in which Haemonchus contortus is endemic. Other ubiquitous sheep and goat parasites commonly reported as showing resistance, i.e., Trichostrongylus and Ostertagia spp., are not as pathogenic to all classes of stock as H. contortus, and outbreaks of clinical parasitism due to drug-resistant worms have been less common. Nevertheless, subclinical production loss resulting from ineffective anthelmintic treatment against resistant Trichostrongylus and Ostertagia spp. as well as costs in terms of wasted time and labor are likely to be substantial.

Resistance evolved in step with the commercial release of the broad-spectrum anthelmintics; it thereby appeared in chronological sequence to phenothiazine, the benzimidazoles, and levamisole and morantel tartrate. Resistance has also been reported to phenothiazine and the benzimidazoles in the cyathastome parasites of horses (reviewed by Donald, 1983a), but there has been no unequivocal evidence of anthelmintic resistance in nematode parasites of cattle.

Phenothiazine has virtually disappeared from the marketplace because the newer drugs are more efficacious, safer, and easier to use. They have been grouped on the basis of their apparent modes of action, structure, and efficacy against resistant nematode populations (Prichard et al., 1980) and are commonly referred to as group 1 (the benzimidazoles and probenzimidazoles) and group 2 (levamisole and morantel tartrate). Once resistance has been recorded in a parasite population to one anthelmintic in either group, resistance to all others in the same group, termed side resistance, tends to occur rapidly. There have been only a few published reports of multiple resistance (resistance across anthelmintic groups) (Sangster et al., 1979; Green et al., 1981; Hall et al.,

1981*b*). However, recent surveys, particularly of goat farms, in Australasia indicate that this form of resistance is increasing at an alarming rate (Green *et al.*, 1982; Anonymous, 1983; Kettle *et al.*, 1983).

The first reports of resistance were made largely on farms involved in parasitological research where anthelmintics were often used intensively, and the effects of treatment were monitored either indirectly by fecal egg counts or directly by necropsy of animals following treatment (reviewed by Kelly and Hall, 1979; Prichard *et al.*, 1980; Donald, 1983*a*). Such methods could detect incipient resistance in parasite populations that would otherwise go unnoticed. These cases were often considered no more than parasitological curiosities, with their potential significance overlooked. Meantime, on commercial properties, particularly in *H. contortus*-endemic areas in Australia, resistance was not diagnosed, and continued use of anthelmintics from the same group increased the frequency of resistant individuals until ultimately there were major failures in control (Blanch, 1984). The current status of anthelmintic resistance is described in Sections 3.1–3.5.

3.1. Australia

The greatest single problem involves *Haemonchus contortus* resistance against the benzimidazole anthelmintics. Surveys on sheep properties on the Northern Tablelands of New South Wales (Webb *et al.*, 1979), southeastern Victoria (N. J. Campbell, personal communication), and southwest Western Australia (G. C. de Chaneet, personal communication) and on goat farms on the central and northern coast of New South Wales (Anonymous, 1983) and southern Queensland (Green *et al.*, 1982) show that resistance to benzimidazoles is widespread, at a high level, and likely to extend over the entire geographic range of this parasite. Resistance to levamisole and morantel tartrate in *H. contortus* was slow to evolve under field conditions, with the first report of failure of these two anthelmintics, as well as to thiabendazole, made by Green *et al.* (1981). However, multiple resistance in *H. contortus* now seems to be a common occurrence on goat farms (Green *et al.*, 1982; Anonymous, 1983; N. J. Campbell, personal communication).

Similar to *H. contortus*, benzimidazole resistance in *Ostertagia* and *Trichostrongylus* spp. is both widespread and common (Anonymous, 1983; N. J. Campbell, personal communication; G. C. de Chaneet, personal communication). By contrast, early reports of resistance to levamisole and morantel tartrate were just as frequent as those to the benzimidazoles (for review, see Donald, 1983*a*). Multiple resistance has also been recorded for these two species from varying localities (Sangster *et al.*, 1979; Hall *et al.*, 1981*b*; R. J. Dobson, A. D. Donald, and P. J. Waller, unpublished observations).

A survey of anthelmintic resistance in horse parasites (Kelly *et al.*, 1981*b*) showed a close association between incidence of resistance in small strongyles and frequent exclusive use of benzimidazoles. Those farms that used these drugs less often than every 3 months, or in combination with piperazine, or alternated drugs with different modes of action had no problem with resistance.

3.2. New Zealand

No country has been surveyed for anthelmintic resistance as comprehensively as New Zealand. These surveys showed that on a significant number of sheep properties, low-level benzimidazole resistance was present in *Haemonchus contortus* and/or *Trichostrongylus* spp. populations (Kemp and Smith, 1982) but unlikely to cause treatment failure (Kettle *et al.*, 1981). However, more recent reports indicate that the magnitude of the problem is increasing, with control failures attributed to highly resistant *Ostertagia* spp. (Hughes and Seifert, 1983) in an intensive lamb-producing system, and one field report of high-level benzimidazole resistance in *Nematodirus* spp. (Middleburg and McKenna, 1983). This is an addition to the range of important helminth pathogens showing benzimidazole resistance.

In common with the goat industry in Australia, goat farmers are confronted with a major problem of resistance in *H. contortus*, *Trichostrongylus* spp., and *Ostertagia* spp. (Kettle *et al.*, 1983). As many as 78% of farms surveyed by the FECD test had problems with resistance, with approximately one-half showing resistance to both group 1 and group 2 anthelmintics.

3.3. North America

Despite the fact that the initial reports of anthelmintic resistance were made in the United States, there have been no published surveys on the extent and level of resistance in sheep and goat flocks. These early reports of resistance, first to phenothiazine and then to thiabendazole in Kentucky by Drudge and co-workers and by Colglazier and associates in Maryland to thiabendazole, were confined exclusively to *Haemonchus contortus* on research farms in these localities (for review, see Donald, 1983*a*).

The Kentucky workers were also the first to report benzimidazole resistance in the small strongyles of horses (Drudge and Lyons, 1965). Further studies (Drudge *et al.*, 1979) established that resistance occurred in five species of small strongyles, whereas 19 others were susceptible, as were the large strongyles (*Strongylus vulgaris* and *S. edentatus*). On the basis of published reports and veterinary practitioner feedback, Herd *et al.* (1981) consider horses on many farms in the United States to be infected with resistant populations of strongyles. Benzimidazole resistance in small strongyles of horses has also been reported in Canada (Slocombe and Cote, 1977).

The reduced efficacy of levamisole against *Ostertagia ostertagi* infections in cattle, also found by the Kentucky workers (Lyons *et al.*, 1981), was interpreted as possibly due to resistance, making this the first report in cattle parasites. However, doubts arise as to whether this is true, because only small numbers of cattle, with low worm burdens, were used in their trial.

3.4. Britain

Two surveys indicate low levels of resistance exist in nematode parasites of sheep. First, Britt (1982) reported a reduced efficacy of benzimidazoles on a small number of farms, and from one of these he isolated a thiabendazole-resistant strain of *Ostertagia circumcincta*. Second, a survey of 52 farms in southeast England showed *Haemonchus contortus* populations in seven flocks to have a variable resistance to thiabendazole (Cawthorne and Cheong, 1984). Benzimidazole resistance has also been reported in small strongyles of horses (Round *et al.*, 1974).

3.5. Other Countries

To our knowledge, no surveys of anthelmintic resistance have been published in other countries. Isolated reports of resistance have been made elsewhere, establishing at least the ubiquitous, albeit patchy, distribution of resistant parasite populations. For example, benzimidazole resistance in *Haemonchus contortus* has been reported in Switzerland (Jordi, 1980) and in the Netherlands (Boersema *et al.*, 1982). In common with New Zealand and Britain, most of the land used for grazing in Europe has a climate normally very favorable for the survival of free-living stages on pasture that will not be subjected to anthelmintic selection. This may largely account for the lower incidence of resistance as compared with Australia where, except in *H. contortus*-endemic areas, the frequency of anthelmintic usage is unlikely to be greater.

There are few reports of resistance in South America and Africa, which have similar climate, nematode parasite problems, and animal management practices to those of Australia. Reports have been made of thiabendazole resistance (Santos and Franco, 1967) and levamisole resistance (Santiago *et al.*, 1978) in *H. contortus* in Brazil. Benzimidazole resistance in this species has also been found in South Africa by Berger (1975) and van Wyck and Gerber (1980). The latter investigators comment that little work has been done on anthelmintic resistance in South Africa, and the problem is likely to be much more common than would appear from published reports.

4. LABORATORY STUDIES ON ANTHELMINTIC RESISTANCE

Apart from field surveys, studies on anthelmintic resistance have largely been confined to laboratory experiments. These results are often extrapolated to the field to explain the reason for existing resistance problems or the likely course of events if certain control programs are adopted. Although laboratory experiments are of value in obtaining precise information about certain qualitative aspects of resistance, with the added virtue of providing relatively prompt results, there is a danger that certain conclusions, either unsupported or backed by tenuous evidence, will become established as dogma.

For example, it is now generally accepted that rapid alternation between anthelmintic groups hastens the selection for multiple resistance by exposing worms to a range of drugs within the same generation. This warning was based largely on the studies by Le Jambre and co-workers. Donald and Waller (1982) did not find their evidence convincing, however. In selection studies using thiabendazole, morantel tartrate, and levamisole, either separately or in combination against different lines of *Haemonchus contortus* (Le Jambre *et al.*, 1976), *Ostertagia circumcincta* (Le Jambre *et al.*,

Table 1. Percentage Efficiency of Anthelmintics at Recommended Dose Rate against Laboratory-Selected Parasite Lines[a,b]

Parasite species	Anthelmintic(s) used in selection	Percentage efficiency at recommended dose rate			References
		TBZ[a]	MT[a]	LEV[a]	
Haemonchus con-	TBZ	0	>99	>99	Le Jambre et al. (1976)
tortus	TBZ + MT[b] (3rd gen.)	—	75	—	
	TBZ + MT[b] (4th gen.)	9	90	>99	
	Unselected (Field)	24.5	>99	>99	
Ostertagia cir-	TBZ	9.5	—	—	Le Jambre et al. (1977)
cumcincta	LEV	—	—	97.3	
	MT	—	98.4	—	
	0	99.9	99.9	99.9	
	TBZ + LEV + MT[c] (Field)	87	97.9	98.7	
Ostertagia cir-	TBZ	12.5	—	—	Le Jambre et al. (1978a)
cumcincta	LEV	—	—	95.4	
	MT	—	98.1	—	
	TBZ + MT + LEV[c]	23	94.4	86.2	
	0	99.9	99.9	99.3	
Trichostrongylus	TBZ	60.3	—	—	Le Jambre et al. (1978b)
colubriformis	MT	—	67.4	99.9	
	TBZ + MT[b]	18.2	66.5	99.9	
	0	50.3	76.5	99.9	

[a]Abbreviations: LEV, levamisole; MT, morantel tartrate; TBZ, thiabendazole.
[b]TBZ + MT: both drugs used in each generation.
[c]TBZ + LEV + MT: three drugs used in each generation.

1977, 1978a), and *Trichostrongylus colubriformis* (Le Jambre et al., 1978b), and in which pronounced resistance to thiabendazole existed prior to the commencement of selection, only very slight resistance developed to levamisole and morantel (see Table I). In contrast, the results of field selection (Le Jambre et al., 1977) suggest the opposite. Alternation every 7–10 days among thiabendazole, morantel tartrate, and levamisole for 3 years resulted in an *Ostertagia* population remaining highly susceptible to both morantel tartrate and levamisole, with only a marginal loss of efficiency of thiabendazole (see Table I). This observation is supported by the findings of Donald et al. (1980), where frequent alternation of drenches was used to produce worm-free lambs on pasture. The standard procedure used for 8 years was to give thiabendazole and levamisole at twice recommended dose rate alternately every 2 weeks. Periodic fecal egg counts and slaughter of lambs showed only negligible numbers of parasites.

From a model of pesticide resistance, Comins (1977) concluded that the use of two compounds within the same generation may be a good general policy. This is because, depending on the genetic system involved, selection for multiple resistance will be no faster, and in some cases delayed, than if one compound is used until it fails before switching to the other. In the management of acaricide resistance in the cattle tick, *Boophilus microplus*, Sutherst and Comins (1979) suggest the use of mixtures of acaricides with different modes of action to delay resistance. If this is combined with fewer treatments, the risk of successful multiple-resistance alleles will be very small. Similar considerations may apply to the use of anthelmintics, particularly if they are given at high dose rates to ensure the death of heterozygous resistant individuals.

Another commonly held belief is that anthelmintic-resistant genotypes exhibit superior fitness as compared with susceptible genotypes. This view was initially expressed by Kelly *et al.* (1978), who compared the physiological characteristics of various strains of *H. contortus*. However, there are a number of inconsistencies in their data that deserve closer examination. First, in a preliminary experiment, superior infectivity was recorded for the resistant field (48%) and laboratory-selected (70%) lines than for the McMaster-susceptible line (19%). This is based on the mean worm counts of three sheep per line and is abnormally low for the susceptible isolate, which routinely shows 60–80% establishment in previously worm-free lambs. In addition, these workers should have paid heed to their own previously published data for the susceptible isolate (Kelly *et al.*, 1977), in which a 77% establishment rate was recorded. Effects on the host were compared between a TBZ laboratory-selected strain and another recently isolated from the field that was considered "susceptible" to TBZ; however, it had a LD_{50} of 64 mg/kg, approximately 1.5 times the recommended dose rate of the drug (Kelly *et al.*, 1978). The laboratory-passaged line was shown to be superior in causing the greatest effects on the parameters measured; however, the comparison was not between a resistant and susceptible line but between two lines exhibiting different levels of resistance. Based on data of the above experiment, Kelly and Hall (1979) advanced the proposition that there is a direct correlation between the degree of anthelmintic resistance and infectivity and pathogenicity, i.e., the more resistant the strain, the greater its infectivity and effects on the host. Subsequent papers (Hall *et al.*, 1981a; Kelly *et al.*, 1981a) claim support for the proposal, showing higher establishment rates in the most resistant lines. However, a comprehensive examination of trials conducted by Hall and Kelly and co-workers shows the evidence to be far less convincing (see Table II). Apparently there is substantial variation in the establishment of each isolate, irrespective of resistance status. This may be partly attributed to the small group sizes (three sheep/group) and comparative interactions between *H. contortus* and *O. circumcincta* when both species are given to the same animal. Also, in direct conflict with the claim of increased pathogenicity of resistant lines, a study that also involved these workers (Prichard *et al.*, 1978) demonstrated that susceptible *H. contortus* and *T. colubriformis* caused deaths in one-third of the sheep and clinical parasitism in the remainder, whereas resistant worms cultured similarly, of the same age prior to infection, and administered at the same dose rate, caused no obvious clinical signs.

4.1. Limitations of Laboratory Studies

Before embarking on any laboratory studies it is prudent to consider their limitations and departures from conditions that exist in the field. These include small gene pool, anthelmintic dose rates, and the use of discrete generations.

Table II. Degree of Infectivity of Different Strains of Benzimidazole-Resistant and -Susceptible Parasites

Strain	Resistance status	Percentage establishment	Reference
Haemonchus contortus			
McMaster	Susceptible	13–20	Kelly *et al.* (1981*a*)
		19	Kelly *et al.* (1978)
		77	Kelly *et al.* (1977)
		60–80	Laboratory trials[c]
VRSG	Resistant	10	Gunawan *et al.* (1979)
		17	Hall *et al.* (1978)
		9[a]; 29[b]	Hall *et al.* (1981*a*)
		14–25	Kelly *et al.* (1981*a*)
		44	Hogarth-Scott *et al.* (1976)
		48	Kelly *et al.* (1977)
		48	Hall *et al.* (1981*c*)
		70	Kelly *et al.* (1978)
Ostertagia circumcincta			
McMaster	Susceptible	65–70	Laboratory trials[c]
VRSG	Susceptible	19–35	Kelly *et al.* (1981*a*)
PF5	Resistant	13–20	Sangster *et al.* (1980)
		30	Whitlock *et al.* (1980*a*)
		22–24	Kelly *et al.* (1981*a*)
Glenfield	Resistant	23[a]; 38[b]	Hall *et al.* (1981*a*)
Trichostrongylus colubriformis			
McMaster	Susceptible	49–57	Kelly *et al.* (1981*a*)
		87	Kelly *et al.* (1977)
		65–70	Laboratory trials[c]
PF4	Resistant	28–30	Sangster *et al.* (1980)
		28	Whitlock *et al.* (1980*a*)
		57–66	Kelly *et al.* (1981*a*)
VRSG	Resistant	44	Kelly *et al.* (1977)
		54	Gunawan *et al.* (1979)
		60	Hall *et al.* (1978)
		86	Hogarth-Scott *et al.* (1976)

[a]Generation 1 establishment.
[b]Generation 5 establishment.
[c]Percentage establishment expected for single infections given to young worm-free sheep.

4.1.1. Small Gene Pool

In studies on insecticide resistance in arthropods, Brown and Pal (1971) recognized that small populations will have limited potential for selection for resistance, and therefore laboratory strains often fail to respond to selection as strongly as field strains. Consequently, when selection in the laboratory leads to the development of resistance, it can be concluded that the parent strain in the field has the potential to develop resistance. Little can be concluded, however, if a laboratory selected strain fails to develop resistance. Furthermore, the absolute or relative rates of the development of resistance in the field cannot be predicted on the basis of laboratory selection.

4.1.2. Anthelmintic Dose Rates

Laboratory studies aimed at selecting for resistance from an apparently susceptible population usually involve discriminating dose rates, which are usually much less than the recommended dose rate, and would therefore greatly increase the chance of heterozygotes surviving. In addition, dose rates are carefully controlled and administered, often intraruminally, according to individual sheep weights, whereas in the field the flock or herd is treated as a whole, with dose rates generally based on average animal weight.

In relation to these differences between field and laboratory investigations, the studies by McKenzie *et al.* (1980) and Whitten *et al.* (1980) on the development of insecticide resistance in the Australian sheep blowfly, *Lucilia cuprina,* are of interest. These investigators showed that under field conditions, the large variation that invariably occurs in the level of insecticide dose to which individuals are exposed leads to selection for resistance involving single, major allelic substitutions, whereas in laboratory studies on *L. cuprina* a uniform dose is applied favoring individuals whose polygenic makeup is above the threshold for mortality of the major genotypes. Therefore, they argue, laboratory selection discriminates in favor of individuals whose polygenic nature makes them slightly more resistant than average, conditions that would rarely exist in the field. Such principles may well apply to the genetics of selection for anthelmintic resistance in the laboratory.

4.1.3. The Use of Discrete Generations

In laboratory studies, each generation is invariably composed entirely of progeny derived from survivors of anthelmintic treatment of the previous generation. In the field, however, substantial overlapping of generations is common because of the iteroparity of adult female nematodes and prolonged survival of free-living stages on pasture. In addition, the progeny of survivors of an anthelmintic treatment have to contend with environmental conditions on pasture before being acquired by a host of variable nematode resistance status and before they can contribute to the evolution for drug resistance by passing their resistance alleles on to the next generation.

In an attempt to study the effect of environmental factors on the rate of development of resistance in the laboratory, Martin *et al.* (1981) examined the effect of refugia (where a certain proportion of the population escapes exposure to the drug) on the development of benzimidazole resistance in *H. contortus.* This study was based on the model of Georghiou and Taylor (1977) for insecticide resistance. Although the delay in the development of resistance showed direct correlation with the proportion of the population in refugia, all treatments responded faster than predicted. However, the design did not permit the effects of selection, and of the proportion in refugia initially, to influence the rate of infection in the next generation. In addition, the effects of generation overlap that usually occur under field conditions were not considered.

Although the principles of selection and counterselection within and between different classes of anthelmintics can be tested more rapidly in the laboratory, it is vital that hypotheses resulting from these studies be validated under field conditions where other natural selective agencies can be expressed with anthelmintic selection, as there are likely to be complex interactions between them.

5. FIELD STUDIES ON ANTHELMINTIC RESISTANCE

Apart from being expensive and slow to yield results, field studies have been criticized for lacking general applicability. This is because the parasite populations involved may simply be ecotypes with limited distribution, so that results do not necessarily apply to other populations of the same species unless verified by similar studies in widely separated localities. Nevertheless, the genetic diversity of parasite populations exposed to field selection is likely to be much greater than in isolates used in laboratory studies, and the complexities of the natural host–parasite–environment relationship, which are impossible to simulate in the laboratory, are allowed to operate.

Although nematodes possess the necessary genetic variability to develop resistance to anthelmintics, the evolution of such resistance in the field has been slow compared with insecticide resistance in certain arthropod pests. This may be partly attributed to the fact that animals are often treated in response to clinical signs of infection, at which point larval availability on pasture is usually very high. Therefore, the major portion of the parasite biomass escapes anthelmintic selection, estimated to be as high as 97% during a haemonchosis outbreak in sheep (Le Jambre, 1978).

The intensity of anthelmintic selection also depends on the opportunity of the free-living stages that escaped anthelmintic exposure to reproduce, compared with the opportunity available to resistant parasitic stages that actually survived treatment. This in turn is determined by the interval between treatments relative to the prepatent period of the parasite, the rate of development and transmission of free-living stages, and the survival time of the parasitic stages in the host (Donald, 1983b).

As the interval between anthelmintic treatment is reduced to approach the prepatent period (approximately 3 weeks for most GI nematodes), selection pressure increases greatly. This is because susceptible worms would be removed every time providing little, if any, contribution to the next generation, while permitting the resistant worms to remain *in situ*, continuing to reproduce. This was confirmed in a grazing experiment by Martin *et al.* (1982), in which the level of benzimidazole resistance that developed in *Ostertagia* spp. in sheep was shown to be proportional to the frequency of treatment.

On the other hand, the effects of anthelmintic selection may be retarded by conditions that extend the parasite generation interval. For example, during periods of adverse environmental conditions such as cold winters or hot, dry summers, any preferential contamination of pasture by drug-resistant worms will yield negligible numbers of infective larvae while favoring the survival of those already present on pasture that had developed at an earlier, but more favorable, time. Such conditions existed during the course of a field experiment described by Donald *et al.* (1980) and Waller *et al.* (1983); the lack of change in resistance levels over a 5-month period in *Ostertagia* spp. populations exposed to monthly anthelmintic treatment was attributed to the cold, dry winter at the experimental site. There is clearly a need to consider the rate of change in the frequency of resistant individuals among the infective larval population, which may at times lag well behind the rate of change of resistance of parasitic stages within the host. Seasonal hypobiosis and host-induced arrested development also extend the parasite generation interval and may be expected to retard the rate of development of anthelmintic resistance.

In addition, factors that determine the regulation of parasite populations within the host are likely to have an important bearing on the development of resistance. For worm populations regulated by a rapid, density-dependent turnover of adults, as described by Michel (1963, 1969) for *Ostertagia ostertagi*, the importance of survivors of an anthelmintic treatment is slight, as their contribution to the next generation is minimal. By contrast, *Trichostrongylus* spp. populations seem to be regulated by an accumulation of adult worms limited first by a reduction in the establishment of incoming larvae (reviewed by Donald and Waller, 1982). For a variable period after establishment has virtually ceased there is no loss of adults; any survivors of a previous anthelmintic treatment would have a disproportionately high contribution to the development of resistance.

These factors clearly illustrate the complexities of the natural host–helminth parasite relationship that need to be considered in the evolution of anthelmintic resistance. They also highlight the need for care in extrapolating findings of laboratory studies to the field.

6. GENETICS OF RESISTANCE

In comparison with insect species, little is known of the genetics of resistance in nematodes, largely because of their inherent biological complexity, the impossibility of determining the sex of free-living stages, and the difficulties of breeding experiments that need to be done within the host. These limitations virtually restrict genetic analysis studies to mass matings, making it difficult to distinguish genetic from environmental variation unless homozygous resistant and susceptible strains derived originally from the same source are used.

Le Jambre et al. (1976) concluded that thiabendazole resistance in *H. contortus* is probably attributable to a single gene. Two later studies on the genetics of benzimidazole resistance in *H. contortus* (Le Jambre et al., 1979; Herlich et al., 1981) judged that resistance is inherited through alleles at several loci. However, in the study by Le Jambre et al. (1979) it appeared to be inherited as an autosomal semidominant trait, whereas Herlich et al. (1981) concluded that resistance is not sex linked and is probably inherited as a multigenic recessive trait. Although these investigations produced conflicting conclusions on the mode of inheritance of benzimidazole resistance in *H. contortus*, Donald (1983a) pointed out that the parasite isolates used for these studies were not ideal. The resistant and susceptible strains used by Le Jambre et al. (1979) were of entirely different origin and perhaps exhibited intrastrain mating preferences or different genetic backgrounds for the expression of resistance/susceptibility. In the strain used by Herlich *et al.* (1981) resistance was still evolving. It is also possible for resistance to the same class of drug to vary in dominance hierarchy in different ecotypes of the same nematode species (Le Jambre, 1982), especially if resistance is polygenic.

Polygenic resistance has also been reported in the free-living nematode *Caenorhabditis elegans* to levamisole (Lewis *et al.*, 1980). These workers attributed resistance to 13 genes in levamisole-resistant mutants.

The relatively low absolute levels of anthelmintic resistance attained in selection studies on nematodes compared with the situation in insects, as well as the nonpersistent nature of anthelmintics, led Le Jambre (1982) to suggest that the resistances developed so far are a form of vigor tolerance. This may be attributed to the accumulation of alleles that confer slight survival advantage in the offspring, leading to the development of polygenic resistance. He also suggested that if anthelmintics are incorporated into devices permitting their continuous release over an extended period of time, they would be effectively converted into the equivalent of persistent pesticides. To survive such continuous exposure, parasite populations would have to evolve different survival mechanisms, likely to involve a major change in a physiological process under the control of a single, principle gene, analogous to most field cases of insecticide resistance. However, Le Jambre's hypothesis does not preclude the development of monogenic resistance under conventional anthelmintic usage, and recent studies by Waller *et al.* (1985) suggest that this form of resistance developed in a strain of *Trichostrongylus* spp. selected by levamisole under field conditions.

7. MECHANISMS OF RESISTANCE

Knowledge of the biochemical basis of anthelmintic resistance is almost entirely confined to benzimidazole resistance. Initial investigations on the mode of action of benzimidazoles demonstrated that thiabendazole exerted its action on carbohydrate metabolism via inhibition of fumarate reductase activity in benzimidazole-susceptible, but not benzimidazole-resistant, strains of nematodes (Malkin and Camacho, 1972; Prichard, 1973; Romanowski *et al.*, 1975). These studies suggested that resistance involves a direct change in this enzyme. However, more recent work by Bennet (1981) and Rew *et al.* (1982) clearly indicates that resistant strains show more generalized effects on carbohydrate metabolism.

An alternative hypothesis suggested by Coles (1977) attributing thiabendazole resistance to reduced uptake of drug in resistant strains was subsequently examined by Prichard *et al.* (1978), Rew *et al.* (1982), Sangster and Prichard (1984), and Weston *et al.* (1984), all of whom were unable to detect significant differences between the uptake of drug in susceptible and resistant strains. As uptake of benzimidazoles appears to be a passive process (Sangster and Prichard, 1984; Weston *et al.*, 1984), such a mechanism is unlikely to be a significant factor in resistance.

Recently, R. S. Rew, R. K. Prichard, and E. Lacey (unpublished observations) found uptake of 3-*O*-methylglucose by *H. contortus* and *T. colubriformis* to be more sensitive to inhibition by benzimidazoles in susceptible than in resistant strains. However, it is particularly interesting that these workers as well as R. K. Prichard, E. Lacey and A. Darwish (unpublished observations) have found both 3-0-methylglucose uptake and fumarate reductase activity in *H. contortus* to be inhibited by the tubulin-specific drug, colchicine, and that these inhibitions are more marked in benzimidazole-sensitive than resistant strains. Tubulin, a ubiquitous structural protein in eukaryotic cells, has been found to be a constituent of plasma and mitochondrial membranes (Bernier-Valentin and Rousset, 1982; Bernier-Valentin *et al.*, 1983).

The role of tubulin in the mode of action of benzimidazoles and the mechanism of benzimidazole resistance has been made clear by the findings of Sangster *et al.* (1985). These workers found benzimidazole treatment to produce greater effects on microtubule-dependent secretion of AChE, the presence of microtubules in intestinal cells, and colchicine binding in susceptible, as compared with benzimidazole-resistant *T. colubriformis*. In addition, the binding of thiabendazole, parbendazole, and oxibendazole was markedly reduced in crude tubulin extracts from the latter strain. Subsequent studies (E. Lacey and R. K. Prichard, unpublished observations) using tritium-labeled benzimidazoles have confirmed the reduced affinity of benzimidazoles for crude tubulin extracts of resistant strains of *H. contortus*, *O. circumcincta*, and *T. colubriformis*, demonstrating the generality of this mechanism for nematode resistance.

On the basis of these studies, the primary effect of benzimidazoles appears to relate to their action on nematode tubulin, whether it is free, polymerized as microtubules, or in cell membranes. Also, tubulin in benzimidazole-resistant nematodes has a lower affinity for these drugs. Because of the many roles of tubulin in cells, the binding of benzimidazoles by tubulin will express itself in a multitude of different physiological functions, and this effect will be modulated by other factors controlling these physiological functions.

The only biochemical work on levamisole resistance in nematodes has been performed on the free-living nematode *C. elegans* (Lewis *et al.*, 1980). These workers found that mutants of *C. elegans*, which were resistant to levamisole and morantel, had fewer ACh binding sites at which these cholinergic drugs could act.

8. RESISTANCE IN RELATIONSHIP TO WORM-CONTROL PRACTICES

Current worm-control practices fall into two broad categories: those that rely solely on regular or timed anthelmintic treatment and those that integrate anthelmintics with some form of grazing management. Both kinds of systems are capable of removing most of the production losses produced by helminth infection but are threatened by the development of resistance related directly to the degree to which they rely on high anthelmintic efficiency.

In animals grazing the same pastures continuously, the relationship between frequency of anthelmintic treatment and selection for resistance is unlikely to be linear. The occasional curative treatment, given when symptoms of clinical helminthiasis appear, results in only a low selection pressure, as treatment usually coincides with maximum numbers of larvae on pasture that escape exposure to the drug (Le Jambre,

1978), giving susceptible worms ample opportunity to infect the host and reproduce. As the number of treatments increase, with anthelmintics having the same mode of action, selection pressure is likely to increase at a greater rate because resistant worms are able to continue uninterrupted reproduction and may also accumulate in the host, whereas after each treatment the susceptibles acquired by new infection will produce no progeny for at least the prepatent period of the parasite. Monthly dosing of young sheep, which was shown by Johnstone et al. (1979) to be profitable, has been adopted by farmers in many parts of the world. This procedure is likely to be a strong selector for resistance, because susceptible worms acquired after each treatment are allowed only about 1 week in 4 to produce progeny. Unless resistant worms are substantially less fit, this must result in a steady increase in the frequency of resistant larvae on pasture.

Analysis of published reports of resistance shows an overwhelming association with its occurrence and the frequent use of drugs with the same mode of action (Donald, 1983a). At one end of the spectrum are the goat farms in Australasia, where very high levels of multiple resistance have emerged (Green et al., 1982; Anonymous, 1983; Kettle et al., 1983). On these farms, high stocking rates on permanent pasture are practiced, favoring very heavy nematode infection, which until now was kept in check by intensive anthelmintic treatment. Some of these farms now have no option but to abandon goat farming. In the process, there is the danger of dispersing stock harboring multiple resistant worms throughout the grazing industry rather than being consigned to the abattoir. At the other extreme is the absence of any genuine resistance in nematode parasites of cattle. This is most unlikely to be due to a lack of genetic variation in cattle parasites, with no parasite populations possessing alleles which confer resistance to anthelmintics, and may be attributed to such factors as the less frequent use of anthelmintics in cattle.

Whether it is desirable to alternate the use of anthelmintics with different modes of action, and if so at what frequency, is still a matter of speculation. There is no good evidence that a regular rotation will enhance the development of resistance to any one of them (Donald and Waller, 1982). Rotation of anthelmintic groups, promoted by Prichard et al. (1980), may not reliably delay resistance either, but at least in horse management, practices such as rotation and the use of anthelmintic combinations have been markedly more successful in delaying the occurrence of anthelmintic resistance than the use of a single anthelmintic class (Kelly et al., 1981b). Rotation, perhaps on an annual basis, is unlikely to be harmful and may in fact prevent resistance to one drug group from reaching very high levels before detection, thereby reducing losses from poor nematode control.

An appreciation of the epidemiology and species succession has also led to a more enlightened approach to anthelmintic usage. For example, Prichard et al. (1980) recommend the use of narrow-spectrum drugs to control H. contortus in endemic areas, to reduce selection pressure on broad-spectrum anthelmintics, and to save on costs. Similarly, when Trichostrongylus spp. are likely to cause problems, an organophosphate anthelmintic could be used.

A recent development in the use of anthelmintics has been their incorporation into sustained-release devices. Following deposition into the rumen by oral dosing, these devices release the anthelmintic for extended periods of time. This technique is an extension of the principle of low-level administration of anthelmintics either in drink-ing water, licks, or blocks, but whose major deficiency is the voluntary, and therefore variable, intake of the drug by animals. A bolus releasing morantel for 60 days or more has been developed and marketed for use in cattle in Europe (Jones, 1981), and a device releasing oxfendazole has been tested successfully in sheep and cattle in Australia (Anderson and Laby, 1979; Anderson *et al.*, 1980).

Sustained-release devices have the same effect in preventing the establishment and reproduction of susceptible parasites as do individual anthelmintic treatments given at intervals of 2 weeks or less during the lifetime of the device. Theoretically they can select strongly for resistance, but a number of factors may reduce this hazard, as suggested by Donald (1983*b*): (1) the total release time should be less than the max-imum life-span of the parasite free-living stages, (2) the device should be used infre-quently, (3) the release rate must be maintained at a constant high level sufficient to produce a very high parasite kill, and (4) the release rate must decline rapidly to zero when the device becomes exhausted.

Misgivings have also been expressed about selection for resistance in integrated control schemes (Le Jambre, 1978; Michel *et al.*, 1983). The basic argument advanced is that a single strategic anthelmintic treatment combined with a movement of treated animals to pastures carrying few infective larvae may select strongly for resistance because the survivors of the treatment will make a major contribution to the next generation. This warning must not go unchallenged because (1) it undermines the whole concept of integrated control and thus the confidence of those promoting such shemes, and (2) it has not been verified under field conditions. The extent to which this practice will produce strong selection will depend on the frequency with which animals are dosed and moved to prepared pasture, the "cleanliness" of the pasture, and the opportunity for the progeny of the worms that survived the anthelmintic to contribute to future generations of the parasite. At the practical level, a consideration of integrated control schemes for cattle and sheep that have been advocated and practiced for nearly two decades in Europe suggests that resistance is currently of little importance. In addition, it has been shown that high levels of production can be obtained in young sheep where not all pasture changes are accompanied by anthelmintic treatment (Don-ald and Waller, 1982).

Most integrated control schemes rely on only a few anthelmintic treatments each year, and their effectiveness can be further safeguarded if the recommendations made by Donald (1983*b*) are adopted: (1) high dose rates of drugs should be used, leaving few if any survivors and thus retarding the development of resistance by restricting genetic variability; and (2) an annual change to a drug with a different mode of action would further reduce the risk.

9. NEW DEVELOPMENTS OF NEMATODE CONTROL

9.1. *Nonchemotherapeutic*

Major constraints have been associated with the research and development of alternative, nonchemical methods of helminth control, because in the final analysis they have to compete favorably with the cheap, effective, reliable control afforded by anthelmintics. However, the development of alternative control schemes has been given greater impetus by the emergence of anthelmintic resistance as a serious problem. Exploitation of the immune response of the host offers greatest promise in this area. Failure to immunize effectively against helminths in animals under natural grazing conditions has generally been attributed to a deficiency in the immunogenicity of vaccines. However, recent research points to a failure in a genetically determined component of the host's resistance mechanism. For this reason the approach to vaccination and exploitation of immunological control focuses not only on the detection and isolation of protective antigens, but also on manipulation of the host's genetic constitution (for reviews see Dineen and Outteridge, 1984; Dineen and Wagland, 1982).

9.2. Chemotherapeutic

Despite recent advances made in nonchemotherapeutic control, anthelmintics will continue to dominate helminth control, certainly in the immediate and short-term future. Ivermectin (Campbell et al., 1983) represents a new kind of broad-spectrum anthelmintic, apparently unaffected by cross-resistance. However, there is no reason to assume that resistance to this drug could not develop, and it behooves all those involved in its use to consider carefully how that risk might be minimized. This is particularly important, as it is unlikely that there will be a steady stream of highly effective anthelmintics with novel forms of action appearing on the marketplace, because of the enormously high development costs.

Rather than continually searching for new classes of compounds, Prichard (1978) considered that better anthelmintics may be developed and at less cost by manipulating the pharmacokinetic behavior of existing drugs. Significant progress in this area has been made. For example, combinations of drugs have resulted in synergistic increases in efficacy (Bennet et al., 1980). Chemical modification of the benzimidazole molecule to improve solubility and permit its administration by injection (Hennessy et al., 1983), as well as alteration of the metabolism and elimination of anthelmintics (Hennessy et al., 1985) have both been shown to extend the systemic availability and efficacy of currently available drugs.

Considerable progress has been made in the control of various arthropod pests of grazing ruminants with compounds other than conventional insecticides. These include analogues of juvenile hormone, chitin inhibitors, and metabolic products of bacteria. Studies in the United States (Harris et al., 1973, 1974; Miller et al., 1976, 1977) have shown these compounds to be potent at very low concentrations in inhibiting the development of certain dipteran larvae in cattle feces and offer a practical alternative form of control (Beadles et al., 1975). Similar compounds have also been shown to possess biological activity against nematodes, by delaying hatching or inhibiting exsheathment of infective larval stages in vitro (Rogers, 1973, 1978; Boisvenue, et al., 1977). It is therefore reasonable to expect that certain of these compounds may affect the production and viability of eggs from established nematode infections or may affect developing infections by delaying or inhibiting moults. In this way effective compounds could substitute for conventional anthelmintics in sustained-release devices; they would not contribute to the loss of potent anthelmintics by selection for resistance and would provide good levels of worm control.

10. CONCLUSION

Although anthelmintic resistance is apparently not widespread globally and is currently limited to the nematode parasites of sheep, goats, and horses, there is no reason to expect that it will not appear in other species of nematode parasites of the same or different classes of livestock or that resistance to other commercially developed anthelmintics will not arise. Anthelmintic resistance remains a threat to the main form of control and constitutes the single most important problem confronting the control of nematode parasites of livestock in the near future.

There is an urgent need to provide advice to users of anthelmintics on practices they should adopt to minimize the selection for resistance or to overcome an existing resistance problem. Recommendations should be based on the results of studies both in the laboratory and in the field. Both approaches are complementary and are most probably essential if a thorough understanding of the problem is to be achieved. Laboratory studies are of value in providing precise information about certain qualitative aspects of resistance, whereas field studies are necessary because the complexities of the natural host–parasite–environment relationship are difficult or impossible to simulate in the laboratory.

In general, the more effective a control system is, and the more its effectiveness depends on anthelmintic efficiency, the greater the potential for the development of anthelmintic resistance. This is made clearly apparent by the close association between reports of resistance and a high frequency of anthelmintic treatments with drugs having the same mode of action.

It is therefore important to recognize and avoid those practices that select strongly for resistance in order to conserve the existing efficiency of the available anthelmintics. Helminth control should be based on these considerations, where high levels of animal production can be obtained by methods that are not heavily dependent on the use of only a few highly efficient anthelmintic groups.

REFERENCES

Anderson, N., and Laby, R. H., 1979, Activity against *Ostertagia ostertagi* of low doses of oxfendazole continuously released from intraruminal capsules in cattle, *Aust. Vet. J.* 55:244–246.

Anderson, N., Laby, R. H., Prichard, R. K., and Hennessy, D., 1980, Controlled release of anthelmintic drugs: A new concept for prevention of helminthosis in sheep, *Res. Vet. Sci.* 29:333–341.

Anonymous, 1983, *Worms in Sheep and Goats on the N.S.W. North Coast*, No. 3: *Results of Drench Resistance Survey*, Information from Department of Agriculture, New South Wales.

Beadles, M. L., Miller, J. A., Chamberlain, W. F., Eschle, J. L., and Harris, R. L., 1975, The hornfly: Methoprene in drinking water of cattle for control, *J. Econ. Entomol.* 68:781–785.

Bennet, E. M., 1981, Biochemical studies on the nature of benzimidazole resistance in *Haemonchus contortus* (Rudolphi, 1803), Ph.D. thesis, Australian National University, Canberra.

Bennet, E. M., Behm, C., Bryant, C., and Chevis, R. A. F., 1980, Synergistic action of mebendazole and levamisole in the treatment of benzimidazole-resistant *Haemonchus contortus* in sheep, *Vet. Parasitol.* 7:207–214.

Berger, J., 1975, The resistance of a field strain of *Haemonchus contortus* to five benzimidazole anthelmintics in current use, *J. South Afr. Vet. Assoc.* 46:369–372.

Bernier-Valentin, F., and Rousset, B., 1982, Interaction of tubulin with rat liver mitochondria, *J. Biol. Chem.* 257:7092–7099.

Bernier-Valentin, F., Aunis, D., and Rousset, B., 1983, Evidence for tubulin-binding sites on cellular membranes: plasma membranes, mitochondrial membranes and secretary granule membranes, *J. Cell Biol.* 97:209–216.

Blanch, L., 1984, Resistance to wormers in sheep. A sheep breeder's experience, *Aust. Rural Chem. Mag.* 1:28–31.

Boersema, J. H., Leweng-van der Wiel, P. J., and Borgsteede, F. H. M., 1982, Benzimidazole resistance in a field strain of *Haemonchus contortus* in The Netherlands, *Vet. Rec.* 110:203–24.

Boisvenue, R. J., Emmick, T. L., and Galloway, R. B., 1977, *Haemonchus contortus:* Effects of compounds with juvenile hormone activity on the *in vitro* development of infective larvae, *Exp. Parasitol.* 42:67–72.

Britt, D. P., 1982, Benzimidazole-resistant nematodes in Britain, *Vet. Rec.* 110:343–344.

Brown, A. W. A., and Pal, R., 1971, *Insecticide Resistance in Arthropods*, 2nd ed., World Health Organization, Geneva, Switzerland.

Campbell, W. C., Fisher, M. H., Stapley, E. O., Albers-Schönberg, G., and Jacob, T. A., 1983, Ivermectin: A potent new antiparasitic agent, *Science* 221:823–827.

Cawthorne, R. J. G., and Cheong, F. H., 1984, Prevalence of anthelmintic resistant nematodes in south-east England, *Vet. Rec.* 114:562–564.

Coles, G. C., 1977, The biochemical mode of action of some modern anthelmintics, *Pesticide Sci.* 8:536–543.

Coles, G. C., and Simpkin, K. G., 1977, Resistance of nematode eggs to the ovicidal activity of benzimidazoles, *Res. Vet. Sci.* 22:386–387.

Comins, H. N., 1977, The management of pesticide resistance, *J. Theoret. Biol.* 65:399–420.

Dineen, J. K., and Outteridge, P. M., 1984, *Immunogenetic Approaches to the Control of Endoparasites with Particular Reference to Parasites of Sheep*, C.S.I.R.O. Division of Animal Health, Melbourne, Australia.

Dineen, J. K., and Wagland, B. M., 1982, Immunoregulation of parasites in natural host–parasite systems—With special reference to the gastrointestinal nematodes of sheep, in: *Biology and Control of Endoparasites* (L. E. A. Symons, A. D. Donald, and J. K. Dineen, eds.), pp. 297–329, Academic Press, Sydney, Australia.

Dobson, R. J., Donald, A. D., Waller, P. J., and Snewdon, K. L., 1985, An egg-hatch assay for resistance to levamisole in trichostrongyloid nematode parasites, *Vet. Parasitol.* (in press).

Donald, A. D., 1983*a*, The development of anthelmintic resistance in nematodes of grazing animals, in: *Facts and Reflections. IV. Resistance of Parasites to Anthelmintics* (F. H. M. Borgsteede, Sv. Aa. Henriksen, and H. J. Over, eds.), pp. 15–28, Central Veterinary Institute, Lelystad, The Netherlands.

Donald, A. D., 1983*b*, Anthelmintic resistance in relation to helminth control and grazing systems, in: *Facts and Reflections. IV. Resistance of Parasites to Anthelmintics* (F. H. M. Borgsteede, Sv. Aa. Henriksen, and H. J. Over, eds.), pp. 187–198, Central Veterinary Institute, Lelystad, The Netherlands.

Donald, A. D., and Waller, P. J., 1982, Problems and prospects in the control of helminthiasis in sheep, in: *Biology and Control of Endoparasites* (L. E. A. Symons, A. D. Donald, and J. K. Dineen, eds.), pp. 157–186, Academic Press, Sydney, Australia.

Donald, A. D., Waller, P. J., Dobson, R. J., and Axelsen, A., 1980, The effect of selection with levamisole on benzimidazole resistance in *Ostertagia* spp. of sheep, *Int. J. Parasitol.* 10:381–389.

Drudge, J. H., and Lyons, E. T., 1965, Newer developments in helminth control and *Strongylus vulgaris* research, *Proc. Am. Assoc. Equine Pract.* 115:381–389.

Drudge, J. H., Lyons, E. T., and Tolliver, S. C., 1979, Benzimidazole resistance of equine strongyles—Critical tests of six compounds against Population B, *Am. J. Vet. Res.* 40:590–594.

Foot, M. A., 1980, Nematicide resistance in plant-parasitic nematodes, *N. Z. J. Zool.* 7:599.

Georghiou, G. P., and Taylor, C. E., 1977, Genetic and biological influences in the evolution of insecticide resistance, *J. Econ. Entomol.* 70:319–323.

Green, P. E., Forsyth, B. A., Rowan, K. J., and Payne, G., 1981, The isolation of a field strain of *Haemonchus contortus* in Queensland showing multiple anthelmintic resistance, *Aust. Vet. J.* 57:79–84.

Green, P. E., Murphy, M. L., and O'Sullivan, B. M., 1982, Anthelmintic resistance studies in goats in south-east Queensland, *Aust. Adv. Vet. Sci.* 181–183.

Gunawan, M., Sangster, N. C., Kelly, J. D., Griffin, D., and Whitlock, H. V., 1979, The efficacy of fenbendazole and albendazole against immature and adult stages of benzimidazole-resistant sheep trichostrongylids, *Res. Vet. Sci.* 27:111–115.

Hall, C. A., Kelly, J. D., Campbell, N. J., Whitlock, H. V., and Martin, I. C. A., 1978, The dose response of several benzimidazole anthelmintics against resistant strains of *Haemonchus contortus* and *Trichostrongylus colubriformis* selected with thiabendazole, *Res. Vet. Sci.* 25:364–367.

Hall, C. A., Kelly, J. D., Whitlock, H. V., Martin, I. C. A., McDonell, P. A., and Gunawan, M., 1981a, Five generations of selection with benzimidazole and non-benzimidazole anthelmintics against benzimidazole resistant strains of *Haemonchus contortus* and *Ostertagia* spp. in sheep, *Res. Vet. Sci.* 30:138–142.

Hall, C. A., Ritchie, L., and McDonell, 1981b, Investigations for anthelmintic resistance in gastrointestinal nematodes from goats, *Res. Vet. Sci.* 31:116–119.

Hall, C. A., Kelly, J. D., Martin, I. C. A., Whitlock, H. V., McDonnell, P. A., and Gunewan, M., 1981c, Changes in response to a benzimidazole resistant strain of *Haemonchus contortus* sheep after passing through calves, *Res. Vet. Sci.* 30:143–146.

Harris, R. L., Frazer, E. D., and Younger, R. L., 1973, Horn flies, stable flies and house flies: development in feces of bovines treated orally with juvenile hormone analogues, *J. Econ. Entomol.* 66:1099–1102.

Harris, R. L., Chamberlain, W. F., and Frazer, E. P., 1974, Horn flies and stable flies: Free-choice feeding of methoprene mineral blocks to cattle for control, *J. Econ. Entomol.* 67:384–386.

Hennessy, D. R., Lacey, E., and Prichard, R. K., 1983, Pharmacokinetic behaviour and anthelmintic efficacy of 1-n-butyl carbamoyl oxfendazole given by intramuscular injection, *Vet. Res. Commun.* 6:177–187.

Hennessy, D. R., Lacey, E., Pritchard, R. K., and Steel, J. W., 1984, Potentiation of the anthelmintic activity of oxfendazole by parbendazole, *Journal of Veterinary Pharmacological Ther.* (in press).

Herd, R. P., Miller, T. B., and Gabel, A. A., 1981, A field evaluation of pro-benzimidazole, benzimidazole and non-benzimidazole anthelmintics in horses, *J. Am. Vet. Med. Assoc.* 179:686–691.

Herlich, H., Rew, R. S., and Colglazier, M. L., 1981, Inheritance of cambendazole resistance in *Haemonchus contortus*, *Am. J. Vet. Res.* 42:1342–1344.

Hogarth-Scott, R. S., Kelly, J. D., Whitlock, H. V., Ng, B. K. Y., Thompson, H. G., James, R. E., and Mears, F. A., 1976, The anthelmintic efficacy of fenbendazole against thiabendazole-resistant strains of *Haemonchus contortus* and *Trichostrongylus colubriformis* in sheep, *Res. Vet. Sci.* 21:232–237.

Hughes, P. L., and Seifert, D. A., 1983, Field comment on anthelmintic resistance of sheep nematodes, *N. Z. Vet. J.* 31:183–184.

Johnstone, I. L., Darvill, F. M., Bowen, F. L., Butler, R. W., Smart, K. E., and Pearson, I. G., 1979, The effect of four schemes of parasite control on production in Merino wether weaners in two environments, *Aust. J. Exp. Agr. Husb.* 19:303–311.

Jones, R. M., 1981, A field study of the morantel sustained release bolus in the seasonal control of parasitic gastroenteritis in grazing calves, *Vet. Parasitol.* 8:237–251.

Jordi, R., 1980, Untersuchungen zur Anthelminthika Resistanz von Trichostrongyliden des Schafes, *Schweiz. Arch. Tierheilkd.* 122:679–694.

Kelly, J. D., and Hall, C. A., 1979, Anthelmintic resistance in nematodes. 1. History, present status in Australia, genetic background and methods for field diagnosis, *N. S. W. Vet. Proc.* 15:19–31.

Kelly J. D., Hall, C. A., Whitlock, H. V., Thompson, H. G., Campbell, N. J., and Martin, I. C. A., 1977, The effect of route of administration on the anthelmintic efficacy of benzimidazole anthelmintics in sheep infected with strains of *Haemonchus contortus* and *Trichostrongylus colubriformis* resistant or susceptible to thiabendazole, *Res. Vet. Sci.* 22:161–168.

Kelly, J. D., Whitlock, H. V., Thompson, N. G., Hall, C. A., Martin, I. C. A., and Le Jambre, L. F., 1978, Physiological characteristics of free-living and parasitic stages of strains of Haemonchus contortus, susceptible or resistant to benzimidazole anthelmintics, Res. Vet. Sci. 25:376–385.

Kelly, J. D., Whitlock, H, V., Gunawan, M., Griffin, D., Porter, C. J., and Martin, I. C. A., 1981a, Anthelmintic efficacy of low-dose phenothiazine against strains of sheep nematodes susceptible or resistant to thiabendazole, levamisole and morantel tartrate: Effect on patent infections, Res. Vet. Sci. 30:161–169.

Kelly, J. D., Webster, J. H., Griffin, D. L., Whitlock, H. V., Martin, I. C. A., and Gunawan, M., 1981b, Resistance to benzimidazole anthelmintics in equine strongyles. 1. Frequency, geographical distribution and relationship between occurrence, animal husbandry procedures and anthelmintic usage, Aust. Vet. J. 57:163–171.

Kemp, G. K., and Smith, C. F., 1982, Anthelmintic resistance survey in New Zealand, N. Z. Vet. J. 30:141–144.

Kettle, P. R., Vlassoff, A., Lukers, J. M., Ayling, J. M., and McMurtry, L. W., 1981, A survey of nematode control measures used by sheep farmers and of anthelmintic resistance on their farms. Part 1: North Island and the Nelson region of the South Island, N. Z. Vet. J. 29:81–83.

Kettle, P. R., Vlassoff, A., Ayling, J. M., McMurtry, L. W., Smith, S. W., and Watson, A. J., 1982, A survey of nematode control measures used by sheep farmers and of anthelmintic resistance on their farms. Part 2: South Island excluding the Nelson region, N. Z. Vet. J. 30:79–81.

Kettle, P. R., Vlassoff, A., Reid, T. C., and Horton, C. T., 1983, A survey of nematode control measures used by milking goat farmers and of anthelmintic resistance on their farms, N. Z. Vet. J. 31:139–143.

Le Jambre, L. F., 1976, Egg hatch as an in vitro assay of thiabendazole resistance in nematodes, Vet. Parasitol. 2:385–391.

Le Jambre, L. F., 1978, Anthelmintic resistance in gastrointestinal nematodes of sheep, in: The Epidemiology and Control of Gastrointestinal Parasites of Sheep in Australia (A. D. Donald, W. H. Southcott, and J. K. Dineen, eds.), pp. 109–120, C.S.I.R.O. Division of Animal Health, Melbourne, Australia.

Le Jambre, L. F., 1982, Genetics and the control of trichostrongylid parasites of ruminants, in: Biology and Control of Endoparasites (L. E. A. Symons, A. D. Donald, and J. K. Dineen, eds.), pp. 53–80, Academic Press, Sydney, Australia.

Le Jambre, L. F., Southcott, W. H., and Dash, K. M., 1976, Resistance of selected lines of Haemonchus contortus to thiabendazole, morantel tartrate and levamisole, Int. J. Parasitol. 6:217–222.

Le Jambre, L. F., Southcott, W. H., and Dash, K. M., 1977, Resistance of selected lines of Ostertagia circumcincta to thiabendazole, morantel tartrate and levamisole, Int. J. Parasitol. 7:473–479.

Le Jambre, L. F., Southcott, W. H., and Dash, K. M., 1978a, Development of simultaneous resistance in Ostertagia circumcincta to thiabendazole, morantel tartrate and levamisole, Int. J. Parasitol. 8:443–447.

Le Jambre, L. F., Southcott, W. H., and Dash, K. M., 1978b, Effectiveness of broad spectrum anthelmintics against selected strains of Trichostrongylus colubriformis, Aust. Vet. J. 54:570–574.

Le Jambre, L. F., Royal, W. M., and Martin, P. J., 1979, The inheritance of thiabendazole resistance in Haemonchus contortus, Parasitology 78:107–119.

Lewis, J. A., Wu, C. H., Levine, J. H., and Berg, H., 1980, Levamisole-resistant mutants of the nematode Caenorhabditis elegans appear to lack pharmacological acetylcholine receptors, Neuroscience 5:967–989.

Lyons, E. T., Tolliver, S. C., Drudge, J. H., Hemken, R. W., and Button, F. S., 1981, Efficacy of levamisole against abomasal nematodes and lungworms in dairy calves: Preliminary tests indicating reduced activity for Ostertagia ostertagi, Am. J. Vet. Res. 42:1228–1230.

Malkin, M. F., and Camacho, R. M., 1972, The effect of thiabendazole on fumarate reductase from thiabendazole-sensitive and resistant Haemonchus contortus, J. Parasitol. 58:845–846.

Martin, P. J., and Le Jambre, L. F., 1979, Larval paralysis as an in vitro assay of levamisole and morantel tartrate resistance in Ostertagia, Vet. Sci. Commun. 3:159–164.

Martin, P. J., Le Jambre, L. F., and Claxton, J. H., 1981, The impact of refugia on the development of thiabendazole resistance in Haemonchus contortus, Int. J. Parasitol. 11:35–41.

Martin, P. J., Anderson, N., Jarrett, R. G., Brown, T. H., and Ford, G. E., 1982, Effects of a preventive and a suppressive control scheme on the development of thiabendazole resistance in Ostertagia spp., Aust. Vet. J. 58:185–190.

McKenzie, J. A., Dearn, J. M., and Whitten, M. J., 1980, Genetic basis of resistance to diazinon in Victorian populations of the Australian sheep blowfly, *Lucilia cuprina, Aust. J. Biol. Sci.* 33:85–95.

Michel, J. F., 1963, The phenomena of host resistance and the course of infection of *Ostertagia ostertagi* in calves, *Parasitology* 53:63–84.

Michel, J. F., 1969, Some observations on the worm burdens of calves infected daily with *Ostertagia ostertagi, Parasitology* 59:575–595.

Michel, J. F., Cawthorne, R. J. G., Anderson, R. M., Armour, J., Clarkson, M. J., and Thomas, R. J., 1983, Resistance to anthelmintics in Britain: husbandry practices and selective pressure, in: *Facts and Reflections. IV. Resistance of Parasites to Anthelmintics* (F. H. M. Borgsteede, Sv. Aa. Henriksen, and H. J. Over, eds.), pp. 41–59, Central Veterinary Institute, Lelystad, The Netherlands.

Middleberg, A., and McKenna, P. B., 1983, Oxfendazole resistance in *Nematodirus spathiger, N. Z. Vet. J.* 31:65–66.

Miller, J. A., Chamberlain, W. F., Beadles, M. L., Pickens, M. O., and Gingrich, A. R., 1976, Methoprene for control of horn flies: Application to drinking water of cattle via a tablet formulation, *J. Econ. Entomol.* 69:330–332.

Miller, J. A., Beadles, M. L., Palmer, J. S., and Pickens, M. O., 1977, Methoprene for control of the horn fly: A sustained-release bolus formulation for cattle, *J. Econ. Entomol.* 70:589–591.

Powers, K. G., Wood, I. B., Eckert, J., Gibson, T., and Smith, H. J., 1982, World Association for the Advancement of Veterinary Parasitology. Guidelines for evaluating the efficacy of anthelmintics in ruminants (Bovine and ovine), *Vet. Parasitol.* 10:265–284.

Prichard, R. K., 1973, The fumarate reductase reaction of *Haemonchus contortus* and the mode of action of some anthelmintics, *Int. J. Parasitol.* 3:409–417.

Prichard, R. K., 1978, Sheep anthelmintics, in: *The Epidemiology and Control of Gastrointestinal Parasites of Sheep in Australia* (A. D. Donald, W. H. Southcott, and J. K. Dineen, eds.), pp. 75–107, C.S.I.R.O. Division of Animal Health, Melbourne, Australia.

Prichard, R. K., Kelly, J. D., and Thompson, H. G., 1978, The effects of benzimidazole resistance and route of administration on the uptake of fenbendazole and thiabendazole by *Haemonchus contortus* and *Trichostrongylus colubriformis* in sheep, *Vet. Parasitol.* 4:243–255.

Prichard, R. K., Hall, C. A., Kelly, J. D., Martin, I. C. A., and Donald, A. D., 1980, The problem of anthelmintic resistance in nematodes, *Aust. Vet. J.* 56:239–251.

Rew, R. S., Smith, C., and Colglazier, M. L., 1982, Glucose metabolism of Haemonchus *contortus* adults: Effects of thiabendazole on susceptible versus resistant strain, *J. Parasitol.* 68:845–850.

Rogers, W. P., 1973, Juvenile and moulting hormones from nematodes, *Parasitology* 67:105–113.

Rogers, W. P., 1978, The inhibitory action of insect juvenile hormone on the hatching of nematode eggs, *Comp. Biochem. Physiol.* 61A:187–190.

Romanowski, R. D., Rhoads, M. L., Colglazier, M. L., and Kates, K. C., 1975, Effect of cambendazole, thiabendazole and levamisole on fumarate reductase in cambendazole-resistant and sensitive strains of *Haemonchus contortus, J. Parasitol.* 61:777–778.

Round, M. C., Simpson, D. J., Haselden, C. S., Glendenning, E. S. A., and Barkerville, R. E., 1974, Horse strongyles' tolerance to anthelmintics, *Vet. Rec.* 95:517–518.

Sangster, N. C., and Prichard, R. K., 1984, Uptake of thiabendazole and its effects on glucose uptake and carbohydrate levels in thiabendazole-resistant and susceptible *Trichostrongylus colubriformis, Int. J. Parasitol.* 14:121–126.

Sangster, N. C., Whitlock, H. V., Russ, I. G., Gunawan, M., Griffin, D. L., and Kelly, J. D., 1979, *Trichostrongylus colubriformis* and *Ostertagia circumcincta* resistant to levamisole, morantel tartrate and thiabendazole: Occurrence of field strains, *Res. Vet. Sci.* 27:106–110.

Sangster, N. C., Kelly, J. D., Whitlock, H. V., Gunawan, M., and Porter, C. J., 1980, *Trichostrongylus colubriformis* and *Ostertagia* sp. resistant to levamisole, morantel tartrate and thiabendazole: Infectivity, pathogenicity and drug efficacy in two breeds of sheep, *Res. Vet. Sci.* 29:26–30.

Sangster, N. C., Pritchard, R. K., and Lacey, E., 1985, Tubulin and benzimidazole-resistance in *Trichostrongylus colubriformis* (Nematoda), *J. Parasitol.* (in press).

Santiago, M. A. M., da Costa, U., and Benevenga, S. F., 1978, Anthelmintic activity of dl-Tetramisole and thiabendazole on a levamisole resistant strain of *Trichostrongylus colubriformis*, *Rev. Centro Ciencias Rurais* 8:257–261.

dos Santos, V. T., and Franco, E. B. O., 1967, A parecimento de *Haemonchus* resistene AO radical benz-imidazole EM Uruguaiana, *Proceedings of the First Latin-American Congress of Parasitology, Santiago, Chile,* p. 105.

Slocombe, J. O. D., and Cote, J. F., 1977, Small strongyles of horses with cross-resistance to benzimidazole anthelmintics and susceptibility to unrelated compounds, *Can. Vet. J.* 18:212–217.

Suthurst, R. W., and Comins, H. N., 1979, The management of acaricide resistance in the cattle tick, *Boophilus microplus* (Canestrini) (Acari:Ixodidae), in Australia, *Bull. Entomol. Res.* 69:519–537.

Turton, J. A., and Clark, C. J., 1974, The effect of natural worm loss on the estimate of anthelmintic activity in an anthelmintic test with *Haemonchus contortus*, *Parasitology* 69:191–196.

van Wyck, J. A., and Gerber, H. M., 1980, A field strain of *Haemonchus contortus* showing slight resistance to rafoxanide, *Onderstepoort J. Vet. Res.* 47:137–142.

Waller, P. J., Dobson, R. J., and Donald, A. D., 1983, Further studies of the effect of selection with levamisole on a benzimidazole resistant population of *Ostertagia* spp. of sheep, *Int. J. Parasitol.* 13:463–468.

Waller, P. J., Dobson, R. J., Donald, A. D., Griffiths, D. A., and Smith, E. F., 1985, Selection studies on anthelmintic resistant and susceptable populations of *Trichostrongylus colubriformis* of sheep, *International Journal of Parasitology* (in press).

Webb, R. F., McCully, C. H., Clarke, F. L., Greentree, P., and Honey, P., 1979, The incidence of thiabendazole resistance in field populations of *Haemonchus contortus* on the Northern Tablelands of New South Wales, *Aust. Vet. J.* 55:422–426.

Weston, K. M., O'Brien, R. W., and Prichard, R. K., 1984, Respiratory metabolism and thiabendazole susceptibility in developing eggs of *Haemonchus contortus*, *Int. J. Parasitol.* 14:159–164.

Whitlock, H. V., Sangster, N. C., Gunawan, M., Porter, C. J., and Kelly, J. D., 1980a, *Trichostrongylus colubriformis* and *Ostertagia* sp. resistant to levamisole, morantel tartrate and thiabendazole: Isolation into pure strain anthelmintic titration, *Res. Vet. Sci.* 29:31–35.

Whitlock, H. V., Kelly, J. D., Porter, C. J., Griffin, D. L., and Martin, I. C. A., 1980b, In vitro field screening for anthelmintic resistance in strongyles of sheep and horses, *Vet. Parasitol.* 7:215–232.

Whitten, M. J., Dearn, J. M., and McKenzie, J. A., 1980, Field studies on insecticide resistance in the Australian sheep blowfly, *Lucilia cuprina*, *Aust. J. Biol. Sci.* 33:725–735.

IV

Trematodes

18

Chemistry of Antitrematodal Agents

HELMUT MROZIK

1. INTRODUCTION

The overwhelming attention of medicinal chemists and parasitologists concerned with trematode infections was directed toward schistosomiasis, a common plague of man in certain tropical or subtropical regions, and fascioliasis, a disease afflicting sheep and cattle with important economic implications. The lancet fluke (*Dicrocoelium dentriticum*) was subjected at one time to a systematic effort in search of new chemotherapeutic agents, which resulted in a specific drug for this infection.

The chemotherapy of trematode infections has been periodically reviewed in detail (Islip, 1979; Robertson, 1977; Miller, 1976; Laemmler, 1968). The latest developments were summarized in the yearly editions of the *Annual Reports in Medicinal Chemistry* (Ginger, 1982). Short abstracts of the more widely used drugs can be found in the *Merck Index* (Windholz, 1983). It is the purpose of this chapter to describe in short the history leading to the important classes of drugs for these infections and to provide more details only for the more recent and useful therapeutics.

Since both schistosomiasis and fascioliasis are systemic infections that occur outside the gastrointestinal (GI) tract, the chemicals must be delivered to the parasites through the bloodstream of the host. The effective agents must interfere lethally with an important function of the parasite without doing any substantial harm to the host. It is therefore perhaps not surprising that practically all the early drugs used in the therapy of these infections showed some serious toxic side effects either immediately, because of a low therapeutic index, or are now, after more careful studies, suspect of mutagenic or carcinogenic properties. The search for drugs that are highly effective as parasiticides and at the same time well tolerated by their hosts is still continuing. Selective toxicity toward a parasite enzyme target, different affinities to host and parasite receptors, metabolic activation of prodrugs or rapid metabolic detoxification of the drug by the host are some of the mechanisms by which the more desirable antiparasitic agents

HELMUT MROZIK • Merck Sharp & Dohme Research Laboratories, Rahway, New Jersey 07065.

accomplish their specific effects. Schistosome and liver fluke worms occur in different parts of the host body. Despite their close biological relationship, few chemicals have useful activities against both worms, and even compounds effective against all three schistosome species are rare. It is therefore logical to treat the two infections separately.

2. CHEMISTRY OF ANTISCHISTOSOMAL AGENTS

2.1. Antimony Compounds

Salts of arsenic, such as arsphenamine (Salvarsan), discovered by Ehrlich in 1909, and of antimony played an important role in early chemotherapy. Antimony potassium tartrate (tartar emetic) 1a was introduced as the earliest drug used against schistosomal infections nearly 70 years ago. Trivalent antimony salts of tartaric acid (antimony sodium tartrate), gluconic acid (antimony sodium gluconate, Triostam), 4,5-di-hydroxy-1,3-benzenedisulfonic acid (stibophen, Fuadin), mercaptosuccinic acid (Anthiolimine), or 2,3-dimercaptosuccinic acid (stibocaptate, TWSb] long remained the only effective chemotherapeutic agents for all three species of schistosomes, although severe side effects sometimes required discontinuation of treatment.

$$
\begin{array}{c}
\text{O} \\
\backslash \\
\text{C—O} \\
| \qquad \backslash \\
\text{HC—O—Sb} \\
| \qquad / \\
\text{HC—O} \\
| \\
\text{C—OK} \\
/ \\
\text{O}
\end{array}
$$

1a
Antimony potassium tartrate

2.2. The Miracils

A series of synthetic chemical compounds with 1-amino-4-methyl xanthone and thioxanthone structures related to the antimalarial quinacrine, which cured schistosome infections in experimental animals, were described in 1946 (Kikuth et al., 1946). Miracil D, 2a, one of the group of compounds to become known as the miracils, was selected for clinical trials in man. It was subsequently used as the first orally active and first metal-free drug under the generic name lucanthone hydrochloride in the treatment of S. haematobium and S. mansoni. An extensive chemical effort modifying these structures resulted in the preparation of many potent analogues. Their activities in experimentally infected animals demonstrated the necessity of the 4-aminotoluene structure part (2b) for biological activity. Further modifications and simplifications of the lucanthone structure led to a series of p-toluidene derivatives such as Mirasan (2c) and

Hoechst S-688 (**2d**) with very high antischistosomal activities in mice, but much lower in monkeys and none at all in man.

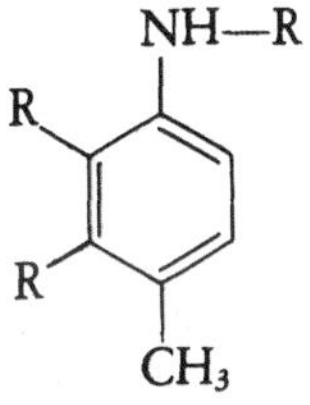

2b
4-Aminotoluene (R = H)

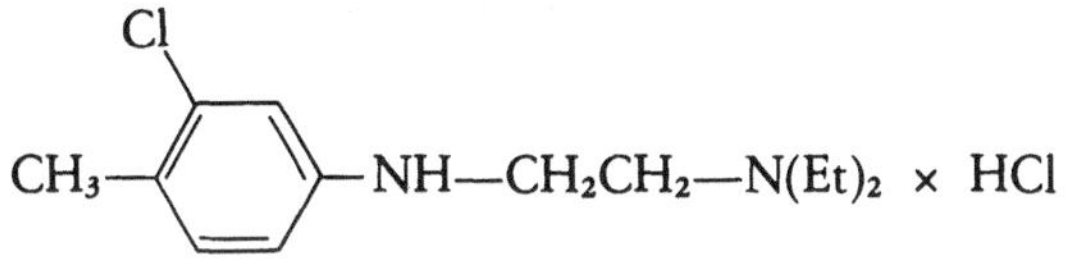

2c
Mirasan

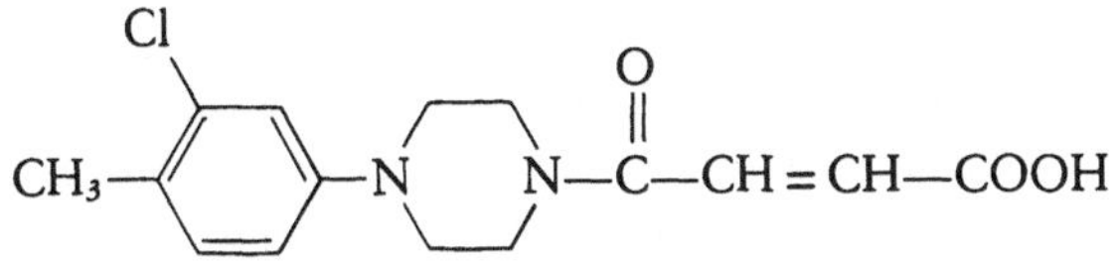

2d
Hoechst S-688

This curious property of varying potencies in different hosts together with the knowledge of rapid metabolism led to the speculation of host-specific metabolic activation of these miracil drugs, although a metabolite could not be isolated and identified. Eventually in 1965, a new compound was obtained through microbial hydroxylation of the methyl group of lucanthone with high activities in a wide range of host animals (Rosi *et al.*, 1965). This compound, hycanthone (**2e**), could then be shown to be identical with the evasive metabolically activated lucanthone derivative, suggesting that the methyl groups necessary for activities in all the compounds of this series must be metabolically hydroxylated and that this metabolism proceeds at different rates in different hosts. Another version of a synthetic *p*-aminobenzyl alcohol derivative in current use is the quinoline compound oxaminiquin (**2f**). High mutagenic activity in the Ames test was shown by hycanthone, although much less for some equally antiparasitic and closely related structures, especially the N-oxide version (**2g**).

2.3. Bisanilino Compounds (or Aminophenols)

A new structural class of bisanilino compounds was discovered through a mouse screen against *S. mansoni* in 1952 and further modified extensively by chemical synthesis of structures of the general formula 3a at May and Baker, and at Wellcome. These compounds, however, failed to be of practical therapeutic value because of inherent serious toxic side effects.

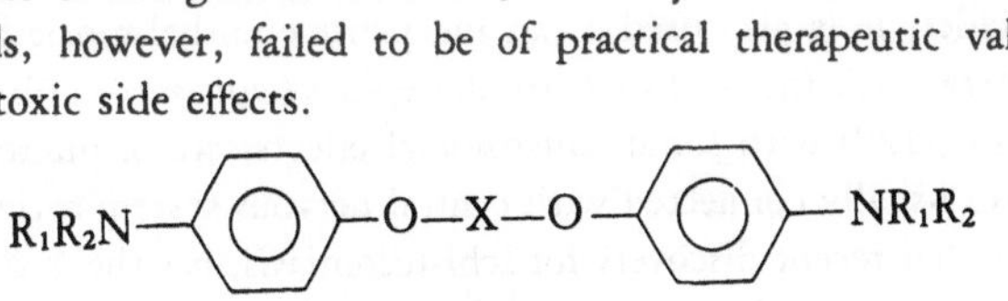

3a
R_1, R_2 = H, alkyl, acyl
X = $(CH_2)_n$, *etc.*

Structurally, the recently synthesized amoscanate (3b) with good activities against all three human schistosome species is closely related to this group of compounds. Exploitation of the bisanilino lead for liver fluke chemotherapy is treated later in this chapter (Section 3.5).

2.4. Nitroheterocyclic Compounds

Certain nitrothiazoles have been known for some time to possess moderate anti-schistosomal activities. In the more recent past, the synthetic modification of this lead afforded niridazole (4a) as a potent drug that occasionally causes serious disturbances of the CNS in the form of convulsions, especially in patients in whom a diseased liver does not allow rapid metabolic detoxification. This prevented the use of niridazole as a mass treatment suitable for the poor areas of the world where the disease is endemic.

Nitrofurans are mainly known as antibacterials, although there are examples with antischistosomal activities exemplified by the furan compound (4b) (Hulbert et al., 1973). Unfortunately the mutagenic potential of nitroheterocyclic compounds as shown by nearly all compounds of this group in the Ames test makes their future pursuit as drugs questionable (Cantelli-Forti et al., 1983).

$$O_2N \underset{O}{\diagdown} CH = CH - \underset{N}{\overset{N-O}{\diagdown}} NH_2$$

4b

2.5. Praziquantel

The most significant advance in recent chemotherapy of schistosomal infections is the discovery of praziquantel (5), which is active against all three species of human schistosomes, is well tolerated and free of potential mutagenic problems. It also has excellent activity against tapeworms and is therefore discussed in detal in Chapter 22.

2.6. Miscellaneous Substances

Trichlorfon (6a) is one of many hundreds of organophosphates originally synthesized as insecticides; it is also used as an inexpensive anthelmintic agent despite its rather narrow therapeutic index. Two benzodiazepines (clonazepam 6b and its 3-methyl derivative RO 11-3128) with some schistosomal effects, are of interest as representatives of structures usually connected with central nervous system actions in mammals. Oltipraz, 6c, another recent discovery for schistosomiasis, has the 1,2-dithiol-3-thione as a new structure type. It has no toxic effects on the cardiovascular, respiratory, or nervous systems and is devoid of mutagenic or immunosuppressive properties. Many urinary metabolites have been detected that result from further oxidation after opening of the dithiol ring and formation of a substituted pyrrolo[1,2-*a*]pyrazine ring system **6d**, a reaction that also can be carried out by treatment of the drug with Na_2S and aqueous DMSO, followed by an alkylation reaction.

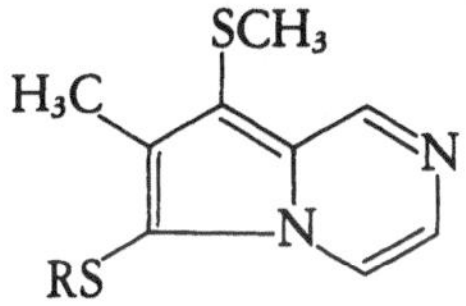

6d

LUCANTHONE HYDROCHLORIDE

CARN: 548-57-2
$C_{20}H_{25}ClN_2OS$ mol. wt. 376.94
1-[[2-(diethylamino)ethyl]amino]-4-methyl-9*H*-thioxanthen-9-one, monohydrochloride
Synonyms: RP3735, Miracil D, Nilodin.

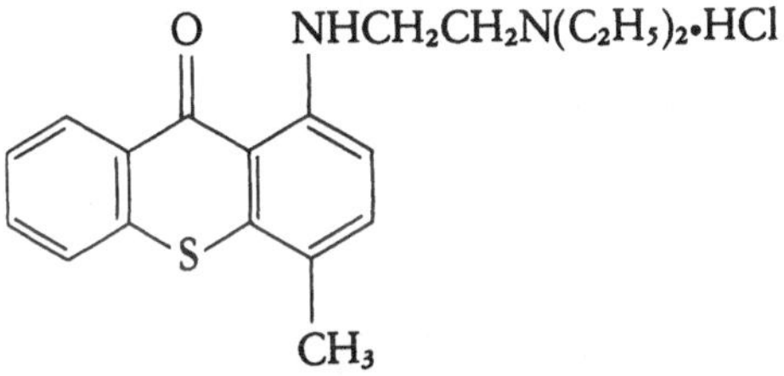

2a

Solubility: water-soluble as hydrochloride, as free base soluble in organic solvents; active metabolite is hycanthone.
Preparation: Mauss (1948).

HYCANTHONE

CARN: 3105-97-3
$C_{20}H_{24}N_2O_2S$ mol. wt. 356.48
1-[[2-(diethylamino)ethyl]amino]-4-(hydroxymethyl)-9*H*-thioxanthen-9-one
Synonyms: etrenol (= mesylate salt).

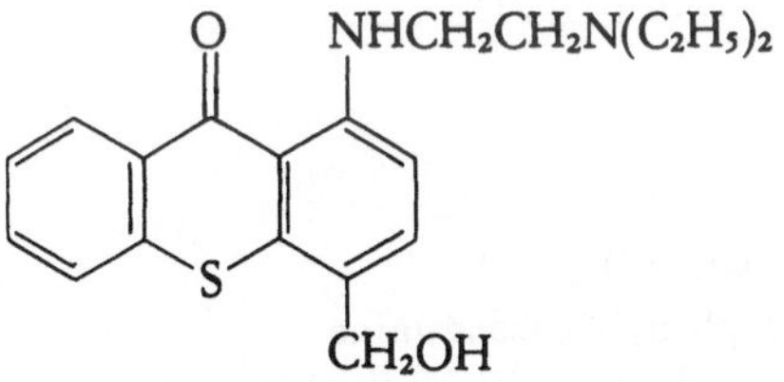

2e

Acid sensitive, must be injected intramuscularly.

Mutagenicity: Highly mutagenic to *Salmonella typhimurium* strains (Ames test) and hepatocarcinogenic after a single-dose administration to mice infected with *S. mansoni.* A newer chloroimidazole analogue and its *N*-oxide (2 g) are equally potent but are only mildly mutagenic (Batzinger and Bueding, 1977).

Preparation: Rosi *et al.* (1967).

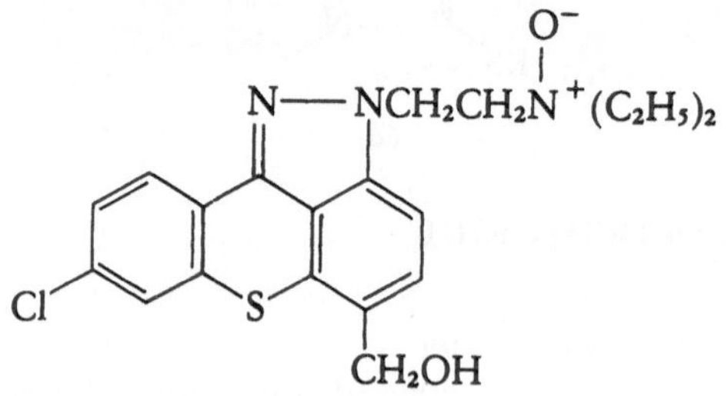

2g

OXAMNIQUINE

CARN: 21738-42-1

$C_{14}H_{21}N_3O_3$ mol. wt. 279.34

1,2,3,4-tetrahydro-2-[[1-methylethyl)amino]methyl]-7-nitro-6-quinolinemethanol

Synonyms: Mansil, Vansil, UK 4271.

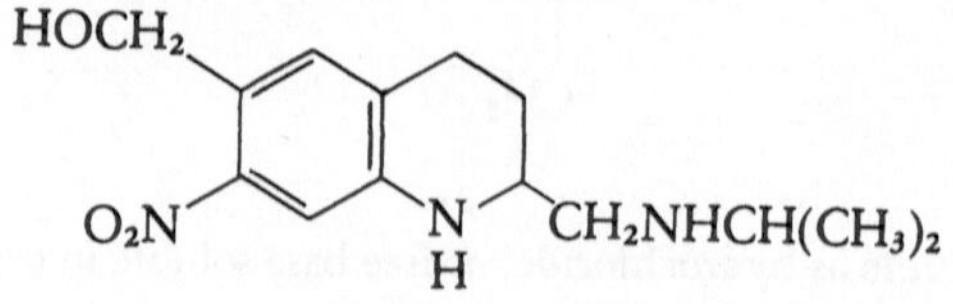

2f

Metabolism: 70–90% of drug metabolized after 4 hr in mice (Woolhouse and Kaye, 1977).

Toxicity: LD_{50} in mice, rabbits: >800 mg/kg.

Mutagenicity: Mutagenic to *Salmonella typhimurium* strains (Ames test), especially in the host-mediated assay (Batzinger and Bueding, 1977).

Toxicology: No evidence of carcinogenicity was observed at dose levels up to 150 mg/kg in chronic studies in mice and hamsters (Chvedoff *et al.,* 1984).

Preparation: Baxter and Richards (1972).

AMOSCANATE

CARN: 26328-53-0

$C_{13}H_9N_3O_2S$ mol. wt. 271.30

4-Isothiocyanato-*N*-(4-nitrophenyl)benzeneamine

Synonyms: Isothiocyanic acid *p*-(*p*-nitroanilino)-phenyl ester, 4-nitro-4'-isothiocyanatodiphenylamine, 4-isothiocyanato-4'-nitrodiphenyl-amine, C9333-GO, CGP-4540, nithiocyamine.

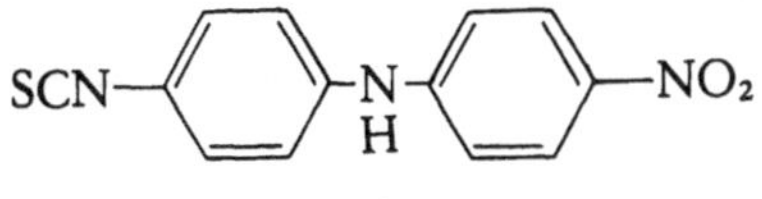

$$SCN-\text{⟨⟩}-\underset{H}{N}-\text{⟨⟩}-NO_2$$

3b

Solubility: insol. in water and most organic solvents; sol. in polyethylene glycol 400 or dimethylacetamide.

Formulation: Reduction of particle size diameter from 30 to 0.5 μm permitted reduction of single dose from 200–300 mg/kg to as low as 10 mg/kg in mice (Bueding *et al.*, 1976).

Mutagenecity: No mutagenic activity detected *in vitro* in *Salmonella* tester strains (Ames test) in the absence or presence of liver microsome preparations, but a mutagenic metabolite was observed in the host mediated assay system and in the urine of drug treated mice. Simultaneous application of a sulfa antibacterial drug decreased these urinary mutagenic metabolites markedly, which suggests a role of intestinal bacteria in the formation of mutagenic metabolites (Bueding *et al.*, 1976).

NIRIDAZOLE

CARN: 61-57-4
$C_6H_6N_4O_3S$ mol. wt. 214.22
1-(5-Nitro-2-thiazolyl)-2-imidazolidinone
Synonyms: Ambilhar, CIBA 32644-Ba.

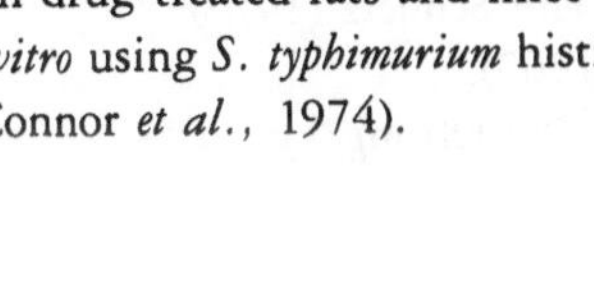

$$O_2N-\text{⟨thiazole⟩}-N-\underset{O}{\overset{}{C}}-NH$$

4a

Metabolism: Extensively metabolized to unknown metabolites by *S.* mansoni; 4-keto-niridazole isolated from drug-treated rats and mice (Catto *et al.*, 1984).

Mutagenicity: Mutagenic *in vitro* using *S. typhimurium* histidine auxotrophs (Ames test); frameshift mutagen (Connor *et al.*, 1974).

TRICHLORFON

CARN: 52-68-6
$C_4H_8Cl_3O_4P$ mol. wt. 257.45
(2,2,2-Trichloro-1-hydroxyethyl)phosphonic acid, dimethyl ester
Synonyms: Metrifonate, dipterex, neguvon, chlorofos.

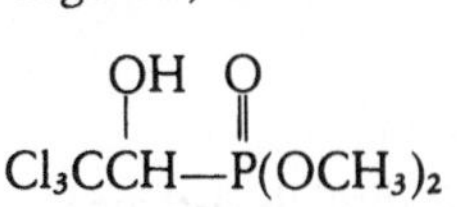

$$\underset{Cl_3CCH}{\overset{OH}{|}}-\underset{}{\overset{O}{\underset{||}{P}}}(OCH_3)_2$$

6a

Solubility: sol. in water and ether.

Toxicity: LD_{50} orally in female rats: 560 mg/kg.

Metabolism: (Lange, 1980).

Mutagenicity: Low mutagenic activity in *Salmonella typhimurium* strains (Ames test) but higher in the host-mediated assay (Batzinger and Bueding, 1977).

PRAZIQUANTEL

CARN: 55268-74-1

See Chapter 22.

CLONAZEPAM

CARN: 1622-61-3

$C_{15}H_{10}ClN_3O_3$ mol. wt. 315.72

5-(2-Chlorophenyl)-1,3-dihydro-7nitro-2H-1,4-benzodiazepin-2-one

Synonym: RO 5-4023.

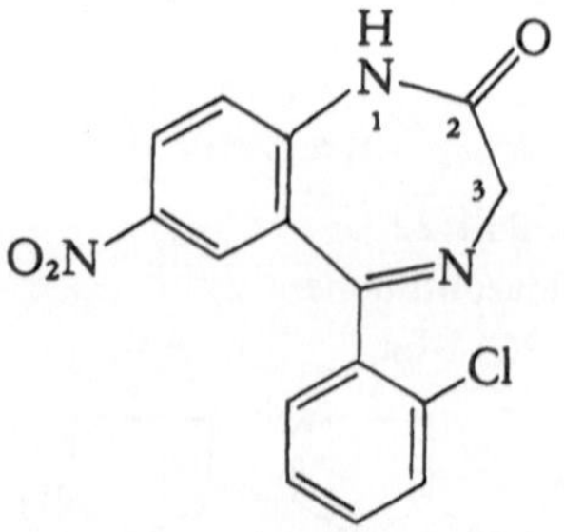

6b

Solubility: v. low water solubility; sol. in acetone and methanol.

Toxicology: Blum *et al.* (1973).

Analysis and Metabolites: Ebel and Schuetz (1977).

Preparation: Sternbach *et al.* (1963).

Toxicity: LD_{50} orally in mice: >4000 mg/kg.

RO 11-3128

CARN: 67027-56-9

This is the 3-methyl analogue of clonazepam.

OLTIPRAZ

CARN: 64224-21-1

$C_8H_6N_2S_3$ mol. wt. 226.34

4-Methyl-5-(2-pyrazinyl)-3H-1,2-dithiole-3-thione

Synonym: RP 35972.

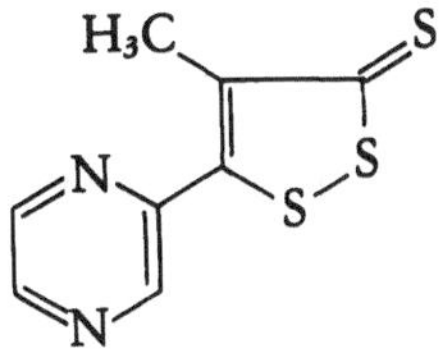

6c

Metabolism: Bieder *et al.* (1983).
Analytical method: Ali *et al.* (1984).
Preparation: Leroy *et al.* (1978).

3. CHEMISTRY OF FASCIOLICIDES

3.1. Halogenated Hydrocarbons

The chemotherapy of fascioliasis was carried out during the 1920s with male fern extract or the two halogenated hydrocarbons carbon tetrachloride (7a) and hexachloroethane (7b). Until very recently, the latter was the only agent approved for veterinary medicine in the United States but is no longer used because of the mutagenic properties observed with a number of polyhalogenated hydrocarbons. Related compounds such as difluorotetrachloroethane (Freon 112) or 1,4-bistrichloromethylbenzene (hetol) (7c) have been used to a limited extent. Hetol was also proposed for human *Chlonorchis sinensis* infections but was later withdrawn because of serious side effects.

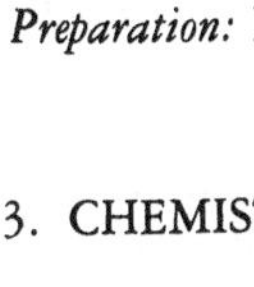

7a

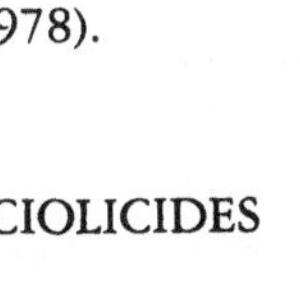

7b

Hetol

7c

3.2. Halogenated Phenols and Bisphenols

Hexachlorophene (8a) was used since the 1940s as an anti-infective topical agent and was included in germicidal soaps. It was introduced in the late 1950s as the first member of this new group of compounds effective against mature *F. hepatica* infections. Subsequently, a number of chemicals with similar structure were tested and advanced as fasciolicides with varying degrees of potency. Bithionol (8b) has a sulfur bridge between the two phenol rings; the corresponding sulfoxide (8c) is also known as a fasciolicide. Menichlopholan (8d) is a bisphenol in which the two phenol rings are attached directly *via* a carbon–carbon bond. Two monophenols substituted by electron-withdrawing substituents such as halogen, nitro, or cyano groups with fasciolicidal activities are disophenol (8e) and nitroxynil (8f). A closer look at the structures suggests that two such substituents are necessary in at least the ortho- and para-positions of the phenol and that the other ortho-position of the phenol must also be substituted in order to show fasciolicidal activity. A similar structure–activity relationship applies to the salicylanilides, which can be regarded as close analogues of the bisphenols containing a carboxamide group to join the two aromatic rings.

3.3. Salicylanilides

In 1963 Lienert discovered the fasciolicidal activity of Diaphene, a mixture containing 3,4′,5-tribromosalicylanilide (tribromsalane) (9a) as major component and active principle, and 4′,5-dibromosalicylanilide (9b), which was used as a germicide. This new lead was actively pursued by several research laboratories and, within the next 10 years, a number of modified salicylanilides were developed as new fasciolicides (9c–9h). The major achievement resulting from this research activity was the increased potency against adult and particularly the more refractive immature flukes accompanied by an increased safety margin, which for the first time permitted mass treatment of sheep and cattle with good efficacy against the young flukes down to 6 and 4 weeks of age. Introduction of highly lipophilic groups such as iodine, chlorophenoxy, or tert-, butyl-substituents was particularly beneficial for high activities. The plasma half-life of active fasciolicidal salicylanilides is 2–4 days and that of the most potent ones, including rafoxanide and bromoxanide, extends to 5–6 days (Lee, 1973). This is reflected in slow excretion and persistent drug residues, requiring several weeks of withdrawal periods before slaughter. The drug residue levels in milk exclude the use of most salicylanilides as well as phenol-type fasciolicides from use in milk-producing animals (Heeschen et al., 1972). Halogenated phenols and salicylanilides are known to be uncouplers of oxidative phosphorylation (Campbell and Montague, 1981). Their safety margin as a group is narrow; lethal levels are often only slightly higher than effective dose levels, especially at the increased doses required for effectiveness against immature F. hepatica infections (Boray, 1969).

Toxic manifestations caused by sublethal doses of salicylanilides include depression, anorexia, diarrhea, peripheral neuropathy, cerebral edema, blindness, and vacuolation of the white matter of the CNS, papilledema, equatorial cataracts, optic neuropathy, and extensive vacuolation of the white matter of the brain and spinal cord (Brown et al., 1972).

3.4. Benzimidazoles

Although thiabendazole, the first of a series of broad-spectrum anthelmintic agents, displayed activity at high doses against the lancet fluke Dicrocoelium dentriticum, it has, as with nearly all benzimidazole broad-spectrum anthelmintics, no effect on liver flukes. Albendazole, however, a more recent analogue in the benzimidazole series, has an anthelmintic spectrum that includes at least mature F. hepatica in sheep and cattle, although at higher doses as is required for its nematocidal activities.

A very recent addition to the group of benzimidazoles is triclabendazole (10a), which is very well tolerated, with a wide safety margin and good activity against *F. hepatica* in sheep and cattle from the earliest age through the fully mature stages. It does not, however, possess a broad spectrum against nematodes, and it probably acts by a mechanism different from that of the structurally related benzimidazole anthelmintics.

3.5. Bisanilino Compounds

The bisanilino compounds were originally pursued for their antischistosomal activities. This group represents so far the only chemical class of compounds with members active against both of the two major flatworms. An extensive research program, including many mono- as well as bisanilino structures, resulted in a number of very potent fasciolicides that could not be used, however, because of serious toxic side effects at use levels, such as visual disturbances, including blindness (Laemmler and Loewe, 1962). Only much later was diamfenetide (11a) introduced as a fasciolicide in the form of a bisacetylated prodrug that originated from 4-tert-butoxcyacetanilide and 4-allyloxyacetanilide as an early lead (Harfenist, 1973). Although this diacetate must be metabolized *in vivo* to the bisanilino compound 11b, which is the active principle, the serious side effects in the host associated with bisanilino compounds are avoided, presumably because of the slow release of the active principle combined with its rapid metabolism. The metabolic deacetylation proceeds rapidly in liver extracts of sheep, slowly in liver extracts of rabbits, mice, and cattle, and not at all in rats. As a consequence, diamfenetide is more effective in sheep than in cattle (Coles, 1976). In contrast to almost all other fasciolicides, diamfenetide is much more effective against the immature than mature *F. hepatica*.

3.6. Benzene Sulfonamides

Compounds of this class have provided highly successful drugs for a number of diseases ever since the discovery of antibacterial activities for sulfanilamide. Recently fasciolicidal activity of halogenated sulfanilamide derivatives was discovered; extensive chemical modification of this lead produced clorsulon (12a), with good activities against flukes from the age of 4 weeks with low toxicity and rapid excretion, making it very suitable for use in meat-producing animals.

4. AGENT EFFECTIVE AGAINST *DICROCOELIUM DENTRITICUM*

The discovery of hetolin 13a, a new structural type with specific activity against this rather rare parasite, resulted from the screening and chemical modification of the lead compound (Schorr *et al.*, 1964).

NITROXYNIL

CARN: 1689-89-0

$C_7H_3IN_2O_3$ mol. wt. 290.03

4-Hydroxy-3-iodo-5-nitrobenzonitrile

Synonyms: Dovenix, Trodax (*N*-ethylglucamine salt, $C_{15}H_{22}IN_3O_8$, mol. wt. 290.03)

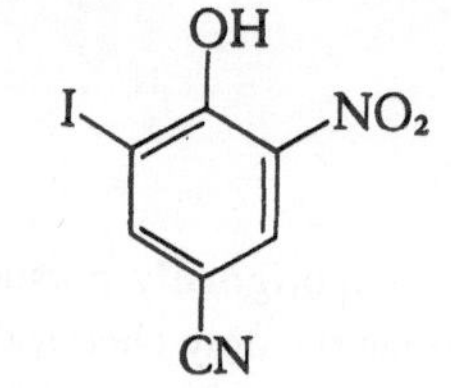

8f

Solubility: Low water solubility; soluble in organic solvents.

N-Ethylglucamine salt (Trodax) freely sol. in water; aq. soln. is stable.

Tissue residue analysis: Parnell (1970).

Milk residue analysis: Takeshita *et al.* (1980); Bluethgen *et al.* (1982).

BISPHENOLS

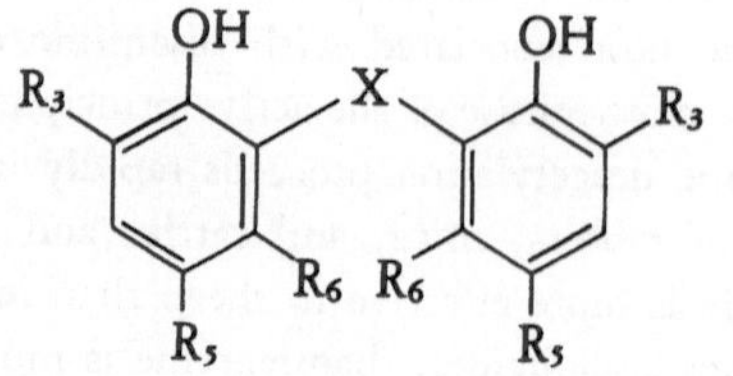

		R_3	R_5	R_6	X
8a	Hexachlorophene	Cl	Cl	Cl	CH_2
8b	Bithionol	Cl	Cl	H	S
8c	Bithionol sulfoxide	Cl	Cl	H	SO
8d	Menichlopholan	NO_2	Cl	H	Direct bond

HEXACHLOROPHENE

CARN: 70-30-4

$C_{13}H_6Cl_6O_2$ mol. wt. 406.92

2,2'-Methylenebis[3,4,6-trichloro]phenol

Synonyms: Bilevon, pHisohex.

Solubility: pract. insol. in water; sol. in alcohol, acetone, ether, propylene glycol.

Notes: Used mainly in germicidal soaps; use regulated by FDA due to potential neurotoxicity.

BITHIONOL

CARN: 97-18-7

$C_{12}H_6Cl_4O_2S$ mol. wt. 356.07

2,2'-Thiobis[4,6-dichloro]phenol

Forms a sodium salt.

Solubility: pract. insol. in water; sol. in acetone, dimethylacetamide; low solubility in propylene glycol and ethanol.

Note: Banned by FDA from use in cosmetics.

Sulfoxide

$C_{12}H_6Cl_4O_3S$ mol. wt. 372.07

Synonym: Bitin-S.

MENICHLOPHOLAN

CARN: 10331-57-4

$C_{12}H_6Cl_2N_2O_6$ mol. wt. 345.09

5,5'-Dichloro-3,3'-dinitro-[1,1'-biphenyl]-2,2'-diol

Synonyms: Niclofolan, Bayer 9015, Me3625, Bilevon-M.

Solubility: insol. in water; sol. in organic solvents.

Milk residue analysis: Bluethgen *et al.* (1982).

SALICYLANILIDES

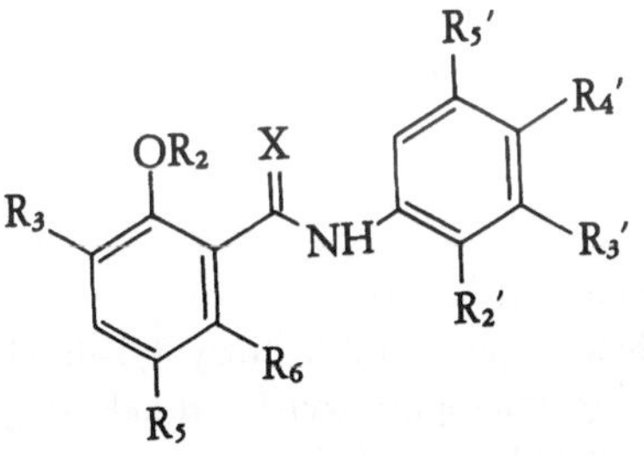

		R_2	R_3	R_5	R_6	X	$R_{2'}$	$R_{3'}$	$R_{4'}$	$R_{5'}$
9a	Tribromsalan	H	Br	Br	H	O	H	H	Br	H
9b		H	H	Br	H	O	H	H	Br	H
9c	Oxyclozanide	H	Cl	Cl	Cl	O	OH	Cl	H	Cl
9d	Clioxanide	COCH$_3$	I	I	H	O	H	H	Cl	H
9e	Rafoxanide	H	I	I	H	O	H	Cl	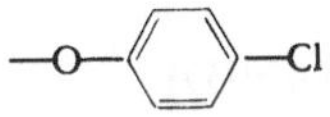 —O—⬡—Cl	H
9f	Brotianide	COCH$_3$	Br	Cl	H	S	H	H	Br	H
9g	Bromoxanide	H	C(CH$_3$)$_3$	NO$_2$	CH$_3$	O	CF$_3$	H	Br	H
9h	Closantel	H	I	I	H	O	CH$_3$	H	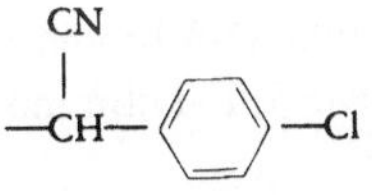 —CH(CN)—⬡—Cl	Cl

TRIBROMSALAN

CARN: 87-10-5

$C_{13}H_8Br_3NO_2$ mol. wt. 449.96

3,5-Dibromo-*N*-(4-bromophenyl)-2-hydroxybenzamide

Synonyms: 3,4',5-Tribromosalicylanilide, major component and active ingredient in Diaphene and Hilomide (in mixture with 4',5-dibromosalicylanilide, **9b**)

Solubility: pract. insol. in water; sol. in organic solvents like hot acetone; v. sol. in DMF.

Note: Used as a bacteriostat in detergents; banned by FDA from use in cosmetics.

OXYCLOZANIDE

CARN: 2277-92-1

$C_{13}H_6Cl_5NO_3$ mol. wt. 401.48

2,3,5-Trichloro-*N*-(3,5-dichloro-2-hydroxyphenyl)-6-hydroxybenzamide

Synonyms: 3,3',5,5',6-Pentachloro-2'-hydroxysalicylanilide, Zanil.

Solubility: insol. in water, sol. in DMF.

Milk residue analysis: Bluethgen *et al.* (1982).

CLIOXANIDE

CARN: 14437-41-3

$C_{15}H_{10}ClI_2NO_3$ mol. wt. 541.54

2-(Acetyloxy)-*N*-(4-chlorophenyl)-3,5-diiodobenzamide

Synonyms: 2-Acetoxy-4'-chloro-3,5-diiodobenzanilide, Tremerad.

Solubility: insol. in water; sol. in DMF, acetone, methanol.

Toxicity: LD_{50} by ruminal application in sheep: 420 mg/kg.

RAFOXANIDE

CARN: 22662-39-1

$C_{19}H_{11}Cl_2I_2NO_3$ mol. wt. 626.01

N-[3-Chloro-4-(4-chlorophenoxy)phenyl]-2-hydroxy-3,5-diiodobenzamide

Synonyms: 3'-Chloro-4'-(*p*-chlorophenoxy)-3,5-diiodosalicylanilide,   MK-990, Bovanide, Duofas, Flukanide, Ranide.

Solubility: pract. insol. in water; sol. in acetone, methanol, DMF.

Analytical procedures: Talley *et al.* (1971); Fink (1981).

Metabolism and residue: Dedek *et al.* (1977, 1978).

Determination of milk residues: Gabrio *et al.* (1978).

Preparation: Mrozik *et al.* (1969).

BROTIANIDE

CARN: 23233-88-7

$C_{15}H_{10}Br_2ClNO_2S$ mol. wt. 463.59

2-(Acetyloxy)-3-bromo-*N*-(4-bromophenyl)-5-chlorobenzenecarbothioamide

Synonyms: 3,4'-Dibromo-5-chlorothiosalicylanilide acetate, BAY 4059, Dirian.

BROMOXANIDE

CARN: 41113-86-4

$C_{19}H_{18}BrF_3N_2O_4$ mol. wt. 475.27

N-[4-Bromo-2-(trifluoromethyl)phenyl]-3-(1,1-dimethylethyl)-2-hydroxy-6-meth-
yl-5-nitrobenzamide
Synonyms: None.

CLOSANTEL

CARN: 57808-65-8
$C_{22}H_{14}Cl_2I_2N_2O_2$ mol. wt. 663.08
N-(5-Chloro-4-[(4-chlorophenyl)cyanomethyl]-2-methylphenyl)-2-hydroxy-3,5-
diiodobenzamide
Synonyms: None.

ALBENDAZOLE

CARN: 54965-21-8
See Chapter 11.

TRICLABENDAZOLE

CARN: 68786-66-3
$C_{14}H_9Cl_3N_2OS$ mol. wt. 501.80
5-Chloro-6-(2,3-dichlorophenoxy)-2-(methylthio)1H-benzimidazole
Synonyms: CGA 89317, Fasinex.

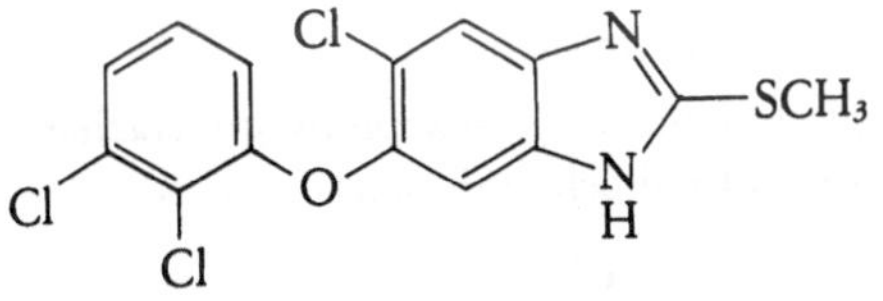

10a

Note: Water-based drench formulations tolerated in sheep at 150–200 mg/kg.

DIAMFENETIDE

CARN: 36141-82-9
$C_{20}H_{24}N_2O_5$ mol. wt. 372.42
N,N'-[Oxybis(2,1-ethanediyloxy-4,1-phenylene)]bisacetamide
Synonyms: Diamphenetide, Coriban

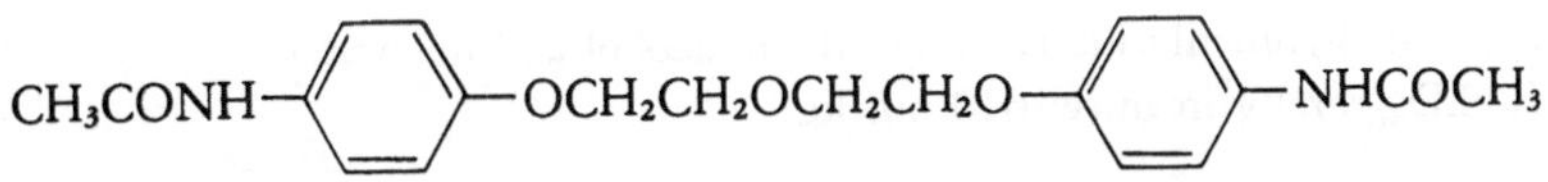

11a

Toxicity: LD$_{50}$ in rodents: >3000 mg/kg orally.

Active metabolite:

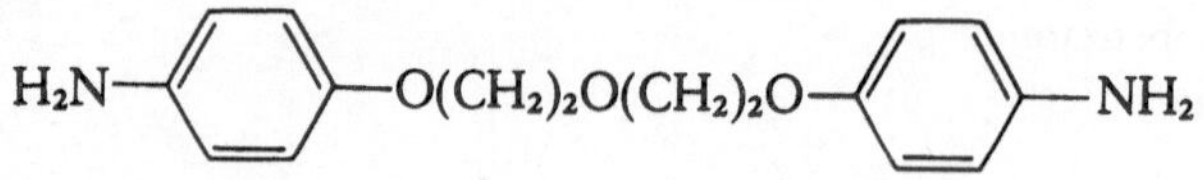

$$H_2N-\bigcirc-O(CH_2)_2O(CH_2)_2O-\bigcirc-NH_2$$

11b

CLORSULON

CARN: 60200-06-8
$C_8H_8Cl_3N_3O_4S_2$ mol. wt. 380.66
4-Amino-6-(trichloroethenyl)-1,3-benzenedisulfonamide
Synonyms: L-631,529, MK-401.

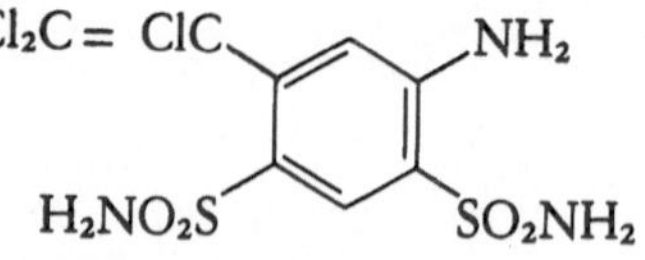

$$Cl_2C=ClC\diagdown\quad\diagup NH_2$$
$$H_2NO_2S\diagup\quad\diagdown SO_2NH_2$$

12a

Solubility: sol. in hot water, alcohol, ethyl acetate, ether, DMF; insol. in $CHCl_3$.
Analytical method: Vanden Heuvel *et al.* (1977).
Preparation: Mrozik *et al.* (1977).

HETOLIN

CARN: 2390-22-9
$C_{26}H_{25}Cl_3N_2O$ mol. wt. 487.85
1-Methyl-4-[3,3,3-tris(4-chlorophenyl)-1-oxopropyl]piperazine
Synonyms: LZ-544, Dicroden (hydrochloride salt).

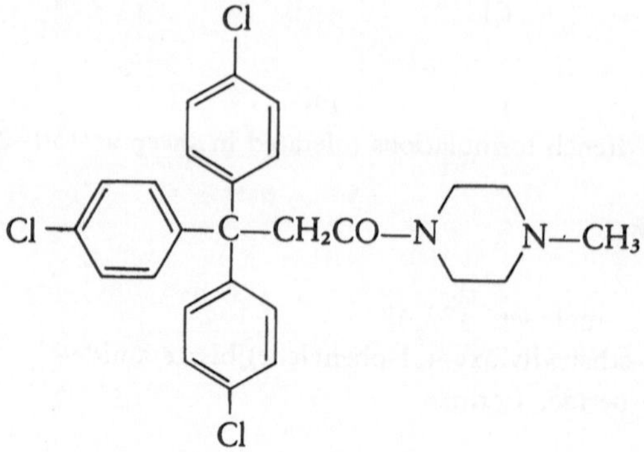

$$Cl-\bigcirc-\overset{\displaystyle\bigcirc-Cl}{\underset{\displaystyle\bigcirc-Cl}{C}}-CH_2CO-N\diagup\quad\diagdown N-CH_3$$

13a

Solubility: The hydrochloride is freely sol. in alcohol and hot water.
Toxicity: LD_{50} orally in mice: 610 mg/kg.

EMETINE

CARN: 483-18-1
$C_{29}H_{40}N_2O_4$ mol. wt. 480.63
6',7',10,11-Tetramethoxyemetan

14a

Solubility: sol. in organic solvents (alcohols, acetone, ethyl acetate, ether); sl. sol. in water, emetine dihydrochloride; freely sol. in water and alcohol.

Toxicity: LD_{50} in rats ip: 12 /mg/kg; LD_{50} of dihydrochloride in mice po: 30 mg/kg

Note: Major use as an amebicide.

REFERENCES

Ali, H. M., Bennett, J. L., Sulaiman, S. M., and Gaillot, J., 1984, Method for the determination of oltipraz, a new antischistosomal agent in blood, *J. Chromatogr.* 305:465–469.

Batzinger, R. P., and Bueding, E., 1977, Mutagenic activities *in vitro* and *in vivo* of five antischistosomal compounds, *J. Pharmacol. Exp. Ther.* 200:1–9.

Baxter, C. A. R., and Richards, H. C., 1972, Schistosomicides. 2. Derivatives of 2,3,4,4a,5,6-hexahydro-1H-pyrazino[1,2-a]quinoline, *J. Med. Chem.* 15:351–356.

Bieder, A., Decouvelaere, B., Gaillard, C., Depaire, H., Heusse, D., Ledoux, C., Lemar, M., LeRoy, J. P., Raymond, L., Snozzi, C., and Gregoire, J., 1983, Comparison of the metabolism of oltiptraz in the mouse, rat, monkey and in man, *Arzneimittelforsch.* 33:1289–1297.

Bluethgen, A., Heeschen, W., and Nijhuis, H., 1982, Gas chromatographic determination of fasciolicide residues in milk, *Milchwissenschaft* 37:206–211.

Blum, J. E., Haefely, W., Jalfre, M., Pole, P., and Schaerer, K., 1973, Pharmacology and toxicology of the antieliptic drug clonazepam, *Arzneimittelforsch.* 23:377–389.

Boray, J. C., 1969, Experimental fascioliasis in Australia, in: *Advances in Parasitology* (B. Dawes, ed.), Vol. 7, pp. 95–210, Academic Press, New York.

Brown, W. R., Rubin, L. Hite, M., and Zwickey, R. E., 1972, Experimental papilledema in the dog induced by a salicylanilide, *Toxicol. Appl. Pharmacol.* 21:532–541.

Bueding, E., Batzinger, R., and Petterson, G., 1976, Antischistosomal and some toxicological properties of a nitrodiphenylaminoisothiocyanate (C9333-Go/CGP4540), *Experientia* 32:604–606.

Campbell, A. J., and Montague, P. E., 1981, A comparison of the activity of uncouplers of oxidative phosphorylation against the common liver fluke *Fasciola hepatica*, *Mol. Biochem. Parasitol.* 4:139–147.

Cantelli-Forti, G., Aicardi, G., Guerra, M. C., Barbaro, A. M., and Biagi, G. L., 1983, Mutagenicity of a series of 25 nitroimidazoles and two nitrothiazoles in *Salmonella typhimurium*, *Terat. Carcin. Mutagen.* 3:51–63.

Catto, B. A., Tracy, J. W., and Webster, L. T., Jr., 1984a, 1-Thiocarbamoyl-2-imidazolidinone, a metabolite of niridazole in *Schistosoma mansoni*, *Mol. Biochem. Parasitol.* 10:111–120.

Catto, B. A., Valencia, C. I., Hafez, K., Fairchild, E. H., and Webster, L. T., Jr., 1984b, 4-Ketoniridazole: A major niridazole metabolite with central nervous system toxicity different than niridazole, *J. Pharmacol. Exp. Ther.* 228:662–668.

Chvedoff, M., Faccini, J. M., Gregory, M. H., Hull, R. M., Monro, A. M., Perraud, J., Quinton, R. M., and Reinert, H. H., 1984, The toxicology of the schistosomicidal agent oxamniquin, *Drug Dev. Res.* 4:229–235.

Coles, G. C., 1976, The inactivity of diamphenetide against liver fluke in certain species of mammals, *Res. Vet. Sci.* 20:110–111.

Connor, T., Stoeckel, M., and Legator, M. S., 1974, Niridazole, a direct acting frameshift mutagen not affected by microsomal enzyme preparation which can be detected in the host-mediated assay, *Mutat. Res.* 26:456–457.

Dedek, W., Schwarz, H., and Liebaug, E., 1977, Degradation and residue dynamics of the anthelmintic 131I-rafoxanide in blood, milk, meat and fat following different dosages in cattle, *Arch. Exp. Veterinaermed.* 31:365–368.

Dedek, W., Grahl, R., Schwarz, H., and Ludwig, P., 1978, Metabolism, residues, and excretion of the anthelmintic 131I-rafoxanide in blood, milk, meat and urine of tbe lactating cow, *Arch. Exp. Veterinaermed.* 32:951–955.

Ebel, S., and Schuetz, H., 1977, Studies on the detection of clonazepam and its main metabolites with regard to the thin-layer chromatographic separation of nitrazepam and its major metabolic products, *Arzneimittelforsch.* 27:325–337.

Fink, D. W., 1981, Spectrophotometric quantification of the salicylanilide anthelmintic rafoxanide based on the charge-transfer absorbance of its iron (III) complex, *Anal. Chim. Acts* 131:281–285.

Gabrio, T., Konrad, H., Scheybal, A., Dedek, W., and Schwarz, H., 1978, Determination of rafoxanide and hexachloro-p-xylene residues in milk after administration of these fasciolicides, *Nahrung* 22:409–414.

Ginger, C. D., 1982, Antiparasitic agents, *Annu. Rep. Med. Chem.* 17:129.

Harfenist, M., 1973, Diamphenetide—A new fasciolicide active against immature parasites, *Pestic. Sci.* 4:871–882.

Heeschen, W., Tolle, A., and Bluethgen, A., 1972, Fasciolicides in milk, *Arch. Lebensmittelhyg.* 23:1–7.

Hulbert, P. B., Bueding, E., and Robinson, C. H., 1973, Structure and antischistosomal activity in the nitrofuran series, *J. Med. Chem.* 16:72–78.

Islip, P. J., 1979, Anthelmintic agents, in: *Burger's Medicinal Chemistry* (M. E. Wolf, ed.), 4th ed., Part II, p. 481, Wiley, New York.

Kikuth, W., Goennert, R., and Mauss, H., 1946, Miracil, a new chemotherapeutic compound against intestinal bilharziosis, *Naturwissenschaften* 33:253.

Laemmler, G., 1968, Chemotherapy of trematode infections, in: *Advances in Chemotherapy* (A. Goldin, F. Hawking, and R. J. Schnitzer, eds.), Vol- 3, p. 153, Academic Press, New York.

Laemmler, G., and Loewe, H., 1962, Die Chemotherapie der Fasciolose, *Arzneimittelforsch.* 12:15–21, 164–168.

Lange, C., 1980, Identification of a metabolite of trichlorfon, *Z. Chem.* 20:446–447.

Lee, R. M., 1973, The relationship between biological action and structure for some fasciolicidal salicylanilides, *Parasitology* 67:xiii–xiv.

Leroy, J. P., Barreau, M., Cotrel, C., Jeanmart, C., Messer, M., and Benazet, F., 1978, Laboratory studies of 35972 R.P., a new schistosomicidal compound, *Curr. Chemother.* 1:148–150

Mauss, H., 1948, Über basisch substituierte Xanthon- und Thioxanthon- Abkömmlinge; Miracil, ein neues Chemotherapeutikum, *Chem. Ber.* 81:19.

Miller, M. J., 1976, Protozoan and Helminth parasites—A review of current treatment, *Progr. Drug Res.* 20:433–464.

Mrozik, H., Jones, H., Friedman, J., Schwartzkopf, G., Schardt, R. A., Patchett, A. A., Hoff, D. R., Yakstis, J. J., Riek, R. F., Ostlind, D. A., Plishker, G. A., Butler, R. W., Cuckler, A. C., and Campbell, W. C., 1969, A new agent for the treatment of liver fluke infection (Fascioliasis), *Experientia* 25:883.

Mrozik, H., Bochis, R. J., Eskola, P., Matzuk, A., Waksmunski, F. S., Olen, L. E., Schwartzkopf, G., Jr., Grodski, A., Linn, B. O., Lusi, A., Wu, M.-T., Shunk, C. H., Peterson, L. H., Milkowski, J. D., Hoff, D. R., Kulsa, P., Ostlind, D. A., Campbell, W. C., Riek, R. F., and Harmon, R. E., 1977, 4-Amino-6-(trichloroethenyl)-1,3-benzenedisulfonamide, a new, potent fasciolicide, *J. Med. Chem.* 20:1225–1227.

Parnell, M. J., 1970, Determination of nitroxynil residues in sheep and calves, *Pestic. Sci.* 1:138–143.

Robertson, E. L., 1977, Anticestodal and Antitrematodal Drugs, in: *Veterinary Pharmacology and Therapeutics* (L. M. Jones, N. H. Booth, and L. E. McDonald, eds.), 4th ed., p. 1064; Iowa State University Press, Ames, Iowa.

Rosi, D., Peruzotti, G., Dennis, E. W., Berberian, D. A., Freele, H. W., and Archer, S., 1965, A new, active metabolite of miracil D, *Nature (Lond.)* 208:1005–1006.

Rosi, D., Dennis, E. W., Berberian, D. A., Freele, H. W., Tullar, B. F., and Archer, S., 1967, Hycanthone, a new active metabolite of lucanthone, *J. Med. Chem.* 10:867–876.

Schorr, M., Loewe, H., Juergens, E., Weber, H., and Laemmler, G., 1964, Carbonsaurepiperazide mit chemotherapentischer Wirkung gegen Dicrocoelium dentriticum, *Arzneimittelforsch.* 14:1151–1156.

Sternbach, L. H., Fryer, R. I., Keller, O., Metlesics, W., Sach, G., and Steiger, N., 1963, Quinazolines and 1,4-benzodiazepines. X. Nitro-substituted 5-phenyl-1,4-benzodiazepine derivatives, *J. Med. Chem.* 6:261–265.

Takeshita, Y., Kishi, T., Seki, M., Fujiyama, K., Otsuka, G., and Ahiko, K., 1980, Analysis of nitroxynil (fasciolicide) in milk and dairy products, *Milchwissenschaft* 35:133–135.

Talley, C. P., Trenner, N. R., Downing, G. V., Jr., and VandenHeuvel, W. J. A., 1971, Gas chromatographic determination of rafoxanide [3'-chloro-4'-(4-chlorophenoxy)-3,5-diiodosalicylanilide] in plasma by electron capture detection of its trimethylsilyl derivative, *Anal. Chem.* 43:1379–1382.

Vanden Heuvel, W. J. A. III, Gruber, V. F., Walker, R. W., and Wolf, F. J., 1977, Gas-liquid chromatographic determination of 4-amino-6-(trichloroethenyl)-1,3-benzenedisulfonamide, a new anthelmintic, in biological fluids, *J. Agric. Food Chem.* 25:389–392.

Windholz, M., ed., 1983, *The Merck Index*, 10th ed., Merck and Co., Rahway, New Jersey.

Woolhouse, N. M., and Kaye, B., 1977, Uptake of [14C] oxamniquine by *Schistosoma mansoni*, *Parisitology* 75:111–118.

19

Trematode Infections of Man

WILLIAM C. CAMPBELL and EDITO G. GARCIA

1. INTRODUCTION

A consideration of the chemotherapy of trematode infections of man will invariably be unevenly distributed with respect to the parasites involved. The great preponderance of attention must be devoted to the blood flukes or schistosomes, because of their great medical importance and because so much is known about their treatment. The remaining flukes, having various degrees of medical importance and having a lesser body of therapeutic lore, can be covered more briefly.

2. SCHISTOSOMIASIS

2.1. General Principles

Until recently, the treatment of human schistosomiasis was highly unsatisfactory. Drugs are now available that are both effective and safe, although these attributes are by no means absolute or to be taken for granted.

Since the pathogenesis of schistosomiasis is attributable to schistosome eggs rather than to the worms themselves, a treatment that blocked reproduction could prevent tissue damage and thereby prevent or halt the clinical manifestations of infection. Some of the standard schistosomicidal drugs interfere with reproduction before killing the worms, but some compounds appear to have a specific effect on the reproductive system. These include 4,4'-dinitrocarbanilide in the form of nicarbazin (Campbell and Cuckler, 1967; Pellegrino and Katz, 1969; Warren, 1970; Campbell and Rogers, 1971), ethylenedimethane sulfonate, and hexamethylphosphoramide (Jackson *et al.*,

WILLIAM C. CAMPBELL • Merck Institute for Therapeutic Research, Rahway, New Jersey 07065.   EDITO G. GARCIA • Department of Parasitology, Institute of Public Health, University of the Philippines, Ermita, Manila 2801, Philippines.

1968). None of these is used in medical practice. Indeed, unless chemosterilization were irreversible, treatment would have to be continued for a matter of years—so such treatments are not likely to be introduced. Rather, all the current drugs are used for the purpose of reducing or eliminating the worm population and, since the worms cannot multiply within the human host, total eradication of worms from the patient is not a prerequisite of clinical benefit. A major consideration in the treatment of schistosomiasis is the severity of the disease and its effect on efficacy and safety of the drug being used. This is especially true in infections of *Schistosoma mansoni* and *S. japonicum,* in which severe liver disease is likely to affect drug metabolism and detoxification.

Some drugs have been shown to be prophylactically effective when applied to the skin of laboratory animals. These include various vegetable oils, especially cedarwood oil (Campbell and Cuckler, 1961), various terpenes (Gilbert *et al.,* 1970), and amoscanate, which permits penetration by cercariae but blocks migration to the lungs (Greene *et al.,* 1983). The topical chemoprophylaxis of human schistosomiasis is not likely to become practicable, except perhaps in very unusual circumstances.

While causal prophylaxis may not be feasible, drugs can be used to achieve clinical prophylaxis in infections that are diagnosed before significant damage has been done. Furthermore, treatment can be expected to result in improvements in the form and function of organs that have been damaged by infection. For example, young people with hepatosplenomegaly due to *S. mansoni* showed progressive reduction in the size of the affected organs after treatment (Mahmoud *et al.,* 1983). In older patients such reductions may not occur, but clinical improvement may be marked and further tissue damage can be averted. There have also been reports of post-treatment regression of advanced lesions of the urinary tract attributable to *S. haematobium.* It has been pointed out by Davis (1982) that the prognosis of uncomplicated schistosomiasis is very good, providing that specific chemotherapy is given, and that "the advent of well-tolerated, highly effective new drugs has given physicians flexibility and opportunities to alleviate any chronic complications which were, in the past, therapeutic nightmares."

While there is no doubt that patients with moderate or severe clinical manifestations should be given curative treatment, there is some debate about the treatment of asymptomatic and mildly symptomatic infections. In the past this view was partly dictated by the available drugs, mostly antimonials, which required prolonged administration and were associated with numerous side effects, without any guarantee of cure. Also, on the basis of inadequate knowledge of resistance to reinfection, it was presumed that every treated individual in endemic areas invariably became reinfected. There is now evidence indicating that a significant proportion of treated individuals in endemic areas, although reexposed, are not readily reinfected; and in those that do become reinfected the proportion of infecting parasites that becomes established is less. With the new drugs, every new infection, whether asymptomatic or not, should be treated because schistosomiasis is a long-drawn infection with insidious cumulative pathological damage. One cannot predict the eventual clinical outcome of an early infection.

In endemic areas where available physicians are mostly employed in the government health service, priorities for treatment should be established if there is a lack of sufficient government funds for drugs. If funds are not sufficient for mass chemotherapy, priority should be given to (1) any individual with acute or severe clinical manifestations, (2) patients with high excretal egg output and, (3) patients whose way of life does not entail risks of reinfection or reexposures.

Since schistosomiasis is a public health problem in many tropical and some subtropical countries, chemotherapy is employed not only as a clinical tool but, more importantly, as a public health measure for control. Mass treatment is used as the principal method of control in many endemic areas, and such measures as snail control, proper disposal of human excreta and health education are relegated to secondary roles. The objectives are to reduce or prevent disease, to lower prevalence and, as a substitute for sanitary disposal of schistosome-egg-bearing excreta, to reduce or stop transmission. Since cost is a major consideration in control, ways of saving on drug costs in keeping with the epidemiological situations should be studied. This may be effected by limiting treatment only to cases with high excretal egg-output, or by using reduced dosage of the drug and determining the optimal interval between population treatments for keeping excretal egg output markedly depressed. For further discussion of the relationships between treatment campaigns and other means of control, see Webbe and Jordan (1982) and Warren and Mahmoud (1976).

2.2.   Methods

Several species of laboratory animal can be infected with schistosomes and used for chemotherapeutic studies, but mice are the most commonly used. The evaluation of efficacy has not been easy, and various criteria have been used in the attempt to develop assays with the desired degree of technical simplicity and reproducibility of results. The criteria that have been employed include reduction in fecal egg count, reduced miracidial hatch from eggs in feces and liver, the presence of dead worms or reduction in the number of living worms, altered distribution of living worms or "hepatic shift," decreased mortality rate of the hosts, reduction in macroscopic liver damage, reduction in the number of egg lesions in the host tissues, qualitative changes in the distribution of developmental stages in the eggs in host tissues (oogram), impairment of metabolism or mitosis of worms or developmental stages *in vitro*, and immobilization of worms or larvae *in vitro*.

For a review of these methods and references to the original papers, see Standen (1963), Pellegrino and Katz (1968), and Katz and Pellegrino (1974). Not included in those reviews are the methods used by Muftic (1970), based on inhibition of metabolism or cell division and the more recent account by Campbell *et al.* (1978) of a simple method of using gross inspection of liver pathology as an indicator of drug efficacy.

Methods for evaluating the efficacy of drugs in human schistosomiasis are available, although by no means ideal. Four categories have been reviewed by Davis (1982) and might be summarized as follows:

1. *Clinical examination of the patient:* Assessment of weight gain, reduction in enteral symptoms, and regression of hepatosplenomegaly in *S. mansoni* and *S.*

japonicum infections, as well as reduction in urinary signs and symptoms (especially haematuria) in *S. haematobium* infections are included in the clinical examination.

2. *Direct parasitological examination:* Qualitative or quantitative assessment of the passage of worm eggs in urine or feces or their presence in rectal biopsy specimens is part of the direct parasitological investigation. Care must be taken to use reliable laboratory techniques, live eggs must be distinguished from dead eggs, and examinations must be performed regularly for at least 1 year after treatment to enable the investigator to distinguish between cure and temporary cessation of egg production.

3. *Indirect parasitological examination:* Immunodiagnostic techniques are used to determine the status of infection before and after treatment. Early attempts to correlate changes in antibody level with post-treatment changes in infection were not encouraging, but newer methods are being investigated.

4. *Ancillary clinical examinations:* The post-treatment regression of lesions may be followed by means of clinical techniques such as radiography, endoscopy or fiberoptic colonoscopy.

2.3. Antischistosomal Drugs

For information on the chemistry and mode of action of antischistosomal drugs, see Chapters 18 and 21; for a general review, see Bennett and Depenbusch (1984).

2.3.1. Praziquantel (Biltricide, Bayer AG; Pyquiton)

The discovery of praziquantel represents a major breakthrough in the treatment of schistosomiasis. It is generally safe yet is highly active against the three major schistosome species as well as the minor species *S. mekongi* and *S. intercalatum.*

2.3.1a. Formulation and Dosage. Praziquantel is prepared as 600-mg tablets, scored for breaking into pieces of 150 mg each; it is given orally. Since the drug is relatively new, the recommended dosages may undergo some adjustment, but the following dosages have been used successfully: for *S. haematobium* infection 40 mg/kg as a single dose, for *S. japonicum* and *S. mekongi* infection 20 mg/kg tid (three doses at 4-hr intervals) or 50 mg/kg as a single dose, and for *S. mansoni* infection 40 mg/kg (light infections) or 25 mg/kg repeated after 4 hr.

2.3.1b. Efficacy. Early reports on the efficacy of praziquantel against various schistosome species in mice, hamsters, and nonhuman primates (Gonnert and Andrews, 1977; Pellegrino *et al.,* 1977; Webbe and James, 1977; James *et al.,* 1977) were soon followed by reports of high efficacy in man (Davis and Wegner, 1979; Davis *et al.,* 1979; Katz *et al.,* 1979; Ishizaki *et al.,* 1979; Santos *et al.,* 1979). Subsequent studies further confirmed the high chemotherapeutic efficacy of praziquantel for schistosomiasis. A single dose of 40 mg/kg for *S. haematobium* resulted in a cure rate of

91%, which was better than that obtained with other treatments (Pugh and Teesdale, 1984; McMahon, 1983). A single dose of 40–50 mg/kg resulted in a very high cure rate of *S. mansoni* infections that had not responded to oxamniquine (de Souza Dias *et al.*, 1982), while two doses of 25 mg/kg also gave very satisfactory results (Katz *et al.*, 1981). Against *S. japonicum*, a single dose of 40–50 mg/kg, or 25 mg/kg in two doses, or a dose as low as 10 mg/kg given three times a day for 2 days, provided very satisfactory efficacy (Fu *et al.*, 1983; Santos *et al.*, 1984). A dosage of 30 mg/kg, given after breakfast and repeated after lunch, was used in trials involving more than 6000 patients with light to moderate *S. japonicum* infections, and gave a cure rate of almost 90% (Santos *et al.*, 1984). Generally a single larger dose has the same efficacy as several smaller doses given at intervals of several hours. However, the frequency of side effects is greater with a large single dose. Using rigorous criteria of cure, praziquantel has been estimated to give cure rates of 80–100% against most schistosome infections. In patients not fully cured, the passage of worm eggs is almost completely eliminated. Even such serious complications as colonic polyposis in *S. mansoni* infection and hepatosplenic disease in both *S. mansoni* and *S. japonicum* improve after treatment. The value of praziquantel in the practical control of *S. haematobium* infection has been demonstrated in large-scale trials (Delolme *et al.*, 1983; Pugh and Teesdale, 1984). In a small but rigorously controlled trial, the cure rate for *S. mekongi* was 91%, side effects were mild though common, and hepatomegaly was diminished (Nash *et al.*, 1982). The efficacy of the drug against schistosomes and other trematodes was summarized by Wegner (1984).

2.3.1c. Side Effects. The incidence of side effects with praziquantel varies among ethnic groups, and is often high, but the side effects are generally mild and transitory. Typical side effects are abdominal pain and discomfort, nausea, diarrhea, headache, rash, and fever. In a retrospective survey of 25,693 *S. japonica* patients treated with praziquantel in China, only 0.47% had what were considered relatively serious side effects. Neuropsychiatric reactions occurred in 0.15% of cases, cardiovascular reactions in 0.14%, hepatic changes in 0.02%, dermatological reactions in 0.07%, and delayed fatigue and inability to work in 0.11%. It was concluded that side effects are minimal, but that caution should be taken in chronic cases complicated by heart disease, ascites, poor hepatic compensation or renal failure (Minggang *et al.*, 1984). In trials involving more than 6000 cases in the Philippines, mild to moderate side effects were seen in 68%, while severe reactions were recorded in 1.2%. The safety of the drug has also been demonstrated in trials in Japan (Ishizaki *et al.*, 1979). The toxicological and pharmacological aspects of praziquantel have been reviewed by Frohberg (1984) and Wegner (1984).

2.3.2. Oxamniquine (Mansil, Vansil; Pfizer)

2.3.2a. Formulation and Dosage. Oxamniquine is prepared as capsules of 250 mg or as syrup containing 50 mg oxamniquine/ml. It is given orally. Dosages must take account of geographical origin as well as species of parasite. For some African *S. mansoni* infections, 15 mg/kg twice daily for 3 days may be used; in South America and parts of Africa, a single dosage of 15–20 mg/kg is sufficient. (It is not recommended for species other than *S. mansoni.*)

2.3.2b. Efficacy. Cure rates for *S. mansoni* with oxamniquine are in the range of 70–95%, and egg output is suppressed to a similar degree (Katz *et al.*, 1977; Abaza *et al.*, 1978; Pitchford and Lewis, 1978; Sleigh *et al.*, 1981; Kilpatrick *et al.*, 1982; Lambertucci *et al.*, 1982; Lapierre *et al.*, 1983). Oxamniquine has been used extensively with success in Brazil for mass chemotherapy to reduce disease prevalence and transmission, usually being given as a single dose of 12.5–15 mg/kg for adults and 20 mg/kg for children, repeated every 6 months. It is much less effective in some geographical locations than in others, and these regional differences in efficacy are attributable to differences in parasite strain, not to differences in pharmacological mechanisms in the human host. Drug resistance has been demonstrated experimentally and clinically (de Souza Dias *et al.*, 1982). The drug is essentially inactive against *S. haematobium* in man and against *S. japonicum* in laboratory animals (McMahon, 1976; Foster and Cheetham, 1973).

2.3.2c. Side Effects. Usually mild and transient, side effects of oxamniquinine include dizziness, drowsiness, and headache. Occasionally vomiting and diarrhea have been reported. Abnormal encephalograms were recorded in six of 34 treated patients whose pretreatment encephalograms were normal, and in rare cases epileptic seizures have been reported in treated patients, usually, but not always, in patients with a history of seizure (Krajden *et al.*, 1983). Its use in mass treatment campaigns provides very strong evidence of the safeness of this drug.

2.3.3. Niridazole (Ambilhar; Ciba-Geigy)

2.3.3a. Formulation and Dosage. This drug consists of scored orange-colored tablets of 100 or 500 mg, to be given orally. The dosage is 25 mg/kg per day for 5–10 days. The daily allotment of drug may be divided into two or three separate doses. Dosages of 12.5–15 mg/kg per day have been used to lessen side effects in cases of *S. mansoni* infection (Kilpatrick *et al.*, 1982).

2.3.3b. Efficacy. Niridazole is effective (80–100% cure rates) in *S. hematobium* infections but is much less effective against *S. mansoni* or *S. japonicum*. At a dose of 25 mg/kg, divided in two or three doses and given for 7 days (or 35 mg/kg given for 5 days), niridazole gave a cure rate of 80–94% in *S. haematobium* infection (Davis and Bailey, 1969); the single dose of 35 mg/kg per day for 5 days was very effective, but toxic reactions were frequent.

2.3.3c. Side Effects. Usually few and not serious in *S. hematobium* infections, side effects may be frequent and serious in other infections. Side effects include abdominal pain, nausea, vomiting, diarrhea, and headache. Urine acquires a brown color. The most serious limitation is the occurrence of mental and neurological side effects, especially in patients with severe liver damage or portocaval shunt (due to failure to metabolize drug quickly enough to prevent toxic level of drug in central blood). These side effects include depression, mania, convulsions, and coma. Niridazole is thus contraindicated in patients with severe liver disease, mental illness, or epilepsy. It is also contraindicated in patients receiving isoniazid or in those with severe heart disease (Davis, 1982). The urinary metabolites have been reported to be mutagenic in laboratory test systems (Legator et al., 1975).

2.3.4. Metrifonate (Bilarcil; Bayer AG)

Metrifonate has been widely used as an insecticide under the generic name triclorfon.

2.3.4a. Formulation and Dosage. Metrifonote is prepared as tablets of 100 mg. The drug is given orally. For S. hematobium infections, the dosage is 7.5–10 mg/kg, repeated three or more times at intervals of a few weeks. It is not used against other schistosome species.

2.3.4b. Efficacy. Metrifonate is highly effective against S. hematobium infection but has no useful efficacy against other schistosome species. Against S. hematobium, a dosage of 7.5–10 mg/kg, given three times with a 2-week interval, gives a cure rate of 81–91% (Davis and Bailey, 1969; Saif et al., 1973; Omer and Teesdale, 1978). The difference in susceptibility of the species does not seem to be a function of differences in the susceptibility of their AChEs, to the inhibitory effect of the drug; indeed, the low-grade urinary excretion of S. mansoni eggs in combined S. mansoni and S. haematobium infection can be suppressed by metrifonate treatment (Feldmeier et al., 1982). The differences may relate to differences in anatomical location within the host, but this unusually pronounced variation in susceptibility between species has not been convincingly explained. Although cure rates in S. haematobium infections may be low, especially in heavy infections, egg output is greatly reduced and clinical benefit is achieved (Feldmeier et al., 1981; Mason and Tswana, 1984). Furthermore, administration of metrifonate just three or four times over a 2-year period reduced both the level of parasitism and the severity of disease in schoolboys living under hyperendemic conditions (Doehring et al., 1984).

2.3.4c. Side Effects. Metrifonate has very few side effects mostly mild GI disturbances. Being an organophosphate, metrifonate depresses cholinesterase levels in blood and erythrocytes of treated patients, but these changes are not associated with overt toxic effects (Plestina et al., 1972). To reduce the danger of synergistic toxicity, caution must be exercised in treating patients, especially agricultural workers, who may be exposed to organophosphate insecticides (Davis, 1982).

2.3.5. Miscellaneous Drugs

Amoscanate and oltipraz are new antischistosomal compounds that have shown promising efficacy in clinical trials (Delolme *et al.*, 1983; Kern *et al.*, 1984; Lapierre, *et al.*, 1983; Pieron *et al.*, 1984; Zhou, 1983). These, as well as a few other experimental antischistosomal drugs, have been reviewed in detail by Bennett and Depenbusch (1984); their mode of action is discussed in Chapter 21. Amoscanate, one of the isothiocyanates, is active when given orally or parenterally and is active against all the major species of *Schistosoma* in experimentally infected laboratory animals. It has been widely tested against human schistosomiasis in China, where a dosage of 7 mg/kg per day for 3 days was apparently highly effective. There is evidence that enteric bacteria cause the production of a mutagenic metabolite that is excreted in the urine of amoscanate-treated animals. As with most antischistosomal drugs, young schistosomes are less susceptible than mature worms. Oltipraz at 20–40 mg/kg is effective against *S. mansoni* and *S. haematobium* but has been dropped from further consideration because of toxicity. The qinghaosu derivative artesunate is active against *S. japonicum* in mice and rabbits (Le *et al.*, 1983).

Drugs of former importance in the treatment of schistosomiasis include the antimonials (especially tartar emetic and astiban) lucanthone and hycanthone. Antimonial compounds are not acceptably safe, but if the new drugs are not available satisfactory results may be obtained with sodium antimony dimethylcystine tartrate given at 6–10 mg/kg per day, or every 2 days for a total of four doses. Astiban (sodium antimony dimercaptosuccinate) may be given in five intramuscular injections of 6–8 mg/kg given daily or every other day. After the second injection, the patient should be closely watched for side effects; and if side effects appear these drugs should be given every other day. Hycanthone had the advantage of being effective as a single intramuscular injection but, since it is not as safe as more modern drugs, its use cannot generally be justified. For further information on drugs previously considered important in clinical or experimental schistosomiasis, see reviews by Islip (1973), Lammler (1968), Friedheim (1973), and Katz and Pellegrino (1974).

3. OTHER TREMATODE INFECTIONS

3.1. General Principles and Methods

The chemotherapy of human trematode infections other than schistosomiasis has until recently been notably unsatisfactory. The advent of praziquantel has reversed that situation with respect to most of the infections.

Drug trials can be carried out against natural infections of *Opisthorchis felineus* in cats. Dogs, cats, guinea pigs, rabbits, and especially hamsters can be infected experimentally, and a technique for screening compounds in hamsters has been worked out (Lammler, 1968). Infections of *Clonorchis sinensis* can be established in dogs, cats, guinea pigs, rabbits, and to some extent in rats (Wykoff, 1958). Drug tests against

Paragonimus westermani are commonly done in naturally infected dogs, but experimental infections of *P. ohirai* in laboratory animals can also be used. Yokogawa and Miyazaki and others have shown that mice, rats, cats, and dogs are suitable hosts for such purposes (Lammler, 1968). The methodology for testing drug against *Fasciola* sp. is more appropriately considered in Chapter 20 of this volume. Because of the marked differences in habitat and pathogenesis of these flukes, there are few common points in the methods used for the assessment of drug efficacy against these flukes in man.

3.2. The Drugs

3.2.1. Drugs Used against Intestinal Flukes

3.2.1a. Infection with Fasciolopsis buski. The drug of choice is praziquantel. In a trial conducted in schoolchildren in Thailand, this drug was 100% effective when given as a single dose at 15 mg/kg (Harinasuta *et al.*, 1984). Side effects occurred in 21% of children but were mild and transient; sleepiness was the most common side effect. Hexylresorcinol, bephenium, dichlorophen, and tetrachlorenthylene were previously used for this infection.

3.2.1b. Infection with Echinostoma *sp.* Praziquantel is effective at 40 mg/kg, or 25 mg/kg bid (Radomyos *et al.*, 1982).

3.2.1c. Infection with Metagoninus *sp.* Studies by Rim and colleagues (cited by Cho *et al.*, 1984) indicate that praziquantel is highly effective against *M. yokogawai* in man at dosages of 10–20 mg/kg, given once or twice. Previously used drugs (bithionol, niclosamide) suppressed egg production but gave a low cure rate.

3.2.2. Drugs Used against Liver Flukes

3.2.2a. Infection with Fasciola *sp.* Despite past usage of emetine and chloroquine, there is no persuasive evidence that these drugs are effective. Bithionol (30–50 mg/kg, orally, on alternate days for 2 or 3 weeks) and hexachloroparaxylene (25–35 mg/kg, orally, twice daily after food) are probably effective (Yoshida *et al.*, 1962; Rim, 1973). Anecdotal reports of the efficacy of praziquantel against *Fasciola* in man must be accepted with caution because of the inactivity of this drug against the parasite in other animals (Wegner, 1984). Clinical trials are being conducted to settle this matter.

3.2.2b. Infection with Clonorchis *sp.* It has recently been found that praziquantel provides an excellent treatment for clonorchiasis. In 34 patients, a dosage of 25 mg/kg, three times daily for 2 days, was 100% effective on the basis of 1-year follow-up evaluation (Chen and Hsieh, 1984). The same dosage given in the space of 1 day was not quite so effective (Chen and Hsieh, 1984; Soh, 1984; Kuang *et al.*, 1984). Complete cure has also been obtained with 14 mg/kg tid for 5 days (Wegner, 1984). For mass-treatment purposes, a single dose at 40 mg/kg has been recommended (Lee, 1984].

Laboratory studies with praziquantel and *C. sinensis* have been reviewed by Soh (1984). The drug causes vacuolization of the tegument in *C. sinensis* as it does in schistosomes. In experimental infections in rats, worms less than 1 day old can be removed by praziquantel at 300–600 mg/kg. Worms 4–7 days old can be eliminated by a dosage of 50 mg/kg bid for 5 days.

Various antitrematodal drugs had previously been used in the treatment of clonorchiasis, but none was found satisfactory. In the case of hexachloroparaxylol, complete cure could be achieved, but the drug was withdrawn from human use because of toxicological considerations (Rim, 1984).

3.2.2c. Infection with Opisthorchis *sp.* Mebendazole at 30 mg/kg per day has been reported effective, but praziquantel is the drug of choice. Trials with praziquantel, using various dosages and involving nearly 5000 patients, were summarized by Bunnag *et al.* (1984), who concluded that a cure rate of 100% could be achieved with a dosage of 25 mg/kg, twice daily, for 1 or 2 days. A high cure could also be obtained with a single dose of 40–50 mg/kg. Side effects were mild and transient and more common at higher dosages. Gallbladder dysfunction caused by *O. viverrini* infection was found to be reversible with treatment, the rapidity of recovery being inversely proportional to the degree of dysfunction (Dhiensiri *et al.*, 1984). The efficacy and safety of praziquantel in the treatment of *O. viverrini* (and *O. felineus*) infection have also been reported by Supahvanich *et al.* (1981), Ambroise-Thomas *et al.* (1984), and Wegner (1984). In a mass-treatment campaign, the use of a single 40-mg/kg dose was highly satisfactory (Sormani *et al.*, 1984). Studies in hamsters indicated that young flukes are more susceptible than adults and that intracardiac injection of liposome-encapsulated praziquantel provides efficacy at much lower dosages than conventional treatment (Ruenwongsa and Thamavit, 1983).

3.2.3. Drugs Used against Lung Flukes

3.2.3a. Infection with Paragonimus *sp.* For both the Asiatic species (*P. westermani*) and the African species (*P. uterobilateralis*), the drug of choice is praziquantel. In one study a dosage of 25 mg/kg tid for 2 days was sufficient to give 100% cure of *P. westermani* infection (Vanijanonta *et al.*, 1984), while in another study a 3-day course was required (Rim, 1984). In a third study, 2 out of 22 patients were not cured with the 3-day course but were cured with niclofolan therapy (Cao *et al.*, 1984). Good efficacy against *P. westermani* was also reported by Horstmann *et al.* (1981) and Spitalny *et al.* (1982). In these studies, treatment generally provided clinical benefit and was well tolerated except for minor and transient side effects. Against *P. uterobilateralis*, praziquantel at 25 mg/kg tid for 3 days was fully effective (Monson *et al.*, 1983). Preliminary evidence indicates that praziquantel is effective against *P. heterotremus* (Vanijanonta *et al.*, 1984). When *P. westermani* was exposed to praziquantel *in vitro* at 100 μg/ml, only a few vacuoles were formed in the tegument; but flukes recovered from treated dogs showed extensive vacuolization and erosion of the tegument (Rim, 1984).

Various drugs were tried against *P. westermani* before the advent of praziquantel. These drugs have been reviewed by Yokogawa (1984), and only two are worth mentioning here. Yokogawa himself discovered the marked efficacy of bithionol against encysted metacercariae *in vitro* and subsequently demonstrated efficacy in laboratory animals and man. The drug became the treatment of choice and was even safe enough to be used in mass treatment programs (Yokogawa, 1984). The usual dosage was 30–40 mg/kg given every other day for 10–15 doses, and the inconvenience of this regimen was largely responsible for replacement of bithionol by praziquantel in the treatment of paragonimiasis. Niclofolan was found active as a single oral dose, at 2.0 mg/kg, against both *P. westermani* and *P. uterobilateralis* (Rim and Chang, 1980; Monson *et al.*, 1983), but it too has given way to praziquantel (primarily on the basis of safety).

REFERENCES

Ambroise-Thomas, P., Goullier, A., and Peyron, F., 1984, Therapeutic results in opisthorchiasis with praziquantel in a reinfection-free environment in France, *Arzneimittelforsch.* 34(II):1177–1179.

Abaza, H. H., Hammouda, N., Abd Rabbo, H., and Shafei, A. Z., 1978, Chemotherapy of schistosomal colonic polyposis with oxamniquine, *Trans. R. Soc. Trop. Med. Hyg.* 72:602–604.

Bennett, J. K., and Depenbusch, J. W., 1984, The chemotherapy of schistosomiasis, in: *Parasitic Diseases,* Vol. 2: *The Chemotherapy* (J. M. Mansfield, ed.), pp. 73–131, Dekker, New York.

Bunnag, D., Pungpark, S., Harinasuta, T., Viravan, C., Vanijanonta, S., Suntharasamai, P., Migasena, S., Charoenlarp, P., Riganti, M., and LooAreesuwan, S., 1984, *Opisthorchis viverrini:* Clinical experience with praziquantel in hospital for tropical diseases, *Arzneimittelforsch.* 34(II):1173–1174.

Campbell, W. C., and Cuckler, A. C., 1961, The prophylactic effect of topically applied cedarwood oil on infection with *Schistosoma mansoni* in mice, *Am. J. Trop. Med. Hyg.* 10:712–715.

Campbell, W. C., and Cuckler, A. C., 1967, Inhibition of egg production of *Schistosoma mansoni* in mice treated with nicarbazin, *J. Parasitol.* 53:977–980.

Campbell, W. C., and Rogers, E. F., 1971, Effect of nitrocarbanilides on *Schistosoma mansoni, J. Parasitol.* 57:1372–1373.

Campbell, W. C., Bartels, E., and Cuckler, A. C., 1978, A method for detecting chemotherapeutic activity against *Schistosoma mansoni* in mice, *J. Parasitol.* 64:69–77.

Cao, W. J., He, L. Y., Zhong, H. L. (Chung, H. L.), Xu, Z. S., Bi, Y. C., Yu, G. T., Zhang, Q. C., Li, K. C., Yang, E. V., She, G., and Li, H. J., 1984, Paragonimiasis: Treatment with praziquantel in 40 human cases and in 1 cat, *Arzneimittelforsch.* 34(II):1203–1204.

Chen, C. Y., and Hsieh, W. C., 1984, *Clonorchis sinensis:* Epidemiology in Taiwan and clinical experience with praziquantel, *Arzneimittelforsch.* 34(II):1160–1162.

Chen, M. G., Hua, X. J., Wan, Z. R., Weng, Y. Q., Wang, M. J., Zhu, P. J., He, B. Z., and Xu, M. Y., 1983, Praziquantel in 237 cases of clonorchiasis sinensis, *Chin. Med. J.* 96:935–940 (English transl.).

Cho, S. Y., Kang, S. Y., and Lee, J. B., 1984, Metagonimiasis in Korea, *Arzneimittelforsch.* 34(II):1211–1213.

Davis, A., 1982, Manage of the patient in schistosomiasis, in: *Schistosomiasis* (P. Jordan and G. Webbe, eds.), pp. 184–226, Heineman Medical Books, London.

Davis, A., and Bailey, D. R., 1969, Metrifonate in urinary schistosomiasis, *Bull. WHO* 41:209–224.

Davis, A., and Wegner, D. H. G., 1979, Multicenter trials of praziquantel in the treatment of human schistosomiasis: Designs and techniques, *Bull. WHO* 57:767–772.

Davis, A., Biles, J. E., and Wrich, A. M., 1979, Initial experience with praziquantel in the treatment of human infection due to *Schistosoma haematobium, Bull. WHO* 57:773–780.

Delolme, H., Cot, M., Cavallo, A., Kouka-Bemba, D., and Sentilhes, L., 1983, Réflexions sur le traitement de masse des bilharzioses à *Schistosoma haematobium* dans les états membres de l'Organisation de Coordination pour la lutte contre les Endémies en Afrique Centrale (OCEAC), *Bull. Soc. Pathol. Exot Fil.* 76:534–541.

de Souza Dias, L. C. S., Pedro, R. V., and Deberaldini, E. R., 1982, Use of praziquantel in patients with schistosomiasis mansoni previously treated with oxamniquine and/or hycanthone: Resistance of *Schistosoma mansoni* to schistosomicidal agents, *Trans.'R. Soc. Trop. Med. Hyg.* 76:652–659.

Dhiensiri, T., Eua-Ananta, Y., Bunnag, D., Harinasuta, T., and Schelp, P. F., 1984, Roentgenographically controlled healing of gallbladder lesions in opisthorchiasis after praziquantel treatment, *Arzneimittelforsch.* 34(II):1175–1177.

Doehring, E., Feldmeier, H., Dafalla, A. A., Ehrich, J. H., Vester, U., and Poggensee, U., 1984, Intermittent chemotherapy with trichlorfon (metrifonate) reverses proteinuria, hematuria, and leukocyturia in urinary schistosomiasis: Results of a three-year field study, *J. Infect.Dis.* 149:615–620.

Feldmeier, H., Doehring, E., Daffala, A. A., Omer, A. H. S., and Dietrich, M., 1981, Efficacy of metrifonate in urinary schistosomiasis in light and heavy infections, *Tropenmed. Parasitol.* 33:102–106.

Feldmeier, H., Doehring, E., Daffala, A. A., Omer, A. H. S., and Dietrich, M., 1982, Efficacy of metrifonate in urinary schistosomiasis: Comparison of reduction of *Schistosoma haematobium* and *S. mansoni* eggs, *Am. J. Trop. Med. Hyg.* 31:1188–1194.

Foster, R., and Cheetham, B. L., 1973, Studies with the schistosomicide oxamniquine (UK4271) I, *Trans. R. Soc. Trop. Med. Hyg.* 67:674–684.

Friedheim, E. A. H., 1973, Chemotherapy of schistosomiasis, in: *Chemotherapy of Helminthiasis* (R. Cavier and F. Hawking, eds.), pp. 29–144, Pergamon Press, Oxford.

Frohberg, H., 1984, Results of toxicological studies on praziquantel, *Arzneimittelforsch.* 34(II):1137–1144.

Fu, S., Zhou, X. Z., and Fan, Y., 1983, Comparative study on different dose schedules of praziquantel in the treatment of schistosomiasis japonica, *J. Parasitol. Parasitic Dis.* 1:32–36.

Gilbert, B., DeSouza, J. P., Fortes, C. C., DosSantos, F., DoPrado Seabra, A., Kitagawa, M., and Pellegrino, J., 1970, Chemoprophylactic agents in schistosomiasis: Active and inactive terpenes, *J. Parasitol.* 56:397–398.

Gonnert, R., and Andrews, P., 1977, Praziquantel, a new broad-spectrum antischistosomal agent, *Z. Parasitenk.* 52:129–150.

Greene, L. K., Grenan, M. M., Davidson, D. E., Jr., Jones, D. H., and Shedd, T. R., 1983, Amoscanate as a topically applied chemical for prophylaxis against *Schistosoma mansoni* infections in mice, *Am. J. Trop. Med. Hyg.* 32:1356–1363.

Harinasuta, T., Bunnag, D., and Radomyos, P., 1984, Efficacy of praziquantel on fasciolopsiasis, *Arzneimittelforsch.* 34(II):1214–1215.

Horstmann, R. D., Feldheim, W., Feldmeier, H., and Dietrich, M., 1981, High efficacy of praziquantel in the treatment of 22 patients with *Clonorchis/Opisthorchis* infections, *Tropenmed. Parasitol.* 32:157–160.

Ishizaki, T., Kamo, E., and Boelone, E., 1979, Double-blind studies of tolerance to praziquantel in Japanese patients with *Schistosoma japonicum* infection, *Bull. WHO* 57:787–792.

Islip, P. J., 1973, Progress in the experimental chemotherapy of helminth infections, *Fortschr. Arzneimittelforsch.* 17:241–319.

Jackson, H., Davies, P., and Bock, M., 1968, Chemosterilization of *Schistosoma mansoni*, *Nature (Lond.)* 218:977.

James, C., Webbe, G., and Nelson, G. S., 1977, The susceptibility to praziquantel of *Schistosoma haematobium* in the baboon (*Papio anubis*) and of *S. japonicum* in the vervet monkey (*Cercopithecus aethiops*), *Z. Parasitenk.* 52:1179–1194.

Johnson, R. J., Dunning, S. B., Minshew, B. H., and Jong, E. C., 1983, Successful praziquantel treatment of paragonimiasis following bithionol failure, *Am. J. Trop. Med. Hyg.* 32:1309–1311.

Katz, N., and Pellegrino, J., 1974, Experimental chemotherapy of schistosomiasis mansoni, *Adv. Parasitol.* 12:369–390.

Katz, N., Zicker, F., and Pereira, J. P., 1977, Field trials with oxaminiquine in schistosomiasis mansoni-endemic area, *Am. J. Trop. Med. Hyg.* 26:234–237.

Katz, N., Rocha, R. S., and Chaves, A., 1979, Preliminary trials with praziquantel in human infections due to *Schistosoma mansoni*, *Bull. WHO* 57:781–786.

Katz, N., Rocha, R. S., and Chaves, A., 1981, Clinical trials with praziquantel in *Schistosoma mansoni*, *Rev. Inst. Med. Trop. Sao Paulo* 23:72–78.

Kern, P., Burchard, G. D., and Deitrich, M., 1984, Comparative study of oltipraz versus praziquantel for treatment of schistosomiasis with intestinal manifestation in the Gabon (*Schistosoma intercalatum* and *S. haematobium*), *Tropenmed. Parasitol.* 35:95–99.

Kilpatrick, M. E., El Masry, N. A., Bassily, S., and Farid, Z., 1982, Oxamniquine versus niridazole for treatment of uncomplicated *Schistosoma mansoni* infection, *Am. J. Trop. Med. Hyg.* 31:1164–1167.

Krajden, S., Keystone, J. S., and Glenn, C., 1983, Safety and toxicity of oxamniquine in the treatment of *Schistosoma mansoni* infections, with particular reference to electroencephalographic abnormalities, *Am. J. Trop. Med. Hyg.* 32:1344–1346.

Kuang, Q. H., Zhou, Y. T., Lei, S. Z., Cao, W. J., and Zhong, H. L. (Chung, H. L.), 1984, Clonorchiasis: Treatment with Praziquantel in 50 cases, *Arzneimittelforsch.* 34:(II):1162–1163.

Lambertucci, J. R., Greco, D. B., Pedroso, E. R. P., Rocha, M. O. D., Salazar, H-M, and DeLima, D. P., 1982, A double blind trial with oxamniquine in chronic schistosomiasis mansoni, *Trans. R. Soc. Trop. Med. Hyg.* 76:751–755.

Lammler, G., 1968, Chemotherapy of trematode infections, in: *Advances in Chemotherapy* (A. Goldin, F. Hawking, and R. J. Schnitzer, eds.), pp. 153–251, Academic Press, New York.

Lapierre, J., Keita, A., Faurant, C., Heyer, F., Tourte-Schaefer, C., Ancelle, T., and Dupouy-Camet, J., 1983, Treatment of 700 cases of bilharziasis with the new drugs oxamniquine, oltipraz, praziquantel, *Bull. Soc. Pathol. Exot. Fil.* 76:526–533.

Le, W. J., You, J. Q., and Mei, J. Y., 1983, Chemotherapeutic effect of artesunate in experimental schistosomiasis, *Yao Hsueh Hsueh Pao* 18:619–621.

Lee, S. H., 1984, Large scale treatment of *Clonorchis sinensis* infections with praziquantel under field conditions, *Arzneimittelforsch.* 34(II):1227–1230.

Legator, M. S., Connor, T. H., and Stoeckel, M., 1975, Detection of mutagenic activity of metronidazole and niridazole in body fluids of humans and mice, *Science* 188:1118–1119.

Mahmoud, A. A. F., Siongok, T. K. A., Ouma, J., Houser, H. B., and Warren, K. S., 1983, Effect of targeted mass treatment on intensity of infection and morbidity in schistosomiasis mansoni, *Lancet* 1:849–851.

Mason, P. R., and Tswana, S. A., 1984, Single-dose metrifonate for the treatment of *Schistosoma haematobium* infection in an endemic area of Zimbabwe, *Am. J. Trop. Med. Hyg.* 33:599–601.

McMahon, J. E., 1976, Oxamniquine (UK4271) in *Schistosoma haematobium* infections, *Ann. Trop. Med. Parasitol.* 70:121–122.

McMahon, J. E., 1983, A comparative trial of praziquantel, metrifonate and niridazole against *Schistosoma haematobium*, *Am. Trop. Med. Parasitol.* 77:139–142.

Minggang, C., Sui, F., Xiangjin, H., and Huimin, W., 1984, A retrospective survey on side effects of praziquantel among 25693 cases of schistosomiasis japonica, *Southeast Asian J. Trop. Med. Publ. Health* 14:495–500.

Monson, M. H., Koenig, J. W., and Sachs, R., 1983, Successful treatment with praziquantel of six patients infected with the African lung fluke, *Paragonimus uterobilateralis*, *Am. J. Trop. Med. Hyg.* 32:371–375.

Muftic, M., 1970, New methods for testing schistosomicidal drugs, *J. Trop. Med. Hyg.* 73:232–234.

Nash, T. E., Hofstetter, M., Cheeves, A. W., and Ottesen, E. A., 1982, Treatment of *Schistosoma mekongi* with praziquantel: A double-blind study, *Am. J. Trop. Med. Hyg.* 31:977–982.

Omer, A. H. S., and Teesdale, C. H., 1978, Metrifonate trial in the treatment of various presentations of *Schistosoma haematobium* and *Schistosoma mansoni* infections in the Sudan, *Ann. Trop. Med. Parasitol.* 12:145–150.

Pellegrino, J., and Katz, N., 1968, Experimental chemotherapy of schistosomiasis mansoni, *Adv. Parasitol.* 6:233–290.

Pellegrino, J., and Katz, N., 1969, Experimental chemotherapy of schistosomiasis, part 4: oogram studies with nicarbazin, an egg suppressive agent, *Rev. Inst. Med. Trop. Sao Paulo* 11:215–221.

Pellegrino, J., Lima-Costa, F. F., Carlos, M. A., and Mello, R. T., 1977, Experimental chemotherapy of schistosomiasis mansoni XIII, Z. Parasitenk. 52:151–168.

Pieron, R., Mafart, Y., Lesobre, B., Grivaux, M., and Lancastre, F., 1984, L'oltipraz en traitement bref de la schistosomose à S. haematobium. Trois prises en un jour ou une seule prise, Therapie 39:167–176.

Pitchford, R. J., and Lewis, A. M., 1978, Oxamniquine in the treatment of various schistosome infections in South Africa, South Afr. Med. J. 53:677–680.

Plestina, R., Davis, A., and Bailey, D. R., 1972, Effect of metrifonate on blood cholinesterases in children during the treatment of schistosomiasis, Bull. WHO 46:747–759,

Pugh, R. N., and Teesdale, C. H., 1984, Long-term efficacy of single-dose oral treatment in schistosomiasis haematobium, Trans. R. Soc. Trop. Med. Hyg. 78:55–59.

Radomyos, P., Bunnag, D., and Harinasuta, T., 1982, Echinostoma ilocanum infection in man in Thailand, Southeast Asian J. Trop. Med. Publ. Health 13:265–269.

Rim, H. J., 1973, Chemotherapy of trematode infection excluding schistosomiasis, in: Proceedings of the Tenth SEAMEO-TROPMED Seminar: Symposium on Chemotherapy in Tropical Medicine of Southeast Asia and the Far East, October 26–30, 1972, Bangkok.

Rim, H. J., and Chang, Y. S., 1980, Chemotherapeutic effect of niclofolan and praziquantel in the treatment of paragonimiasis, Korea Univ. Med. J. 17:113–126.

Rim, H. J., Lyu, K. S., Lee, J. S., and Koo, K. H., 1981, Clinical evaluation of therapeutic effect of praziquantel (Embay 8440) against Clonorchis sinensis infection, Ann. Trop. Med. Parasitol. 75:27.

Rim, H. J., 1984, Paragonimiasis: Experimental and clinical experience with praziquantel in Korea, Arzneimittelforsch. 34(II):1197–1203.

Ruenwongsa, P., and Thamavit, W., 1983, Increased efficacy of liposomes—Encapsulated praziquantel in treatment of opisthorchiasis in hamsters, Southeast Asian J. Trop. Med. Publ. Health 14:501–504.

Saif, M., Koura, M., and Abdel-Fattah, F., 1973, The oral treatment of S. haematobium infection with metrifonate, J. Egypt. Med. Assoc. 56:527–531.

Santos, A. T., Blas, B. L., Nosenas, J. S., Portillo, G. P., Ortega, D. M., Hayashi, M., and Boehme, K., 1979, Preliminary clinical trials with praziquantel in Schistosoma japonicum infections in the Philippines, Bull. WHO 57:593–900.

Santos, A. T., Blas, B. L., Portillo, G. P., Nosenas, J. S., Poliquit, O., and Papasin, M., 1984, Phase III clinical trials with praziquantel in S. japonicum infections in the Philippines, Arzneimittelforsch. 34(II):1221–1223.

Sleigh, A. C., Mott, K. E., and Franca Silva, J. T., 1981, A three-year follow-up of chemotherapy with oxamniquine in a Brazilian community with endemic schistosomiasis, Trans. R. Soc. Trop. Hyg. 75:234–238.

Soh, C. T., 1984, Clonorchis sinensis: Experimental and clinical studies with praziquantel in Korea, Arzneimittelforsch. 34(II):1156–1159.

Sornmani, S., Schelp, F. P., Vivatanasesth, P., Patihatakorn, W., Impand, P., Sitabutra, P., Worasan, P., and Preuksaraj, S., 1984, A pilot project for controlling O. viverrini infection in Nong Wai, Northeast Thailand, by applying praziquantel and other measures, Arzneimittelforsch. 34(II):1231–1234.

Spitalny, K. C., Senft, A. W., Meglio, F. D., Morgan, J., and Peter, G., 1982, Treatment of pulmonary paragonimiasis with a new broad-spectrum anthelmintic, praziquantel, J. Pediatr. 101:144–146.

Standen, O. D., 1963, Chemotherapy of helminthic infections, in: Experimental Chemotherapy (R. J. Schnitzer and F. Hawking, eds.), Vol. 1, pp. 701–892, Academic Press, New York and London.

Supanvanich, S., Supavonich, K., and Pawabut, P., 1981, Field trial of praziquantel in human opisthorchiasis in Thailand, Southeast Asian J. Trop. Med. Publ. Health 12:598–602.

Vanijanonta, S., Bunnag, D., and Harinasuta, T., 1984, Paragonimus heterotremus and other Paragonimus spp. in Thailand: Pathogenesis, clinic and treatment, Arzneimittelforsch. 34(II):1186–1188.

Warren, K. S., 1970, Suppression of hepatosplenic schistosomiasis mansoni in mice by nicarbazin, a drug that inhibits egg production by schistosomes, J. Infect. Dis. 121:514–521.

Warren, K. S., and Mahmoud, A. A. F., 1976, Targeted mass treatment. A new approach to the control of schistosomiasis, Trans. Assoc. Am. Physicians 89:195–204.

Webbe, G., and James, C., 1977, A comparison of the susceptibility of praziquantel of Schistosoma *haematobium, S. japonicum, S. mansoni, S. intercalatum* and *S. mattheei* in hamsters, *Z. Parasitenk.* 52:169–177.

Webbe, G., and Jordan, P., 1982, Control, in: *Schistosomiasis* (P. Jordan and G. Webbe, eds.), pp. 293–349, Heinemann Medical Books, London.

Wegner, D. H. G., 1984, The profile of the trematodicidal compound praziquantel, *Arzneimittelforsch.* 34(II):1132–1136.

Wykoff, D. E., 1958, Studies on *Clonorchis sinensis.* III, *J. Parasitol.* 44:461–466.

Yokogawa, M., 1984, Experimental chemotherapy of paragonimiasis, *Arzneimittelforsch.* 34(II):1193–1196.

Yoshida, Y., Miyake, T., Nakaniski, Y., Nishido, K., Yamanashi, Y., Ishikawa, T., Fujisoka, K., Tanaka, A., and Embara, S., 1962, Cases of human infection with *Fasciola* sp. and treatment with Bithionol, *Jpn. J. Parasitol.* 11:41–43.

Zhou, G. X., 1983, Clinical observation on schistosomiasis japonica treated with amoscanate and phenithionate in a hyperendemic area, *Chung Hua Nei Ko Tsa Chih* 22:634–645

20

Trematode Infections of Domestic Animals

J. C. BORAY

1. INTRODUCTION

Although some earlier attempts had been made to develop an effective treatment for fascioliasis (see Chapter 1), experimental chemotherapy for trematode infections of domestic animals began between 1921 and 1926 with the discovery of the anthelmintic effect of carbon tetrachloride and hexachloroethane (Hall, 1921; Ernst, 1925; Thienel, 1926; Montgomery, 1926). Before the discovery of these remedies, survival of sheep and cattle depended on the individual judgment of stockmen during normal years, and catastrophic destruction of millions of animals was observed during wet years (Taylor, 1964). Despite their variable efficacy and relatively high toxicity, both drugs served the animal industry for many years, and appreciable advances in the chemotherapy of trematode diseases, producing safer and more efficient compounds, were only achieved during the past 20 years.

2. METHODS

2.1. Primary Screening in the Laboratory

Some simple *in vitro* techniques have been employed, with questionable results, in laboratory studies for testing candidate compounds for their potential anthelmintic efficacy (Leiper, 1963). A semi-*in vivo* technique of subcutaneously implanting fluke was tested and found to have limited application for primary screening (Lienert, 1963). In recent times, successful *in vitro* culture of helminths directed attention to the possibility of economic screening of a large number of compounds using various stages of nematodes, cestodes, and *Fasciola*. The effect of anthelmintics on the motility of

J. C. BORAY • Department of Agriculture, New South Wales, Central Veterinary Laboratory, Glenfield, New South Wales 2167, Australia.

Fasciola hepatica has been tested in an *in vitro* isometric transducer system (Fairweather *et al.*, 1983, 1984), but the validity of the tests has to be assessed with caution. The use of a free-living nematode *Caenorhabditis elegans* was also proposed (Simpkin and Coles, 1979). These workers detected efficacy of compounds known to be effective against nematodes, cestodes, or trematodes. However, *in vitro* activity against certain helminths could not always be correlated with activity in sheep; also, compounds were not specific to various helminths and some were found to be active only when metabolized by the host. The most efficient screen for candidate drugs would be in target hosts, a financially prohibitive approach. Consequently, laboratory rodents are commonly used.

The most efficient and economic laboratory model for *Fasciola hepatica* is the albino rat. Since the fluke can reach maturity in the rat and establish residence in the bile ducts, this host can be used for studies on the anthelmintic efficacy against both the mature and immature stages of the infection. Because of a competitive inhibition of development, only a few adult fluke will be found in the enlarged main bile duct, so it is a simple matter to count them and record their condition; drug activity can be determined by egg counts (Lämmler, 1959; Thorpe, 1965*a;* Boray *et al.* 1967*b*). The counting of immature *Fasciola* in the host liver is labor intensive, and the practice of postponing necropsy for several weeks to permit maturation and examination of mature fluke is too slow. Examination of fresh liver squashes under a dissecting microscope is commonly employed, particularly for mice, but is made difficult by the highly vascular nature and size of the rat liver. Thorpe (1965*b*) and Campbell and Barry (1970) showed that the concentration of serum glutamic oxaloacetic transaminase (SGOT) is elevated in infected rats, and the latter investigators described a method of exploiting this for screening compounds against the immature phase of infection. Boray *et al.* (1967*b*) showed that the most appropriate time for testing drugs against immature fluke is 4 weeks after infection before severe tissue damage occurs; against adult fluke, it is 18 weeks after infection, when the tissue change is resolved. Under certain circumstances, mice and guinea pigs may be used for primary screening, but in these hosts only efficacy against the immature stages can be studied because of the high pathogenic effect of the fluke if infection is prolonged. Similarly, experimental infections of mice with *F. gigantica* may provide a screening model for detecting compounds effective against early immature stages of *Fasciola* spp. However, not all drugs active against *Fasciola* spp. in sheep could be detected in rodents, and dose rates much higher than those effective in sheep had to be used (Boray, 1969*a;* Coles, 1975). The problems regarding primary screening of anthelmintics against fluke infections have been extensively reviewed (Boray 1963, 1969*a;* Lämmler 1964, 1968; Standen, 1963; Hayes *et al.*, 1973; Coles, 1975). Recently the guinea pig was found to be a suitable laboratory animal for *Fascioloides magna* (Foreyt, 1979), and comparative screening can be carried out under laboratory conditions. However, it is unlikely that specific screening for that species would be economically justified.

Screening for therapeutical agents against members of the Dicrocoeliidae family can be carried out in the golden hamster or in rabbits artificially infected with metacercariae of *Dicrocoelium dendriticum* (Krull, 1956; Hohorst and Lämmler, 1963). C. Eichler and J. C. Boray (1971, unpublished data) found that, irrespective of the age of the hamsters, the recovery rate was 40–73%; for regular screening of anthelmintics, these investigators recommended a dose of 25 metacercariae, preferably in male animals. The establishment of the life cycle in the laboratory, which requires a terrestrial snail and ants, is very difficult. However, collection of metacercariae from the field by harvesting cataleptic ants from endemic areas or from experimental plots in which infection is artificially maintained, is a relatively simple procedure. The metacercariae can be stored in infected ants at 4°C for a considerable time (C. Eichler and J. C. Boray, 1971, unpublished data.

There are no laboratory animal models for testing anthelmintic efficacy against immature or adult paramphistomes. Some drugs exhibiting activity against other trematodes have been tested in sheep experimentally infected with metacercariae of *Paramphistomum microbothrium* (Horak, 1971). Trials can also be carried out during severe outbreaks of paramphistomosis in sheep or cattle naturally infected in the field and moved to the laboratory for treatment (Boray, 1969b).

The medical importance of schistosomiasis has led to testing of large numbers of drugs, using mainly laboratory rodents or dogs (see Chapter 18). Some of these drugs have subsequently been tested against schistosomes in field-infected sheep and cattle.

2.2. Secondary Screening

In order to achieve comparable and reproducible results for both efficacy and toxicity, the use of standardized controlled tests has been proposed for *Fasciola* spp. (Boray, 1963, 1969a). These tests can be adapted to other trematode infections; trematode-free sheep or calves should be artificially infected with metacercariae to produce a medium-level infection. The drugs should be applied with a standardized technique, such as intraruminal injection for ruminants, particularly during the initial stage of dose titration. Treatments are carried out progressively against early immature to adult stages of the fluke. The animals are killed when all fluke have reached maturation in the bile ducts and the fluke recovered and counted. If the monitoring of early drug action against immature fluke is required, the recovery of fluke is difficult. The recovery process can be facilitated by perfusing the liver with a slightly basic trypsin solution to disrupt the integrity of the liver tissue (Ostlind et al., 1972).

Toxicological tests for anthelmintics in the target animal have to be carried out in animals exposed to different stress factors. The most important stress is produced by a heavy infection with the fluke. For drugs used against *F. hepatica*, the maximum tolerated dose has been determined in adult sheep weighing about 40 kg, infected with 1000 metacercariae and treated 8 weeks after infection. Since the pathological changes in the host may depend on the age and size of the animal, in recent tests 25 metacercariae per kilogram body weight were used for the test in younger sheep (Boray et al., 1983). Using the above technique, the safety index (maximum tolerated dose divided by the efficient dose) of drugs can be evaluated in order to select the dose rate that can be used in the field with confidence.

In further tests, the efficacy of drugs must be confirmed in animals heavily infected with the target parasites, resulting in considerable tissue damage and retardation of growth in the fluke, which in turn may influence the metabolism or efficacy of drugs (Boray *et al.*, 1969; Edwards and Parry, 1972; Kendall and Parfitt, 1975). The efficacy of the drugs should also be tested in the field, where multiple infections with fluke of different age are often present. Large variations in development occur in heavy and multiple infections. The physiological development and the size of the fluke may be just as important for susceptibility to drugs as their age (Boray, 1969; Kendall and Parfitt, 1973).

Secondary screening for the efficacy of drugs against *D. dendriticum* in the target hosts can be carried out in sheep infected with about 1000 metacercariae or in naturally infected sheep using the controlled test (Hohorst and Lämmler, 1963). The recovery of fluke at necropsy can be assisted by a liver-perfusion technique (Wolff *et al.*, 1969).

3. GENERAL PRINCIPLES

3.1. *Application Techniques for Trematode Control*

Most anthelmintics against trematode infections are administered orally, but some are effective only by the parenteral route (e.g., nitroxynil). Parenteral application of the same drug often results in higher efficacy than the oral route (Schröder *et al.*, 1977). For practical reasons, oral drenching is the most acceptable method for treatment of sheep and goats, whereas a subcutaneous or intramuscular injection is more convenient for cattle. Some drugs may be mixed with food concentrates (Danek *et al.*, 1979) or incorporated into controlled-release devices, as suggested by Rew and Knight (1980) and Rew *et al.* (1980). For those methods of application only very safe drugs can be used, but uniform intake and high efficacy may be difficult to achieve.

The physiology of the host may have an important role in the absorption and efficacy of the compounds, particularly in the treatment of ruminants, in which the esophageal groove reflex may influence the efficacy of some drugs (Boray and Roseby, 1969). The efficacy of compounds could also be influenced by particle size and the formulation of compounds (Campbell *et al.*, 1970; Boray, 1971). It is important that the efficacy and safety of the final commercial formulation of a newly developed drug be confirmed in the target hosts, using standard techniques.

3.2. *Principles of Chemotherapy*

An anthelmintic agent for efficient fluke control must be highly effective against both immature and mature fluke in order to prevent or alleviate the damage caused by the parasites and to eliminate pasture contamination with eggs. The optimum agent should be inexpensive, easy to apply to large numbers of animals, and nontoxic and should not leave chemical residues in milk and tissues. A very high therapeutic effect and even chemoprophylaxis may be achieved with modern drugs, but the control of trematode infections is often a compromise because of either the limited availability of optimum compounds or economic considerations in some countries. Drugs must be used strategically, depending on the epidemiology of the disease, and integrated into farm management.

3.3. Specificity in Chemotherapy of Trematodes

There are thousands of digenetic trematodes parasitizing domestic and wild animals, but only a few cause serious economic loss and require regular treatment. This chapter presents data on the chemotherapy of members of the Fasciolidae, Dicrocoeliidae, Paramphistomoidea, and Schistosomatidae that occur in herbivorous animals, particularly in ruminants. Some intestinal trematodes of birds and mammals occasionally cause death, but infection with these parasites is economically insignificant. Efficacy against one trematode does not necessarily apply to other species. Most drugs that are highly effective against F. hepatica have no activity at all against members of the Dicrocoeliidae, and specific compounds effective against D. dendriticum are inactive against Fasciola. With few exceptions, drugs effective against Fasciola spp. are not active against schistosomes or paramphistomes. Since the efficacy of drugs depends on the specific metabolic pathways of the parasites and the biochemical action of drugs, a specific screening procedure is necessary to select a highly effective and safe compound for the treatment of different trematode infections. Very often specific testing of anthelmintics is not warranted on economic grounds for many trematode infections. Drugs are normally tested against Dicrocoelium or paramphistome infections if they have been found efficient for Fasciola spp., gastrointestinal nematodes, or cestodes. There is a better chance of finding a suitable anthelmintic for the treatment of schistosomes in ruminants because of the large number of drugs being tested for the control of human infection.

An example of highly specific efficacy is the new benzimidazole compound, triclabendazole. This agent is active against all stages of Fasciolidae spp. and has a high safety margin. The mode of action of the drug is unknown, but it may be speculated that triclabendazole acts against a specific enzyme system, vital for the metabolism of Fasciola spp. and absent or insignificant in other parasites or mammals. Even at high dose rates, triclabendazole does not affect D. dendriticum, paramphistomes, members of the Opisthorchidae family, or nematodes.

4. THE DRUGS AND THEIR USES

4.1. Fasciolidae

4.1.1. Fasciola hepatica

Table I shows the comparative efficacy of older or not commonly used drugs against Fasciola spp. The efficacy of those drugs is based mainly on tests carried out by standardized techniques for their activity and safety in sheep (Boray et al., 1967a; Boray

Table I. *Comparative Efficiency of Drugs against Fasciola spp.: Older or Not Commonly Used Compounds*

Anthelmintic	Route of application[a]	Recommended dose rate[b] (mg/kg) Sheep	Recommended dose rate[b] (mg/kg) Cattle	Max tolerated dose in sheep (mg/kg)	Safety index at recommended dose rate in sheep	Minimum age of fluke in weeks, efficiency ≥90% Sheep	Minimum age of fluke in weeks, efficiency ≥90% Cattle
Carbon tetrachloride	Oral	80	40	160–800	2–10 (erratic)	12	>12
	im	80–160	80–160	—	—	12–10	>12
Hexachloroethane	Oral	250–300	300	1200	4.0	12	>12
Hexachlorophene	Oral	15	20	40	2.6	12	12
Tribromsalan	Oral	20	20	60	3.0	12	12
Bithionol	Oral	75	30	75	1	>12	>12
Hexachloroparaxylene	Oral	150	130	600	4.0	12	12
Bromophenophos	Oral	16	12	50	3.0	12	>12
Disophenol	sc	10	10	25	2.5	>12	>12
Clioxanide	Oral	20	NR	100	5.0	12	NR
Nitroclofene	im	NR	3	?	?	NR	>12

[a] im, intramuscular; sc, subcutaneous.
[b] NR, not recommended.

and Happich, 1968; Edwards and Parry, 1972). Some of the data are also derived from a large number of publications summarized by Gibson (1975) and from unpublished data on work carried out by the present author. Detailed information on the efficient dose rates against various stages of fluke may be found in reviews (Boray, 1969a, 1971, 1982a). In this table the minimum age of fluke is listed when efficacy is 90% or higher at commercially recommended dose rates and the safety of the drugs is recorded. It is shown that those drugs are effective only against sexually mature fluke at tolerated dose rates. Some of those compounds may be effective against advanced immature fluke aged 8–10 weeks at dose rates approaching the toxic level, and a high efficacy against earlier immature fluke can be achieved only at highly toxic doses. These compounds are not suitable for strategic control of fascioliasis or for the treatment of an outbreak of the acute disease. They remain in use in some countries because of economic considerations. However, they fail to prevent serious losses and provide reasonable control only by frequent application of the drugs. Table II provides data on more frequently used or recently developed compounds.

Some of the information is also based on comparative efficacy studies mentioned above with additional information derived from work carried out more recently. Table III shows the spectrum of efficacy of some drugs at recommended dose rates against *F. hepatica*. As a result of experimental work over the past 20 years, anthelmintics have been developed with different efficiency spectrums when given at safe dose rates. One group that includes most of the earlier drugs listed in Table I are effective only against sexually mature fluke. Some of the new benzimidazole compounds used for control of nematodes have marginal effect against adult *Fasciola hepatica* at increased dose rates (Düwel *et al.*, 1975; Kelly *et al.*, 1975; Čorba *et al.*, 1979). From the benzimidazoles, only albendazole has been recommended for use against fascioliasis, but its activity is erratic and restricted to fully grown adult fluke (Knight and Colglazier, 1977; Van Schalkwyk *et al.*, 1979; Johns and Dickeson, 1979; Theodorides and Freeman, 1980; Malone *et al.*, 1982). It must be emphasized that albendazole is unsuitable for the treatment of acute fascioliasis and for the efficient strategic control of the disease. Rew and Knight (1980) applied albendazole as a premix in the feed for a period of 6 weeks with good results. However, this method of treatment is not reliable and would require the application of a slow-release device. From the group of compounds that are effective only against adult fluke at recommended doses, oxyclozanide and niclofolan are the most widely used in both sheep and cattle. Consequently, an overall reduction of prevalence of the disease cannot be expected until more effective drugs are employed.

Another group of compounds, which includes nitroxynil, rafoxanide, and closantel, display good activity against immature fluke aged 6–8 weeks and older but are not effective against earlier stages (Lucas, 1967; Boray and Happich, 1968; Ross, 1970; Armour and Čorba, 1970; Annen *et al.*, 1973; Boray *et al.*, 1973; De Keyser, 1980). Nitroxynil and closantel in sheep are slightly less effective than rafoxanide against immature fluke at recommended dose rates. All are highly active against adult fluke and, as in the case of rafoxanide, the drugs also are active against some nematodes, particularly *Haemonchus contortus*. Both rafoxanide and closantel are active against the nasal bot of sheep, *Oestrus ovis*. From this group of compounds, nitroxynil is mainly used

Table II. Comparative Efficiency of Drugs against Fasciola spp.: Currently Used or Recently Developed Compounds

Anthelmintic	Route of application[a]	Recommended dose rate[b] (mg/kg)		Max. tolerated dose in sheep (mg/kg)	Safety index at recommended dose rate in sheep	Minimum age of fluke in weeks, efficiency ≥90%	
		Sheep	Cattle			Sheep	Cattle
Oxyclozanide	Oral	15	13–15	60	4.0	12	>14
Niclofolan	Oral	4	3	12	3.0	12	>12
	sc	NR	0.8	?	?	NR	>12
Nitroxynil	sc	10	10	40	4.0	8	10
Brotianide	Oral	5.6	NR	27	4.8	12	NR
Rafoxanide	Oral	7.5	7.5	45	6.0	6	12
	sc	NR	3	?	?	NR	12
Closantel	Oral	7.5–10	NR	40?	4.0?	8–6	NR
	sc	NR	3	?	?	NR	>12
Diamphenetide (ace-midophene, U.S.S.R.)	Oral	80–120	100	400	3.3–5.0	1 day to 6 weeks	1 day to 7 weeks
Albendazole	Oral	4.75	10	30	8	17	>12
Triclabendazole	Oral	10	12	200	20–40	1	1
Clorsulon[c]	Oral	20	7	100	5	6	8
	sc	?	7				8

[a]sc, subcutaneous.
[b]Not recommended.
[c]Not yet available for sheep.

Table III. Efficiency Spectrum of Drugs at Recommended Dose Rates against F. hepatica in Sheep

Drug	Time postinfection (in weeks)													
	1	2	3	4	5	6	7	8	9	10	11	12	13	14
CCl₄, Hexachloroethane, Hexachlorophene, Bromsalans, Bromophenophos, Oxyclozanide, Niclofolan, Albendazole									50–90%			91–99%		
Nitroxynil, Closantel							50–90%			91–99%				
Rafoxanide, Clorsulon					50–90%					91–99%				
Triclabendazole		90–99%							99–100%					
Diamphenetide		100–91%							90–50%					

for beef cattle and nonlactating dairy cattle at the dose rate of 10 mg/kg as a subcutaneous injection. This drug exhibits good but erratic activity against fluke aged 6–8 weeks and is highly active 10 weeks postinfection. In sheep, more than 90% efficacy is achieved 8 weeks postinfection (Lucas, 1967).

When the dose rate of rafoxanide was increased from the normally recommended 7.5 mg/kg to 10–15 mg/kg, it was highly active against fluke aged 4 weeks or older (Armour and Čorba, 1970; Edwards and Parry, 1972). Strategic treatment with rafoxanide at increased dose rates for a period of 2–4 years was very successful in the field for the control of fascioliasis in sheep. The chemoprophylactic treatment reduced pasture contamination to such a low level that no anthelmintic treatment was considered necessary for several years after the program (Armour et al., 1973; Whitelaw and Fawcett, 1977, 1981).

Another anthelmintic, diamphenetide, is highly effective against early immature fluke aged 1 day to 6 weeks, but it has progressively lower activity against the parasites as they develop to maturity (Dickerson et al., 1971; Armour and Čorba, 1972; Annen et al., 1973; Rew et al., 1978). Its relatively low activity against the mature stages is a great disadvantage, and the drug has to be applied at high dose rates with a low safety index. When the drug was applied strategically, however, a chemoprophylactic effect was achieved (Rowlands, 1973; Enzie et al., 1980). Rew et al. (1980) suggested that diamphenetide may be useful for administration in a controlled-release device to achieve chemoprophylaxis.

Recently a new drug, triclabendazole, which is highly specific to Fasciolidae, showed high efficacy against all ages of fluke at the low dose rate of 10–12 mg/kg. The compound showed high activity against F. hepatica from 1 day after infection and was 100% active against fluke aged 6 weeks or older. The maximum tolerated dose was found to be 200 mg/kg, giving a high safety index of 20 (Boray et al., 1981, 1983; Wolff et al., 1983; Dorchies et al., 1983; Smeal and Hall, 1983; Turner et al., 1984). Similarly, high efficacy of triclabendazole was reported in cattle (Boray, 1982b). The efficacy of the compound was shown not to be affected by the operation of the esophageal groove reflex. It was also found that the few fluke that survived treatment during the early liver migration phase were retarded in their growth, and the prepatent period was extended. When the drug was used at intervals of 8–10 weeks (within the prepatent period), elimination of fascioliasis could be achieved (Boray et al., 1985). Triclabendazole may prove the most suitable drug for the treatment of acute fascioliasis and for efficient chemoprophylaxis.

Few comparative trials have been carried out on the efficacy of fluke-anthelmintics in cattle. It has been recognized that cattle are more resistant to Fasciola spp. than sheep, producing a vigorous tissue reaction to infection. It has also been shown that F. hepatica in cattle is less susceptible to anthelmintic treatment than in sheep of comparable age (see Tables I and II), particularly with heavy or repeated infections when the severe tissue reaction results in retarded growth (Boray, 1969a; Kendall and Parfitt, 1975). It has been concluded that if production loss is to be prevented, treatment should be carried out in cattle against the immature infection at the time when the highest pickup of metacercariae is expected. However, most drugs used for the treatment of *F. hepatica* in cattle are effective only against fluke aged 8 weeks and older, at which point severe pathological damage has already occurred. The most commonly used drug against *F. hepatica* in beef or nonlactating cattle is nitroxynil, but its efficacy is erratic at 6 and 8 weeks after infection and higher efficacy can only be expected when the fluke develop to maturity (Dobbins and Wellington, 1982). The efficacy of oxyclozanide, another commonly used anthelmintic in beef and dairy cattle, is lower and more than 90% efficacy can be achieved only against fluke aged 14 weeks or older. The most convenient treatment of cattle is the parenteral application of drugs and, in addition to nitroxynil, which is always given by injection, injectable formulations of rafoxanide, closantel, and brotianide have been developed. At the recommended dose rates, however, they are only active against adult fluke and the activity is very low against *F. hepatica* aged 6–8 weeks (Dobbins and Wellington, 1982). The new benzimidazole compound, triclabendazole, may prove the most effective and safe drug for the treatment of cattle, with more than 90% efficacy against fluke aged 1 week and approaching 100% efficacy against fluke aged 8 weeks or older at the recommended dose rate of 12 mg/kg (Boray, 1982*b*).

The high efficacy of a benzene sulfonamide compound, clorsulon, has been reported (Ostlind *et al.*, 1977). It appears that this drug is more effective in cattle than in sheep. The efficacy was more than 90% against adult fluke given as a subcutaneous injection at a dose rate of 2 mg/kg (Wyckoff and Bradley, 1983). Similarly, high efficacy was achieved subcutaneously at a dose rate of 4–8 mg/kg against fluke aged 8 weeks and with the oral dose of 7 mg/kg against adult fluke with a high margin of safety (Malone *et al.*, 1984). The drug should prove a useful treatment for fascioliasis in cattle, particularly in the United States, where no other anthelmintics are currently registered for that purpose.

4.1.2. F. gigantica

The data presented in Tables I–III are generally applicable for the treatment of *F. gigantica*. In sheep at comparable dose rates, the efficacy of niclofolan, tribromsalan, and oxyclozanide against *F. gigantica* aged 8 weeks was similar to that previously found against *F. hepatica* aged 6 weeks (Hildebrandt, 1968*a,b*; Hildebrandt and Ilmolelian 1968; Boray and Happich, 1968). Rafoxanide at a dose rate of 7 mg/kg was 94% and 50% effective against 6-week-old *F. hepatica* and *F. gigantica*, respectively, but 8 weeks after infection the drug was 100% effective against *F. gigantica* (Boray *et al.*, 1973). Similarly, rafoxanide was more effective against advanced immature *F. gigantica* than against *F. hepatica* of comparable age. At a dose rate of 2.5 mg/kg, rafoxanide was more effective against adult *F. gigantica* than against adult *F. hepatica* aged 12 weeks (Boray *et al.*, 1973). In cattle, higher efficacy was achieved against adult *F. gigantica* than against *F. hepatica* with injectable rafoxanide (Schröder *et al.*, 1977). In general, the data presented for the efficacy of drugs against *F. hepatica* can be considered valid for *F. gigantica*, but at the early immature stage *F. gigantica* may be less susceptible to treatment at comparable dose rates, while higher activity of drugs can be expected against adult *F. gigantica* (Horak *et al.*, 1972).

4.1.3. Integrated Control

Control of fascioliasis should be preventive rather than curative (1) by eliminating the parasite from the host by regular strategic anthelmintic treatment, thereby minimizing pasture contamination; (2) by reducing the number of intermediate host snails by drainage or chemical control; and (3) by reducing the chances of infection by keeping stock away from contaminated areas. Many of the proposed control measures involving farm management have been reviewed, and several recommendations have been made (Boray, 1969a, 1982a). Some of the methods, such as pasture rotation, would offer good preventive control even with older remedies effective only against adult fluke. However, such control requires a great deal of involvement in farm management as well as some initial financial investment. In spite of all these possibilities, a decrease in the overall prevalence of fascioliasis has only been evident since the use of drugs that have higher efficacy against the immature parasite. It now appears that with the most recent development of new anthelmintic compounds, improved chemotherapy of the disease will offer more efficient control and even eradication from certain areas.

4.1.4. Fascioloides magna

Fascioloides magna is a common trematode afflicting deer in North America that may cause serious disease in sheep, goats, and cattle as well. With its introduction into European countries and South Africa, more attention has been paid to the chemotherapy of the disease. It is particularly important that some of the drugs that are normally effective only in the bile ducts would not be effective for the prevention of disease in sheep and goats, in which continuous tissue migration of the fluke cause the eventual death of the host. Most anthelmintics used for the treatment of F. hepatica and F. gigantica so far tested proved efficient against F. magna. It is crucial to achieve 100% efficacy in sheep and goats, because even a single migrating fluke can kill the host. Oxyclozanide at 15 mg/kg was found effective against adult fluke in the white-tailed deer, but it was not effective against immatures (Foreyt and Todd, 1973). In cattle, rafoxanide was 100% effective against both immature and mature F. magna at dose rates of 10 or 15 mg/kg, but oxyclozanide at 15 mg/kg showed only partial activity against either immature or mature fluke in that host (Foreyt and Todd, 1974). In a 2-year program, bithionol sulfoxide at a dose rate of 40–50 mg/kg given to cattle with feed reduced the prevalence of the disease (Chroustova et al., 1980). More recently, the efficacy of albendazole was tested, but high dose rates of 11–54 mg/kg had only a 38% efficacy against the parasite in the white-tailed deer (Foreyt and Drawe, 1978). High doses of 15–45 mg/kg of albendazole were 90% effective against the parasite in cattle (Ronald et al., 1979). Foreyt and Foreyt (1980) found albendazole at 15 mg/kg to be 91% effective in goats infected with F. magna aged 8–14 weeks. Stromberg et al. (1984) treated artifically infected sheep 10 weeks after infection with increasing dose rates of albendazole from 5 to 15 mg/kg or two doses of 7.5 mg/kg, and an overall reduction of worm burden of 70% was observed. However, these workers found the efficacy unsatisfactory, since a single fluke can kill a sheep. Irrespective of the dose regimen, only 40–50% of treated animals were protected.

At various stages of its development, F. magna may be less susceptible to anthelmintic treatment than *F. hepatica;* also, because 100% efficacy in sheep and goats is crucial, the newer and more effective anthelmintics should be tested for the elimination of the disease. Clorsulon at a dose rate of ≥15 mg/kg should be tested in cattle, and triclabendazole at increased dose rates of 20–25 mg/kg should be effective against the fluke both in sheep and in cattle. Stromberg *et al.* (1984) reported that closantel at 20 mg/kg was 100% effective against 8-week-old *F. magna* in sheep.

4.2. Dicrocoeliidae

Although the economic loss due to members of the Dicrocoeliidae family are not comparable to that of Fascioliidae, considerable attention has been paid to the chemotherapy of the disease caused by *Dicrocoelium dendriticum* and *D. hospes.* Table IV summarizes the efficacy of several compounds. Most of these experimental studies were carried out in naturally infected animals, using the controlled test. It is interesting to note that very few drugs are represented in the list that are effective against *Fasciola* spp. as well, but some of the drugs that display activity against nematodes and cestodes are also active against *Dicrocoelium.* Very few compounds have good activity against this parasite at dose rates that are tolerated and that would result in elimination of pasture contamination and efficient control. The specific compound, Hetolin 1,1,1-tris(*p*-chlorophenyl)propionic acid-4-methylpiperazide hydrochloride has an erratic efficacy at dose rates lower than 60 mg/kg in sheep and cattle. The efficacy of 80–90% was achieved only at high dose rates with a low safety margin. The drug is not available commercially. Hexachloroparaxylene (Hetol) is widely used in the U.S.S.R. at a dose rate approaching toxic levels and with a relatively low efficacy. Some of the benzimidazoles are effective at very high dose rates, and the application of these drugs against *Dicrocoelium* may not be economically feasible. Praziquantel was reported effective against the parasite, but a very high dose of 50 mg/kg is required, which may not be economically feasible either. The same applies to diamphenetide, which even at very high and nearly toxic dosages was not better than many of the other drugs.

If treatment is carried out, it should be done when the highest infection of grazing animals occurs, usually in early spring and autumn, and other control measures should support the treatment. *Dicrocoelium hospes* in Africa is closely related to *D. dendriticum* and, although no specific data are available, the chemotherapy of dicrocoeliosis in Africa should be similar to that for *D. dendriticum.*

Li *et al.* (1983) successfully treated sheep infected with *Eurytrema pancreaticum* with praziquantel at a dose rate of 50–70 mg/kg. No other data are available on the chemotherapy of the pancreatic fluke, but other drugs that have been proved effective against *D. dentriticum* should be tested against this parasite.

For the treatment of *Platynosomum fastosum,* the liver fluke of cats, which is found in Asia, South America, Caribbean Islands, southern United States, and the Pacific area, nitroscanate at a dose rate of 100 mg/kg or praziquantel at 20 mg/kg were found effective, but diamphenetide at 200 mg/kg and thiabendazole at 500 mg/kg three times with 7-day intervals were not effective (Evans and Green, 1978). Nitroscanate is not recommended for the treatment of cats, as it has toxic side effects, but praziquantel at high dose rates should provide good results. The efficacy of the new benzimidazoles in multiple doses should also be tried.

Table IV. Efficiency of Drugs against Adult Dicrocoelium dendriticum in Sheep Evaluated by Controlled Tests

Anthelmintic	Dose rate (mg/kg)	Efficiency (%)	Safety index	Reference
Hexachloroparaxylene (Hetol)	300	80	2	Fetisov (1964)
1,1,1-tris(*p*-chlorophenyl) pro-	15–25	80–100	5	Lämmler (1963, 1964)
pionic acid-4-methyl-	66	90	2	Kassai and Holló (1970)
piperazide hydrochloride	<60	Erratic		Gibson (1975)[b]
(Hetolin)	15–40	Erratic in cattle		Gibson (1975)[b]
Cambendazole	25	78	7	Šibalić *et al.* (1971), Fetisov
	50	95	3	(1976), Foix (1977), Čorba *et al.* (1978)
Diamphenethide (acemido-	160	93	2.5	Gundlach *et al.* (1982)
phene, U.S.S.R.)	200	91	2	Calamel *et al.* (1979)
	240	85	1.6	Čorba *et al.* (1978)
	220–330	>90		Devillard and Villemin (1976)
Thiabendazole	200–300	96–98	4	Gibson (1975)
	200–300	52		Reinhardt (1978)
Mebendazole	20	70	>30	Reinhardt (1978)
Fenbendazole	150	90	4	Düwel *et al.* (1975)
	5 × 20 daily	90	>5	Čorba *et al.* (1979)
	100	90	5	Čorba *et al.* (1978)
Febantel	25	64		
	50	91		
	100	93		Čorba (1981)
Albendazole[a]	10	Nil	3	Tharaldsen (1981)
	2 × 10–12 (week's interval)	90	3	Tharaldsen and Wethe (1980)
	15	99	2	Cordero del Campillo *et al.* (1982)
	20	98	1.5	Himonas and Liakos (1980)
Praziquantel	20	73		Güralp *et al.* (1977)
	30	52		Wolff and Eckert (1979)
	40	76	>4	
	50	98		

[a]At these high dose rates, the drug is not recommended in the first month of pregnancy.
[b]Literature for sheep is reviewed under hexachloroparaxylene by error (Gibson, 1975).

4.3. Paramphistomata

Although many papers have been published on the chemotherapy of natural infections with paramphistomes, very few results are based on controlled experiments. Table V summarizes most of the data reported in the literature (Lämmler *et al.*, 1969; Boray, 1969*b*, 1982*a*; J. C. Boray, 1979, unpublished data; Horak, 1971; Gibson, 1975;

Table V. Efficiency of Drugs against Immature and Adult Paramphistomes Evaluated by Controlled Tests

Anthelmintic	Dose rate (mg/kg)	Efficiency (%)		Matures in rumen
		Immatures in small intestine		
		Sheep or goat	Cattle	Sheep and cattle
Hexachloroethane	300	0	0	+ [a]
Hexachlorophene	20	0	0	+ + [b]
Hexachloroparaxylene	400	0	0	80
Bithionol	100–200	99	—	73
	25–100	99–100	—	+ + [b]
	25– 35	—	99–100	+ [a]
	75	100	—	—
Bithionol sulfoxide	40	?	?	97–100
Niclofolan	6	76–95	0	0
Niclosamide	50	94–99	0	0
	90	99.9	—	—
	100	—	0–96	0
Oxyclozanide alone or with levamisole	15	80–92	60	73–90
Resorantel	65	80–99	80–99	85–100
Brotianide	15	?	85	87–90
Rafoxanide	15	92	0	0
Clioxanide	20	0	0	0
Pyrantel	25	0	0	0
Nitroxynil	10	0	0	0
Praziquantel	10	0	0	0

[a] +, some activity.
[b] + +, moderate activity.

Schillhorn Van Veen and Bida, 1975; Chhabra *et al.*, 1977; Prasad, 1983; P. F. Rolfe and J. C. Boray, 1984, unpublished data). The availability of a highly effective and safe drug for the treatment of an acute outbreak, caused by the migrating immature worms in the small intestine, is very limited, and none of the drugs that show high efficacy against adult fluke is active enough to be used for the elimination of pasture contamination. Bithionol, which is available only in some African and Asian countries, seems to be highly effective against both immature infection and the adult fluke in the rumen, but the effective dose rate is toxic. Nevertheless, it could be used for treating an outbreak if other drugs are not available and if a large proportion of the animals would likely be lost through the disease. The most effective and safe compound for the control of an outbreak in sheep is niclosamide, which yields spectacular results at dose rates of 50–100 mg/kg. Niclosamide is not absorbed from the small intestine and is very safe. Recovery in sheep occurs within a few days. Unforutnately, the drug has an erratic effect in calves at dose rates as high as 150 mg/kg. Niclosamide is not effective against adult paramphistomes in both sheep and cattle. Niclofolan is highly effective at a dose rate of 6 mg/kg against the immature paramphistomes in sheep; it can also be useful against concurrent infection with *Fasciola* spp. Unfortunately, the drug has no efficacy against either the immature or adult paramphistomes in cattle. Resorantel is a specific drug that has slightly erratic but good efficacy against immature and mature paramphistomes in sheep, goats, and cattle at the relatively high dose of 65 mg/kg. It is also effective against adult worms but can be disappointing in cattle.

Favorable reports were published on the effect of oxyclozanide alone or in combination with levamisole against both immature and mature paramphistomes (Schillhorn Van Veen and Bida, 1975; Chhabra *et al.*, 1977; Prasad, 1983). Oxyclozanide was highly effective against the pathogenic immature forms in sheep or goats at a dose rate of 15 mg/kg, and many reports from Eastern Europe or the U.S.S.R. confirm the efficacy of the drug against the adult parasites in both sheep and cattle. In controlled trials at the Central Veterinary Laboratory, Glenfield, Australia, oxyclozanide, at 15 mg/kg, was highly effective against the ruminal stage of advanced immature fluke in cattle. The drug showed a reasonable overall efficacy (58%) against the intestinal stage of immature paramphistomes in calves, but its effect was erratic in some animals (P. F. Rolfe and J. C. Boray, 1984, unpublished data). It appears that in an outbreak of acute intestinal paramphistomosis in calves, oxyclozanide may be the most suitable drug to use, particularly when concurrent infection with adult *Fasciola* spp. is also present. However, niclosamide may also control the clinical disease at high dose rates. Both drugs are highly effective against immature paramphistomes in sheep and goats.

In an outbreak of intestinal paramphistomosis, animals should be removed from infected pastures and treated. Control measures should concentrate on keeping susceptible livestock, particularly young animals, away from habitats of the intermediate host snails, particularly when high rainfall favors increased snail populations and production of metacercariae.

4.4. Schistosomatidae

Schistosomes infect sheep, goats, cattle, and buffalo in India, Africa, and China. The species involved are *Schistosoma bovis, S. mattheei, S. nasalis, S. indicum, S. spindale,* and *S. japonicum.* In contrast to vast research efforts dealing with chemotherapy of human schistosomiasis (see Chapter 18), relatively little reliable information is available on the treatment of ovine or bovine infections. Table VI summarizes the literature, showing the complicated dose regimens and noting the efficacy and safety of the treatments. The efficacy and relative safety are often difficult to determine from various trials because, apart from the toxic side effects of the drugs, the destroyed fluke may also cause pathological damage to the hosts. Van Wyk *et al.* (1974) warned that even with highly effective drugs, treatment should be carried out cautiously, particularly in heavily infected animals, in which large numbers of disintegrating parasites may produce emboli, occlusion of the portal system, or liver infarction.

Antimony preparations are toxic at effective dosages; the same is true for newer compounds, such as lucanton, hycanton, and niridazole. Variable results and toxic side effects have been reported following oral administration of the organophosphorous compound trichlorophon. However, it appears that small and steadily increasing intramuscular doses of trichlorophon may produce clinical recovery of affected animals (Van Wyk et al., 1974). The efficacy of haloxon varies from animal to animal and toxic side effects can also be expected. A new drug, amoscanate, which is under development for the treatment of human schistosomiasis in a micronized form, has shown high efficacy in laboratory tests (Bueding et al., 1976; Striebel, 1976). Quin et al. (1982) reported the use of the drug in an intravenous injection in a 2% suspension; satisfactory results were obtained against S. japonicum in cattle and buffalo. Amoscanate (nithiocyanamide), has been manufactured in China for some time and used for the treatment of human schistosomiasis.

According to the most recent literature, the most promising compound for the treatment of human schistosomiasis is praziquantel (see Chapter 18). Tested in cattle by Bushara et al. (1982) against S. bovis, this drug was found to be highly effective and safe. It required only two treatments at a dose rate of 20 mg/kg. Praziquantel may become the drug of choice for the treatment of schistosomiasis in ruminants.

If a highly effective drug can be used economically in a strategic control program, the use of the newly developed compounds could play an important role in reducing economic loss and contamination of the environment. Under certain conditions, domestic animals can maintain the contamination of endemic areas with schistosome eggs, which become available for human infection. Human infection may occur with S. mattheei, but the most important zoonotic schistosomiasis is caused by S. japonicum, which is commonly found in ruminants, dogs, cats, and other animals in the field. Strategic treatment of these animals may assist in the economic control of the disease in man.

4.5. Intestinal Trematodes of Birds and Mammals

Members of Echinostomatidae, Psilostomatidae, Strigeidae, Notocotylidae, Heterophyidae, and Troglotrematidae may cause infection in the intestinal tract of birds and some mammals. Those infections are economically insignificant. Nevertheless, individual animals may suffer from the infection in wildlife sanctuaries or zoological gardens, and treatment should be attempted in certain cases. Tetrachlorethylene and carbon tetrachloride have been used against these infections (Malek, 1980). However, less toxic and more effective compounds such as niclosamide, oxyclozanide, rafoxanide, or praziquantel are now available. Successful treatments of strigeid infections in falcons, using rafoxanide, praziquantel, or niclosamide, were reported (Greenwood et al., 1984). Infections of dogs and cats and occasionally other animals by Opisthorchidae (Opisthorchis felineus, O. viverrini, and Clonorchis sinensis) are common in East Asia. Regular treatment of animals may not be economical or practical but, in view of potential zoonotic conditions, treatment of animals in certain environments may be desirable. For the treatment of Opisthorchidae, repeated high doses of hexacloroparaxylene may be effective. Good efficacy was achieved by repeated doses of niclofolan and praziquantel (Rim and Lee, 1979; and Rim et al. (1981). Praziquantel is well tolerated by animals and should be tested in repeated doses of 20–25 mg/kg.

Table VI. Efficiency of Anthelmintics against Schistosoma spp. in Ruminants

Anthelmintic	Species (host)	Dose regimen[a]	Efficiency	Safety	Reference
Antimony potassium tartrate	S. nasalis cattle, sheep	2 mg/kg per day 6×; 3.5 mg/kg every 2nd day 6× iv	81–88%	Toxic side effects	Gibson (1975)
Antimony sodium tartrate	S. nasalis cattle	1.5 mg/kg per day or 2 mg/kg every 2nd day 6×; 8.5 mg/kg per day, 6 equal doses for 2 days, iv	Clinical improvement, relapse; 100%	Toxic side effects; Toxic side effects	Gibson (1975)
Sodium antimony dimercaptosuccinate	S. japonicum cattle	20–35 mg/kg im	High	Less toxic than tartar emetic	Shi (1981)
Stibophene	S. mattheei sheep	5 mg/kg per day 5× im; 10 mg/kg per day 5× im; 15 mg/kg per day 5× im	Inefficient	Tolerated	Lawrence (1968)
	S. mattheei cattle	4.5 mg/kg, alternate days 10× im; 6.5 mg/kg per day 10× im; 7.5 mg/kg per day 6× im; 10 mg/kg per day 3× im	High clinical improvement	Tolerated	Lawrence and Schwartz (1969)
Lucanthone	S. mattheei sheep	20 mg/kg per day 3× oral; 40 mg/kg per day 3× oral; 60 mg/kg over 5 days oral; 180 mg/kg daily 3× oral	Inefficient; 4 of 6 satisfactory	Tolerated; Tolerated	Lawrence (1968)
Hycanthone	S. mattheei sheep	6 mg/kg single dose im	High 98–100%	1 of 4 died; Local tissue reaction	Lawrence and McKenzie (1970)

Drug	Species/animal	Dose	Efficacy	Side effects	Reference
Niridazole	S. nasalis cattle	25–50 mg/kg oral	Inefficient	75 mg/kg fatal	Muraleedharan et al. (1977)
	S. mattbei sheep and goats	100 mg/kg daily 3× oral	100%	Toxic side effects	Hurter and Potgieter (1967)
		100 mg/kg single dose oral	1–98%	Toxic side effects	Hurter and Potgieter (1967)
		150 mg/kg single dose oral	Inefficient	One sheep died	Hurter and Potgieter (1967)
		35 mg/kg per day 5× oral	Inefficient	Well tolerated	Lawrence (1968)
		30–40 mg/kg per day 3× oral	Low	Toxic side effects	Gibson (1975)
Trichlorphon	S. nasalis cattle	25 mg/kg 3 × 3-day interval oral + 50 mg/kg 3 × 3-day interval oral	Nil	Not reported	Bushara et al. (1982)
	S. bovis cattle	50–75 mg/kg 4–6 × 3-day interval oral	Satisfactory	Tolerated	Dinnik (1967)
	S. mattbei cattle	75 mg/kg 2 × 3-day interval oral	Satisfactory	2 of 5 died	Lawrence and Schwartz (1969)
	S. mattbei sheep and goats	100–120 mg/kg 4 × 3–4 day interval oral	Satisfactory	Tolerated	Medda (1969), Medda et al. (1969)
	S. mattbei cattle (outbreak)	Increasing dose rate 8–20 mg/kg 8×, or 8–15 mg/kg 8–11×, 3–4-day intervals i.m.	75% reduction, clinical recovery	Toxic side effects but tolerated	Van Wyk et al. (1974)
Haloxon	S. mattbei goats	300 mg/kg 2× oral	30–100%	Tolerated	Hurter and Potgieter (1967)
Nithiocyanamine (Chinese name for Amoscanate)	S. japonicum cattle, buffalo	1.5–2 mg/kg single iv as a suspension (2%)	Satisfactory	Not reported	Quin et al. (1982) In experimental animals: Bueding et al. (1976), Striebel (1976)
Praziquantel	S. bovis cattle	20 mg/kg at 9th and 14th days after infection, oral	99%	Well tolerated	Bushara et al. (1982)

[a]im, intramuscular; iv, intravenous.

419

Paragonimus spp., or lung fluke, may also occur in dogs and cats; treatment with bithionol should be attempted when necessary. The drug is used routinely to treat the infection in man (Malek, 1980). For more detailed data on the treatment of Opisthorchidae and *Paragonimus* spp., see Chapter 18.

REFERENCES

Annen, J. M., Boray, J. C., and Eckert, J., 1973, Prüfung neuer Fasziolizide: II. Wirksamkeitsvergleich von Rafoxanid und Diamphenthid bei subakuter und chronischer Fasziolose des Schafes. *Schweiz. Arch. Tierheilk.* 115:527–538.

Armour, J., and Čorba, J., 1970, The anthelmintic activity of rafoxanide against immature *Fasciola hepatica* in sheep, *Vet. Rec.* 87:213–214.

Armour, J., and Čorba, J., 1972, The anthelmintic efficiency of diamphenethide against *Fasciola hepatica* in sheep, *Vet. Rec.* 91:211–213.

Armour, J., Čorba, J., and Bruce, R. G., 1973, The prophylaxis of ovine fascioliasis by strategic use of rafoxanide, *Vet. Rec.* 92:83–89.

Boray, J. C., 1963, Standardization of techniques for pathological and anthelmintic studies with *Fasciola* spp., in: *Proceedings of the First International Conference of the World Association for the Advancement of Veterinary Parasitology, Hannover 1963* (E. J. L. Soulsby, ed.), pp. 34–45, Merck and Co., Inc., Rahway, New Jersey.

Boray, J. C., 1969a, Experimental fascioliasis in Australia in: *Advances in Parasitology* (B. Dawes, ed.), Vol. 7, pp. 95–210, Academic Press, London and New York.

Boray, J. C., 1969b, Studies on intestinal paramphistomosis in sheep due to *Paramphistomum ichikawai* Fukui, 1922, *Vet. Med. Rev.* No. 4:290–308.

Boray, J. C., 1971, Fortschritte in der Bekämpfung der Fasciolose, *Schweiz. Arch. Tierheilk.* 113:361–386.

Boray, J. C., 1982a, Fascioliasis, in: *Handbook Series in Zoonoses*, Section C: *Parasitic Zoonoses* (J. H. Steele, G. V. Hillyer, and C. E. Hopla, eds.), Vol. III, pp. 71–88, CRC Press, Boca Raton, Florida.

Boray, J. C., 1982b, Chemotherapy of fasciolosis, *New South Wales Vet. Proc.* 18:42–47.

Boray, J. C., and Happich, F. A., 1968, Standardised chemotherapeutical tests for immature and mature *Fasciola hepatica* infections in sheep, *Aust. Vet. J.* 44:72–78.

Boray, J. C., and Roseby, F. B., 1969, The effect of the route of administration on the efficiency of clioxanide against immature *Fasciola hepatica* in sheep, *Aust. Vet. J.* 45:363–365.

Boray, J. C., Happich, F. A., and Andrews, J. C., 1967a, Comparative chemotherapeutical tests in sheep infected with immature and mature *Fasciola hepatica*, *Vet. Rec.* 80:218–224.

Boray, J. C., Happich, F. A., and Andrews, J. C., 1967b, Studies on the suitability of the albino rat for testing anthelmintic activity against *Fasciola hepatica*, *Ann. Trop. Med. Parasitol.* 61:104–111.

Boray, J. C., Happich, F. A., and Jones, W. D., 1969, Chemotherapeutical tests for heavy immature *Fasciola hepatica* infections in sheep, *Aust. Vet. J.* 45:94–96.

Boray, J. C., Wolff, K., and Trepp, H. C., 1973, Prüfung neuer Fasziolizide: I. Wirksamkeit und Toxizität von Rafoxanid bei künstlich mit *Fasciola hepatica* oder *F. gigantica* infizierten Schafen, *Schweiz, Arch. Tierheilk.* 115:367–371.

Boray, J. C., Strong, M. B., Schellenbaum, M., and von Orelli, M., 1981, Chemoprophylaxis of fasciolosis in sheep and cattle, in: *Prooceedings of the Ninth International Conference of the World Association for the Advancement of Veterinary Parasitology, Budapest, 1981*, abstract, p. 234, Egyetemi Nyomda, Budapest.

Boray, J. C., Crowfoot, P. D., Strong, M. B., Allison, J. R., Schellenbaum, M., von Orelli, M., and Sarasin, G., 1983, Treatment of immature and mature *Fasciola hepatica* infections in sheep with triclabendazole, *Vet. Rec.* 113:315–317.

Boray, J. C., Jackson, R., and Strong, M. B., 1985, Chemoprophylaxis of fascioliasis with triclabendazole, *N. Z. Vet. J.* 33 (in press).

Bueding, E., Batzinger, R., and Patterson, G., 1976, Antischistosomal and some toxicological properties of a nitro-diphenyl-aminoisothiocyanate (C 9333-Go/CGP), *Experientia* 32:604–605.

Bushara, H. O., Hussein, M. F., Majid, M. A., and Taylor, M. G., 1982, Effects of praziquantel and metrifonate on *Schistosoma bovis* infections in Sudanese cattle, *Res. Vet. Sci.* 33:125–126.

Calamel, M., Villemin, D., and Leimbacher, F., 1979, Efficacy of diamphenethide in the treatment of dicrocoeliasis of sheep, *Rec. Med. Vet.* 155:37–46.

Campbell, W. C., and Barry, T. A., 1970, A biochemical method for the detection of anthelmintic activity against liver fluke (*Fasciola hepatica*), *J. Parasitol.* 56:325–331.

Campbell, W. C., Ostlind, D. A., and Yakstis, J. J., 1970, The efficacy of 3,5-diiodo-3'-chloro-4-(p-chloro-phenoxy)-salicylanilide against immature *Fasciola hepatica* in sheep, *Res. Vet. Sci.* 11:99–100.

Chhabra, R. C., Gill, B. S., and Dutt, S. C., 1977, Fatal amphistomiasis in sheep and goats and its control in Punjab, in: *Proceedings of the First National Congress of Parasitology, Baroda, India,* p. 44, Indian Society for Parasitology.

Chroustova, E., Hulka, J., and Jaros, J., 1980, Prevention and therapy of *Fascioloides* infection in cattle with bithionol sulphoxide, *Vet. Med. (Praha)* 25:557–563.

Coles, G. C., 1975, Activity of commercial fasciolicides in small laboratory mammals, *J. Parasitol.* 61:54–58.

Čorba, J., 1981, Efficacy of febantel (Rintal®) against some important helminthiases of sheep and cattle, *Vet. Med. Rev.* No. 1:15–24.

Čorba, J., Legeny, J., Stoffa, P., Krupicer, I., and Pacenovsky, J., 1978, The effect of pharmacological preparations on dicrocoeliasis in ruminants, *Veterinarstvi,* 28:274–275.

Čorba, J., Lietava, P., Düwel, D., and Reisenleiter, R. 1979, Efficiency of fenbendazole against the most important trematodes and cestodes of ruminants, *Br. Vet. J.* 135:318–323.

Cordero del Campillo, M., Rojo Vazquez, F. A., Diez Banos, P., and Chaton-Schaffner, M., 1982, Efficacité de l'albendazole contre une infestation naturelle a *Dicrocoelium dendriticum* chez le mouton, *Rev. Med. Vet.* 133:41–49.

Danek, J., Strosova, Z., Kinsa, H., Kinkorova, J., and Čorba, J., 1979, Helmisan premix: Another form of a combined anthelmintic preparation for sheep and cattle, *Biol. Chem. Zivocisne Vyroby Vet.* 15:553–566.

De Keyser, H., 1980, Die Aktivität von Closantel auf Jugendformen von Fasciola, in: *Proceedings: Symposium Parasitosen der Wiederkäuer, November 1980, Rothenburg ob der Tauber, Bonn,* pp. 25–29.

Devillard, J. P., and Villemin, P., 1976, Treatment of *Dicrocoelium* infection of the goat with diamphenetide, *Bull. Mens. Soc. Vet. Prat. Fr* 60:563–576.

Dickerson, G., Harfenist, M., and Kingsbury, P. A., 1971, A chemotherapeutic agent for all stages of liver fluke disease in sheep. *Br. Vet. J.* 127:XI.

Dinnik, N. N., 1967, The effect of neguvon on *Schistosoma bovis* in naturally infected cattle, *Vet. Med. Rev.* No. 1:76–78.

Dobbins, S. E., and Wellington, A. C., 1982, Comparison of the activity of some fasciolicides against immature liver fluke in calves, *Vet. Rec.* 111:177–178.

Dorchies, P., Franc, M., and De Lahitte, J. D., 1983, Étude de l'activité du triclabendazole (DCI) sur *Fasciola hepatica* chez l'agneau, *Rev. Med. Vet.* 134:231–234.

Düwel, D., Kirsch, R., and Reisenleiter, R., 1975, The efficacy of fenbendazole in the control of trematodes and cestodes, *Vet. Rec.* 97:371.

Edwards, C. M., and Parry, T. O., 1972, Treatment of experimentally-produced acute fascioliasis in sheep, *Vet. Rec.* 90:523–526.

Enzie, F. D., Rew, R. S., and Colglazier, M. L., 1980, Chemoprophylaxis with diamphenetide against experimental infections of *Fasciola hepatica* in ruminants, *Am. J. Vet. Res.* 41:179–182.

Ernst, P., 1925, Leberegelheilmittel, *Berl. Munch. Tierarztl. Wochenschr.* 76:1109–1117.

Evans, J. W., and Green, P. E., 1978, Preliminary evaluation of four anthelmintics against the cat liver fluke, *Platynosomum concinnum, Aust. Vet. J.* 54:454–455.

Fairweather, I., Holmes, S. D., and Threadgold, L. T., 1983, *Fasciola hepatica:* A technique for monitoring *in-vitro* motility, *Exp. Parasitol.* 56:369–380.

Fairweather, I., Holmes, S. D., and Threadgold, L. T., 1984, *Fasciola hepatica:* Motility response to fasciolicides *in vitro, Exp. Parasitol.* 57:209–224.

Fetisov, V. I., 1964, Hexachloroparaxylol, hetol and hetolin tested against dicrocoeliasis, *Veterinariya,* 41:47–48.

Fetisov, V. I., 1976, Investigation of anthelmintics for efficacy against *Dicrocoelium, Biull. Vsesoiuznogo Inst. Gelmintol.* 18:96–100.

Foix, J., 1977, Traitement de la dicrocoeliose par le cambendazole, *Rev. Med. Vet.* 128:1111–1119.

Foreyt, W. J., 1979, *Fascioloides magna:* Development in selected nonruminant mammalian hosts, *Exp. Parasitol.* 47:292–296.

Foreyt, W. J., and Drawe, D. L., 1978, Anthelmintic activity of albendazole in White-Tailed Deer, *Am. J. Vet. Res.* 39:1901–1903.

Foreyt, W. J., and Foreyt, K. M., 1980, Albendazole treatment of experimentally induced *Fascioloides magna* infections in goats, *Vet. Med. Small Anim. Clin.* 75:1441–1444.

Foreyt, W. J., and Todd, A. C., 1973, Action of oxyclozanide against adult *Fascioloides magna* (Bassi, 1875) infections in White-Tailed Deer, *J. Parasitol.* 59:208–209.

Foreyt, W. J., and Todd, A. C., 1974, Efficacy of rafoxanide and oxyclozanide against *Fascioloides magna* in naturally infected cattle, *Am. J. Vet. Res.* 35:375–377.

Gibson, T. E., 1975, *Veterinary Anthelmintic Medication,* 3rd ed., Commonwealth Agricultural Bureau, Slough, England.

Greenwood, A. G., Furley, C. W., and Cooper, J. E., 1984, Intestinal trematodiasis in falcons (order Falconiformes), *Vet. Rec.* 114:477–478.

Gundlach, J. L., Furmaga, S., Uchacz, S., and Sadzikowski, A., 1982, Chronic dicrocoeliasis in sheep and its treatment, *Med. Wet.* 38:204–206.

Güralp, N., Oguz, T., and Zybek, H., 1977, *Dicrocoelium dendriticum* 'la tabii enfekte koyunlarda Embay 8440 (praziquantel, Droncit) ile tapilan tedavi deneyleri, *Vet. Fak. Dergisi* 24:85–89.

Hall, M. C., 1921, Carbon tetrachloride for the removal of parasitic worms, especially hookworms, *J. Agric. Res.* 21:157–175.

Hayes, T. J., Bailer, J., and Mitrovic, M., 1973, Murine fascioliasis: Laboratory model for the detection of fasciolicidal activity of chemical compounds, *J. Parasitol.* 59:314–318.

Hildebrandt, J., 1968a, Die Wirksamkeit von Bilevon M gegen unreife und geschlechtsreife Stadien von *Fasciola gigantica* in künstlich infizierten Schafen, *Berl. Munch. Tierarztl. Wochenschr.* 81:66–69.

Hildebrandt, J., 1968b, Dibromosalicylanilide tribromosalicylanilide effect against immature and mature stages of *Fasciola gigantica* in artifically infected sheep, *Vet. Rec.* 82:699–700.

Hildebrandt, J., and Ilmolelian, L. L., 1968, Die Wirksamkeit von Zanil gegen unreife und geschlechtsreife Stadien von *Fasciola gigantica* in künstlich infizierten Schafen, *Berl. Munch. Tierarztl. Wochenschr.* 81:178–180.

Himonas, C. A., and Liakos, V., 1980, Efficacy of albendazole against *Dicrocoelium dendriticum* in sheep, *Vet. Rec.* 107:288–289.

Hohorst, W., and Lämmler, G., 1963, Experimentelle Dicrocoeliose-Studien Z. *Tropenmed. Parasitol.* 13:377–397.

Horak, I. G., 1971, Paramphistomiasis of domestic ruminants, in: *Advances in Parasitology* (B. Dawes, ed.), Vol. 9, pp. 33–72, Academic Press, London and New York.

Horak, I. G., Snijders, A. J., and Louw, J. P., 1972, Trials with rafoxanide 5. Efficacy studies against *Fasciola hepatica, Fasciola gigantica, Paramphistomum microbothrium* and various nematodes in sheep, *J. S. Afr. Vet. Assoc.* 43:397–403.

Hurter, L. R., and Potgieter, L. N. D., 1967, Schistosomiasis in small stock in the Potgietersrus veterinary area, *J. S. Afr. Vet. Med. Assoc.* 38:444–446.

Johns, D. R., and Dickeson, S. J., 1979, Efficacy of albendazole against *Fasciola hepatica* in sheep, *Aust. Vet. J.* 55:431–432.

Kassai, T., and Holló, F., 1970, Tapasztalatok a juh-dicrocoeliosis Hetolin 50-nel és Hetolin 75-tel végzett gyógykezeléséröl, *Magy. Allatorv. Lap.* 25:30–32.

Kelly, J. D., Chevis, R. A. F., and Whitlock, H. V., 1975, The anthelmintic efficacy of mebendazole against adult *Fasciola hepatica* and a concurrent mixed nematode infection in sheep, *N. Z. Vet. J.* 23:81–84.

Kendall, S. B., and Parfitt, J. W., 1973, The effect of diamphenetide on *Fasciola hepatica* at different stages of development, *Res. Vet. Sci.* 15:37–40.

Kendall, S. B., and Parfitt, J. W., 1975, Chemotherapy of infection with *Fasciola hepatica* in cattle, *Vet. Rec.* 97:9–12.

Knight, R. A., and Colglazier, M. L., 1977, Albendazole as a fasciolicide in experimentally infected sheep, *Am. J. Vet. Res.* 38:807–808.

Krull, W. H., 1956, Experiments involving potential definitive hosts of *Dicrocoelium dendriticum* (Rudolphi 1819) Looss, 1899: Dicrocoeliidae, *Cornell Vet.* 46:511–525.

Lawrence, J. A., 1968, Treatment of *Schistosoma mattheei* infestation in sheep, *J. S. Afr. Vet. Med. Assoc.* 39:47–51.

Lawrence, J. A., and McKenzie, R. L., 1970, Treatment of *Schistosoma mattheei* infestation in sheep: Further observations, *J. S. Afr. Vet. Med. Assoc,* 41:298–306.

Lawrence, J. A., and Schwartz, W. O. H., 1969, Treatment of *Schistosoma mattheei* infestation in cattle, *J. S. Afr. Vet. Med. Assoc.* 40:129–136.

Lämmler, G., 1959, Die Chemotherapie der Fasciolose. III. Ueber die experimentelle *Fasciola hepatica* Infektion der Albino-Ratte, *Z. Tropenmed. Parasitol.* 10:379–384.

Lämmler, G., 1963, Die experimentelle Chemotherapie der Dicrocoeliose mit Hetolin®, *Berl. Munch. tierarztl. Wochenschr.* 70:373–377.

Lämmler, G., 1964, Die experimentelle Chemotherapie der Trematoden-Infektionen und ihre Problematik. 2, *Z. Tropenmed. Parasitol.* 15:164–199.

Lämmler, G., 1968, Chemotherapy of trematode infections, *Adv. Chemother.* 3:153–251.

Lämmler, G., Sahai, B. N., and Herzog, H., 1969, Anthelmintic efficacy of 2,6-dihydroxy benzoic acid-4′-bromanilide (Hoe 296 V) against mature and immature *Paramphistomum microbothrium* in goats, *Acta Vet. Acad. Sci. Hung.* 19:447–451.

Leiper, J. W. G., 1963, The evaluation of potential anthelmintics by in-vitro techniques, in: *Proceedings of the First International Conference of the World Association for the Advancement of Veterinary Parasitology, Hannover, 1963* (E. J. L. Sousby, ed.) pp. 14–17, Merck and Co., Rahway, New Jersey.

Li, J. Y., Wang, F. Y., Huo, X. C., and Chen, Y. J., 1983, Treatment of pancreatic flukes in sheep with praziquantel, *Chin. J. Vet. Med.* 9:15.

Lienert, E., 1963, The evaluation of anthelmintics for trematodes in domestic animals, in: *Proceedings of the First International Conference of the World Association for the Advancement of Veterinary Parasitology, Hannover, 1963* (E. J. L. Sousby, ed.) pp. 62–73, Merck and Co., Rahway, New Jersey.

Lucas, J. M. S., 1967, 4-cyano-2-iodo-6-nitrophenol, M & B 10, 755. I. Activity against experimental fascioliasis in rabbits, sheep and calves, *Br. Vet. J.* 123:198–211.

Malek, E. A., 1980, *Snail-Transmitted Parasitic Diseases,* Vol. II, CRC Press, Boca Raton, Florida.

Malone, J. B., Smith, P. H., Loyacano, A. F., Hembry, F. G., and Brock, L. T., 1982, Efficacy of albendazole for treatment of naturally acquired *Fasciola hepatica* in calves, *Am. J. Vet. Res.* 43:879–881.

Malone, J. B., Ramsey, R. T., and Loyacano, A. F., 1984, Efficacy of clorsulon for treatment of mature naturally acquired and 8 week old experimentally induced *Fasciola hepatica* infections in cattle, *Am. J. Vet. Res.* 45:851–854.

Medda, A., 1969, Il neguvon nella terapia della schistosomiasi ovina, *Atti. Soc. Ital. Sci. Vet.* 23:898–901.

Medda, A., Reinhardt, S., and Muscas, L., 1969, Neguvon Bayer in the treatment of goat schistosomiasis, *Vet. Ital.* 20:403–412.

Montgomery, R. F., 1926, Carbon tetrachloride in liver rot of sheep, *J. Comp. Pathol.* 39:113–131.

Muraleedharan, K., Kumar, S. P., Hegde, K. S., and Alwar, V. S., 1977, Comparative efficacy of neguvon, ambilhar and sodium antimony tartrate against nasal schistosomiasis in cattle, *Ind. Vet. J.* 54:703–708.

Ostlind, D. A., Hartman, R. K., Yakstis, J. J., and Campbell, W. C., 1972, A technique for the recovery of immature *Fasciola hepatica* from sheep liver, *Vet. Rec.* 90:370.

Ostlind, D. A., Campbell, W. C., Riek, R. F., Baylis, P., Cifelli, S., Hartman, R. K., Lang, R. K., Butler, R. W., Mrozik, H., Bochis, R. J., Eskioa, A., Matzuk, A., Waksmunski, F. S., Olen, L. E., Schwartzkopf, G., Grodski, A., Linn, B. O., Lusi, A., Wu, M. T., Shunk, C. H., Peterson, L. H., Milkowski, sJ. D., Hoff, D. R., Kulsa, P., and Harmon, R. E., 1977, The efficacy of 4-amino-6-tricholroethenyl-1,3-benzenedisulphonamide against liver fluke in sheep and cattle, *Br. vet. J.* 133:211–214.

Prasad, K. D., 1983, Anthelmintic efficacy of terenol and zanil against experimental paramphistomiasis in goats, *Ind. J. Vet. Med.* 3:27–32.

Quin, L. R., Liu, Z. L., Chen, Y. Z., Ma, L. H., Zeng, X. G., and Xu, M. G., 1982, Treatment. of *Shistosoma japonicum* infestation in farm cattle with nithiocyanamin, *Chin. J. Vet. Med.* 8:2–6.

Reinhardt, P., 1978, Untersuchungen zur medikamentellen Metaphylaxe bei der Dikrozöliose des Schafes, *Montasschr. Vet. Med.* 33:898–901.

Rew, R. S., and Knight, R. A., 1980, Efficacy of albendazole for prevention of fascioliasis in sheep, *J. Am. Vet. Med. Assoc.* 176:1353–1354.

Rew, R. S., Colglazier, M. L., and Enzie, F. D., 1978, Effect of diamfenetide on experimental infections of *Fasciolia hepatica* in lambs: Anthelmintic and clinical investigations, *J. Parasitol.* 64:290–294.

Rew, R. S., Enzie, F. D., and Colglazier, M. L., 1980, Diamphenetide as a controlled-release prophylactic fasciolicide in sheep: Daily oral doses, continual infusion and serum drug levels, *Int. Goat and Sheep Res.* 1:96–103.

Rim, H. J., and Lee, S. I., 1979, Chemotherapeutic effect of Niclofolan (Bayer 9015, Bilevon) in the treatment of *Chlonorchiasis sinensis, Korea Univ. Med. J.* 16:167–182.

Rim, H. J., Lyu, K. S., Lee, J. S., and Joo, H. K., 1981, Clinical evaluation of the therapeutic efficacy of praziquantel (Embay 8440) against *Clonorchis sinensis* infection in man, *Ann. Trop. Med. Parasitol.* 75:27–33.

Ronald, N. C., Craig, T. M., and Bell, R. R., 1979, A controlled evaluation of albendazole against natural infections with *Fasciola hepatica* and *Fascioloides magna* in cattle, *Am. J. Vet. Res.* 40:1299–1300.

Ross, D. B., 1970, Treatment of experimental *Fasciola hepatica* infection of sheep with rafoxanide, *Vet. Rec.* 87:110–111.

Rowlands, D. T., 1973, Diamphenetide—A drug offering a fresh approach to the treatment of liver fluke disease in sheep, *Pesticide Sci.* 4:883–889.

Schillhorn Van Veen, T., and Bida, S. A., 1975, Acute paramphistomiasis in sheep in Zaria, *Proceedings of the Twentieth Wold Veterinary Congress, Summaries, Thessaloniki, Greece,* Vol. 1, pp. 202–203.

Schröder, J., Honer, M. R., and Louw, J. P., 1977, Trials with rafoxanide 8. Efficacy of an injectable solution against trematodes and nematodes in cattle, *J. S. Afr. Vet. Assoc.* 48:95–97.

Shi, S. K., 1981, Clinical observation on the treatment of 100 cases of bovine schistosomiasis with Sb-58, *Chin. J. Vet. Med.* 7:16–18.

Šibalić, S., Lepojev, O., and Miklijan, S., 1971, Effect of cambendazole on *Dicrocoelium dendriticum* in naturally infected sheep, *Vet. Glasnik* 25:835–839.

Simpkin, K. G., and Coles, G. C., 1979, A new *in-vitro* test for anthelmintics *Parasitology* 79:XIX

Smeal, M. G., and Hall, C. A., 1983, The activity of triclabendazole against immature and adult *Fasciola hepatica* infections in sheep, *Aust. Vet. J.* 60:329–331.

Standen, O. D., 1963, Chemotherapy of helminthic infections, in: *Experimental Chemotherapy* (R. J. Schnitzer and F. Hawking, eds.), Volume 1, pp. 701–892, Academic Press, New York.

Striebel, H. P., 1976, 4-Isothiocyanato-4'-nitrodiphenylamine (C 9333-Go/CGP 4540), an anthelmintic with an unusual spectrum of activity against intestinal nematodes, filariae and schistosomes, *Experientia* 32:457–458.

Stromberg, B. E., Schlotthauer, J. C., and Conboy, G. A., 1983, Efficacy of albendazole against *Fascioloides magna* in sheep, *Am. J. Vet. Res.* 45:80–82.

Stromberg, B. E., Schlotthauer, J. C., and Conboy, G. A., 1984, The efficacy of closantel against *Fascioloides magna* in sheep, *J. Parasitol.* 70:446–447.

Taylor, E. L., 1964, *Fascioliasis and the Liver Fluke,* Food and Agricultural Organization of the United Nations Agricultural Studies No. 64, Rome.

Tharaldsen, J., 1981, Further trials with albendazole against *Dicrocoelium lanceolatum* in sheep, in: *Proceedings of the Ninth International Conference of the World Association for the Advancement of Veterinary Parasitology, Budapest,* 1981, abst., p. 236, Egyetem: Nyomda, Budapest.

Tharaldsen, J., and Wethe, J. A., 1980, A field trial with albendazole against *Dicrocoelium lanceolatum* in sheep, *Nord. Vet. Med.* 32:308–312.

Theodorides, V. J., and Freeman, J. F., 1980, Efficacy of albendazole against *Fasciola hepatica* in cattle, *Vet. Rec.* 106:78–79.

Thienel, M., 1926, Neue Arbeiten zur medikamentösen Bekämpfung der Leberegelseuche, *Berl. Munch. Tierarztl. Wochenschr.* 77:771–772.

Thorpe, E., 1965a, Chemotherapy of experimental fascioliasis in the albino rat, *J. Comp. Pathol.* 75:45–53.

Thorpe, E., 1965b, Liver damage and the host–parasite relationship in experimental fascioliasis in the albino rat, *Res. Vet. Sci.* 6:498–509.

Turner, K., Armour, J., and Richards, R. J., 1984, Anthelmintic efficacy of triclabendazole against *Fasciola hepatica* in sheep, *Vet. Rec.* 114:41–42.

Van Schalkwyk, P. C., Geyser, T. L., Recio, M., and Erasmus, F. P. G., 1979, The anthelmintic efficacy of albendazole against gastrointestinal roundworms, tapeworms, lungworms and liver flukes in sheep, *J. S. Afr. Vet. Med. Assoc.* 50:31–35.

Van Wyk, J. A., Bartsch, R. C., Van Rensburg, L. J., Heitmann, L. P., and Goosen, P. J., 1974, Studies on schistosomiasis. 6. A field outbreak of bilharzia in cattle, *Onderstepoort J. Vet. Res.* 41:39–50.

Whitelaw, A., and Fawcett, A. R., 1977, A study of a strategic dosing programme against ovine fascioliasis on a hill farm, *Vet. Rec.* 100:443–447.

Whitelaw, A., and Fawcett, A. R., 1981, Further studies on the control of ovine fascioliasis by strategic dosing, *Vet. Rec.* 109:118–119.

Wolff, K., and Eckert, J., 1979, The efficiency of praziquantel against the lancet fluke, *Dicrocoelium dendriticum* in sheep, in: *Proceedings of the Ninth Symposium of the Scandinavian Society for Parasitology, Abo, Finland, 1979*, p. 54.

Wolff, K., Ruosch, W., and Eckert, J., 1969, Perfusionstechnik zur Gewinnung von *Dicrocoelium dendriticum* aus Schaf-und Rinderlebern, *Z. Parasitenk.* 33:85–88.

Wolff, K., Eckert, J., Schneiter, G., and Lutz, H., 1983, Efficacy of triclabendazole against *Fasciola hepatica* in sheep and goats, *Vet. Parasitol.* 13:145–150.

Wyckoff, J. H., and Bradley, R. E., 1983, Efficacy of a benzenedisulfonamide against experimental *Fasciola hepatica* infections in calves, *Am. J. Vet. Res.* 44:2203–2204.

21

Mode of Action of Antitrematodal Agents

JAMES L. BENNETT and DAVID P. THOMPSON

1. MODE OF ACTION OF TREMATOCIDAL AGENTS

Chemotherapeutic agents exert their effect by interference with physiological or biochemical mechanisms essential for the functional integrity or the reproduction of the invading organism. Many compounds are capable of altering a multitude of biochemical reactions or physiological responses, especially when used in concentrations far above those that are chemotherapeutically effective. The problems of which if any of the observed effects is responsible for the trematocidal action of a given drug requires careful and critical analysis. To this end, attention has been directed, in the present discussion of trematocidal agents, toward several important criteria outlined in a classic paper by Hunter and Lowry (1956). Furthermore, the question must be examined whether an observed biochemical or physiological change is the primary cause, rather than the result, of the functional damage produced by the drug. In at least one instance—the antischistosomal action of trivalent organic antimonials—trematocidal activity can be ascribed to an inhibitory effect of the drug on a single enzyme. On the other hand, in the case of the action of piperazine on *Ascaris*, inhibition of the formation of succinate has been found to be the result, rather than the cause, of paralysis of the parasite (Del Castillo *et al.*, 1964).

In the following summaries of trematocidal drug actions, the focus is primarily on agents active against *Schistosoma* sp. and *Fasciola* sp.—trematodes of paramount medical and economic importance. We have not attempted to review all the relevant literature, but rather to present information on proposed mechanisms which, based on current knowledge, appear most plausible.

JAMES L. BENNETT and DAVID P. THOMPSON • Department of Pharmacology and Toxicology, Michigan State University, East Lansing, Michigan 48824.

1.1. Modes of Action of Schistosomicidal Agents

The long-term survival of schistosomes *in vivo* appears to depend on their ability to remain *in situ* within species-dependent veins of predilection. Since maintenance of position within the host requires coordinated neuromuscular activity, any agent that interferes with neuronal signaling and/or excitation-contraction coupling in the parasite may possess schistosomicidal activity. Possible selective bases for drugs that affect neuromuscular activity in schistosomes, such as metrifonate and praziquantel, include the presence of an acetylcholinesterase (ACh), which is at least 10 times more sensitive to inhibition by organophosphorus compounds than that of the host (Bueding *et al.*, 1972; Senft and Hillman, 1973) and of a low-resistance pathway between the tegument and muscle fibers, which permits any perturbation of ionic conductance at the parasite's surface to affect the underlying muscle fibers directly (Bricker *et al.*, 1982; Thompson *et al.*, 1982).

Since adult schistosomes derive most of their energy anaerobically by the fermentation of glucose to lactate (Bueding, 1950; Bueding and Fisher, 1982), their glycolytic pathway represents another potentially specific target for anthelmintic attack. At least one important class of schistosomicidal compounds, the trivalent organic antimonials, owe their selectivity to the differential host—parasite sensitivity of phosphofructokinase (Bueding and Fisher, 1966), the rate-limiting enzyme of glycolysis. Other metabolic differences between the parasites and their vertebrate hosts, such as the absence in schistosomes of *de novo* pathways for the synthesis of purines (Senft *et al.*, 1972) or steroids (Meyer *et al.*, 1970), represent additional sites for selective chemotherapeutic intervention, which may be relevant to the undefined mechanisms of other schistosomicidal compounds.

1.1.1. Oxamniquine and Hycanthone

Among the effects attributed to oxamniquine are reductions in schistosome ornithine-δ-transaminase activity (Goldberg *et al.*, 1980), ATPase content (Nechay *et al.*, 1980), vitelline gland vitality (Popiel and Erasmus, 1982) and fecundity (Foster and Cheetham, 1973), as well as vacuolization of parenchymal and muscle regions (Kohn *et al.*, 1979) and stimulation of motor activity (Chavasse *et al.*, 1979). On the basis of the dose and time dependencies of these changes, however, as well as their apparent unrelatedness, it is likely that many of these represent secondary responses to an alternative perturbation of the parasite.

Recent studies show that exposure to therapeutic levels of oxamniquine *in vitro*, for periods as brief as 30 min, causes irreversible inhibition of nucleic acid and protein synthesis in adult *S. mansoni* (Pica-Mattoccia and Cioli, 1984). This effect is also seen *in vivo* after administration of a single oral dose of oxamniquine to infected mice. Under all conditions examined, irreversible inhibition of labeled amino acid incorporation is highly correlated with subsequent parasite mortality. Furthermore, male parasites, which show a higher level of oxamniquine-induced mortality than is found in females, also show a higher level of inhibition of protein synthesis. Conversely, protein synthesis in immature parasites and hycanthone-resistant strains of *S. mansoni* is only transiently inhibited by oxamniquine during *in vitro* and *in vivo* studies, findings consistent with the high level of refractoriness also shown by these parasites to the lethal effects of the drug.

Hycanthone, like the structurally related oxamniquine, is reported to affect a number of processes in the schistosome. At therapeutic levels, the drug stimulates motor activity and partially blocks the inhibitory effects of carbachol and physostigmine (Hillman and Senft, 1975), implicating an antagonistic interaction with the putative inhibitory cholinergic component of the parasite's nervous system. These observations are consistent with the results of metabolic studies, showing a transient stimulation of glycogenolysis in hycanthone-treated parasites (Rogers and Bueding, 1971), as an increase in energy demand would be expected to accompany cholinergic disinhibition. However, because these changes are also found in hycanthone-resistant parasites, appear only after a hepatic shift has occurred, and are not observed after administration of schistosomicidal structural analogues of hycanthone, it is likely that they represent secondary effects, indirectly related to the primary mode of action of hycanthone (Tomosky-Sykes and Bueding, 1977).

An alternative mechanism of action for hycanthone has recently been proposed, which, like that derived from studies on oxamniquine, involves inhibition of schistosome nucleic acid synthesis (Neame *et al.*, 1978). *In vitro* studies indicate that incorporation of [^{3}H]amino acid is significantly inhibited after a 1-hr incubation in 10 μM hycanthone. Because a similar effect on incorporation also occurs in hycanthone-resistant schistosomes, it was originally concluded that a different mechanism of action must account for the schistosomicidal activity of the drug (Neame *et al.*, 1978). However, results recently obtained by Pica-Mattoccia and Cioli (1984) from *in vitro* and *in vivo* studies show that although synthesis of macromolecules in insensitive strains of *S. mansoni* is only transiently inhibited by hycanthone (or oxamniquine), sensitive strains show irreversible changes that could account for their susceptibility to the lethal effects of these compounds.

1.1.2. Metrifonate

Most evidence indicates that metrifonate is converted nonenzymatically *in vivo* to dichlorvos (Nordgren *et al.*, 1981), which phosphorylates the active site of acetyl-cholinesterase (AChE), thereby inactivating the enzyme (Bueding *et al.*, 1972). Pharmacokinetic studies indicate that the peak serum concentration of dichlorvos obtained 1 hr after a single therapeutic dose of metrifonate is 0.3 μM (Nordgren *et al.*, 1981), a level that significantly depresses schistosome AChE activity within 15 min *in vitro* (Reiner, 1981). Inhibition of AChE induces a flaccid paralysis of schistosomes, presumably by potentiating inhibitory cholinergic effects on the parasite's musculature (Barker *et al.*, 1966). With their musculature inhibited, schistosomes are swept away from their predilected blood vessesl to sites that are predominantly species dependent. Inhibition of AChE may not fully account for the hepatic shift observed in *S. mansoni* infections, however, as Bloom's (1981) results indicate that AChE activity is equally reduced in parasites not shifted to the liver and recovered from the mesenteric veins.

Whereas the inhibitory potency of metrifonate on AChE and motility are similar for *S. mansoni* and *S. haemotobium* (Bueding *et al.*, 1972), the chemotherapeutic effects of the drug are restricted to infection by *S. haematobium*. This observation may be explained on the basis that AChE of *S. haematobium* is more sensitive to dichlorvos than that of *S. mansoni* (Bueding *et al.*, 1972) and the fact that the two species occupy different locations with the host organism (Forsyth, 1965). Whereas *S. mansoni* shift from their normal location in the mesenteric veins to the liver in response to metrifonate exposure, most *S. haematobium* in primates are swept from the vesical plexus to the lungs (James *et al.*, 1972; James and Webbe, 1974). After the drug effects on motility subside, *S. mansoni* are able to migrate back into the mesenterics, while *S. haematobium* are apparently unable to return from the lungs, where they are sequestered and eventually destroyed by host-immune effectors. Direct support for the lung-shift hypothesis for the differential susceptibility of *S. mansoni* and *S. haematobium* to metrifonate was obtained in recovery studies of infected baboons (James and Webbe, 1974). Furthermore, recent field studies have shown that Sudanese patients with concomitant *S. mansoni* and *S. haematobium* infections that also excrete eggs of both species in their urine exhibit identically high levels of metrifonate-induced reductions in urinary egg burdens for both species, while fecal excretion of *S. mansoni* eggs is only slightly reduced (Omer and Teesdale, 1978; Feldmeier *et al.*, 1982). These results corroborate the view that both *Schistosoma* sp. are intrinsically susceptible to AChE inhibition by dichlorvos but that only parasites occupying the vesical plexus are permanently affected by the drug.

1.1.3. Antimonials

There is considerable evidence of a causal relationship between the inhibition of phosphofructokinase (PFK) activity, the rate-limiting reaction in schistosome glycolysis (Bueding and Mansour, 1957), and the schistosomicidal action of the trivalent organic antimonials. First, the hepatic shift induced by administration of these drugs occurs rapidly and coincides with a reduction in lactate excretion and a marked increase in the ratio (G6P + F6P)/(FDP + triose phosphates) (Bueding and Fisher, 1966). Second, exogenous rabbit muscle PFK protects schistosome homogenates from inhibition by antimonials, indicating that the drug may directly affect the rate-limiting step in schistosome glycolysis, i.e., the rate of PFK reaction (Bueding and Fisher, 1966). Finally, the return of sugar phosphate levels to normal coincides with the return of surviving *S. mansoni* to the mesenteric veins (Fisher *et al.*, 1966).

Inhibition of PFK and the subsequent energy depletion may not, however, fully account for the schistosomicidal activity of the antimonial compounds. The results reported by Coles and Chappell (1979) indicate that antimony-induced toxicity *in vivo* in immature (21-day) worms is lower than that of adults, even though similar amounts of drug are accumulated and similar changes in sugar phosphate ratios are obtained. However, the reduced antimonial sensitivity observed by those investigators in immature schistosomes may also be attributable to a lower metabolic requirement (they remain primarily in the liver, and do not yet attach themselves to the inner wall of the mesenteric veins) or to the availability of an alternate (oxidative) pathway of energy production not available to the adult worms. The age-related changes in *in vivo* toxicity to antimony could also be a consequence of differential secondary responses to the drug. That is, after shifting to the liver in a reduced energy state, adult parasites may become susceptible to host-immune effectors to a greater extent than occurs in immature parasites. This effect could be produced by drug-induced lesions of the tegument (Otubanjo, 1981), which may become increasingly susceptible to disruption as the parasite matures (Simpson and McLaren, 1982; Catto *et al.*, 1984). Tegumental disruption could also lead to exposure of reactive parasite antigens, which are normally disguised. In this context, recent studies by Doenhoff and Bain (1978) indicate that the efficacy of antimonials in mice depends on T-cell components, the suppression of which results in a marked reduction in antimonial-induced parasite toxicity.

1.1.4. Niridazole

Niridazole is another slow-acting schistosomicide for which the precise mechanism of action has been difficult to determine. Recent studies show that 85–90% of the drug bound by schistosomes is covalently associated with the protein fraction and that this binding depends on nitroreductive metabolic activation within the parasite (Tracy *et al.*, 1983).

Most experimental evidence indicates that the major action of niridazole is on glycogen metabolism in schistosomes. Parasites obtained from mice 18 hr after administration of therapeutic doses of niridazole show significant glycogen depletion and, after three such doses given at daily intervals, glycogen levels are reduced by 50%. Depletion is primarily from the musculature of the parasite and appears to result from direct inhibition of phosphorylase phosphatase with the subsequent potentiation of phosphorylase a activity (Bueding and Fisher, 1970). The significance of glycogen depletion to the schistosomicidal action of niridazole, however, has not been firmly established. The drug does not affect the rate of glycolysis, so one would predict that most energy needs of the organism could be met by readily available plasma glucose from the host (Bueding and Fisher, 1970). However, Bueding and Fisher (1970) suggested that in some cell compartments of the schistosome glycogen may be an obligatory substrate either for energy production or for maintaining the structural or functional integrity of the organism.

Administration of niridazole-*in vivo* has also been shown to cause structural damage to the reproductive system of female parasites (Bueding and Fisher, 1970), which bind twice as much drug per milligram protein (Tracy *et al.*, 1983) and show a higher level of toxicity (Striebel, 1969) than do males. However, these changes appear to coincide with glycogen depletion and may represent a secondary response to that effect.

Another possible mechanism for the action of niridazole on schistosomes involves the capacity shared by numerous nitroheterocyclic compounds to inhibit DNA synthesis (Edwards, 1981). Preliminary studies by Sin-Xing (1976) showing reduced DNA content in niridazole-treated *S. japonicum* are consistent with this possible mode of action. Additional support for an effect by niridazole on nucleic acids comes from studies demonstrating that this drug, like hycanthone, possesses mutagenic and carcinogenic activities in numerous other organisms (Urman et al., 1975).

1.1.5. Praziquantel

The molecular mechanism(s) underlying the schistosomicidal activity of praziquantel (PZ) have not been determined, although most evidence implicates the muscle and tegumental systems of susceptible parasites as important sites of action (Andrews and Thomas, 1983). Schistosomes exposed in vitro to therapeutic doses (1 μM) of PZ exhibit an almost instantaneous sustained contraction of their longitudinal musculature, with a half-maximal effect occurring in less than 12 sec (Pax et al., 1978). This tetanic contraction results in paralysis of the parasites and probably accounts for the hepatic shift observed in vivo, which may be 95% complete in mice within 5 min after a single oral dose of the drug (Melhorn et al., 1981). The effect does not appear to result from a direct interaction with the parasite's nervous system, as it is not blocked by carbachol, dopamine, serotonin, or other agents acting at putative neuroreceptive sites in S. mansoni (Pax et al., 1978).

The effects of PZ on muscle tension may result from the drug's ability to alter the distribution of ions across muscle membranes in the schistosome. In vitro electrophysiological studies by Bricker et al. (1982) indicate that 1 μM PZ significantly depolarizes muscle fibers in S. mansoni within 5–10 min. Since the muscle depolarization induced by PZ occurs with a slower time course than the tension change, it is unlikely that ion fluxes mediating the voltage change mediate the initial phase of the contracture as well. Muscle membrane potential changes induced by the drug may, however, be important in sustaining the contracture, perhaps by maintaining high levels of intramuscular Ca^{2+}.

An important role of Ca^{2+} in the parasite's mechanical response to PZ is now well established. Results obtained from altered-ion experiments indicate that schistosomes preincubated in medium containing a low $Ca^{2+} : Mg^{2+}$ ratio exhibit only a transient increase in muscle tension upon addition of PZ (Pax et al., 1978; Fetterer et al., 1980b), while elimination of Ca^{2+} from the recording medium results in a pronounced attenuation of this response. Similar attenuation of the response is not observed in the presence of reduced levels of Na^+, K^+, or Cl^- (Pax et al., 1978).

Although PZ does not possess the characteristics of an ionophore (Chubb et al., 1978), it does stimulate Ca^{2+} influx into the schistosome, and the inotropic effect of the drug is partially mimicked by the Ca^{2+} ionophore A-23187 (Pax et al., 1978). The Ca^{2+}-dependent effects of PZ do not appear to be mediated by membrane channels specific for Ca^{2+}, however, as neither voltage dependent (e.g., D-600, nifedipine, cinnarizine) nor voltage independent (amrinone) Ca^{2+} channel blockers antagonize the response (Fetterer et al., 1980a; J. W. Depenbusch, personal communication).

A role for Ca^{2+} has also been implicated in the second major effect of PZ on schistosomes, that being a pronounced structural disruption of the parasite's tegument (Becker et al., 1980; Melhorn et al., 1983). Extensive vacuolization of the tegumental syncytium concurrent with evaginations or "blebbing" of the surface membrane appear after incubations as brief as 30 sec in 1 μM PZ (Bricker et al., 1983). In Ca^{2+}-free medium, these lesions are attenuated (Bricke et al., 1983; Xiao et al., 1984), and the response is even more inhibited in the presence of elevated levels of Mg^{2+}, but not other multivalent cations (Bricker et al., 1983).

Whereas tegumental disruption may contribute to the anthelmintic potential of PZ, it is not itself lethal to the parasites. This is evidenced by the results of in vivo studies showing that extensive tegumental damage induced by subcurative doses of PZ are tolerated by schistosomes (Shaw and Erasmus, 1983). Furthermore, in vitro studies reveal that tegumental disruption analogous to that attributed to PZ may be induced by a number of compounds which do not possess anthelmintic properties (Bricker et al., 1983); and in the absence of PZ, the contractility of muscle fibers in S. mansoni is not abolished after complete removal of the tegument with Triton X-100 (Depenbusch et al., 1983).

PZ is reported to be therapeutically more effective against adult than against immature stages of S. mansoni (Gonnert and Andrews, 1977). Attempts to delineate the basis for developmental changes in susceptibility reveal that all stages of the schistosome are equally susceptible to the effect on muscle tension induced by PZ; immature stages, however, require 10-fold increase in drug concentration for induction of tegumental disruption (Catto et al., 1984). These results, together with those that show tegumentally disrupted worms exposed to low levels of PZ can survive in vivo, suggest that the schistosomicidal action of PZ may require both effects. That is, it is possible that the paralysis induced by PZ augments the effectiveness of intrinsic protective mechanisms in the host, such as cell-mediated immune effectors observed to attach to the parasite and penetrate drug-induced lesion sites in the tegument as early as 4 hr after PZ administration (Melhorn et al., 1981). In this context, Xiao (1981) report the appearance of previously undetected surface antigens of S. japonicum within 30 min after treatment of infected mice with PZ. The suggestion of a possible synergy between PZ and the immune system is further supported by studies showing that S. mansoni worm burdens are less reduced by the drug in immunosuppressed mice than in controls (Doenhoff et al., 1982).

1.1.6. Amoscanate

There is little currently known of the molecular mechanisms underlying the schistosomicidal actions of this compound. Amoscanate binds irreversibly to amino groups of amino acids and proteins to form thiourea derivatives (Striebel, 1984). By virtue of its isothiocyanate moiety, it is likely that the drug could act by inhibiting a wide range of enzymes that require thiol groups for their catalytic activities. One expected consequence of thiol interference would be inhibition of PFK and of the glycolytic sequence (Gilbert, 1982). In vivo studies of the cestode H. diminutia (Nelson and Saz, 1983), as well as the nematodes B. pahangi and L. carinii (Nelson and Saz, 1984) showing reductions in lactate, succinate, and acetate following administration of amoscanate, support that possibility. However, results of the second study suggest that the initial effect of short-term amoscanate exposure may be inhibition of glucose uptake.

Morphological studies indicate that amoscanate also induces extensive swelling, wrinking and erosion of the tegument of *S. mansoni* (Voge and Bueding, 1980; Irie and Yasuraoka, 1982). The extent to which these effects may contribute to the schistosomicidal activity of the drug is unknown; however, the lesions are apparent within 1 hr of *in vivo* exposure to subcurative doses of amoscanate and they persist, to some degree, for at least 3 months after treatment. On the basis of these observations, Voge and Bueding (1980) suggest that amoscanate may act to inhibit processes that mediate synthesis and repair of tegumental membrane. The capacity for amoscanate to inhibit amino acid incorporation in *S. mansoni* (Wooder and Wright, 1981) is consistent with that hypothesis. However, reduced amino acid incorporation could also be explained on the basis of transport inhibition (Nelson and Saz, 1984) that might accompany tegumental lesions. Furthermore, the fact that parasites survive in spite of extensive lesioning induced by subcurative doses of the drug argues against the notion that amoscanate-induced surface lesions by themselves represent a sufficient lethal effect.

1.1.7. Oltipraz

Oltipraz is an extremely slow-acting drug *in vivo* that requires up to 2 months for its full schistosomicidal effects to become evident (Bueding *et al.*, 1982). To date, published evidence for a molecular mechanism of action for oltipraz is limited primarily to the findings of Bueding *et al.*, which show administration of the drug to cause a marked reduction in parasite glutathione (GSH) levels. The significance of GSH depletion to the schistosomicidal capacity of oltipraz is evidenced indirectly by the fact that a dose-dependent hepatic shift induced by the drug is always preceded by a significant drop in GSH levels within the parasite. Furthermore, among structural analogues of oltipraz, there is a positive correlation between schistosomicidal activity and depression of GSH levels. It has not been determined, however, whether other agents expected to deplete GSH (e.g., diamide or diethyl maleate) or to inhibit the γ-glutamyl cycle (e.g., buthionine sulfoximine) are also schistosomicidal or whether, in fact, they reduce a hepatic shift. Administration of buthionine sulfoximine to mice infected with *Trypanosoma brucei* rapidly reduces GSH levels and induces a lethal lysis of these parasites. In this case, toxicity is attributed to the parasite's reduced capacity for handling endogenous oxidant stress due to H_2O_2 accumulation (Arrick *et al.*, 1981). Whereas the potential for oxidant stress should be low in schistosomes, the effects of GSH perturbations on other cellular processes, particularly the glycolytic pathway (Gilbert, 1982), could form the basis for the toxicity associated with GSH depletion in oltipraz-treated *S. mansoni*.

On the basis of *in vivo* studies, there appears to be a link between the efficacy of oltipraz, changes in GSH levels that it induces, and the presence of high levels of L-cysteine. That is, Bueding *et al.* (1982) show enhancement of GSH depletion and the schistosomicidal activity of oltipraz by coadministration of L-cysteine and suggest that the synergistic action may be attributable to competition between this amino acid and a GSH precursor, such as glutamylcysteine. An alternative basis for the enhancement of the schistosomicidal capacity of oltipraz by L-cysteine comes from a recent study that shows coadministration of L-cysteine markedly increases the rate and extent of the drug's bioavailability in green monkeys (Ali *et al.*, 1984).

1.2. Mode of Action of Fasciolicidal Agents and Agents Effective against Less Common Trematodes

In addition to predilections for occupying different locations within different mammalian hosts, *Fasciola* sp. and *Schistosoma* sp. are distinguishable on the basis of numerous biochemial and physiological characteristics. These differences are reflected in the anthelmintics developed for each genus which overlap only recently with the development of praziquantel.

1.2.1. Diamfenetide

Diamfenetide is a prodrug deacylated in the liver to an active form, the diamfenetide amine (DPT-FA) (Harfenist, 1973). Consistent biochemical effects induced by DPT-FA on *F. hepatica* include inhibition of glucose uptake (Edwards *et al.*, 1981a) and elevation of malate levels within the parasite, both of which occur within 6 hr of exposure (Edwards *et al.*, 1981a; Rew and Fetterer, 1984). The close association between fasciolicidal activity and the accumulation of malate induced by DPT-FA is strengthened by observations that *in vitro* both effects are antagonized by L-DOPA, dopamine, epinephrine, and, to a lesser extent, serotonin (Edwards *et al.*, 1981b). The mechanism by which catecholamines afford protection from the harmful effects of DPT-FA is unknown. Edwards *et al.* suggest that the drug and the protective agents may exert antagonistic effects at the level of solute and fluid transport across membranes of the parasite.

The results of recent *in vitro* studies by Rew and Fetterer (1984) indicate that DPT-FA induces dose- and time-dependent increases in several end products of glucose metabolism, including acetate, propionate, lactate, and CO_2, whereas ATP levels in the parasite decline. These results suggest that DPT-FA may stimulate glucose catabolism by uncoupling the flow of carbon from ATP generation. Such an effect would not be inconsistent with the accumulation of malate which, by itself, would not account for the fasciolicidal activity of this drug.

An alternative mechanism by which DPT-FA may exert fasciolicidal effects is obtained from *in vitro* physiological studies (Rew *et al.*, 1983) that show *F. hepatica* exposed to DPT-FA exhibit rapid changes in membrane function that precede significantly the metabolic changes noted above. Immature and adult stages of the parasite exhibit dose-dependent increases in longitudinal muscle tension, as well as reductions in contraction amplitudes after 1–3 hr incubations in the drug. These effects, in turn, may be explained on the basis of specific membrane conductance changes induced by DPT-FA, evidenced during microelectrode recordings from the parasite as a rapid depolarization of the tegumental membrane concomitant with Na^+ accumulation. A causal link between the observed membrane conductance changes and inhibition of glucose uptake as well as tegumental disruption, which is also observed to occur (Rew et al., 1983), may be inferred. Whether these changes induce the metabolic changes indicative of uncoupling secondarily remains unknown.

1.2.2. Albendazole and Triclabendazole

These drugs are relatively new members of a class of compounds, the benzimidazoles, which possess a purinelike molecular structure; they have been shown to affect a variety of processes in helminth parasites (Vanden Bossche, 1976; Rahman and Bryant, 1977). Much less is known of the specific biochemical effects of albendazole or triclabendazole than of earlier benzimidazoles such as thiabendazole or mebendazole, which reduce ATP levels in F. hepatica by interfering with enzymes involved in the production of propionate and acetate (Vanden Bossche, 1972a; Pritchard, 1973; Cornish and Bryant, 1976). Recent studies indicate that some benzimidazoles inhibit microtubule assembly in numerous preparations (Davidse, 1977), including the nematode Ascaris suum (Kohler and Bachmann, 1981); the newer benzimidazoles may owe their fasciolicidal activity to this effect (Vanden Bossche, 1980). Consistent with this view, albendazole and its metabolites, at therapeutic levels, rapidly and markedly inhibit [³H]colchicine binding to homogenates of F. hepatica as well as to whole worms in vitro (Fetterer, 1984). Results that show the drug to have little effect on glucose metabolism of F. hepatica suggest that the effect on tubulin may represent the primary mechanism of drug action.

Whereas inhibition of microtubule function is a plausible mechanism for the fasciolicidal activity of albendazole, it is difficult to extrapolate the results obtained from in vitro studies to the in vivo action of this compound. That is, total [³H]colchicine binding is not reduced in homogenates of F. hepatica recovered from sheep 12 or 24 hr after albendazole treatment (Fetterer, 1984), suggesting that in vivo the effects may be either transient or less pronounced. Furthermore, the reported K_i of mebendazole on colchicine binding with tubulin of Ascaris suum (Kohler and Bachmann, 1981), as well as that derived from the data on albendazole-treated F. hepatica (Fetterer, 1984), suggest that the capacities of these drugs to interact with tubulin of adult stage helminths and host tissue are approximately equal. This low differential affinity of parasite and host tubulin would appear insufficient to account for the selective interaction of these drugs with the parasite.

Triclabendazole, although a potent fasciolicide in sheep (Boray et al., 1983), inhibits neither [³H]colchicine binding to parasite tubulin nor prevents the embryonation of fluke eggs, even at levels 100-fold greater than the effective concentration of albendazole (Fetterer, 1984). Triclabendazole must therefore act on alternative processes in F. hepatica that are presently unknown.

1.2.3. MK-401

MK-401 is a potent sulfonamide fasciolicide (Mrozik *et al.*, 1977) that inhibits two specific glycolytic enzymes in *F. hepatica* (Schulman and Valentino, 1982; Schulman *et al.*, 1982). Metabolic profiles of *F. hepatica* exposed for 1 hr *in vitro* to therapeutic levels of MK-401 reveal a 60% inhibition of [^{14}C]glucose uptake and a marked reduction in acetate and propionate formation. Concomitant with these changes are reduced levels of ATP, phosphoenolpyruvate, G6P and F6P, while glycerol and the free sugars fructose and mannose increase (Schulman *et al.*, 1979). Direct measurements of the effects of MK-401 on glycolytic enzymes reveal that the activities of both phosphoglycerate kinase and phosphoglyceromutase are competitively inhibited in a dose-dependent manner. This inhibition is highly specific, as the drug affects neither the activities of other glycolytic enzymes nor those of analogous enzymes obtained from rat liver homogenate (Schulman *et al.*, 1982). On the basis of computer-generated models of MK-401, it appears likely that the drug's specific inhibitory activity is a result of its remarkably close structural resemblance to the diphosphoglycerates with which it competes (Schulman *et al.*, 1982).

1.2.4. Closantel, Rafoxanide, and Oxyclozanide

The fasciolicidal activity of these three salicylanilides has been linked to their capacity for uncoupling electron-transport-associated phosphorylation and possibly the site-1 phosphorylation of ADP associated with the reduction of fumarate to succinate (Van Miert and Groeneveld, 1969; Corbett and Goose, 1971). Results reported by Campbell and Montague (1981) show a high correlation between uncoupling activity and flukicidal activity *in vitro* over a wide range of uncouplers. These correlations are not always obtained *in vivo*, however, indicating the importance of metabolism and/or distribution of these drugs within the host on drug efficacy.

In vitro and *in vivo* studies show that *F. hepatica* exposed to therapeutic levels of closantel exhibit changes in substrate utilization, end-product formation, and adenine nucleotides, which support the view that uncoupling is the primary mode of action on this parasite. That is, by 3 hr, significant increases in the production of acetic, propionic, and succinic acids are evident, and after 12 hr *in vivo* exposure, the increase in total flux through these organic acids reaches 170% of control. Concurrent with these changes are a depression in ATP levels and an elevation of AMP, with the ATP : ADP ratio falling from 1.2 to 0.77. Furthermore, closantel induces a fivefold increase in the oxaloacetate/malate ratio, which is not mediated by inhibition of succinate decarboxylase activity (Kane *et al.*, 1980).

Recent studies of the effects of closantel on *F. hepatica* show that the drug may reduce the pH and G6P levels in the parasite by 1 hr, before significant changes in ATP levels are detectable (Rorher *et al.*, 1983). Since a reduction in ATP levels would be an expected initial consequence of an uncoupling effect, these preliminary results suggest that the primary effects of closantel may reside in the glycolytic pathway instead of in electron transport. Validation of this hypothesis will require additional studies.

The metabolic profile of *F. hepatica* obtained from rafoxanide-treated sheep indicates that drug-induced changes in energy metabolites (Pritchard, 1978) are qualitatively similar to those induced by closantel. These results are consistent with those obtained from *in vitro* studies on *F. hepatica* (Corbett, 1974; Cornish and Bryant, 1976), as well as from studies using isolated mitochondria from *Ascaris suum* (Vanden Bossche, 1972*b*). As with closantel, the most profound evidence implicating rafoxanide as an uncoupler of oxidative phosphorylation is the capacity for the drug to rapidly change the redox balance of *F. hepatica* toward a more oxidative state, as evidenced by dramatic increases obtained in the ratios [NAD$^+$] : [NADH] and [oxaloacetate] : [malate] (Pritchard, 1978).

Oxyclozanide, while inducing several changes in *F. hepatica* indicative of an uncoupler (Corbett and Goose, 1971), also induces possible neurotoxic effects. That is, *F. hepatica* are paralyzed by therapeutic levels of oxyclozanide *in vitro* long before ATP levels are depressed (Coles, 1975; Fairweather, 1978). The biochemical basis for this effect is unknown. An additional possible mechanism of action for oxyclozanide (as well as rafoxanide) in some *Fasciola* sp. is the direct inhibition of malate dehydrogenase (Lewin and Probert, 1975; Probert *et al.*, 1981). By this mechanism, ATP synthesis would be prevented by limiting the supply of malate to parasite mitochondria.

1.2.5. Praziquantel

Fasciola are one of only two trematodes previously examined that do not show tegumental disruption in response to PZ (Becker *et al.*, 1980). The absence of morphological effects in this case may be attributable to the thickness of the tegument (up to 22 μm, versus 1–3 μm in *Schistosoma*) and the high content of fortifying fibrils (Melhorn *et al.*, 1983). Acute tetanic contraction of the musculature of *F. hepatica* is induced by PZ *in vitro*, but only at concentrations at least 100-fold greater than those required in *S. mansoni* (Terada *et al.*, 1982). Therefore, the molecular mode of action of PZ may be significantly different for these two trematodes.

Most trematodes pathogenic to man are susceptible to the tegument-lesioning effects of PZ. In most cases, tegumental disruption analogous to that observed in *Schistosoma* is apparent within 5 min exposure to therapeutic levels of the drug, both *in vitro* and *in vivo* (Melhorn *et al.*, 1983). Although little is currently known of the effects of PZ on physiological processes in parasites other than *S. mansoni*, it is now established that most susceptible parasites exhibit a tetanic contraction upon exposure to the drug, both *in vitro* and *in vivo* (Melhorn *et al.*, 1983). These observations implicate, once again, the musculature as an important site of action for this drug. Although the role of Ca^{2+} in the morphological or physiological responses of other parasites to PZ has not been well defined, direct measurements show that the drug stimulates $^{45}Ca^{2+}$ uptake in *Opistorchis viverrini*. Furthermore, this uptake is inhibited by 10 mM $MgCl_2$, 2 mM $LaCl_3$, or 1 mM vandadium oxide, suggesting that the action of PZ on less common trematodes and *S. mansoni* may be quite similar (Ruenwongsa *et al.*, 1983).

REFERENCES

Ali, H. M., Sulaiman, S. M., Bennett, J. L., and Homeida, M. M. A., 1984, Effect of cysteine on oltipraz blood levels in green monkeys (*Cercopithecus aethiops*), *Chemotherapy* (in press).

Andrews, P., and Thomas, H., 1983, Praziquantel, *Med. Res. Rev.* 3:147–200.

Arrick, B. A., Griffith, O. W., and Cerami, A., 1981, Inhibition of glutathione synthesis as a chemotherapeutic strategy for trypanosomiasis, *J. Exp. Med.* 153:720–725.

Barker, L. W., Bueding, E., and Timms, A. R., 1966, The possible role of acetylcholine in *Schistosoma mansoni*, *Br. J. Pharmacol.* 26:656–665.

Becker, B., Melhorn, H., Andrews, P., Thomas, H., and Eckert, J., 1980, Light and electron microscopic studies of the effect of praziquantel on *Schistosoma mansoni*, *Dicrocoelium dendriticum* and *Fasciola hepatica* (Trematode) *in vitro*, *Z. Parasitenkd.* 63:113–128.

Bloom, A., 1981, Studies of the mode of action of metrifonate and DDVP in schistosomes: Cholinesterase activity and the hepatic shift, *Acta Pharmacol. Toxicol.* (Suppl. V) 49:109–113.

Boray, J. C., Crowfoot, P. D., Strong, M. D., Allison, J. R., Schellenbaum, M., Von Orelli, M., and Sarasin, G., 1983, Treatment of immature and mature *Fasciola hepatica* infections in sheep with triclabendazole, *Vet. Rec.* 113:315–317.

Bricker, C. S., Depenbusch, J. W., Bennett, J. L., and Thompson, D. P., 1983, The relationship between tegumental disruption and muscle contraction in *Schistosoma mansoni* exposed to various compounds, *Z. Parasitenkd.* 69:61–71.

Bricker, C. S., Depenbusch, J. W., Bennett, J. L., and Thompson, D. P., 1983, The relationship between tegumental disruption and muscle contraction in *Schistosoma mansoni* exposed to various compounds, *Z. Parasitenkd.* 69:61–71.

Bueding, E., 1950, Carbohydrate metabolism of *Schistosoma mansoni*, *J. Gen. Physiol.* 33:475–495.

Buedning, E., Dolan, P., and Leroy, J. P., 1982, The antischistosomal activity of oltipraz, *Res. Commun. Chem. Pathol. Pharmacol.* 37:293–303.

Bueding, E., and Fisher, J., 1966, Factors affecting the inhibition of phosphofructokinase activity of *Schistosoma mansoni* by trivalent organic antimonials, *Biochem. Pharmacol.* 15:1197–1211.

Bueding, E., and Fisher, J., 1970, Biochemical effects of niridazole on *Schistosoma mansoni*, *Mol. Pharmacol.* 6:523–539.

Bueding, E., and Fisher, J., 1982, Metabolic requirements of schistosomes, *J. Parasitol.* 68:208–212.

Bueding, E., and Mansour, J. M., 1957, The relationship between inhibition of phosphofructokinase activity and the mode of action of trivalent organic antimonials on *Schistosoma mansoni*, *Br. J. Pharmacol. Chemother.* 159:165–171.

Bueding, E., Liu, C. L., and Rogers, S. H., 1972, Inhibition by metrifonate and dichlorvos of cholinesterases in schistosomes, *Br. J. Pharmacol.* 46:480–487.

Campbell, A. J., and Montague, P. E., 1981, A comparison of the activity of uncouplers of oxidative phosphorylation against the common liver fluke *Fasciola hepatica*, *Mol. Biochem. Parasitol.* 4:139–147.

Catto, B. A., Xiao, S., and Webster, L. T., 1984, Effects of praziquantel on different development stages of *Schistosoma mansoni in vitro* and *in vivo*, WHO Scientific Working Group on the Biochemistry and Chemotherapy of Schistosomiasis, Geneva, January.

Chavasse, C. J., Brown, M. C., and Bell, D. R., 1979, Activity of *Schistosoma mansoni* over a ten-hour period *in vitro*, and its modification by oxamniquine, *Ann. Trop. Med. Parasitol.* 73:241–249.

Chubb, J. M., Bennett, J. L., Akera, T., and Brody, T. M., 1978, Effects of praziquantel, a new anthelmintic, on electrochemical properties of isolated rat atria, *J. Pharmacol. Exp. Ther.* 207:284–293.

Coles, G. C., 1975, Fluke biochemistry—Fasciola and Schistosoma, *Helminthol. Abstr. Ser. A* 44:147–162.

Coles, G. C., 1977, The biochemical mode of action of some modern anthelmintics, *Pesticide Sci.* 8:536–543.

Coles, G. C., and Campbell, L. H., 1979, *Schistosoma mansoni*: Effects of antimony on immature and adult worms, *Exp. Parasitol.* 47:49–53.

Corbett, J. R., 1974, *The Biochemical Model of Action of Pesticides*, Academic Press, London.

Corbett, J. R., and Goose, J., 1971, A possible mode of action of the fasciolicides nitroxynil, hexachlorophene and oxyclozanide, *Pesticide Sci.* 2:119–121.

Cornish, R. A., and Bryant, C., 1976, Changes in energy metabolism due to anthelmintics in *Fasciola hepatica* maintained *in vitro*, *Int. J. Parasitol.* 6:393–398.

Davidse, L. C., 1977, Mode of action, selectivity and mutagenicity of benzimidazole compounds, *J. Pathol.* 83:135–144.

Del Castillo, J., DeMello, W. C., and Morales, T. A., 1964, The mechanism of the paralyzing action of piperazine in the somatic musculature of *Ascaris lumbricoides*, *Br. J. Pharmacol.* 22:463–477.

Depenbusch, J. W., Thompson, D. P., Pax, R. A., and Bennett, J. L., 1983, Tegumental disruption with Triton X-100 and its effects on longitudinal muscle function in male *Schistosoma mansoni*, *Parasitology* 87:61–73.

Dias, L. C. S., Pedro, R. J., and Debelardini, E. R., 1982, Use of praziquantel in patients with schistosomiasis mansoni previously treated with oxamniquine and/or hycanthone, *Trans. R. Soc. Trop. Med. Hyg.* 76:652–659.

Doenhoff, M. J., and Bain, J., 1978, The immune-dependence of schistosomicidal chemotherapy: Relative lack of efficacy for an antimonial in *Schistosoma mansoni*-infected mice deprived of their T-cells and the demonstration of drug–antiserum synergy, *Clin. Exp. Immunol.* 33:232–238.

Doenhoff, M., Harrison, R., Schath, A., Murare, H., Dunne, D., and Hassounah, O., 1982, Schistosomiasis in the immunosuppressed host: Studies on the host–parasite relationship of *Schistosoma mansoni* and *S. bovis* in T-cell deprived and hydrocortisone-treated mice, in: *Animal Models in Parasitology* (D. G. Owen, ed.), pp. 155–169, Macmillan, New York.

Edwards, D. L., 1981, Mechanisms of toxicity of nitroimidazole drugs, in: *Progress in Medicinal Chemistry* (G. P. Ellis and G. B. West, eds.), Vol. 18, pp. 87–166. Elsevier/North-Holland Biomedical Press, Amsterdam.

Edwards, S. R., Campbell, A. J., Sheers, M., Moore, R. J., and Montague, P. E., 1981a, Studies on the effect of diamphenethide and oxyclozanide on the metabolism of *Fasciola hepatica*, *Mol. Biochem. Parasitol.* 2:323–338.

Edwards, S. R., Campbell, A. J., Sheers, M., Moore, R. J., and Montague, P. E., 1981b, Protection of *Fasciola hepatica* against flukicidal action of the amine of diamphenethide *in vitro*, *Mol. Biochem. Parasitol.* 2:339–348.

Fairweather, L., 1978, *Fasciola hepatica*: Effects of fasciolicides upon *in vitro* motility, *Proc. Br. Soc. Parasitol.* 39.

Feldmeier, H., Doehring, E., Daffala, A. A., Omer, A. H. S., and Dietrich, M., 1982, Efficacy of metrifonate in urinary schistosomiasis: Comparison of reduction of *Schistosoma haematobium* and *S. mansoni* eggs, *Am. J. Trop. Med. Hyg.* 31:1188–1194.

Fetterer, R. H., 1984, The effect of albendazole and triclabendazole on colchicine binding in the liver fluke *Fasciola hepatica*, *J. Vet. Res.* (in press).

Fetterer, R. H., Pax, R. A., and Bennett, J. L., 1980a, Praziquantel, ptoassium and 2,4-dinitrophenol: Analysis of their action on the musculature of *Schistosoma mansoni*, *Eur. J. Pharmacol.* 64:31–38.

Fetterer, R. H., Pax, R. A., Thompson, D., Bricker, C., and Bennett, J. L., 1980b, Praziquantel: Mode of its antischistosomal action, in: *The Host–Invader Interplay* (H. Vanden Bossche, ed.), pp. 695–698, Elsevier/North-Holland Biomedical Press, Amsterdam.

Fetterer, R. H., and Rew, R. S., 1984, Interaction of *Fasciola hepatica* with albendazole and its metabolites, *J. Vet. Pharm. Exp. Ther.* (in press).

Fisher, J., Bruce, J. L., Bourgeois, J. G., Bueding, E., and Sadun, E. H., 1966, Effect of a subcurative dose of TW56 on the levels of phosphate esters in *Schistosoma mansoni*, *Am. J. Trop. Med. Hyg.* 15:507–509.

Forsyth, D. M., 1965, Treatment of urinary schistosomiasis—Practice and theory, *Lancet* 2:354–358.

Foster, R., and Cheetham, B. L., 1973, Studies with the schistosomicide oxamniquine (UK-4271). 1. Activity in rodents and *in vitro*, *Trans. R. Soc. Trop. Med. Hyg.* 67:139–145.

Gilbert, H. F., 1982, Biological disulfides: The third messenger? Modulation of phosphofructokinase activity by thiol/disulfide exchange, *J. Biol. Chem.* 257:12086–12091.

Goldberg, M., Gold, D., Flescher, E., and Lengy, J., 1980, Effect of oxamniquine on *Schistosoma mansoni*: Some biological and biochemical observations, *Biochem. Pharmacol.* 29:838–840.

Gonnert, R., and Andrews, P., 1977, Praziquantel, a new broad-spectrum antischistosomal agent, *Z. Parasitenkd.* 52:129–150.

Harfenist, M., 1973, Diamphenethide—A new fasciolicide active against immature parasites, *Pesticide Sci.* 4:871–882.

Hillman, G. R., and Senft, A. W., 1975, Anticholinergic properties of the antischistosomal drug hycanthone, *Am. J. Trop. Med. Hyg.* 24:827–834.

Hunter, A., and Lowry, O. H., 1956, The effects of drugs on enzyme systems, *Pharmacol. Rev.* 8:89–103.

Irie, Y., and Yasuraoka, K., 1982, Morphological alterations of *Schistosoma japonicum* associated with the administration of amoscanate, *Jpn. J. Exp. Med.* 52:139–148.

James, C., and Webbe, G., 1974, Treatment of *Schistosoma haematobium* in the baboon with metrifonate, *Trans. R. Soc. Trop. Med. Hyg.* 68:4137–417.

James, C., Webbe, G., and Preston, J. M., 1972, A comparison of the susceptibility to metrifonate of *Schistosoma haematobium, S. mattheci* and *S. mansoni* in hamsters, *Ann. Trop. Med. Parasitol.* 66:467–474.

Kane, H. J., Behm, C. A., and Bryant, C., 1980, Metabolic studies on the new fasciolicidal drug, closantel, *Mol. Biochem. Parasitol.* 1:347–355.

Kohler, P., and Bachmann, R., 1981, Intestinal tubulin as possible target for chemotherapeutic action of mebendazole in parasite nematodes, *Mol. Biochem. Parasitol.* 4:325–336.

Kohn, A., Serapiao, C. J., Katz, N., and Dias, E. P., 1979, Effects of oxamniquine on the morphology of *Schistosoma mansoni, Rev. Inst. Med. Trop. Sao Paolo* 21:217–226.

Lewin, T., and Probert, A. J., 1975, Effect of certain fasciolicides on malate dehydrogenase activity in *Fasciola hepatica:* A possible biochemical mode of action of hexachlorophene and oxyclozanide, *Pesticide Sci.* 6:121–128.

Melhorn, H., Becker, B., Andrews, P., Thomas, H., and Frenkel, J. K., 1981, *In vivo* and *in vitro* experiments on the effects of praziquantel on *Schistosoma mansoni, Arzneimforsch.* 31:544–554.

Melhorn, H., Kojina, S., Rim, H. J., Ruenwongsa, P., Andrews, P., Thomas, H., and Bunnag, B., 1983, Ultrastructural investigations on the effects of praziquantel on human trematodes from Asia: *Clonorchis sinensis, Metagonimus yokogawai, Opistorchis viverrini, Paragonismus westermani* and *Schistosoma japonicum, Arzneimforsch.* 33:91–98.

Meyer, F., Meyer, H., and Bueding, E., 1970, Lipid metabolism in the parasitic and free-living flatworms, *Schistosoma mansoni* and *Dugesin dovotocephala, Biochim. Biophys. Acta* 210:257–266.

Mrozik, H., Bochis, R. J., Eskola, P., Matzuk, A., Waksmunski, F. S., Olen, L. E., Schwartzkopf, G., Grodski, A., Linn, B. O., Lusi, A., Wu, M. T., Shunk, C. H., Peterson, L. H., Milkowski, J. D., Hoff, D. R., Kulsa, P., Ostlind, D. A., Campbell, W. C., Riek, R. F., and Harmon, R. E., 1977, 4-Amino-6-(trichloroethenyl)-1,3-benzenedisulfonamide, a new potent fasciolicide, *J. Med. Chem.* 20:1225–1227.

Neame, K. D., Homewood, C. A., Marshall, I., and Jewsburg, J. M., 1978, The effect of hycanthone on nucleic acid synthesis by *Schistosoma mansoni, Ann. Trop. Med. Parasitol.* 72:587–588.

Nechay, B. R., Hillman, G. R., and Dotson, M. J., 1980, Properties and drug sensitivity of adenosine triphosphatases from *Schistosoma mansoni, J. Parasitol.* 66:596–600.

Nelson, N. F., and Saz, H. J., 1983, *Hymenolepis diminuta:* Effects of amoscanate on energy metabolism and ultrastructure, *Exp. Parasitol.* 56:55–69.

Nelson, N. F., and Saz, H. J., 1984, Effects of amoscanate on utilization of glucose by *Brugia pahangi* and *Litomosoides carinii, J. Parasitol.* 70:194–196.

Nordgren, L., Holmstedt, B., Bengtson, E., and Finkel, Y., 1980, Plasma levels of metrifonate and dichlorvos during treatment of schistosomiasis with bilarcil®, *Am. J. Trop. Med. Hyg.* 29:426–430.

Nordgren, L., Bengtsson, E., Holmstedt, B., and Pettersson, B. M., 1981, Levels of metrifonate and dichlorvos in plasma and erythrocytes during treatment of schistosomiasis with bilarcil®, *Acta Pharmacol. Toxicol.* (Suppl. V) 49:79–86.

Omer, A. H. S., and Teesdale, C. H., 1978, Metrifonate trial in the treatment of various presentations of *Schistosoma haematobium* and *S. mansoni* infections in the Sudan, *Ann. Trop. Med. Parasitol.* 72:145–150.

Otubanjo, O. A., 1981, *Schistosoma mansoni:* Astiban-induced damage to tegument and the male reproductive system, *Exp. Parasitol.* 52:161–170.

Pax, R. A., Bennett, J. L., and Fetterer, R. H., 1978, A benzodiazepine derivative and praziquantel: Effects on musculature of *Schistosoma mansoni* and *Schistosoma japonicum, Naunyn-Schmiedeberg's Arch. Pharmacol.* 304:309–315.

Pica-Mattoccia, L., and Cioli, D., 1984, Studies on the mode of action of oxamniquine and related schistosomicidal drugs, *Am. J. Trop. Med. Hyg.* (in press).

Pica-Mattoccia, L., Lelli, A., and Cioli, D., 1982, Sex and drugs in *S. mansoni, J. Parasitol.* 68:347–349.

Popiel, L., and Erasmus, D. A., 1982, *Schistosoma mansoni:* The survival and reproductive status of mature infections in mice treated with oxamniquine, *J. Helminth.* 56:257–261.

Pritchard, R. K., 1973, The fumarate reductase reaction of *Haemonchus contortus* and the mode of action of some anthelmintics, *Int. J. Parasitol.* 3:409–412.

Pritchard, R. K., 1978, The metabolic profile of adult *Fasciola hepatica* obtained from ratoxanide-treated sheep, *Parasitology* 76:277–288.

Probert, A. J., Sharma, R. K., Singh, K., and Saxena, R., 1981, The effect of five fasciolicides on malate dehydrogenase activity and mortality of *Fasciola gigantia, Fasciolopsis buski* and *Paramphistomum explanatum, J. Helminth.* 55:115–122.

Rahman, M. S., and Bryant, C., 1977, Studies of regulatory metabolism in *Moniezia expansa:* Effects of cambendazole and mebendazole, *Int. J. Parasitol.* 7:403–409.

Reiner, E., 1981, Esterases in schistosomes: Reactions with substrates and inhibitors, *Acta Pharmacol. Toxicol.* (Suppl. V) 49:72–78.

Rew, R. S., and Fetterer, R. H., 1984, Effects of diamfenetide on metabolic and excretory functions of *Fasciola hepatica in vitro, Comp. Biochem. Physiol. C* (in press).

Rew, R. S., Fetterer, R. H., and Martin, T. C., 1983, *Fasciola hepatica:* Effects of diamfenetide free amine on *in vitro* physiology, biochemistry and morphology, *Exp. Parasitol.* 55:159–167.

Rogers, S. H., and Bueding, E., 1971, Hycanthone resistance: Development in *S. mansoni, Science* 172:1057–1068.

Rohrer, S. P., Nowak, T., and Saz, H. J., 1983, High resolution ^{31}P-NMR studies of the metabolisms of *Ascaris suum* and *Fasciola hepatica,* in: *Proceedings of Fifty-eighth Annual Meeting, American Society of Parasitology San Antonio, Texas.*

Ruenwongsa, P., Hutadilok, N., and Yuthavong, Y., 1983, Stimulation of Ca^{2+} uptake in the human liver fluke *Opistorchis viverrini* by praziquantel, *Life Sci.* 32:2529–2534.

Schulman, M. D., and Valentino, D., 1982, Purification, characterization and inhibition by MK-401 of *Fasciola hepatica* phosphoglyceromutase, *Mol. Biochem. Parasitol.* 5:321–332.

Schulman, M. D., Valentino, D., Cifelli, S., Lang, R. K., and Ostlind, D. A., 1979, A pharmacokinetic basis for the efficacy of 4-amino-6-trichloethenyl-1,3-benzenedisulfonamide against *Fasciola hepatica* in the rat, *J. Parasitol.* 49:206–215.

Schulman, M. D., Ostlind, D. A., and Valentino, D., 1982, Mechanism of action of MK-401 against *Fasciola hepatica:* Inhibition of phosphoglycerate kinase, *Mol. Biochem. Parasitol.* 5:133–145.

Senft, A. W., and Hillman, G. R., 1973, Effect of hycanthone, miridazole and antimony tartrate on schistosome motility, *Am. J. Trop. Med. Hyg.* 22:734–742.

Senft, A. W., Meich, R. P., Brown, P. R., and Senft, D. G., 1972, Purine metabolism in *Schistosoma mansoni, Int. J. Parasitol.* 2:249–260.

Senft, A. W., Senft, D. G., Hillman, G. R., Polk, D., and Kryger, S., 1976, Influence of hycanthone on morphology and serotonin uptake of *S. mansoni, Am. J. Trop. Med. Hyg.* 25:832–848.

Shaw, M. K., and Erasmus, D. A., 1983, *Schistosoma mansoni:* The effects of a subcurative dose of praziquantel on the ultrastructure of the worms *in vivo, Z. Parasitenkd.* 69:73–90.

Simpson, A. J. G., and McLaren, D. J., 1982, *Schistosoma mansoni:* Tegumental damage as a consequence of lectin binding, *Exp. Parasitol.* 53:105–116.

Sin-Xing, P., 1976, *Annual Report of the Institute of Parasitological Disease,* Shanghai, People's Republic of China, p. 41.

Striebel, H. P., 1969, The effects of niridazole in experimental schistosomiasis, *Ann. N.Y. Acad. Sci.* 160:491–518.

Striebel, H. P., 1984, Amoscanate: Metabolism, pharmacokinetics and mode of action, *WHO Scientific Working Group on Biochemistry and Chemotherapy of Schistosomiasis, Geneva, January.*

Terada, M., Ishui, A. I., Kino, H., Fujiu, Y., and Sono, M., 1982, Studies on chemotherapy of parasitic (IX). Effects of praziquantel on themotility of various parasitic helminths and isolated host tissues, *Experientia* 38:549–553.

Thompson, D. P., Pax, R. A., and Bennett, J. L., 1982, Microelectrode studies of the tegument and subtegumental compartments of male *Schistosoma mansoni:* An analysis of electrophysiological properties, *Parasitology* 85:163–178.

Tomosky-Sykes, T. K., and Bueding, E., 1977, Effects of hycanthone on neuromuscular systems of *Schistosoma mansoni, J. Parasitol.* 63:259.

Tracy, J. W., Catto, B. W., and Webster, L. T., 1983, Reductive metabolism of niridazole by adult *Schistosoma mansoni, Mol. Pharmacol.* 24:291.

Urman, H. K., Bulay, O., Clayson, D. B., and Shubik, P., 1975, Carcinogenic effects of niridazole, *Cancer Lett.* 1:69–74.

Vanden Bossche, H., 1972*a*, Biochemical effects of anthelmintic drug mebendazole, in: *Comparative Biochemistry of Parasites* (H. Vanden Bossche, ed.), pp. 139–157, Academic Press, New York.

Vanden Bossche, H., 1972*b*, Studies on the phosphorylation in *Ascaris mitochondria,* in: *Comparative Biochemistry of Parasites* (H. Vanden Bossche, ed.), pp. 455–468, Academic Press, New York.

Vanden Bossche, H., 1976, The molecular basis of anthelmintic action, in: *Biochemistry of Parasites and Host-Parasite Relationships* (H. Vanden Bossche, ed.), pp. 553–572, Elsevier/North-Holland Biomedical Press, Amsterdam.

Vanden Bossche, H., 1980, Peculiar targets in anthelmintic chemotherapy, *Biochem. Pharmacol.* 29:1981–1990.

Van Miert, A., and Groeneveld, H. W., 1969, Anthelmintic used for the treatment of fascioliasis as uncouplers of oxidative phosphorylation in warm blooded animals, *Eur. J. Pharmacol.* 8:385–388.

Voge, M., and Bueding, E., 1980, Tegumental surface alterations induced by subcurative doses of amoscanate, *Exp. Parasitol.* 50:251–259.

Wooder, M. F., and Wright, A. S., 1981, Alkylation of DNA by organophosphorus pesticides, *Acta Pharmacol. Toxicol.* (Suppl. V):51–53.

Woolhouse, N. M., 1979, Biochemical and pharmacological effects in relation to the mode of action of antischistosomal drugs, *Biochem. Pharmacol.* 28:2413–2418.

Xiao, S. H., 1981, The appearance of surface antigen of *Schistosoma japonicum* recovered from infected mice after treatment with pyguiton, *Shanghai J. Immunol.* 1:9–18.

Xiao, S., Friedman, P. A., Catto, B. A., and Webster, T., 1984, Praziquantel-induced vesicle formation in the tegument of male *Schistosoma mansoni* is calcium dependent, *J. Parasitol.* 70:177–179.

V

Cestodes

22

Chemistry of Anticestodal Agents

PETER ANDREWS and GERHARD BONSE

1. INTRODUCTION

Historically, treatment of cestode infections has long been the domain of natural products. These herbal preparations are difficult to standardize and are but poorly tolerated. The first synthetic cestocide was dichlorophen. It was introduced into veterinary and human medicine in 1946 and 1956, respectively, and was at that time regarded as an important advance in the treatment of infections caused by adult cestodes. Typically, cestodes inhabit the intestinal lumen and thus can be easily reached by orally administered drugs. Whenever their ability to maintain their position in the intestine is impaired they are easily expelled from it. These two characteristics are probably the reason such a startling variety of natural products and synthetic compounds have been employed, or considered for use, as cestocides. Table I provides a list of these compounds, which is by no means complete and which has been compiled from several excellent reviews (de Carneri and Vita, 1973; Islip, 1973; Sharma *et al.*, 1980; Vanden Bossche, 1980).

Several of the anticestodal agents have a wide spectrum of activity and have other major antiparasitic applications besides being used as cestocides. Such compounds are the benzimidazole carbamates, bithionol, metrifonate, and several salicylic acid anilides, and quinacrine, which are treated in the corresponding antinematodal, antitrematodal, and antiprotozoal chapters (Parts II, III, IV).

Six compounds considered important for the control of cestode infections of man, his livestock, and companion animals are treated in alphabetical order in this chapter. Data on the acute toxicity of these agents are compiled in Table II. References to the analytical methods developed to estimate their concentration in biological material are

PETER ANDREWS • Institut für Chemotherapie, Bayer AG, Pharma-Forschungszentrum, D-5600 Wuppertal 1, Bundesrepublik, West Germany.   GERHARD BONSE • Chemische Forschung, Pflanzenschutzzentrum Monheim, D-5090 Leverkusen- Bayerwerk, Bundesrepublik, West Germany.

Table I. Compounds with Anticestodal Effects

Natural organic products: betel nut (arecoline), *Chrysanthemum* flowers (pyrethrin), *Diospyros* berries (diospyrol), *Holarrhena* bark (connessine), kamala (rottlerine), kousso (α- and β-kosin), male fern (aspidine, filicic acid, flavaspidic acid, albaspidine), pomegranate (pelletierenes), pumpkin seed (cucurbitin)

Antibiotics: axenomycin, homomycin, streptotricin, thiamycin

Inorganic compounds: tin dust, copper sulfate, potassium permanganate, arsenates of lead, tin, zinc, copper, and calcium

Organometallic compounds: di-*n*-butyltin maleate, di-*n*-butyltin dilaureate, di-*n*-butyllead diacetate, dicyclohexyllead diacetate

Organophosphorus compounds: cyclophosamide, dichlorovos, diuredosan, fospirate, metrifonate, uredofos

Phenols: hexylresorcinol, *p*-isopropylbromocresol, β-(4-hydroxy-3,5-diiodophenyl)-α-phenyl propionic acid.

Diphenylmethanes: dichlorophen, hexachlorophene

Bisulfides: bithionol, bithionol sulfoxide

Salicylic acidanilides: niclosamide, oxyclozanide, rafoxanide, resorantel

Acridine derivatives: acranil, chloroquine, quinacrine

Isothiocyanates: bitoscanate, nitroscanate

Naphthamidines: bunamidine

Benzimidazole carbamates: albendazole, cambendazole, fenbendazole, mebendazole, oxfendazole, parbendazole

Table II. Acute Toxicity (LD_{50} Values in mg/kg) of Anticestodal Agents

Compound	Animal	Route of administration				
		po	sc	iv	ip	im
Arecoline	Mouse	—	65	36	—	—
	Dog	—	5	—	—	—
Arecoline × HCL	Mouse	—	—	32	154	—
Arecoline × HBr	Mouse	—	—	18	—	—
	Dog	—	5	—	—	—
Bunamidine × HCl	Mouse	540	—	—	—	—
Niclosamide	Mouse	1500	>20,000	—	210	—
	Rat	—	—	—	—	—
	Cat	—	—	>5	—	—
	Dog	>250	—	—	—	—
Niclosamide piperazine salt	Mouse	>5000	—	—	—	—
	Rat	>5000	—	—	—	—
	Dog	>5000	—	—	—	—
Nitroscanate	Mouse	3177	—	—	—	—
	Rat	3503	—	—	2554	—
Paromomycin	Rat	1625	650	156	—	—
Paromomysin sulfate salt	Mouse	2275	423	90	—	—
Praziquantel	Mouse	2454	7172	—	—	>2000
	Rat	2840	>16,000	—	796	>1000

Table III. Analytical Methods Developed for the Determination of Anticestodal Agents in Biological Material

Compound	Technique	Limit of detection (μg/ml)	Reference
Arecoline	Colorimetry, GLC	—	Kovensky and Poole (1970)
Bunamidine	—	—	—
Niclosamide	Colorimetry	0.02	El-Dib and Aly (1972)
	HPLC	0.0001	Muir and Grift (1980)
	GLC	0.00001	Churchill and Ku (1980)
Nitroscanate	—	—	—
Paromomycin	Agar diffusion	0.01	Lentzen *et al.* (1981)
Praziquantel	GLC	0.01	Diekmann (1979)
	Fluorometry	0.01	Pütter (1979)
	HPLC	0.0025	Xiao *et al.* (1983)

found in Table III. The universally applicable radiometric techniques are not mentioned.

2. ANTICESTODAL AGENTS

1. ARECOLINE

CARN: 63-75-2
$C_8H_{13}NO_2$ mol. wt. 155.2
3-Pyridine carboxylic acid-1,2,5,6-tetrahydro-1-methylester
Synonyms: Anthelmin®, Nemural®, Hydarex®.

HCl salt: mp 163°C; HBR salt: mp 172°C (Hydarex); carboxyphenylstibonic acid salt (Anthelmin); 3-acetamido-4-hydroxyphenyl arsenate acid salt (mol. wt. 430.3) (Nemural); b$_{17}$ 106–107°C; n$_D^{20}$ 1.4790.
Solubility: sol. in water (1 : 1) and ethanol (1 : 10).

Notes: The cestofugal properties of betel nut (*Areca catechu*) extracts have long been known; the alcaloid contained in them, arecoline, has been widely used in veterinary medicine since 1921 (Watkins, 1958). Arecoline is rapidly absorbed from the mouth but poorly from the intestine or from sites of injection. It is detoxified by the liver, possibly by demethylation to arecaidine. Side effects are attributable to its parasympathomimetic action and can be relieved by atropine (Forbes, 1964).

Synthesis:

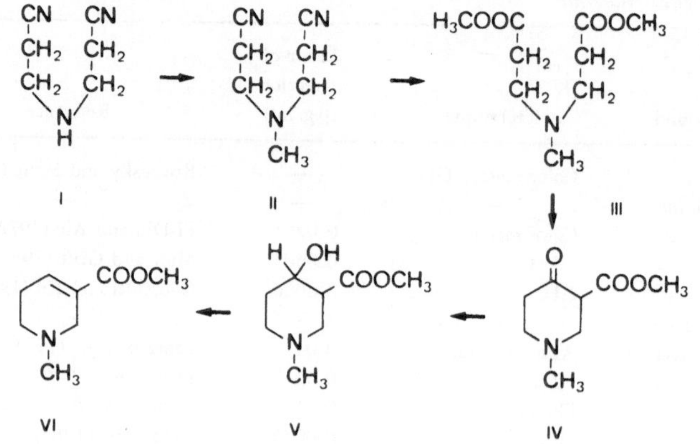

Arecoline VI can be synthesized from bis(β-cyanoethyl)amine I, a by-product of alanine production (Knox, 1950). I is first converted into a tertiary amine II which is then converted to bis(β-carbomethoxyethyl)methylamine III by reaction with acidified methanol. The subsequent Dieckmann condensation gives 1-methyl-3-carboethoxy-4-piperidone IV, which is reduced to the corresponding 4-hydroxy-piperidine V, and then finally dehydrated with thionyl chloride to give arecoline.

Notes: The N-alkyl homologues of arecoline are inactive, and only the propyl member displays slight activity (Preobrazhinskij *et al.*, 1957).

2. BUNAMIDINE HYDROCHLORIDE

CARN: 3748-77-4
$C_{25}H_{38}N_2O \times HCl$ mol. wt. 419.1
N,N-dibutyl-4-(hexyloxy)-1-naphthalene-carboximidamide
Synonyms: Scolaban®

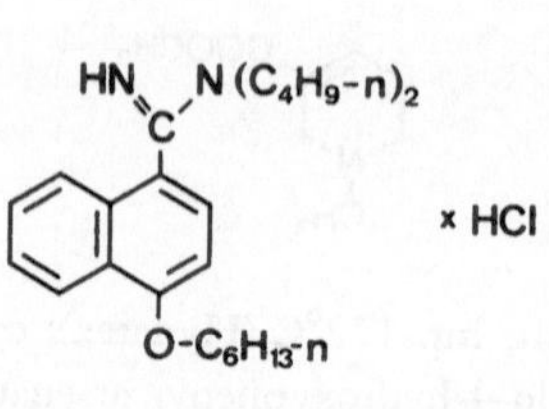

White odorless, crystals.
3-Hydroxy-2-naphthoate salt: mp 169–170°C (Buban®).
Solubility: sol. in methanol and hot water.

Notes: The discovery of bunamidine was announced in 1965 (Baltzly *et al.*, 1965). Bunamidine hydrochloride is apparently absorbed from the intestine. The liver appears to be the main organ of detoxification, as erratic deaths of treated dogs have been related to hepatic dysfunction (Fastier, 1972). In dogs, only 0.5% of an oral dose is excreted by the kidneys (Virji and Laverty, 1972). The free amidine base may be irritating to the skin, and the hydrochloride may be irritating to the mucosal membranes of the mouth and eyes (Harfenist *et al.*, 1971).

Synthesis:

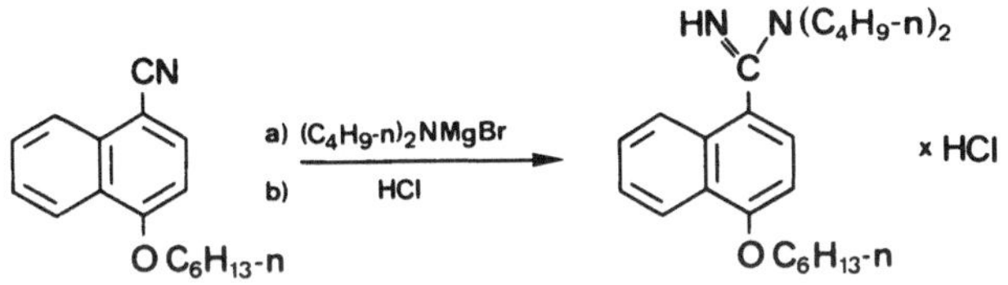

Bunamidine hydrochloride **VIII** is prepared by reaction of 4-hexyloxy-α-naphthonitrile **VII** with di-*n*-butylamino-magnesium bromide (Harfenist and Baltzly, 1966). The free base is then dissolved in ethanol and treated with a slight excess of a concentrated ethanolic HCl solution to give the HCl salt.

Notes: A large number of 4-alkoxy-1-naphthamidines have been prepared in order to establish a structure–activity relationship. The best cestocidal activity was obtained when the total number of carbon atoms of the alkoxy chain and the amidine group was C_{12}–C_{23}. The general pattern, that an improvement of the therapeutic index could be achieved with an increase in the size of the alkoxy and alkyl groups, was more evident in the mouse than in the dog (Harfenist *et al.*, 1971; Burrows *et al.*, 1971).

3. NICLOSAMIDE

CARN: 50-65-7
$C_{13}H_8Cl_2N_2O_4$ mol. wt. 327.1
2′, 5-Dichloro-4′-nitrosalicylanilide
Synonyms: Mansonil-P®, Lintex-M®, Mansonil-M®, Yomesan®.

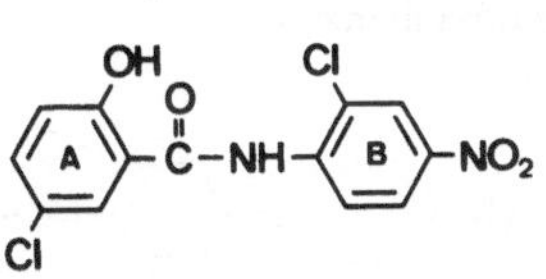

Pale yellow crystals, tasteless.
Solubility: pr. insol. in water (1 : 100,000); sol. in ethanol (1 : 150), sol. in chloroform (1 : 400) and in ether (1 : 350); mp 227–232°C.

Notes: The salicylic acid anilides were investigated as potential drugs because of their structural relationship to dichlorophen, which was the first useful synthetic cestocide during the 1950s. The discovery of niclosamide was announced in 1958 (Gönnert and Schraufstätter, 1959) and its use as a cestocide in 1960 (Gönnert and Schraufstätter, 1960). About one-third of an oral dose of niclosamide is absorbed from the intestine of rats, while 2–25% of the dose is absorbed in man. The absorbed fraction is excreted renally in the form of glucoronide conjugates of niclosamide, its 4′-amino and its 4′-acetamino analogues. The 4′-amino compound is the main metabolite and is devoid of biological activity (Andrews *et al.*, 1983*a*).

Synthesis:

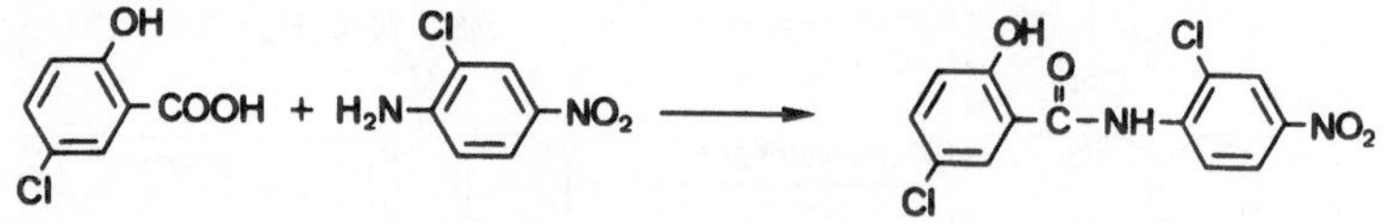

Niclosamide **XI** is easily obtained by heating 5-chlorosalicylic acid **IX** and 2-chloro-4-nitroaniline **X** in xylene in the presence of PCl_3 (Schraufstätter and Gönnert, 1964).

Notes: The following structural parameters for optimal cestocidal activity were derived from the study of a wide range of congeners of niclosamide (Gönnert *et al.*, 1963, Sharma *et al.*, (1980). The most important prerequisite for cestocidal activity is the presence of a phenolic —OH group. Its replacement by —OCH_3 causes loss of activity. The two aromatic rings (A and B) must be connected by an amidic (thioamidic) linkage. Amidine or aminomethyl linkages do not display cestocidal activity. The presence of a chlorine atom at position 5 of ring A plays a vital role in determining cestocidal activity. Introduction of a further chlorine at position 3 of ring A enhances the activity. The chlorine atoms can be replaced by bromo substitution. Electron withdrawing groups at position 4 of ring B are necessary for activity. Electron-donating groups such as —NH_2 result in a loss of biological activity. The presence of a chlorine atom at position 2 of ring B is not an absolute requirement for high cestocidal activity.

4. NITROSCANATE

CARN: 19881-18-6
$C_{13}H_8N_2O_3S$ mol. wt. 272.3
1-Isothiocyanato-4-(4-nitrophenoxy)benzene
Synonyms: Lopatol®, Cantrodifene®.

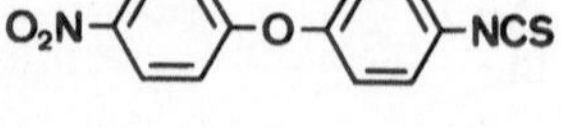

Buff-colored odorless crystals.
Solubility: insol. in water; sol. in org. solvents.

Notes: The discovery of nitroscanate was announced in 1973 (Boray *et al.*, 1979). Pharmacological data on nitroscanate have not appeared in the literature. The observations that small particle size nitroscanate (Lopatol, Cantrodifene) (<5 μm) is more effective than the larger particle size material (10–20 μm) may indicate poor absorption of the drug (Richards and Somerville, 1980).

Synthesis:

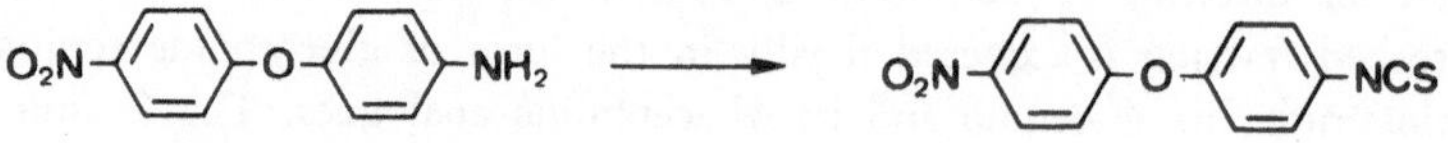

Nitroscanate **XIII** is prepared in good yield from the corresponding amine **XII**, which is easily obtainable from *p*-acetamidophenol and chloronitrobenzene, and from ammonium thiocyanate (Magdanyi *et al.*, 1977). Carbon disulfide (Magdanyi *et al.*, 1979) or thiophosgene (Antos *et al.*, 1970) may be used instead of ammonium thiocyanate.

5. PAROMOMYCIN

CARN: 7542-37-2

$C_{23}H_{45}N_5O_{14}$ mol. wt. 615.7

0-2-Amino-2-deoxy-α-D-glucopyranosyl-0-(0-2.6-diamino-2.6-dideoxy-β-L-ido-pyranosyl-β-D-ribofuranosyl)-2-deoxy-D-streptamine

Synonym: Humatin®.

Amorphous white powder.

Solubility: sol. in water (1 : 1); mod. sol. in methanol; sp. sol. in ethanol; $[\alpha]_D^{25} + 64°$; paromomycin sulfate (Humatin): $[\alpha]_D^{25} + 50.5°$ contains 70% paromomycin.

Notes: Paromomycin was isolated in 1955 (Frohardt *et al.*, 1956) and first used as a cestocide by Ulivelli (1963). Paromomycin is poorly absorbed from the gastrointestinal tract. In man, less than 1% of the oral dose is absorbed from the stomach and the intestine and is subsequently excreted unchanged in the urine (Lentzen *et al.*, 1981).

Paromomycin is a fermentation product of *Streptomyces rimosus* forma *paromomycinus* (Frohardt *et al.*, 1956). It is conveniently isolated from fermentation broths by cation exchange chromatographic procedures and commercially supplied as its neutral sulfate salt.

The little that is known about structure–activity relationship concerns the antibacterial action of paromomycin and not its anticestodal efficacy. Destruction of the basic functions of the molecule, i.e., *N*-acylation of the primary amino groups, results in a complete loss of activity (Fisher and Thompson, 1964).

PAROMOMYCIN II

CARN: 51795-47-2

Notes: 2,6-amino-2.6-dideoxy-D-glucose has replaced the respective L-idose derivative contained in paromomycin. This minor component, obtained from fermentation broths, has less antibacterial activity.

Preparation: Rinehart *et al.* (1962); Reuter *et al.* (1975).

6. PRAZIQUANTEL

CARN: 55268-74-1

$C_{19}H_{24}N_2O_2$ mol. wt. 312.4

2-(Cyclohexylcarbonyl)-1,2,3,6,7,11*b*-hexahydro-4*H*-pyrazino[2, 1*a*]isoquinolin-4-one

Synonyms: Biltricide®, Droncit®, Cesol®, Cestox®, Cisticide®.

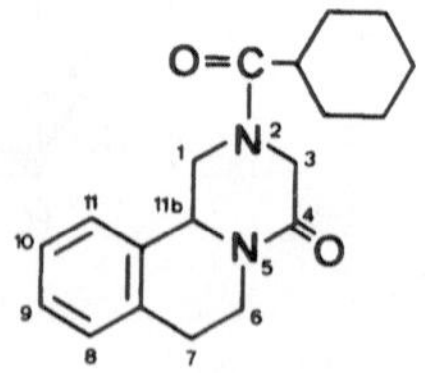

White crystals of bitter taste.

Solubility: sp. sol. in water (1 : 2500); sol. in ethanol (1 : 10) and chloroform (1 : 2).

Notes: The discovery of praziquantel was announced in 1975 (Thomas *et al.*, 1975). Praziquantel is absorbed almost quantitatively from the intestinal tract. It is rapidly and extensively metabolized in the liver. The main metabolite in serum is the 4-hydroxycyclohexyl derivative. No unchanged drug is excreted in the urine, which contains glucoronide conjugates and sulfate esters of metabolites carrying two hydroxyl groups (Andrews *et al.*, 1983*b*).

Synthesis:

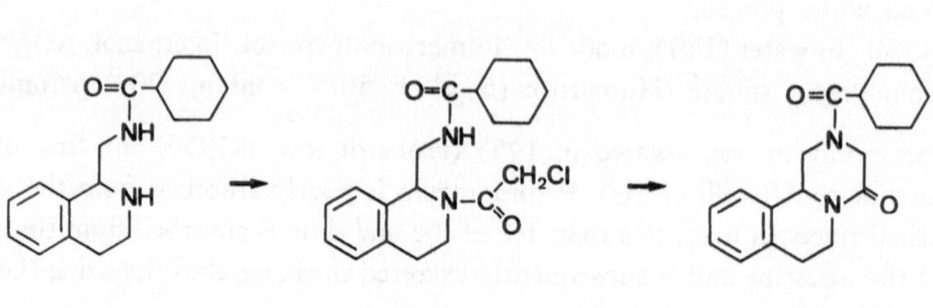

Praziquantel **XVI** can be synthesized starting from the easily available *N*-1.2.3.4-tetrahydroisoquinoly-1-methyl carboxamide **XIV**. Acylation of **XIV** with chloroacetyl chloride to **XV** is followed by ring closure in the presence of a strong base to give **XVI** (Seubert *et al.*, 1977).

Notes: The study of the structure–activity relationship of the pyrazino[2,1-*a*]isoquinolin-4-ones has resulted in the following conclusions (Andrews *et al.* 1983*b*). The oxo group in position 4 is essential for high and broad anthelmintic activity. All derivatives with other substituents at this position lack substantial activity with the exception of the thioanalogue. A further prerequisite for activity is an acyl or thioacyl group in position 2. Within the group of aromatic acyl derivatives, the unsubstituted benzoyl derivative is one of the most active. Further increase in activity is achieved by amino substitution (m,p) and fluoro substitution (o,m). A decrease in activity is caused by ortho substitution (with the exception of o-fluoro) and by di- or polysubstitution. Open-chained aliphatic acyl derivatives are of rather low activity in comparison with the corresponding cyclic analogues. Cyclic derivatives exhibit a dramatic rise in activity in going from the three membered to the six-membered ring (praziquantel) and a decline with further increase in ring size. Positions other than 2,4, and 11b appear to be of minor importance in determining anthelmintic activity.

REFERENCES

Andrews, P., Thyssen, J., and Lorke, D., 1983a, The biology and toxicology of molluscicides, Bayluscide, *Pharmacol. Ther.* 19:245–295.

Andrews, P., Thomas, H., Pohlke, R., and Seubert, J., 1983b, Praziquantel, *Med. Res. Rev.* 3:147–200.

Antos, K., Drobnica, L., Nemec, P., Martvon, A., Kristian P., and Dzurila, M., 1970, Ger. Offen. DE 1 932690, assigned to Ceskosclovenska Akadmie Ved.

Baltzly, R., Burrows, R. B., Harfenist, M., Fuller, K. A., Keeling, J. E. D., Standen, O. D., Hatton, G. J., Nunns, V. J., Rawes, D. A. Blood, B. D., Moya, V., and Lylyveld, J. L., 1965, A series of compounds active against cestodes, *Nature (Lond.)* 206:408–409.

Boray, J. C., Strong, M. B., Allison, J. R., von Orelli, M., Sarasin, G., and Gfeller, W., 1979, Nitroscanate a new broad spectrum anthelmintic against nematodes and cestodes of dogs and cats, *Aust. Vet. J.* 55:45–53.

Burrows, R. B., Hatton, C. J., Lillis, W. G., and Hunt, G. R., 1971, Cestocidal activity of 4-alkoxy-1-naphthamidines against dog and cat tapeworms, *J. Med. Chem.* 14:87–90.

Churchill, F. C., and Ku, D. N., 1980, Extractive alkylation of 5,2′-dichloro-4′-nitrosalicylanilide (niclosamide) for gas–liquid chromatographic analysis, *J. Chromatogr.* 189:375–388.

De Carneri, I., and Vita, G., 1973, Drugs used in cestode diseases, in: *International Encyclopedia of Pharmacology and Therapeutics*, Section 64, Vol. 1 (C. Radouco-Thomas, R. Cavier, and R. Hawking, eds.), pp. 145–213, Pergamon Press, Oxford.

Diekmann, H. W., 1979, Quantitative determination of praziquantel in body fluids by gas liquid chromatography, *Eur. J. Drug. Metab. Pharmacol.* 4:139–141.

El-Dib, M. A., and Aly, O. A., 1972, Colorimetric determination of phenylamide pesticides in natural waters, *J. Assoc. Off. Anal. Chem.* 55:1276–1279.

Fastier, F. N., 1972, Pharmacological aspects of bunamidine dosing of dogs, *N. Z. Vet. J.* 20:148–151.

Fisher, M. W., and Thompson, P. E., 1964, Antibiotics with specific affinities, Part 3: Paromomycin, in: *Experimental Chemotherapy* (R. J. Schnitzer and F. Hawking, eds.), Vol. 3, pp. 329–345, Academic Press, New York.

Forbes, L. S., 1964, The relation between method of administration, route of absorption, inhibitory actions and acute toxicity of arecoline hydrobromide in dogs, *Ann. Trop. Med. Parasitol.* 58:119–131.

Frohardt, R. P., Haskell, T. H., and Ehrlich, J., 1956, Ger. Offen. DE 1 025 578, assigned to Parke Davis and Co.

Gönnert, R., and Schraufstätter, E., 1959, A new molluscicide: Molluscicide Bayer 73, *Proceedings of the Sixth International Congresses on Tropical Medicine and Malaria, Lisbon, Sept. 5–13, 1958,* 2:197–202.

Gönnert, R., and Schraufstätter, E., 1960, Experimentelle Untersuchungen mit N-(2′-chlor-4′-nitrophenyl)-5-chlorsalicylamid, einem neuen Bandwurmmittel, *Arzneimittelforsch.* 10:881–884.

Gönnert, R., Johannis, J., Schraufstätter, E., and Strufe, R., 1963, Konstitution und cestocide Wirkung in der Yomesan-Reihe, *Med. Chem.* 7:540–567.

Harfenist, M., and Baltzly, R., 1966, U.S. Patent 3,290,375, assigned to Burroughs Wellcome and Co.

Harfenist, M., Burrows, R. B., Baltzly, R., Pedersen, E., Hunt, G. R., and Gurbaxani, S., 1971, Synthesis and anthelmintic activity of 4-alkoxy-1-naphthamidines, *J. Med. Chem.* 14:97–103.

Islip, P. J., 1973, Progress in the experimental chemotherapy of helminth infections. Part I. Trematode and cestode infections, *Prog. Drug Res.* 17:241–318.

Knox, L. H., 1950, U.S. Patent 2,506,458, assigned to Nopco Chemical Co.

Kovensky, B. J., and Poole, C. W., 1970, Colorimetric and gas chromatographic analyses of arecoline in capsule preparations, *J. Pharmacol. Sci.* 59:1651–1652.

Lentzen, H., Kölle, E. U., and Daschner, F., 1981, Vergleichende Untersuchung der Serumspiegel und Urinausscheidung nach oraler Gabe von Paromomycin und Neomycin, *Arzneimittelforsch.* 31:1967–1971.

Magdanyi, L., Rakoczy, G., Kovacs, L., Hutak, A., Pallos, L., Magyar, K., Gyenes, J., and Foris, P., 1977, Hung, Teljes HU 12898, assigned to E. Gy. T. Gyogyszervegyeszeti Gyar.

Magdanyi, L., Rakoczy, G., Kovacs, L., Hutak, A., Pallos, L., Magyar, K., Gyenes, J., and Foris, P., 1979, Hung. Teljes HU 16577, assigned to E. Gy. T. Gyogyszervegyeszeti Gyar.

Muir, D. C. G., and Grift, N. P., 1980, Determination of niclosamide (Bayer 2353) in water and sediment samples, *Int. J. Environ. Anal. Chem.* 8:1–14.

Preobrazhenskij, N. A., Malkov, K. M., Maurit, M. E., Vorobev, M. A., and Vlasov, A. S., 1957, Synthesis of alkaloid arecoline and its homologs, *Zh. Obshchei Khim.* 27:3162–3170.

Pütter, J., 1979, A fluorometric method for the determination of praziquantel in blood-plasma and urine, *Eur. J. Drug. Metab. Pharmacol.* 4:143–148.

Reuter, G., Liebermann, B., and Köster, H., 1975, Zur Physiologie und Biochemie der Streptomyceten, 1.Mitteilung: Isolierung, Identifizierung und Untersuchungen zur mikrobiellen Synthese der Stereoisomere im Paromomycin-Komplex, *Pharmazie* 30:733–736.

Richards, R. J., and Somerville, J. M., 1980, Field trials with nitroscanate against cestodes and nematodes in dogs, *Vet. Rec.* 106:32–335.

Rinehart, K. L., Hichens, M., Argoudelis, A. D., Chilton, W. S., Carter, H. E., Georgiadis, M. P., Schaffner, C. P., and Schillings, R. T., 1962, *J. Am. Chem. Soc.* 84:3218–3220.

Schraufstätter, E., and Gönnert, R., 1964, U.S. Patent 3,147,300, assigned to Farbenfabriken Bayer A.G.

Seubert, J., Pohlke, R., and Loebich, F., 1977, Synthesis and properties of praziquantel, a novel broad spectrum anthelmintic with excellent activity against schistosomes and cestodes, *Experientia* 33:1036–1037.

Sharma, S., Dubey, S. K., and Iyer, R. N., 1980, Chemotherapy of cestode infections, *Prog. Drug Res.* 24:217–266.

Thomas, H., Gönnert, R., Pohlke, R., and Seubert, J., 1975, A new compound against adult tapeworms, *Proceedings of the Seventh International Conference of the World Association for the Advancement of Veterinary Parasitology, Thessaloniki*, abstract No. 51.

Ulivelli, A., 1963, Terapia antibiotica della teniasi. Primi favorevoli risultati del trattamento con paromomicina, *Riv. Clin. Pediatr.* 72:3–15.

Vanden Bossche, H., 1980, Chemotherapy of hymenolepiasis, in: *Biology of the Tapeworm Hymenolepis diminuta* (H. P. Arai, ed.), pp. 630–693, Academic Press, New York.

Virji, A. S., and Laverty, R., 1972, Bunamidine uptake and distribution in rats and dogs, *Aust. J. Exp. Biol. Med. Sci.* 50:209–215.

Watkins, T. I., 1958, The Chemotherapy of Helminthiasis, *J. Pharm. Pharmacol.* 10:209–227.

Xiao, S.-H., Catto, B. A., and Webster, L. T., 1983, Quantitative determination of praziquantel in serum by high-performance liquid chromatography, *J. Chromatogr.* 275:127–132.

23

Cestode Infections of Man

G. WEBBE

1. INTRODUCTION

In experimental work directed toward the development of new effective anthelmintics, the cestodes have received far less attention than have the trematodes and nematodes. This may be partly because cestode infections are generally considered of minor importance compared with the much more numerous and pathogenic parasites of the other helminth classes. The tapeworms have a worldwide distribution, but their medical and economic significance is variable (Standen, 1963; Keeling, 1968). The larval stages of *Taenia solium* and *Echinococcus granulosus* may, however, produce serious human disease, and only recently have new broad-spectrum anthelmintics been developed with which treatment of cysticercosis and hydatidosis may now be contemplated.

In reviewing the drugs most commonly used against cestode infections in man and animals, Standen (1963) concluded that despite the availability of a limited range of reasonably effective drugs, improvements were needed. In the treatment of human taeniases there was a requirement for drugs with sufficiently wide margins of safety to obviate the need for special preparation of the patient by prolonged fasting before treatment and the removal of the drug by purgation soon afterward. A number of active anthelmintic substances have now been developed with specific activity against cestodes and even against important larval stages. The substances fall inevitably into different levels of development according to their performance in experimental screens.

2. EXPERIMENTAL METHODS

2.1. Techniques for Drug Testing against Adult Tapeworms in Vivo

Techniques are available for testing potential taeniacides against *Hymenolepis diminuta*, *H. nana*, and *Oöchoristica symmetrica* in the mouse, but the use of these screens has to

G. WEBBE • Department of Medical Helminthology, London School of Hygiene & Tropical Medicine, Winches Farm Field Station, St. Albans, Hertfordshire AL4 OXQ, England.

be supplemented, for development of taeniacides active against the larger tapeworms of man and domestic animals, by tests in a secondary screen. Such a screen would usually involve the testing of selected chemical structures in cats or dogs infected with one of the large well-armed species, such as *Taenia pisiformis, T. hydatigena, T. taeniaeformis*, or *Echinococcus granulosus*, or in sheep infected with *Moniezia expansa*.

2.2. Drug Testing against Adult Tapeworms in Vitro

A technique was described by Sen and Hawking (1960) for testing chemical compounds against *Hymenolepis nana in vitro*, the adult worm being recovered from mice infected 20–40 days previously by perfusion in saline. An *in vitro* screening technique was also developed using appropriate lengths of *Moniezia expansa* suspended in Tyrode's solution at 39–40°C (Duguid and Heathcote, 1950*a,b*). Standen (1963) recorded that Batham (1946) used Baldwin's (1943) techniques for *in vitro* tests on nematodes for similar observations on late mature or gravid proglottids of *T. hydatigena* or *T. pisiformis*. Demonstration of activity *in vitro* is of no value unless it is followed up by *in vivo* tests confirming the validity of the observations. Equally, the demonstration of activity *in vivo* in compounds of unknown potency would establish the validity of the *in vitro* test, while information *in vitro* of activity in substances known to be taenicidal *in vivo* is less useful (Standen, 1963).

2.3. Drug Testing against Larval Tapeworms in Vivo

Mice infected with larval *Taenia taeniaeformis (Cysticercus fasciolaris)* were used to test the efficacy of atebrin, which was considered to affect the viability of the cysts but was much less active when treatment began after the cysts had matured (Cuthbertson and Greenfield, 1941). An indication of the activity of the new compound, praziquantel, against larval cestodes was first determined in mice infected with *Hymenolepis nana*, but immature cysticercoids were only partially susceptible to high doses of the drug (Thomas and Gönnert, 1977).

Similarly, the efficacy of benzimidazoles against larval tapeworms was first demonstrated in laboratory animal assays. The initial observations of efficacy were made in mice, jirds (*Meriones*), and rabbits experimentally infected with larval *Echinococcus granulosus, E. multilocularis, Taenia taeniaeformis, T. pisiformis, T. crassiceps*, and *Mesocestoides corti* (Heath and Chevis, 1974; Heath *et al.*, 1975; Campbell and Blair, 1974*a,b;* Krotov *et al.*, 1974; Thienpont *et al.*, 1974). Rabbits infected with larval *T. pisiformis* under experimental conditions were used to detect the larvicidal activity of closantel (Chevis *et al.*, 1980).

2.4. Drug Testing against Larval Tapeworms in Vitro

Lagrange (1946) described a technique for *in vitro* testing of drugs against cystic larvae of *Taenia hydatigena*. The method is based on exposure of the cysts to solutions of the chemical being tested and on observations on the inhibiting effect of such exposure on the evagination stimulus provided by subsequent exposure to bile. According to Standen (1963) a technique was developed by Ross (1927) for the study of drug action *in vitro* against scolices of *Echinococcus granulosas,* the scolices being obtained aseptically from hydatid cysts and then added to several dilutions of test substances. This technique constituted an approach to the identification of substances likely to be of value against hydatid cysts *in vivo.*

Only after the detection of an active substance by one or more of the experimental methods already discussed and the establishment of a satisfactory ratio of antiparasite activity and mammalian toxicity in exhaustive investigations of acute and chronic toxicity in a wide range of mammalian species can clinical trials be considered in man.

2.5. Clinical Trials

Trials of taeniafugal and taeniacidal compounds, in cases of human taeniasis, are usually conducted by macroscopic and microscopic identification of expelled proglottids. This is because eggs may be present only intermittently in the stools in the case of known infections and because it is desirable to identify the scolex after treatment, to confirm both the status of cure and the species identification (Davis, 1973). It has been pointed out by Davis (1973) that drugs are given after the diagnosis is made on the basis of inspection of stools for the scolex and proglottids; if the former is found, evidence of cure is accepted. If the scolex is not found, the patient is requested to observe the stools for the presence of proglottids for a period of 3 months, the time it usually takes for regeneration of *Taenia.* If the stools are observed to be free of proglottids during this time, a cure is accepted. Examinations of concentrated stools for eggs are occasionally undertaken during the post-treatment period, but quantification is almost unknown and is unlikely to be attempted. It is believed that the routine use of perianal adhesive tape swabs to detect *Taenia* eggs would enhance the stringency of the criteria of cure.

3. TREATMENT OF INFECTIONS DUE TO *TAENIA, DIPHYLLOBOTHRIUM, ECHINOCOCCUS,* AND *HYMENOLEPIS*

3.1. Traditional Remedies

Davis (1973) recorded that the tapeworm remedies that have been used for many years include preparations of kamala, kousso, spigelia, pomegranate bark, and raigan, made from a powdered fungus. These substances are considered of historical interest only; no further reference is made to them in this discussion.

3.2. Old Drugs

3.2.1. Aspidium Oleoresin (Extract of Male Fern)

The active principle of Aspidium oleoresin is known as filicin. Commercially available ether extracts should contain 25% w/w of filicin. It has been widely and successfully used for many years against *Taenia saginata*, *T. solium*, and *Diphyllobothrium*.

3.2.1a. Pharmacology. Aspidium oleoresin is absorbed from the gastrointestinal (GI) tract, and a proportion is excreted unchanged in the urine. A pretreatment fat-free diet is considered essential, since lipids increase absorption. There is pronounced individual variability in absorption. Aspidium has an irritant effect on the GI tract and kidneys. High doses may produce serious toxic effects on the central nervous system (CNS) or on the heart, producing bradycardia and reduced contractile capability. Smooth muscle may be depressed by Aspidium and uterine muscle stimulated. Hänel (1950) summarized the experience of 22,000 treatments for tapeworm infections with extracts of male fern in Germany, recording temporary and permanent blindness as well as intoxication with fatalities.

The drug acts as a taeniafuge, causing temporary relaxation of the worm by paralysis of its muscles. A purge is given following treatment to ensure passage of the worm. It is contraindicated in the debilitated patient, especially the old or very young and also in anemia and pregnancy. A formidable array of side effects has been recorded.

3.2.1b. Dosage. Under the correct conditions, Aspidium oleoresin gives cure rates of 70–90%, and successful treatments tend to be related to careful patient pretreatment preparation and administration. Ideally patients should undergo at least 2 days of preparation with a fat-free semifluid diet and highly saline purges. Originally the drug was given in capsules, together with a draught or emulsion with or without glycerol. The concern that such preparations might cause nausea and vomiting led to the use of a duodenal tube. The dose of drug is 3–6 ml of male fern oleoresin (*International Pharmacopeia*) according to age and weight. If given for *T. solium* infections, the drug should be given by a duodenal tube to reduce any risk of vomiting. Extracts of male fern or related synthetic chemicals were used until recently for the treatment of *T. saginata* infections (Dodian, 1962; Ditzel and Schwartz, 1967; Alterio, 1968), but the high toxicity of these drugs will exclude them from further use.

3.2.2. Hypertonic Solutions

As early as 1932, de Rivas suggested the use of hypertonic solutions, given by duodenal tube, for the treatment of tapeworm infections. In recent years, a hypertonic solution of magnesium sulfate has been used as a taeniafuge, but fatal reactions from duodenal doses in excess of 60 g, due to magnesium intoxication, have been reported from Germany (Rösler, 1952), so that this treatment is no longer recommended (Pawlowski and Schultz, 1972).

3.2.3. Acridine Derivatives

Although there is a risk of intolerance and overdosage, acridine drugs have been widely used. Acridine derivatives other than quinacrine (Mepacrine, Atebrin), i.e.,

Acrichin (Krotov and Rusak, 1964) and Acronil (Beier, 1963; Pawlowski, 1970) have been commonly used against *T. saginata, T. solium,* and *D. latum.*

3.2.3a. Pharmacology. Absorption from the gut is rapid, and peak plasma levels are reached in about 8 hr. Excretion, which takes place mainly in feces and urine, with small amounts in bile, sweat, and saliva, is slow; that is because the compounds have a great affinity for many tissues in which concentrations may be greater than in plasma. Most of the circulating drug is bound to plasma protein and may cross the placenta; and fetal tissue levels may be similar to maternal levels. Mepacrine is readily intercalated with DNA and, like other drugs (4-aminoquinolines and some antibiotics), it acts at the molecular level by arresting protein synthesis. Few pharmacological effects are seen after conventional doses. It may, however, inhibit a number of enzyme systems, including cholinesterase, and high blood levels may depress the respiratory and cardiovascular systems (Davis, 1973). It is considered highly probable that the anthelmintic action is a function of interference with the sucking action of the tapeworm. These drugs intensify both the motility of the tapeworm and the peristaltic movements of the host intestine (Beier, 1965*a*).

3.2.3b. Dosage. The usual dose of an acridine derivative, for an adult, is 0.6–0.8 g. In children, proportionately smaller doses are given, of the order of 15–20 mg/kg. The most effective means of treatment is by intraduodenal tube followed by a saline purge 2 hr later. If given by mouth, it is common practice to give an antiemetic before and sodium bicarbonate concurrently. Cure rates of 70–90% may be achieved, but this is an individual form of treatment and cannot be used for ambulatory outpatients because of necessary pretreatment and post-treatment preparations.

Nausea and vomiting frequently occur during oral use. Dizziness, diarrhea, colic, headache, and urticaria have been recorded. Central nervous system side effects may occur. The use of these drugs should be avoided in elderly patients, in young children, and in patients with skin problems or cardiac, hepatic, or renal disease. The use of mepacrine is contraindicated by concurrent administration of 8-aminoquinolines, since the toxicity of the former is enhanced.

Davis (1973) recorded that uncontrolled trials suggested that the use of intramuscular Pituitrin 1 hr after administration of mepacrine both assisted worm expulsion and minimized the risk of vomiting. Davis emphasized that its use in *T. solium* infections should be by the intraduodenal route, with all the necessary precautions to prevent vomiting.

3.2.4. Tin Compounds

Tin compounds have been used for treatment of tapeworm infections over some centuries. The efficacy of these compounds varies according to the particular drug used. The proprietary preparations are based on mixtures of metallic tin with its oxide or chloride (e.g., Cestodin, Taeniafuge, and Stannotaen). The efficacy of various tin compounds, based on the treatment of 868 outpatients with *T. saginata* infection, was 88.8% (Dufek and Kalivoda, 1969; Pawlowski, 1970).

3.2.4a. Dosage. The precise dosage of tin compounds depends on the particular product, since the ingredients in each one differ. The total number of tablets varies: Cestodin, 15; Stannotaen, 10; and Taenifuge, 90. The drug should be well pulverized, since it probably acts by covering the worm cuticle with a thin layer of active tin particles, rendering the strobila susceptible to digestion. The drug is taken two or three times a day for a period of 5 days despite the fact that the strobila may be evacuated early in the treatment course. A saline purge is given on the third day and at the end of treatment.

Pure metallic tin and tin oxide particles appear to be virtually nontoxic, but the irritative action of tin chloride is probably responsible for the side effects observed in patients treated with tin compounds (Dadlez *et al.*, 1954). The side effects are mostly GI disorders. The contraindications of this group of drugs are pregnancy, GI disorders that produce increased drug absorption, and severe liver and renal disease (Bojanowicz and Pietrowa, 1968). Storage of these compounds for more than 2 years may reduce their efficacy. Variable side effects and the length of treatment required are drawbacks to their usage despite the high cure rates obtained.

3.2.5. Bithionol

Limited treatments have been made with this drug in Japan (Yokagawa *et al.*, 1962). Dufek and Kalivoda (1969) treated 20 patients and cured 18 using 40–55 mg/kg in two doses with an interval of 1 hr, followed 2 hr later by a saline purge. Although clearly active against *T. saginata* and *D. latum* infections, it seems unlikely that this drug will be used further in view of available new compounds.

3.3. New Drugs

3.3.1. Dichlorophen

This drug acts rapidly as a taeniacide, resulting in the elimination of a totally or partially disintegrated worm, but the precise mode of action is unknown. It has been the drug of choice in *T. saginata* infections, and many physicians use it for the treatment of *T. solium* with added precautions despite the theoretical risk of cysticercosis. Dichlorophen is curative in *D. latum* infections and has some effect against *H. nana* (Davis, 1973). For some time the drug has been used for mass treatment in the U.S.S.R, but intolerance to standard doses (6–9 g in adults) has relegated it to use only as an alternative drug.

3.3.1a. Dosage. The recommended dose is 70 mg/kg, but doses ranging from 60–100 mg/kg have been used, with a maximum of 6 g for adults given as a single dose. Variable results have been reported and some workers reported only 50% cure rates. In children, clinical experience has shown that doses of <4.5 mg/kg are ineffective. Preliminary starvation is unnecessary except the night before treatment and, because the drug has a mild laxative action, post-treatment purgation is also unnecessary. Follow-up examinations of stools for proglottids over some 3–4 months after treatment is necessary, since the scolex is rarely seen in post-treatment feces (Lassance *et al.*, 1957; Adams and Seaton, 1959; Schneider, 1959; Seaton, 1960; Turner, 1963; Alterio, 1968; Pawlowski, 1970). Optimum results have been obtained when the drug is given over 2 or 3 days. Krotov *et al.* (1968) used dichlorophen in a very low dose (1.0 g) together with niclosamide (2.0 g), under the name of Dichlosal, which is regarded as highly effective against beef and fish tapeworms in the U.S.S.R. Serious toxic side effects have been reported, however, and it is doubtful that this drug mixture can be considered safe. Toxic side effects of dichlorophen may include nausea and vomiting, diarrhea, and other GI disturbances. Contraindications have not been fully established, but care should be taken in patients with severe heart disease and in liver disease.

3.3.2. Niclosamide

Niclosamide, a chlorinated salicylanilide, is a tasteless, yellowish-white powder that is almost insoluble in water. Introduced by Gönnert and Schraufstätter in 1960, niclosamide has been the drug of choice in cestodiasis for almost 20 years.

3.3.2a. Pharmacology. The drug is not absorbed from the GI tract, and it is a powerful taeniacide on contact. According to Gönnert (1968), investigations with radioactive labeled and unlabeled compound show that 25–30% of orally administered drug is excreted in the urine (the greater part being metabolites), and the remainder is excreted in the feces. There is no accumulation of compound or its metabolites in the whole body or in single organs. Thus the drug is rapidly and quantitatively excreted, clearly the reasons for the good tolerance and safety of niclosamide. It has virtually no pharmacodynamic action. The scolex of the worm and proximal segments are killed on contact and the dead worm may be digested, so that it is not usually possible to identify either the scolex or proglottids in the stools after purging.

Extensive clinical trials have demonstrated the high curative efficacy of niclosamide in the treatment of *T. saginata, T. solium, D. latum,* and *H. nana* (Beier, 1965*b*, 1966; Ahkami and Hadjian, 1969; Perera *et al.*, 1970). High cure rates have been reported in the case of *T. saginata;* for example, Gherman (1968) reported a 93.6% cure rate and Khalil (1969) a 84.6% cure rate. Other investigators have reported a much lower efficacy of niclosamide; for instance, Donkaster *et al.* (1961) reported a 53% cure rate and Nitzulescu *et al.* (1962) a 58% cure rate. Pawlowski (1970) considered certain batches of drug or products used in 1962 to have differential bioavailability and much lower efficacy, probably because the particle size of the compounds was outside the range 2–6 μm necessary for the drug to be active.

3.3.2b. Dosage. According to Davis (1973), there is no conclusive evidence that prior starvation is necessary, but it is considered prudent to restrict the diet to fluids only, commencing on the evening preceding treatment. The standard adult dosage is 2 g, consisting of two 0.5-g tablets being chewed thoroughly and swallowed with as little water as possible. This is repeated after 30 min or 1 hr. Some workers give 2.0 g as a single dose. It must be emphasized that the tablets should be chewed thoroughly and that the minimum amount of water is given to aid swallowing, the object being to achieve the maximum amount of drug in the upper small intestine and duodenum.

In *H. nana* infections, treatment is considered necessary for 5–7 days, because man is both the definitive and intermediate host in the life cycle of this parasite. Onchospheres develop in the jejunal villi and cysticercoids emerge into the intestinal lumen some 4 days later, and there is a stage when the onchospheres have no drug contact, so that a 7-day treatment is optimal. Niclosamide given at a dosage of 60–80 mg/kg for 5 days repeated after 10 days if necessary, is regarded by many as the treatment of choice (Muller, 1975). A generally accepted dose for all but young children is 2 g on day 1, given as described, followed by 1 g on days 2–7, with proportionately less drug being given to young children.

Few undesirable side effects have been reported after treatment, but such symptoms may include malaise, fever, abdominal discomfort or pain, lightheadedness, and pruritus. There are virtually no contraindications to the use of niclosamide and it has been administered to both debilitated and pregnant patients (Gönnert and Schraufstätter, 1960).

Niclosamide represented a major advance in the treatment of cestodiasis. Since it is a taeniacide, follow-up is usually carried out by continued observation of the stools for proglottids over a period of 3–4 months, although it has been recorded that a purge given soon after niclosamide will often produce the scolex (Wright, 1964; Ahkamri and Hadjian, 1969), quoted by Davis (1973). F. Biagi (personal communication), quoted by Webbe (1967), working in Mexico, reported the recovery of intact tapeworms (*T. saginata* and *T. solium*) after therapy using niclosamide, without purgation, and observed that the segments were apparently undamaged.

3.3.3. Paromomycin

Paromomycin sulfate is an antibiotic produced by *Streptomyces rimosus* var. *paromomycinus*. It is not absorbed to any extent from the GI tract, and the nature of its effect on tapeworms is unknown.

3.3.3a. Dosage. Botero (1970), treating *T. saginata* and *T. solium* infections, used two dosage schedules of paromomycin: 40 mg/kg for 5 days in 15 patients and a single dose of 75 mg/kg (max 4 g) in another 15 patients. One treatment failure was reported in each group, and side effects were less common when a single dose was given. Garin *et al.* (1970) tested four oligosaccharide antibiotics in patients infected with *T. saginata* and paromomycin was found to be the most effective curing all 20 patients. Abo-Shady (1980) treated 24 patients with *H. nana* infections using 40 mg/kg per day for 7 days, and obtained a 100% cure rate.

Diarrhea and abdominal pain were commonly reported, and nausea, vomiting, and dizziness were infrequent; one episode of epistasis occurred. Davis (1973) states that the manufacturers' literature cites 273 patients treated with an estimated cure rate of 85%, but in very few cases were scolices recovered. Davis considered that there is little doubt that paramomycin is effective in taeniasis, but its further use would seem to be limited because of the availability of alternative highly effective drugs, the length of treatment required and the frequency of side effects.

3.3.4. Praziquantel

Praziquantel, a new type of acylated isoquinoline-pyrazine, was found highly effective as a single oral or subcutaneous dose against juvenile and adult cestodes (*Hymenolepis* spp.) in mice and rats. It is also effective against cestodes in the bile duct. The onset of the effect of praziquantel *in vivo* is rapid, and within 10 min the parasites are immobilized and contracted, being excreted within a few hours in feces (Thomas and Gönnert, 1977).

3.3.4a. Pharmacology. Praziquantel is rapidly absorbed after oral dosage and, after a marked first-pass biotransformation process, metabolites are excreted mainly in the urine. Maximum serum concentrations are reached in healthy volunteers, in 1–2 hr. Using ^{14}C-labeled praziquantel with an isotope-measuring technique and a specific gas chromatogrphic assay, the elimination half-life of the drug from the serum was $1-1\frac{1}{2}$ hr, and that for praziquantel together with metabolites was 4–5 hr. The renal elimination half-life for praziquantel, together with metabolites, was 4–6 hr, and the cumulative renal excretion of praziquantel within 4 days was more than 80% of the dose, 90% of which was eliminated on the first day (Bühring *et al.*, 1978; Leopold *et al.*, 1978).

Praziquantel is generally well tolerated; early clinical trials produced no changes of biological significance in a series of hematological and biochemical monitoring tests or in serial ECGs or EEGs. Side effects of treatments are generally mild and disappear within 24 hr, and all trials to date have confirmed the absence of toxic effects of the drug on vital organs, systems, and functions. The most frequent symptoms reported are epigastric pain or diffuse abdominal discomfort, nausea, anorexia, loose stools or diarrhea, dizziness, headache, pruritus or urticarial-type skin eruptions, and fever. The proportion of those patients complaining of side effects has been noted to vary with the ethnic origin of the patients. Abdominal pain has occurred in up to 50% of some series but is generally mild and is only rarely accompanied by vomiting (Davis, 1982). Clearly, praziquantel is a major chemotherapeutic advance, being well tolerated with no significant effect on liver, renal, hematopoietic, or other body functions, and is highly effective against a wide range of human and animal cestode and trematode parasites.

3.3.4b. Dosage. In clinical trials, single oral doses of 15–25 mg/kg resulted in parasitological cures of more than 90% of patients infected with *H. nana*. Vacuolization of the tegument of the neck region, showing the direct effect of praziquantel in *H. nana* was reported by Becker *et al.* (1980). Given after breakfast, the drug was well tolerated and was generally considered superior in efficacy to niclosamide. It is highly effective in a single dose of 10 mg/kg against *T. saginata* and *T. solium* (Espejo, 1977; Groll, 1980; Baranski *et al.*, 1980; Schenone, 1980; Rim *et al.*, 1978, 1979). Studies have also shown that praziquantel is as effective as niclosamide against *Diphyllobothrium* infections in man in a single dose of 5–10 mg/kg body weight (Bylund *et al.*, 1977; Lumbreras *et al.*, 1982).

4. TREATMENT OF *TAENIA SOLIUM* INFECTIONS

Patients harboring *T. solium* may possibly develop cysticerocis from "internal autoinfection" (Leukart, 1856). It is therefore considered imperative by many workers that the adult worm be specifically diagnosed early and the worm recovered as soon as possible. The treatment of *T. solium* infection is therefore of special concern because of the risks of cysticercosis associated with proglottid destruction and egg dissemination (Webbe, 1967).

The available drugs include the older so-called taeniafuge compounds, such as male fern or acridine compounds associated with nausea and vomiting, resulting in regurgitation of gravid segments into the gastroduodenal area, subsequent digestion with egg hatching and onchospheral penetration, and development of cysticercosis; and the newer taeniacidal compounds, such as dichlorophen, niclosamide, and praziquantel, which may lead to destruction of gravid segments in the GI tract, and since no taeniacides are ovicidal, an increased risk of cysticercosis developing either through internal autoinfection or as a result of viable eggs being transferred from anus to mouth with subsequent infection. Observations on hatching of ova and activation of the onchospheres of *T. solium* and *T. saginata* were carried out by Gönnert *et al.* (1967) confirming the necessity of an initial peptic digestive process followed by tryptic digestion, for the successful hatching and activation of most onchospheres.

Abrams *et al.* (1963) drew attention to the fact that the lethal action of niclosamide does not extend to the ova contained within the tapeworm segments and considered that this meant that in *T. solium* cases following digestion of dead segments viable ova might be liberated in the lower intestine in large numbers and, therefore, increase the risk of cysticercosis. These authors pointed out however that this is not a contraindication to niclosamide therapy, but in their opinion it does make it mandatory that a powerful purge be given after treatment with niclosamide in order to clear the bowel of all dead segments before they can be digested.

Mody (1964) advocated the use of male fern extract and warned against the use of mepacrine, which may cause nausea with the risk of regurgitation of worm segments into the stomach and, therefore, a possible danger of cysticercosis. Mody also warned against the use of dichlorophen and niclosamide, as both cause destruction of ripe segments within the gut, liberating ova that may find their way to the patient's mouth by way of contaminated fingers, and leading to the development of cysticercosis. Wright (1964) commented that Mody (1964) had rightly drawn attention to the danger of cysticercosis from vomiting induced by mepacrine in the treatment of *T. solium*, but considered that it is doubtful that the passage of ova liberated in the intestine by digestion of worm segments by niclosamide is a real hazard.

The major concerns associated with the use of the new taeniacides against *T. solium* are therefore prevention of vomiting and ensuring the rapid expulsion of disintegrated segments from the gut. Davis (1973) commented that the advent of numerous antiemetics has reduced the probability of vomiting to a remote occurrence, and these drugs usually have the property of inducing drowsiness, a useful adjunct, while post-treatment purgation will remove disintegrating segments and, in some patients, the scolex of the worm may be identified.

The benzimidazole compound, mebendazole, has been reported as effective in the treatment of *T. solium* at a dosage of 300 mg twice daily for 3 days (Pēna-Chavarria *et al.*, 1977). The pharmacology of this compound is discussed together with treatment for hydatidosis.

5. TREATMENT OF HUMAN CYSTICERCOSIS

5.1. Praziquantel

During the past 8 years, it has been shown that praziquantel is effective against the cysticerci of numerous species of cestodes, both *in vitro* and in experimental and natural infections, including the larvae of *Taenia solium* (formerly *Cysticercus cellulosae*) in pigs (Thomas, 1977; Chavarria and Gonzalez, 1978; Thomas *et al.*, 1981).

Clinical trials have shown that praziquantel at a dosage of 25 mg/kg body weight daily for 3 or 4 days is effective in destroying cysticerci, including those in the brain, but the course must be repeated in some cases (Rim *et al.*, 1979; Botero and Castaño, 1981, 1982). The side effects directly attributable to the drug were usually mild and reversible. In cases of cerebral cysticercosis, however, more severe side effects have been recorded that may be minimized by administration of corticosteroids during the course of treatment. Fatalities have also been recorded.

Groll (1981) summarized the results of multicenter clinical trials in Mexico, Colombia, Chile, Brazil, and Korea. The investigators were in substantial agreement about diagnostic procedures, including computer tomography (CT), immunodiagnostic monitoring of treatments, and special neurological examinations. A total of 192 patients were treated; the results were evaluated in 172 cases, the duration of the observation period being too short to allow full evaluation in the other 20 patients. The death of parasites in the CNS as a result of treatment with praziquantel can be related to inflamatory reactions of the surrounding brain tissue, with serious consequences that include perifocal vasogenic edema and endocranial hypertension.

Spina-Franca *et al.* (1981) compared four different praziquantel dosage schemes. In the first three groups, the treatment was repeated with a 1-month interval between the two courses. These investigators concluded that the evaluation of the treatment results greatly depends on the duration of the observation period. Since only 21 of these 40 patients satisfied this requirement, the remaining 10 were evaluated only in relationship to their tolerance of the drug. Robles (1981) treated 100 patients suffering from neurocysticercosis, giving them 50 mg/kg of praziquantel per day divided into three equal doses, for a period of 15 days; 50 patients received additional treatment with dexamethasone. In Chile, Brinck *et al.* (1980) treated nine patients with 25 mg/kg of praziquantel per day, divided into three daily doses, for a period of 6 days. Botero and Castaño (1981, 1982) in Colombia treated 21 patients with praziquantel, administering 30 mg/kg per day in three doses for 6 days and repeated this course after 1–2 months. At the same time, the patients received prednisolone at a dose of 10 mg three times a day, with administration begun 1 day before treatment with praziquantel and continuing for up to 3 days after stopping the latter.

As regards CT scan, in most cases the investigators encountered cysticerci in various stages of development, even in one and the same patient. Most of the cysts and the low-density areas disappeared after the praziquantel treatment, while the calcified lesions remained unchanged. No significant changes were observed in the pictures of hydrocephalus before and after treatment. In cases of multiple cysticercosis the size of the ventricles was found to have decreased as a result of edema. On the other hand, in patients whose cysts showed a mass effect, there was a displacement of the ventricular system, sometimes accompanied by hydrocephalus.

Groll (1981) comments that CT permits an appreciation of the state of the cysticerci before and after the treatment, though up to now it has not been possible to establish a clear correlation between the improvement in the patient's clinical condition and the persistence or disappearance of single or multiple cysts. There have been cases of clinical cures with cysticerci still visible, and of the disappearance of the cysticerci with persistence of the clinical manifestations.

Special mention should be made of the observations made by Robles (1981), who found varying degrees of hyperglycemia in 33 of 100 neurocysticercosis patients treated with praziquantel. This hyperglycaemia was benign in character, lasted while the drug was being administered, and disappeared thereafter, except in one case in which the patient was a diabetic, when the symptoms continued for 5 months after the end of the praziquantel treatment. This hyperglycemic effect was detected only in the series of 100 patients treated by Robles (1981) with 50 mg/day of praziquantel for 15 consecutive days, and not in the 92 patients treated by the other investigators, most of whom used smaller doses and administered them for a shorter time.

An analysis of the praziquantel doses used by various investigators shows that even doses as low as 5–10 mg/kg per day can produce a good effect (Gómez and Mehia, 1980; Gómez *et al.*, 1981), although it is impossible to predict which patient will respond to low doses and which to higher doses. The highest daily doses ranged from 50 to 75 mg/kg and were generally well tolerated. Except for the transitory hyperglycemia found in a group of patients treated with 50 mg/kg per day, a dose characteristic for more than one-half the patients, the side effects observed were not greatly different from those recorded at the other doses used.

Groll (1981) holds that the recommended dose of praziquantel for future cases of neurocysticercosis should be 50 mg/kg per day, divided into three equal administrations, given for 10–14 days. The relatively high proportion of patients who show manifestations of intolerance during the first week makes it imperative to evaluate this parameter in greater depth in future investigations. He further commented that the treatment of neurocysticercosis with praziquantel may possibly replace or reinforce the effects of surgery in a certain percentage of cases. Brinck *et al.* (1980) observed that, of four patients treated with praziquantel and subjected to ventriculoatrial derivation, the valves were functioning and in good condition, suggesting that the drug may well contribute in some way to preventing valve obstruction. Moreover, Groll (1981) believes that praziquantel may be useful in cases in which the cysticerci cannot be extirpated surgically and should be considered whenever surgery is impossible or symptomatic medical treatments are ineffective.

Sotelo *et al.* (1984) reported the treatment of 26 patients with cysticercosis of the brain parenchyma, using praziquantel (50 mg/kg body weight daily for 15 days). A marked inflammatory reaction occurred with increased protein and cells being found in cerebrospinal fluid (CSF). It is reported that, after 3 months, all patients had improved clinically and 13 were asymptomatic. The total number of cysts on CT scans decreased from 152, noted at the beginning of treatment, to 51, the mean diameter of cysts being reduced by 72%.

5.2. Metrifonate

The use of metrifonate has also been reported for the treatment of cysticercosis (Trujillo-Valdés *et al.*, 1981). Metrifonate is an organophosphorous ester that inhibits plasma and erythrocyte acetylcholinesterases in various species at different dose levels. Metrifonate is readily absorbed in the digestive tract, metabolized in the liver, and excreted in the urine. It is widely used in the treatment of *Schistosoma haematobium* infection.

Trujillo-Valdés *et al.* (1981) obtained satisfactory results following oral treatments with metrifonate at 7.5 mg/kg of body weight, daily after breakfast for 5 consecutive days. Cholinergic side effects of the medication were minimized by giving 1 mg of atropine sulfate 30 min before each meal (the dose for children weighing below 40 kg being 0.5 mg) over the 5 days of treatment. The procedure was repeated six times at 2-week intervals. The administration of anticonvulsants and analgesic agents was not suspended during metrifonate treatment. Satisfactory results were obtained in approximately 80% of 100 cases treated and followed for periods of 6 months to 10 years. Trujillo-Valdés and co-workers believe that despite the fact that the disease occasionally remains silent even without treatment, evidence of clinical improvements in the treated patients after chemotherapy together with an increase in negative immunological responses and definite changes in the CT scans suggests that the drug acts directly on the parasite.

Ridaura (1982), however, concluded following extensive general discussion, that there were deficiencies in the methodology used in all the clinical studies reported for both praziquantel and metrifonate, at that time attributable to differences in evaluation criteria, lack of controls, and subjective evaluations. It seems that chemotherapy cannot yet be justified in all cases of human neurocysticercosis; there is an urgent need to intensify research that will define guidelines for the use of such therapy.

5.3. Flubendazole

On the basis of their preliminary observations on *T. solium* cysticerci in swine, Tellez-Giron *et al.* (1984) used flubendazole in 13 human volunteers with neurocysticercosis. The dosage used was 20 mg/kg bid for 10 days. Clinical improvement was observed in all but one patient. Computer tomography indicated a reduction in the size of some cysts and the disappearance of cysts in two patients. The treatment lowered antibody levels and was well tolerated. The concurrent use of corticosteroids in some patients did not appear to affect the result of treatment. The results suggest that further trials with flubendazole are warranted.

6. TREATMENT OF HUMAN HYDATIDOSIS

During the past 5 years, studies have been made of the efficacy of drugs of the benzimidazole carbamate group (including mebendazole, flubendazole, albendazole, and fenbendazole) against the larval stages of *Echinococcus* spp. which cause hydatidosis (Schantz *et al.*, 1982; Roche *et al.*, 1982).

6.1. Pharmacology

Absorption from the GI tract of mebendazole is minimal; plasma levels were found to be highest at 2–4 hr, but the mean percentage of the administered dose was less than 0.3%. The bulk of ^{14}C-labeled drug was excreted unchanged in the feces in 24 hr in two volunteers and within 48 hr in another subject. A small proportion of the drug was excreted as the decarboxylated derivative of mebendazole, some 5–10% of the dose being excreted in the urine. The rapid excretion of the drug, its route of excretion, and the very low plasma levels indicate that there is probably no recirculation by an enterohepatic shunt (Brugmans *et al.*, 1971, cited by Davis, 1973).

6.2. Dosage

Bryceson *et al.* (1982) treated patients with inoperable hydatid disease, with high doses of oral mebendazole, up to 200 mg/kg per day for 16–48 weeks. Toxicity was not encountered but, despite careful assessment, it proved difficult to critically evaluate the efficacy of the treatments. Failure of mebendazole therapy was reported in a series of 16 cases of hepatic hydatidosis in Kenya (Okello and Chemtai, 1981).

In reviewing these drugs, with special references to albendazole, Morris (1983) recommends that, until longer-term results are available, the young patient with uncomplicated hydatid and pulmonary cysts would be better advised to undergo surgery. Albendazole may produce regression of cysts, but it is teratogenic and embryotoxic in experimental animals (Morris *et al.*, 1983). These workers found that the serum concentrations of albendazole were some 100 times better than would be expected with the same dose of mebendazole. They found that mebendazole appears to check proliferation and spread of hydatid cysts but does not terminate infection in experimentally infected *Meriones unguiculatus*. The host reaction to the dead or dying parasite may also be severe (Murray-Lyon and Reynolds, 1979).

Eckert (1985) recorded that *E. granulosus* in rodents and sheep can be severely damaged or killed by long-term treatment with high oral doses (30–50 mg/kg body weight per day) of mebendazole, flubendazole, or fenbendazole. In contrast similar drug treatment of the metacestode stage of *E. multilocularis* in rodents is not parasiticidal, but parasite proliferation is inhibited and the formation of metastases can be prevented.

Bircher (1985) discussed the pharmacokinetics and pharmacodynamics of mebendazole in the treatment of patients with echinococcosis, including important adverse reactions to the drug. The latter included leucopenia, drug-induced hepatitis, and glomerulonephritis.

Pawlowski (1985) recorded the results of WHO multicenter clinical studies on the treatment of human echinococcosis with benzimidazole carbamates. Treatment with mebendazole was considered to be fully successful in 8 out of 85 patients and partially successful in 4 others, with multiple localization of *E. granulosus* cysts. The maximum daily dose of mebendazole was between 3.0 and 4.9 g in the majority of patients (72.9%); it was below 3.0 g in 12.9% and above 5.0 g daily in 14.1% of cases. Patients were generally treated for 3 months. Flubendazole was effective only in one case of lung echinococcosis but not in 5 patients with liver or other organ localizations, using a fixed daily dose of 1.5–4.0 g.

Treatment with albendazole was fully successful in 5 out of 30 patients and partially successful in 4 others, given in a daily dose of 0.8 g in adults and 0.25 g or 0.4 g in children. It was used in treatment cycles of 30 days and repeated two or three times with 2-week breaks between. It is considered that the success of treatment with these benzimidazole carbamates depended much upon the localization of the cyst(s). In patients treated with mebendazole, successful results were observed in 21.4% of lung echinococcosis cases, only 7% of liver echinococcosis cases and 6.9% of cases with other localizations (e.g., bone, peritoneum, spleen). Albendazole was successful in three out of four lung echinococcosis cases, in 21.1% of liver echinococcosis cases, and in 16.7% of cases with other localizations. Successful treatment was indicated by disappearance or significant decrease in the size of *E. granulosus* cysts and/or distinct changes in cyst(s) morphology seen by X-ray, ultrasound, and/or CT examination. In patients with multiple localization partial success was assessed if the treatment was successful in one organ but not in the other.

A further 54 patients with *E. multilocularis* infections were treated with mebendazole in clinical centers in Anchorage, Besançon, and Zürich. Thirty-six of these had undergone previous surgery. The usual daily doses of mebendazole were 3, 4, or 4.5 g. Only 10 patients were treated with mebendazole and observed for less than 1 year; 22 patients were treated and observed for 1 or 2 years and another 22 patients for 3–12 years. Among the 54 patients there were 4 deaths reported (3 within 2 years and 1 after 10 years), and 8 cases in which the infection progressed despite mebendazole treatment. In the majority of patients (70.4%), however, the condition was stabilized and improvements in clinical status and in the titres of serological tests were frequent. A definite reduction in the lesion size was observed in only 4 patients. These coordinated studies have confirmed that mebendazole therapy may arrest the development of *E. multilocularis* in man, irrespective of surgery. A further 20 patients with *E. multilocularis* infection have commenced treatments with albendazole, but it is too early to evaluate the results. It is clear that, while these drugs offer some promise, more investigations are necessary.

7. TREATMENT OF LESS COMMON CESTODE INFECTIONS

Bertiella studeri. Most infections reported have been in children and generally provoke no marked symptoms or digestive disorders (Thompson *et al.*, 1967). Niclosamide and other anthelmintics have been used successfully for treatment (Shoura and Morsy, 1974; Dissanaike *et al.*, 1977).

Inermicapsifer madagascariensis. Niclosamide has been successfully used for treatment (Horstmann *et al.*, 1978; Hira, 1975).

Mesocestoides sp. Niclosamide, quinacrine, and paromomycin have been used to treat these infections (Gleason *et al.*, 1973; Hutchinson and Martin, 1980).

Raillietina celebensis. The mild symptoms reported disappeared after treatment with niclosamide (Rougier *et al.*, 1981).

Dipylidium caninum. Treatment is essentially the same as that recommended for other tapeworm infections, including use of niclosamide or quinacrine (Jones, 1979). During a period of 5 years in the United States, 43 patients were treated successfully with niclosamide at a dosage of 2 g in a single dose for adults; 1.5 g for children weighing >34 kg; and 1 g for children weighing 11–34 kg (Jones, 1979, cited by Beaver *et al.*, 1984).

8. CONCLUSIONS

During the past 20 years, niclosamide has unquestionably been established as the drug of first choice in the treatment of *T. saginata*, *D. latum* and *H. nana* infections in man. It has also been widely and successfully used for *T. solium* infections, but with regrettably far too few positive diagnoses. Inevitably its use for this purpose has continued the controversy with regard to use of taeniacidal compounds, and the possible enhanced risk of developing cysticercosis through autoinfection.

It is unfortunate that bunamidine hydrochloride, which is so effective against large tapeworms of other mammalian species, produces such cardiotoxic and marked neuromuscular effects as to preclude its use in human medicine. Clearly praziquantel is the latest major chemotherapeutic advance in the treatment of human cestodiasis. This taeniacidal compound will certainly compete favorably with niclosamide, but it may be too costly for use in many countries. The use of this compound for treatment of human cysticercosis, and in particular neurocysticercosis, requires further study in order to standardize treatment schedules and evaluation criteria in establishing acceptable guidelines for administration.

The benzimidazole carbamate group of drugs holds some promise for the treatment of hydatidosis, but further investigations are indicated. There is little information about the potential dangers to the host that may arise through the release of antigenic substances from degenerating cysts. Keeling (1968) commented that in both cysticerocis and hydatidosis, a large amount of parasitic material may be present; the risks of releasing substantial quantities of potentially pharmacologically active materials must be considered in advocating the use of chemotherapy.

The special hazards of human infection associated with *E. granulosus* continue to lend emphasis to the need for a compound with good ovicidal activity. A substance that could kill adult cestodes and their eggs would also be invaluable in the treatment of *T. solium* infection as a further safeguard against autoinfection.

REFERENCES

Abo-Shady, A. F., 1980, Paromomycin sulfate in *Hymenolepiasis nana, J. Egypt. Soc. Parasitol.* 10:381–385.

Abrams, G. J., Setfel, H. C., and Heinz, J. J., 1963, The treatment of human tapeworm infections with Yomesan, *S. Afr. Med. J.* 37:6–8.

Adams, A. R. D., and Seaton, D. R., 1959, Treatment of *Taenia saginata* infection with Dichlorophen (Demonstration), *Trans. R. Soc. Trop. Med. Hyg.* 53:5.

Ahkami, S., and Hadjian, A., 1969, The appearance of the scolex of *Taenia saginata* in the stool after the eradication of the parasite by niclosamide, *Z. Tropenmed. Parasitol.* 20:341–345 (in German).

Alterio, D. L., 1968, Tratamento das teniases humans por *T. solium* e *T. saginata* con extrato etéreo de feto machointroduzido através da entubacão duodenal, *Rev. Hosp. Clin. Fac. Med. Univ. Sao Paulo* 23:150–152.

Baldwin, E., 1943, An *in vitro* method for chemotherapeutic investigation of anthelmintic potency, *Parasitology*, 35:89–111.

Baranski, M. C., 1981, Treatment of Dermal Cysticercosis with praziquantel, Paper read at workshop: Praziquantel in Human Cysticercosis, Mexico City, April 25–26, 1981.

Batham, E. J., 1946, Testing arecoline hydrobromide as an anthelmintic for hydatid worms in dogs, *Parasitology* 37:185–191.

Beaver, P. C., Jung, R. C., and Cupp, E. W., 1984, *Clinical Parasitology* 9th ed., pp. 488–543, Lea & Febiger, Philadelphia.

Becker, B., Mehlhorn, H., Andrews, P., and Thomas, H., 1980, Scanning and transmission electron microscope studies on the efficacy of praziquantel on *Hymenolepis nana* (Cestoda) *in vitro, Z. Parasitkd.* 61:121–133.

Beier, A., 1963, Die *Taenia saginata* Infection unde ihre Behandlung mit Acranil und Yomesan, *M.M.W.* 105:2075–2083.

Beier, A., 1965a, Zur Wirkung des Akridin-Derivatas Acranil auf Bandwurmer (*Taenia saginata*), *Z. Tropenmed. Parasitol.* 16:433–436.

Beier, A., 1965b, Zur Behandlung der Bandwurminfektion während der Schwangershaft und im Wochenbett, *Med. Welt. (Stuttg.)* 2:2933–2937.

Beier, A., 1966, Therapeutische Erfahrungen mit Yomesan bei menschlichen Bandwurminfektionen, *Z. Tropenmed. Parasitol.* 17:50–57.

Bircher, J., 1985, Clinical Pharmacology of Benzimidazole Anthelmintics Administered for Systemic Effects, Proceedings of XIII Congresco Internacional de Hidatidologia, pp. 348–350. Madrid, Spain.

Bojanowicz, K., and Peitrowa, R., 1968, Aktunulne leki przeciw pasoyztom przewodu pokarmowego i ich uboczne Dzailanie, *Wiad. Parazytol.* 14:303–311.

Botero, D. R., 1970, Paromomycin as effective treatment of *Taenia* infections, *Am. J. Trop. Med. Hyg.* 19:234–237.

Botero, D., and Castaño, S., 1981, Cisticercosis: Tratamiento con praziquantel, *Trib. Med. Colomb.* 63:31–36.

Botero, D., and Castaño, S., 1982, Treatment of cysticercosis with praziquantel in Colombia, *Am. J. Trop. Med. Hyg.* 31:810–821.

Brinck, G., Schenone, H., Diaz, V., Parra, M., and Corrales, M., 1980, Neurocisticercosis. Tratamiento con praziquantel. Estiudio preliminar, *Bol. Chil. Parasitol.* 35:66–71.

Bühring, K. U., Diekmann, H. W,, Muller, H., Garbe, A., and Nowak, H., 1978, Metabolism of praziquantel in man, *Eur. Metab. Pharmacokinet.* 1:179–190.

Bylund, B. G., Bang, B., and Wikgreen, K., 1977, Tests with a new compound (praziquantel) against *Diphyllobothrium latum, J. Helminthol.* 51:115–119.

Bryceson, A. D. M., Cowie, A. G. A., Macleod, C., White, S., Edwards, D., Smyth, J. D., and McManus, D. P., 1982, Experience with mebendazole in the treatment of inoperable hydatid disease in England, *Trans. R. Soc. Trop. Med. Hyg.* 76(4):510–518.

Campbell, W. C., and Blair, L. S., 1974a, Prevention and cure of hepatic cysticercosis in mice, *J. Parasitol.* 60:1049–1052.

Campbell, W. C., and Blair, L. S., 1974b, Treatment of the cystic stage of *Taenia crassiceps* and *Echinococcus multilocularis* in laboratory animals, *J. Parasitol.* 60:1053–1054.

Chavarria, M., and Gonzalez, D. D., 1978, Droncit en al tratamiento de la Cisticercosis Porcina. *Esp. Vet.* 1:159–165.

Chevis, R. A. F., Kelly, J. D., and Griffen, D. L., 1980, The lethal effect of closantel on the metacestodes of *Taenia pisiformis* in rabbits, *Parasitology* 7:333–337.

Culbertson, J. T., and Greenfield, S. H., 1941, Effect of atebrine upon experimental cysticercosis of mice, *J. Pharmacol. Exptl. Therap.* 73:159–161.

Dadlez, J., Gerwel, Cz., and Kaminski, A., 1954, Zastozowanie mieszaniny cyny metalicznej i jej zwizaków w kuracji przeciwtasiemcowej, *Acta Parasitol.* 2:239–245.

Davis, A., 1973, Drug treatment in intestinal helminthiases. Part II. Drugs for cestodiasis, *WHO,* Geneva, pp. 95–111.

Davis, A., 1982, Management of the patient with schistosomiasis. In: "Schistosomiasis: Epidemiology, Treatment and Control", (P. Jordan and G. Webbe, eds.), Heinemann Medical Books, London, pp. 184–226.

de Rivas, D., 1932, Intestinal parasitism. Diagnosis and treatment, *Am. J. Trop. Med. Hyg.* 12:477–492.

Dissanaike, A. S., Thomas, V., and Nagappan, N., 1977, *Bertiella studeri* (Blanchard, 1891) Stiles and Hassall, 1902, infection in a child—first case from Malasia, *Southeast Asian J. Trop. Med. Publ. Health* 8:421–422.

Ditzel, J., and Schwartz, M., 1967, Worm cure without tears. The effect of niclosamide on taeniasis saginata in man, *Acta Med. Scand.* 182:663–664.

Dodion, L., 1962, Nouvelles recherches dans le traitement de la taeniase. Étude pharmacologique et clinique du dryaspidon, *Ann. Soc. Belg. Med. Trop.* 42:683–695.

Donkaster, R., Donoso, F., Atias, A., Faiguenbaum, J., and Jarpa, A., 1961, Trial therapy of taeniasis with a derivative of salicylamide (Yomesan Bayer). (Preliminary note.), *Bol. Chil. Parasitol.* 16:4–6 (in Spanish).

Doroschchak, O. F., and Kitel, V. S., 1968, Side effects in application of phenasal and dichlorophene, *Med. Parazitol. (Moskva)* 37:110.

Dufek, M., and Kalivoda, R., 1969, Experience with modern treatment of taeniasis, *Rev. Czech. Med.* 15:29–32.

Duguid, A. M. E., and Heathcote, R. St. A., 1950a, The action of drugs *in vitro* on cestodes: I. Anthelmintics, *Arch. Intern. Pharmacodyn.* 82:309–330.

Duguid, A. M. E., and Heathcote, R. St. A., 1950b, The action of drugs *in vitro* on cestodes: II. Nonanthelmintic drugs, *Arch. Intern. Pharmacodyn.* 84:159–175.

Eckert, J., 1985, Chemotherapy of Experimental Echinococcosis as a basis for trials in humans, Proceedings of XIII Congresco Internacional de Hidatidologia, pp. 343–345, Madrid, Spain.

Espejo, H., 1977, Tratiemento de infecciones por *Hymenolepis nana, Taenia solium* y *Diphyllobothrium pacificum* con praziquantel, *Bol. Chil. Parasitol.* 32:39–40.

Garin, J. P., Kalb, J. C., Despeignes, J., and Vincent, G., 1970, Action des antibiotiques oligo-saccharides sur *Taenia saginata, J. Parasitol.* 56:112.

Gherman, I., 1968, Observations sur le traitement du téniasis par le N-2'-chloro-4'-nitrophénil-5-chloro-salicyl amide, *Bull. Soc. Pathol. Exot.* 61:432–434.

Gleason, N. N., Kornblum, R., and Walzer, P., 1973, *Mesocestoides* (Cestoda) in a child in New Jersey treated with niclosamide (Yomesan), *Am. J. Trop. Med. Hyg.* 30:620–624.

Gómez, J. G., and Mehia, A., 1980, Tratamiento de la neurocisticercosis con praziquantel, *Neurologia Col.* 5:503–509.

Gómez, J. G., Peña, G., Patiño, R., and Pradilla, G., 1981, Neurocysticercosis in Colombia, Paper read at workshop: Praziquantel in human cysticercosis, Mexico City, April 25–26, 1981.

Gönnert, R., 1968, Experimental and clinical experiences with Yomesan, *Int. Congr. Trop. Med. Malaria* 8:1088–1089 (abst.).

Gönnert, R., and Schraufstätter, E., 1960, Experimentelle Untersuchungen mit N(2'-chloro-4'-nitrophényl)-5-chlorsalicylamic, einem neuen Bandwormittel. I. Mitteilung; Chemotherapeutische Versuche, *Arzneimittelforsch.* 10:881–884.

Gönnert, R., Meister, G., Strufe, R., and Webbe, G., 1967, Biologische Probleme bei *Taenia solium, Z. Tropenmed. Parasitol.* 18:76–81.

Groll, E., 1980, Praziquantel for cestode infections in man, *Acta Trop.* 37:293–296.

Groll, E., 1981, Human cysticercosis and praziquantel: A survey of first clinical experience, *Bol. Chil. Parasitol.* 36:29–37.

Hänel, L., 1950, Betrag sur Toxikologie der gebrauchlichsten Anthelminthica, *Pharmazie* 5:18–23.

Heath, D. D., and Chevis, R. A. F., 1974, Mebendazole and hydatid cysts, *Lancet* 2:218–219.

Heath, D. D., Christie, M. J., and Chevis, R. A. F., 1975, The lethal effect of mebendazole on secondary *Echinococcus granulosus*, cysticerci of *Taenia pisiformis*, and tetrathyridia of *Mesocestoides corti, Parasitology* 70:273–285.

Hira, P. R., 1975, Human and rodent infection with the cestode *Inermicapsifer madagascariensis* (Davaine, 1870) Baer, 1956, in Zambia, *Ann. Soc. Belg. Med. Trop.* 55:321–325.

Horstmann, R., Bienzle, U., Kern, P., and Voelker, J., 1978, Tapeworm infestation with *Inermicapsifer madagascariensis. Tropenmed. Parasitol.* 29:406–408.

Hutchison, W. F., and Martin, J. B., 1980, *Mesocestoides* (Cestoda) in a child in Mississippi treated with paromomycin sulfate (Humatin), *Am. J. Trop. Med. Hyg.* 29:478–479.

Jones, W. E., 1979, Niclosamide as a treatment for *Hymenolepis diminuta* and *Diplidium canium* infection in man, *Am. J. Trop. Med. Hyg.* 28:300–302.

Keeling, J. E. D., 1968, The chemotherapy of cestode infections, in: *Advances in Chemotherapy*, pp. 109–152, (A. Goldin, F. Hawking, and R. J. Schnitzer, eds.), Vol. 3, Academic Press, New York.

Khalil, H. M., 1969, Treatment of cestode infections with Radeverm, *Trans. R. Soc. Trop. Med. Hyg.* 63:76–78.

Krotov, A. I., and Rusak, L. V., 1964, II. Experimental investigation of Acriquine with novocaine, *Medskaya Parazitol. (Moskva)* 33:408–411 (in Russian).

Krotov, A. I., Prokopenko, L. I., and Bekhli, A. F., 1968, Treatment of *Taenia saginata, Hymenolepis* and *Diphyllobothrium* infections with Phenasal and Dichlosal, pp. 1135–1137, in: *Eighth International Congress of Tropical Medicine Malaria, Teheran, Sept. 7–15, 1968*, Abstract and review.

Krotov, A. I., Tchernaev, A. I., Kovalenko, F. P., Bajandina, D. G., Budanova, I. C., Kuznetsova, O. E., and Voskoboinik, L. V., 1974, Experimental therapy of alveococcosis, *Med. Parazitol. (Mosk.)* 43:314–319. (in Russian with English summary).

Lagrange, E., 1946, A propos de l'action toxique de quelques colorants organiques sur *Cysticercus pisiformis, Compt. Rend. Soc. Biol.* 140:1129,

Lassance, M., Peeters, E., and Grailet, L., 1957, Note sur un taenifuge de masse nouveau, l'Anthiphen, *Ann. Soc. Belg. Med. Trop.* 37:627–630.

Leopold, G., Ungethuem, W., Groll, E., Diekmann, H. W., Nowak, H., and Wegner, D. H. G., 1978, Clinical pharmacology in normal volunteers of praziquantel. A new drug against schistosome and cestodes. *Eur. J. Clin. Pharmacol.* 14:281–291.

Leukart, R., 1856, Die Blasenwurmer und ihre Entwicklung-Zugleich ein Beitrag sur Kenntnis der Cysticercus-Leber, Giessen, p. 162.

Lumbreras, H., Terashima, A., Alvarez, J., Tello, R., and Guerra, H., 1982, Single dose treatment with praziquantel (Cesol R. Embay 8440) of human cestodiasis caused by *Diphyllobothrium pacificum*, *Tropenmed. Parasitol.* 33:5–7.

Mody, V. R., 1964, Treatment of tapeworm infections, *Br. Med. J.* (Suppl. 1) 1:1184.

Morris, D. L., 1983, Chemotherapy of hydatid disease, *J. Antimicrob. Chemother.* 11:6.

Morris, D. L., Dykes, P. W., Dickson, B., Marriner, S., Bogan, J., and Burrows, F., 1983, Albendazole in hydatid disease, *Br. Med. J.* 286:103–104.

Muller, R., 1975, *Worms and Disease. A Manual of Medical Helminthology*, Heinemann Medical Books, London.

Murray-Lyon, I. M., and Reynolds, K. W., 1979, Complications of mebendazole treatment for hydatid disease. *Br. Med. J.* 2:1111–1112.

Nitzulescu, V., Simonescu, O., Lucian, O., Domănescu, N., and Gelber, A., 1962, Unsere Ergebnisse mit Wurmmitteln Yomesan zur Zestodenbehandlung, *Paediatr. Bucuresti* 11:433–441.

Okello, G. B. A., and Chemtai, A. K., 1981, Treatment of hepatic hydatid disease with mebendazole. Report of 16 cases. *East Afr. Med. J.* 58:608–610.

Pawlowski, Z. S., 1970, Inorganic tin compounds as the alternative drug in human taeniarhynchosis, *J. Parasitol.* 56:261.

Pawlowski, Z. S., 1985, Chemotherapy of Human Echinococcosus, Proceedings of the XIII Congreso Internacional de Hidatidologia, pp. 346–347, Madrid, Spain.

Pawlowski, Z., and Schultz, M. G., 1972, Taeniasis and cysticercosis, in: *Advances in Parasitology* (B. Daives, ed.), pp. 269–343, Academic Press, London and New York.

Peña Chavarria, A., Villarejos, V. M., and Zeledón, R., 1977, Mebendazole in the treatment of taeniasis solium and taeniasis saginata, *Am. J. Trop. Med. Hyg.* 26:118–120.

Perera, D. R., Western, K. A., and Schultz, M. G., 1970, Niclosamide treatment of cestodiasis, *Am. J. Trop. Med. Hyg.* 19:610–612.

Ridaura, C., 1982, Clinical aspects, pathology and treatment of human cysticercosis, in: *Cysticercosis. Present State of Knowledge and Perspectives* (A. Flisser *et al.*, eds.), pp. 227–231, Academic Press, London.

Rim, H. J., Park, C. Y., Lee, J. S., Joo, K. H., and Lyu, K. S., 1978, Therapeutic effects of praziquantel (Embay 8440) against *Hymenolepis nana* infection, *Korean J. Parasitol* 16:82–87.

Rim, H-J., Park, S-V., Lee, J. S., and Joo K-H., 1979, Therapeutic effects of praziquantel (Embay 8440) against *Taenia solium* infections, *Korean J. Parsitol.* 17:67–72.

Robles, C., 1981, Resultados preliminaires del tratamiento de la cisticercosis cerebral con praziquantel. Paper read at workshop: Praziquantel in human cysticercosis, Mexico City, April 25–26, 1981.

Roche, G., Canton, P., Gerard, A., Colin, D., Boissel, P., Chaulieu, C., and Dureux, J. B., 1982, Essai de traitement de l'echinococcose alveolaire par le flubendazole. A propos de 7 observations, *Med. Maladies Infect.* 12(4):218–230.

Rösler, O. A., 1952, Neues und altes über die Bandwurmkuren (Zugleich ein Beitrag zur akuten Magnesium sulfuricum Vergiftung bei oraler Verabreichung dieses Mittels), *Wien Klin. Wochenschr.* 64:942–945.

Ross, I. C., 1927, *In vitro* tests of toxicity of certain drugs for hydatid scolices, *Aust. J. Exp. Biol. Med. Sci.* 4:283–288.

Rougier, Y., Legros, F., Durand, J. P., and Cordoliani, Y., 1981, Four cases of parasitic infection by *Raillietina (R.) celbensis* (Kanicki, 1902) in French Polynesia, *Trans. R. Soc. Trop. Med. Hyg.* 79:121.

Schantz, P. M., Vanden Bossche, H., and Eckert, J., 1982, Chemotherapy for larval echinococcosus in animals and humans: Report of a workshop, *Z. Parasitkend.* 67:5–26.

Schenone, H., Ramirez, R., and Roja, A., 1975, Aspectos epidemiologicos de la neurocisticercosis en América Latina, *Bol. Chil. Parasit.*, 28:61–72.

Schneider, J., 1959, Traitment du taeniasis par le 5-5′-dichloro-2,2′-dihydroxy-diphénylmethane, *Therapie (Paris)* 14:63–67.

Seaton, D. R., 1960, On the use of dichlorophen as a taenifuge for *Taenia saginata*, *Ann. Trop. Med. Parasitol.* 54:338–340.

Sen, A. B., and Hawking, F., 1960, Screening of cesticidal compounds on a tapeworm *Hymenolepis nana in vitro*, *Br. J. Pharmacol.* 15:436–439.

Shoura, M. J., and Morsy, T. A., 1974, A case of *Bertiella* infection in an immigrant from Yemen, *J. Kuwait Med. Assoc.* 8:55–56.

Sotelo, J., Escobedo, F., Rodriguez-Carbajal, J., Torres, B., and Rubio-Donnadieu, F., 1984, Therapy of parenchymal brain cysticercosis with praziquantel, *N. Engl. J. Med.* 310:1001–1007.

Spina-Franca, A., Nóbrega, J. F. S., Livramento, J. A., and Machado, L. R., 1981, Administration of praziquantel in neurocysticercosis. Paper read at workshop: Praziquantel in human cysticercosis, Mexico City, April 25–26, 1981.

Standen, O. D., 1963, Chemotherapy of helminthic infections, in: *Experimental Chemotherapy,* (R. J. Schnitzer and F. Hawking, eds.), pp. 701–892, Academic Press, New York.

Tellez-Giron, E., Ramos, M. C., Dufour, L., Montante, M., Tellez, E., Rodriguez, J., Gomez Mendez, F., and Mireles, E., 1984, Treatment of neurocysticercosis with flubendazole, *Am. J. Trop. Med. Hyg.* 33:627–631.

Thienpont, D., Vanparijs, O., and Hermans, L., 1974, Anthelmintic activity of mebendazole against *Cysticercus fasciolaris, J. Parasitol.* 60:1052–1053.

Thomas, H., 1977, Resultados experimentales con praziquantel (Embay 8440) en cestodiasis y cisticercosis, *Bol. Chil. Parasitol.* 32:2–6.

Thomas, H., and Gönnert, R., 1977, The efficacy of praziquantel against cestodes in animals, *Z. Parasitkd.* 52:117–127.

Thomas, H., Andrews, P., and Mehlhorn, H., 1981, New result on the effect of praziquantel in experimental cysticercosis. Paper read at workshop: Praziquantel in human cysticercosis, Mexico City, April 25–26, 1981.

Thompson, C. D., Jelland, C. H., and Buckley, J. J. C., 1967, Human infection with a tapeworm, *Bertiella* sp., probably of African origin. *Br. Med. J.* 3:659–660.

Trujillo-Valdés, V. M., González-Barranco, D., Orozco-Bohne, R., Villaneuva-Diaz, G., and Sandoval-Islas, M. E., 1981, Experimental treatment of cysticercosis and metrifonate, *Arch. Invest. Med. (Mex)* 12:15.

Turner, P. P., 1963, The treatment of tapeworm infestation with Anthiphen, *J. Trop. Med. Hyg.* 66:259–260.

Webbe, G., 1967, The hatching and activation of taeniid ova in relation to the development of cysticercosis in man, *Z. Tropenmed. Parasitol.* 18:354–369.

Wright, F. J., 1964, Treatment of tapeworm infections, *Br. Med. J.* (Suppl.) 1:1378.

Yokogawa, M., Yoshimura, J., Okura, T., and Saito, M., 1962, Treatment of *Taenia saginata* with bithinol. *Jpn. J. Parasitol.* 11:39–44 (in Japanese).

24

Cestode Infections of Domestic Animals

J. H. ARUNDEL

1. INTRODUCTION

The development of cestocidal compounds has generally been neglected. Cobbold (1872) in a series of lectures to medical students gave the most important remedies as male fern, kousso, kamala, turpentine, pumpkin seeds, and pomegranate root bark. Powdered areca nut was acknowledged to be of value but lost strength quickly after crushing. In 1963, Standen listed some of these remedies as still being used in veterinary and human medicine; since then, advances have been more rapid, and none of those listed by Standen for veterinary use is now recommended.

This chapter reviews the more important compounds in use. Older remedies that have been superseded are not discussed, although a few are still used in some countries. Lead arsenate at a standard dose rate of 0.5 g per lamb or 1.0 g per sheep is used either alone or as an additive to thiabendazole. Dichlorophen was commonly used against *Taenia* spp. and *Dipylidium caninum* in dogs, results were variable, probably because it often only removed the strobilus, leaving the scolex to grow new segments during the next 2–3 weeks. This has now been superseded by more efficient drugs but is still available in mixtures with piperazine, toluene, or dithiazanine. Dibutyltin dilaurate is still used occasionally in small poultry flocks and in cage birds, although it has been replaced by niclosamide in larger flocks. Other compounds such as bithionol, mepacrine, copper sulfate, and cupric acetoarsenite are no longer used and have been adequately discussed by Gibson (1975).

On the other hand some newer compounds with cestocidal activity have not been considered. Paromomycin, the axenomycins, diuredosan (Uredofos), fospirate, and resorantel all have cestocidal activity but have not been developed for commercial use because of either insufficient activity or too small a therapeutic ratio.

The following discussion deals with those compounds used in cats and dogs, sheep and cattle, and horses and poultry. Pigs have not been considered, as they are only

---

J. H. ARUNDEL • Veterinary Clinical Centre, University of Melbourne, Werribee, Victoria, Australia 3030.

infected with one species, *Diphyllobothrium latum*. When encountered, bunamidine or praziquantel can be tried at high dose rates.

2. TAPEWORMS OF DOGS AND CATS

2.1. Introduction

Dogs, and to a lesser extent cats, are host to many species of tapeworm, some of which (*Echinococcus* spp., *Dipylidium caninum*, *Diphyllobothrium latum*, and *Spirometra erinacei*) have public health implications. The larval stages of others (*Taenia ovis*, *T. hydatigena*, *E. granulosus*, and *S. erinacei*) are a cause of economic loss because of rejection of meat or offal at the abattoirs.

Dipylidium caninum causes anal irritation as the highly motile segments are passed; the dog may demonstrate discomfort by dragging its anus along the ground (scooting), prompting the owner to seek treatment for the animal. The adults of the other species rarely cause clinical symptoms, but it is important that those species with public health implications (particularly *Echinococcus* spp.) or those causing economic loss be controlled by treatment with an effective cesticidal agent and by subsequently denying the animal access to the larval stages or to the intermediate host. If this is not possible, regular treatments at intervals less than the prepatent period of the parasite may be used to reduce the incidence of infection. The available compounds, their dose rates, and spectrum of activity are shown in Table I.

2.2. Arecoline Hydrobromide

The alkaloid, arecoline, has been used for more than 100 years in human and veterinary medicine. For many years, it was the only compound available that had activity against *Echinococcus granulosus* in the dog. Details of its use, efficacy, and toxicity have been given by Rickard and Arundel (1985). Because of its low efficiency and the severity of its action on the dog, it is no longer recommended as a therapeutic agent. Arecoline hydrobromide paralyzes *Echinococcus* and *Taenia* spp. and has strong parasympathomimetic actions, causing purgation, which removes the paralyzed worms from the bowel. This action makes arecoline a useful diagnostic agent in a control scheme. It is not sufficiently accurate for use in an individual dog but, if used on a group of dogs on a farm, it gives valuable information on whether the dogs are infected and, if so, that they have been fed improperly.

Arecoline hydrobromide is given orally as a 1.5% solution in 15% sucrose at a dose rate of 1–1.5 mg/kg. With this regimen, about 80% of dogs will purge within 2 hr, with a mean purgation time of 30 min (Forbes and Whitten, 1961). If purgation does not occur within this time, a further half-dose may be given. This drug should not be given to pregnant bitches or to pups less than 6 months of age; dogs to be dosed should be fasted for some hours and should not be given bones for the previous 2 days.

Table 1. Recommended Treatments and Their Efficacy in the Dog and Cat[a]

Compound	Dose rates (mg/kg)	Taenia spp.	D. caninum	Spirometra spp.	E. granulosus	Mesocestoides spp.
Arecoline HBr					for diagnostic use only	
Bunamidine	50	+	+	+	+[b]	+
Fenbendazole	50/3 days	±	+	−	−	−
Mebendazole	10/3 days	±	±	−	−	−
Niclosamide	100	+	V	−	−	−
Nitroscanate	50	+	+	−	−	+
Praziquantel	5	+	+	−	+	+

[a] +, high activity; −, poor activity; ±, insufficient data; V, variable activity.
[b] 50 mg/kg repeated in 48hr has high efficiency but will not remove all worms from all dogs.

Arecoline hydrobromide is not recommended for cats and, while arecoline acetarsal has been used, it is now superseded by safer and more effective compounds.

2.3. Bunamidine Hydrochloride

The introduction of bunamidine hydrochloride was a notable advance; it quickly replaced arecoline and dichlorophen for routine treatment against *Taenia* spp., *D. caninum*, *S. erinacei*, and *E. granulosus*.

Against *Taenia* spp., a single oral dose of 25–50 mg/kg was initially recommended. As efficiency against the economically important species *T. hydatigena* decreased when dose rates of <50 mg/kg were used in large-scale field trials in New Zealand (G. A. Thomson, personal communication, 1970), it is now recommended that 50 mg/kg be used routinely against all species other than *E. granulosus*.

Hatton (1965) cleared only 7 of 15 dogs infected with *D. caninum* but reported that Kingsbury had eliminated infection from 12 dogs when doses ranging from 7.5 to 25 mg/kg were given in gelatin capsules. Good results were also obtained by Hromatka *et al.* (1966), Burrows and Lillis (1966), and Roberson (1977). The compound has also been shown effective against *Spirometra mansonoides* (Burrows and Lillis, 1966), *Mesocestoides* lineatus (Hromatka *et al.*, 1966), and *M. corti* (Todd *et al.*, 1978) in dogs, and against *T. taeniaeformis* in cats (Hatton, 1965; Burrows and Lillis, 1966). It is the only compound that is highly effective against *S. erinacei* at normal dose rates.

Initial trials showed high activity against experimental infections of *E. granulosus* of all ages when given as a single oral dose at rates between 50 and 200 mg/kg. Increased activity was obtained against younger worms if the dose was repeated within 48 hr (Gemmell and Shearer, 1968). However, in these experiments, 10 of the 31 dogs retained some degree of infection; this inability to eliminate the worm burden completely was confirmed by Boray *et al.* (1979) and Bankov (1977). Bunamidine hydrochloride was for some years the drug of choice against *E. granulosus* and was used at a dose rate of 50 mg/kg repeated in 48 hr. However, because some worms remained to continue the life cycle after treatment, it was replaced in hydatid control schemes as soon as the high efficiency of praziquantel had been proven.

Bunamidine given as a single oral dose of 50 mg/kg has been shown to cause little toxicity other than slight diarrhea and vomiting (Hatton, 1965; Burrows and Lillis, 1966). However, the proportion of dogs that vomited increased sharply when the dose rate was increased to 100–200 mg/kg (Gemmell and Shearer, 1968). At these dose rates, diarrhea was more common, but it rarely persisted for more than 3 hr. In widespread field usage, about 1 dog in 2000—usually excitable dogs—collapsed and died quickly. It has been shown that in dogs with hepatic dysfunction some bunamidine may pass through the liver and enter the circulation. In excited dogs high levels of epinephrine may then cause ventricular fibrillation in hearts sensitized by bunamidine to endogenous catecholamines (Fastier *et al.*, 1973). Cases of sudden death have occasionally been seen in dogs without evidence of hepatic dysfunction, and it is recommended that excitement and exertion be avoided after treatment (Williams and Keahey, 1976). Reduced spermatogenesis has been reported in dogs, but not in cats, at

4 days and up to 28 days after administration (Roberson, 1977). Bunamidine is an irritant, and if the lactose coating is broken, care should be taken not to carry the drug to the eyes.

2.4. Niclosamide

Niclosamide has been used throughout the world against *Taenia* spp. in dogs and cats at a dose rate of 100 mg/kg and against tapeworms in sheep, horses, and birds. In dogs it lacks activity against *Echinococcus* spp. and is variable against the common *D. caninum*. It has now been withdrawn in favor of praziquantel but may still be available in some countries in proprietary mixtures.

In dogs doses of $\geqslant$100 mg/kg show high efficiency against *Taenia* spp. (Poole *et al.*, 1971), and in widespread field usage in New Zealand regular doses of 125 mg/kg every 6 weeks provided excellent control of *T. ovis* and *T. hydatigena* (G. A. Thomson, personal communication, 1973). Niclosamide is also effective against *T. taeniaeformis* in cats at 100 mg/kg (Westcott, 1967). Repeated treatments are necessary to gain good efficiency against *Mesocestoides corti* (Todd *et al.*, 1978).

Niclosamide has variable activity against the common species, *D. caninum* (Poole *et al.*, 1971; Roberson, 1976), and against *E. granulosus* even when micronized (Gemmell *et al.*, 1977*a*). It is therefore not recommended for use against these species.

The LD_{50} for niclosamide has not been established, but it is known that rats tolerate doses of up to 5000 mg/kg (Hall, 1966). Normal use may cause transient softening of the feces, and a proportion of dogs will vomit (Gemmell *et al.*, 1977*a*). This lack of toxicity is probably related to the poor absorption of the compound (Gregor, 1963) and to the fact that the small fraction that is absorbed is metabolized quickly to the less toxic 4-aminoniclosamide (Strufe and Gonnert, 1967). The compound can be used during pregnancy and lactation as well as in animals with liver disorders, but it should not be used simultaneously with organophosphates unless there is clear evidence that the mixture is safe.

2.5. Substituted Benzimidazoles

The benzimidazoles were introduced to veterinary medicine because of their nematocidal activity. Some have been shown to be active against cestodes; two of them (mebendazole and fenbendazole) have been used widely in dogs because of their broad-spectrum activity and low toxicity. Benzimidazoles interfere with respiration and nutrition of the worm.

Efficiency is enhanced if the parasites are exposed to a threshold level for longer periods. This is easily effected for the less soluble benzimidazoles in ruminants in which the rumen acts as a depot and releases the drug into the abomasum over a few days. In dogs and cats the benzimidazoles must be given daily for 3 days to maintain intestinal fluid and blood levels at high levels for a sufficient time to cause irreversible changes in the parasites and hence give high efficiency.

2.5.1. Mebendazole

Mebendazole was introduced in 1972 with claims for high activity against nematodes and cestodes in man and other mammalian hosts. The discovery that mebendazole was active against secondary cysts of *E. granulosus*, mature and immature cysticerci of *T. pisiformis*, multiplying tetrathyridia of *M. corti*, and larval *T. taeniaeformis* (Heath *et al.*, 1975) spurred great interest, but its use against larval cestodes in animals has been abandoned because of the long course of treatment required and the expense of such treatments.

There is little information on the use of mebendazole against adult cestodes of the dog and cat; few investigators have appreciated the need to use repeated treatments to obtain high efficiency. Gemmell *et al.* (1975) eliminated *T. hydatigena* from a group of 10 dogs when twice the recommended dose of 10 mg/kg was used, but Boray *et al.* (1979), using 20 mg/kg repeated in 48 hr, could only obtain 50% efficiency. It appears that the use of the micronized compound in dogs at the recommended dose rate of 10 mg/kg repeated daily for 3 days requires much more detailed investigation before it can be confidently recommended for use against cestode infections.

2.5.2. Fenbendazole

Fenbendazole is used in dogs at high dose rates (50 mg/kg) for 3 days to give inexpensive but efficient broad-spectrum activity against nematodes. Its use against cestodes is secondary to this purpose, but it has been shown to be effective against the common tapeworms of the dog, other than *E. granulosus* (Duwel, 1978; Gemmell *et al.*, 1977*b*) and against *T. taeniaeformis* in cats (Roberson and Burke, 1980). The efficiency of this dose regimen has given variable results against *D. caninum* and requires further investigation.

Both mebendazole and fenbendazole are very safe compounds, but their toxicity has been examined mostly in farm animals. In dogs mebendazole has been used at 40 mg/kg for 13 weeks without causing any ill effect, while daily doses of 50 mg/kg fenbendazole given to pregnant bitches from 40 days gestation to 10 days after whelping had no effect on the birth weight or growth of the pups (Duwel and Strasser, 1978).

2.6. Nitroscanate

This compound was introduced in 1973 as a broad-spectrum compound for use in dogs against round worms, hook worms, and the cestodes, *Taenia* spp. and *D. caninum*. High dose rates (200 mg/kg repeated in 24 hr) were reported to have high activity against *E. granulosus* and *S. erinacei*, but total elimination of *E. granulosus* was not achieved (Boray *et al.*, 1979). Gemmell *et al.* (1977*c*) reported that micronisation (95% of particles <5 μm) greatly improved efficiency.

Further work with the micronized compound has confirmed that a single dose of 50 mg/kg has high efficiency against *Taenia* spp. and *D. caninum*. Variable results are obtained with *E. granulosus* (Gemmell *et al.*, 1977*c*; Boray *et al.*, 1979; Richards and Somerville, 1980), and it is not recommended against this worm.

The normal dose rate of 50 mg/kg causes vomiting in 10–20% of dogs within 3–5 hr of dosing, but this does not appear to interfere with its activity. Single dose rates up to 10,000 mg/kg do not cause clinical signs other than vomiting, diarrhea, and inappetance (Boray *et al.*, 1979). Vomiting does not appear to be dose dependent and is less frequent with micronized material (Gemmell *et al.*, 1977c). The vomiting is thought to be caused by a CNS effect and can be reduced if the drug is given on an empty stomach to ensure more rapid passage through the intestines. However, this also causes poor absorption and low efficiency. The present recommendation is to give the drug after 12–24 hr of fasting followed immediately by a small quantity of feed (J. C. Boray, personal communication, 1978).

2.7. Praziquantel

The introduction of praziquantel in 1975 made available, for the first time, a safe, highly specific, cestocidal drug active in a single oral, subcutaneous, or intramuscular dose against a broad range of tapeworms. Many reports quickly appeared confirming its activity against juvenile and adult *Taenia* spp., *D. caninum, Joyeuxiella pasqualei, D. latum, S. erinacei,* and *M. corti* (Rommel *et al.*, 1976; Gemmell *et al.*, 1977d; Baldock *et al.*, 1977; Sakamoto, 1977a; Thomas and Gonnert, 1978a). Dose rates of ≤2.5 mg/kg gave complete elimination of *Taenia* spp., *D. caninum,* and *M. corti,* but higher doses were needed against the pseudophyllidean parasites. A dose of 35 mg/kg was needed to remove *D. latum* from dogs, while two doses of 7.5 mg/kg 24 hr apart eliminated *S. erinacei* from cats (Sakamoto, 1977a).

The public health risks of *E. granulosus* and *E. multilocularis* infections and the failure of all other available compounds to remove an infection completely required that the efficacy of praziquantel against these parasites be examined and this was quickly done (Rommel *et al.*, 1976; Gemmell *et al.*, 1977d; Sakamoto, 1977a; Thomas and Gonnert, 1978a; Anderson *et al.*, 1979; Boray *et al.*, 1979; Beck *et al.*, 1980). In all trials a single dose of 5 mg/kg given orally or by injection completely eliminated infection, except in one trial (Sakamoto, 1977a) where one of five dogs remained infected with *E. multilocularis,* but gave a clearance rate of 99.99%. In later work, Gemmell *et al.* (1980) found the compound less active when given subcutaneously. Praziquantel has an ovicidal effect on eggs released from the proglottid but not against those contained in the segment (Thakur *et al.*, 1979). However, the ovicidal action of compounds has little epidemiological value, as the number of eggs remaining in the intestine is small compared with those on the ground.

Praziquantel is very safe given at the recommended dose of 5 mg/kg. The oral LD_{50} in mice and rats is more than 2200 mg/kg, and in rabbits is >1000 mg/kg. The oral toxicity in dogs has not been determined, as doses of >200 mg/kg cause vomiting. The only effect seen when dogs were given doses up to 40 times the recommended dose rate was vomiting, salivation or depression (Baldock and Hopkins, 1977; Shmidl *et al.*, 1981). Repeated treatments of 180 mg/kg per day for more than 4 weeks were tolerated without ill effects (Muermann *et al.*, 1976). Puppies, 4 weeks of age, given five times the recommended dose twice 14 days apart did not show any ill effect or changes in hematology, clinical pathology, or blood cholinesterase levels. The drug was shown to be compatible with the concurrent use of insecticides, anthelmintics, and vaccines, while no effect could be seen on fertility, conception rates, fetal development, or pregnancy (Shmidl *et al.,* 1981).

3. TAPEWORMS OF SHEEP AND CATTLE

3.1. Introduction

Three species, *Moniezia expansa, M. benedini,* and *Thysaniezia giardi,* occur in the small intestine of sheep and to a lesser extent in cattle throughout the world, while *Avitellina* spp. and *Stilesia globipunctata* have a restricted distribution. Two other species, *Stilesia hepatica* and *Thysanosoma actinioides,* which occur in the bile ducts, are found in Africa and the United States, respectively.

None of these species is very pathogenic but, because of their large size, various clinical symptoms have been ascribed to them at times. They are most common in young lambs, which gain infection by eating infected pasture mites (*Oribatidae*). Because lambs may have very large burdens of the intestinal species and pass many segments, which on occasion cover the fecal deposit, they are thought by farmers to be the cause of ill thrift rather than the less obvious nematodes, and treatment is often requested. In these circumstances there is value in using a compound that combines activity against nematodes and cestodes rather than using a specific compound that is unlikely to give an economic return from its use. Older animals are resistant to infection. The compounds used, their dose rates, and spectrums of activity in sheep are shown in Table II.

3.2. Niclosamide

This compound has excellent activity against the intestinal dwelling species *Moniezia* spp., *H. giardi,* and *Avitellina* spp. (Stampa and Terblanche, 1961; Hall,

Table II. Recommended Treatments and Their Efficacy in Sheep

Compound	Dose rate (mg/kg)	Species in	
		Intestine	Bile ducts
Albendazole	3.8	+	+[a]
Bunamidine hydroxynaphthoate	50	+	−
Fenbendazole	5	+	−
Niclosamide	50	+	−
Oxfendazole	5	+	−
Praziquantel	2.5	+	+[b]

[a] Effective at double dose rates.
[b] Effective at three or four times recommended dose rate.

1966; Schalkwyk *et al.*, 1981). The recommended dose rate is 50 mg/kg, with a minimum dose of 1 g (Stampa and Terblanche, 1961). Its action against the bile duct-dwelling species is less satisfactory, doses of 400–600 mg/kg being required against *T. actinioides* (Allen *et al.*, 1967); its action against *S. hepatica* is also poor (Stampa and Terblanche, 1961).

Niclosamide has a very wide margin of safety. Its toxicity has been discussed more fully under tapeworms of dogs and cats, but in sheep and cattle 40 times the normal dose is nontoxic except for some diarrhea. Care should be taken if it is to be used concurrently with an organophosphate.

3.3. Bunamidine Hydroxynaphthoate

This salt is less irritant to mucous membranes than is the hydrochloride and is therefore preferred for use as a drench in ruminants. In sheep and goats doses of 25 mg/kg and 50 mg/kg, respectively, gave good results against natural infections of *M. expansa* (Czipri *et al.*, 1968), and no toxic doses were seen at doses up to 200 mg base/kg. Some transient diarrhea occurred when sheep were given 400 mg base/kg.

3.4. Benzimidazoles

Thiabendazole, which was the first benzimidazole anthelmintic, had no effect on cestodes at normal dosage. Those benzimidazoles developed subsequently had the 5-position blocked to slow down the rate of metabolism and excretion. This allows the compound to persist longer and to have an effect on those parasites only marginally affected by compounds rapidly removed from the body. Campbell (1961) first showed that benzimidazoles had cestocidal action, and sufficient activity was shown by cambendazole for claims to be made against cestodes in sheep. This compound has now been withdrawn.

3.4.1. Mebendazole

Although claims for cesticidal activity in dogs, sheep, and horses are made for this compound, there is little published information on its efficacy against adult parasites in sheep, and its cestocidal use is secondary to its activity against nematodes. The activity of mebendazole against secondary hydatids (Heath *et al.*, 1975) led to great interest in the use of this compound against larval hydatids in man and against larval cestode infections in sheep and cattle. While activity has been demonstrated against larval *E. granulosus, T. hydatigena,* and *T. ovis* in sheep (Heath and Lawrence, 1978), the long course of treatment required and the expense of such treatment preclude its use in animals.

Mebendazole is very poorly absorbed, more than 90% of a dose being excreted in the feces. This makes it a very safe compound, and the LD_{50} for sheep is above 600 mg/kg. No effect on the embryo has been seen when ewes are dosed during pregnancy, and the compound is compatible with other farm chemicals.

3.4.2. Fenbendazole

This compound has been shown to have high efficiency against *Moniezia* spp. in sheep at doses of 5–25 mg/kg (Malan, 1980) and in calves at 10 and 15 mg/kg (Ciordia *et al.*, 1983). At the recommended dose rate of 7.5 mg/kg, it is still 91.7% efficient in calves (Ciordia *et al.*, 1983). This compound is widely used in sheep (5 mg/kg) and cattle because of its excellent activity against nematodes; its cestocidal activity is an added benefit.

Single oral doses of 5000 mg/kg or 30 doses of 45 mg/kg are well tolerated in sheep (Baeder *et al.*, 1974), and no teratogenic effects have been detected in rats, sheep, cattle, or horses (Delatour *et al.*, 1975; Becker, 1975). While fenbendazole can be used simultaneously with flukicides and insecticides in sheep, a serious interaction occurs in cattle when fenbendazole and bromsalans are given together, and deaths occur within 24–48 hr (Borland *et al.*, 1978).

3.4.3. Oxfendazole

This is one of the most active benzimidazoles against nematodes; in sheep, it is active against cestodes as well. At the recommended dose rate of 5 mg/kg, excellent results have been obtained against *Moniezia* spp. in lambs (Michael *et al.*, 1979), but oxfendazole is ineffective against *S. hepatica* infection when given at 3–5 mg/kg(Vester and Marincowitz,1980).

Doses of 20 times the normal therapeutic dose rate are well tolerated by sheep. Repeated dosing of rams from 21 days before the breeding season and of ewes during pregnancy with three times the recommended dose has no effect on the rams, ewes, or lambs. It has also been shown to be safe and to have no teratogenic effect in heifers in early pregnancy (Piercy *et al.*, 1979). Oxfendazole is not compatible with bromalans in cattle and should not be given within 7 days (Prichard, 1978).

3.4.4. Albendazole

This compound is the most recent benzimidazole to be marketed; it has the broadest spectrum of members of this group, with activity against nematodes, trematodes, and cestodes in sheep and cattle. It is highly effective against intestinal cestodes at doses below the recommended dose rates (Schalkwyk *et al.*, 1979; Ciordia *et al.*, 1978), and a double dose (7.5 mg/kg) removes *T. actinioides* from naturally and experimentally infected lambs (Craig and Shepherd, 1980). Albendazole is also effective against larval *T. saginata* in cattle, when given at a dose rate of 50 mg/kg (Lloyd *et al.*, 1978).

Albendazole also has a wide margin of safety. Single oral doses of 37.5 mg/kg produced no ill effect in sheep and 15 mg/kg per day for 3 months did not produce clinical symptoms or histopathological changes. When ewes were treated 28–32 days after the rams were introduced there was no effect on the fetus, and there was no effect on the production or character of sperm when rams were dosed with 15 mg/kg (Johns and Philip, 1977).

3.5. Praziquantel

This specific cestocidal agent has not been widely tested in ruminants probably because its expense inhibits its use. However, 2.5 mg/kg eliminates *Moniezia* spp. (Thomas and Gonnert, 1978*a*), while 8–15 mg/kg eliminates the bile duct parasites *S. hepatica* and *T. actinioides* (Bankov, 1976), a spectrum matched only by albendazole. Praziquantel also has activity against larval *T. hydatigena* in sheep (Thomas and Gonnert, 1978*b*; Heath and Lawrence, 1978; Bankov and Gradinarski, 1982), but high doses are required, and it is not effective against the younger larval stages (Thomas and Gonnert, 1978*b*) or in heavy infections (Heath and Lawrence, 1978).

A compound with activity against larval *Echinococcus* spp. would be of great benefit in veterinary and human medicine. Thomas and Gonnert (1978*b*) found praziquantel to have an effect against protoscolices of *E. multilocularis*, but these workers and others failed to inhibit the growth of cysts of *E. multilocularis* or *E. granulosus* (Sakamoto, 1977*b*; Heath and Lawrence, 1978).

Its activity against *T. saginata* larval stages in cattle is of interest but, while Pawlowski *et al.* (1978) and Walther and Koske (1979) reported high activity in both natural and experimental infections with dose rates of 50–100 mg/kg, the cost of such treatment precludes its use.

4. TAPEWORMS OF THE HORSE

4.1. Introduction

Three species commonly affect the horse: *Anoplocephala perfoliata*, *A. magna,* and *Paranoplocephala mamillana.* The latter two occur in the small intestine, where they cause a catarrhal or rarely a hemorrhagic enteritis, and occasionally in the stomach, while *A. perfoliata* is found in the small intestine, cecum, and more rarely in the colon. It commonly occurs in large numbers near the ileocecal valve and causes edema and ulceration.

Clinical signs associated with tapeworms are uncommon, but occasionally unthriftiness and diarrhea are seen in the late summer and autumn following infections in the spring, when the oribatid mite, the intermediate host, is plentiful. The partial occlusion of the ileocecal valve by granulation tissue may cause a mild colic, while on rare occasions acute colic or sudden death may occur following perforation of the bowel or blockage of the ileocecal valve. Intussusception associated with *A. perfoliata* infection was reported by Barclay *et al.* (1982). The low pathogenicity of tapeworms in horses is reflected by the sparse literature on the efficacy of compounds in this host.

4.2. Niclosamide

High efficiency against anoplocephalids in horses of all ages was obtained by Safaev (1972) when using dose rates of 200–300 mg/kg, while Slocombe (1979) found 50 mg/kg to cause loss of strobila without removing the scolex. Intermediate doses have not been tested, and titration studies are needed. In other species, 100 mg/kg has proved effective, and it is suggested that this dose rate should be used.

Niclosamide is a very safe compound. Its toxicity is discussed under dogs (Section 2.4) and sheep (Section 3.2). In horses care should be taken to avoid its use with trichlorphon or other organophosphates unless there is clear evidence that the combination is safe.

4.3. Pyrantel Pamoate

This compound and its 1-methyl analogue, morantel, are widely used to treat nematode infections. Pyrantel pamoate at the standard dose rate (6.6 mg pyrantel base/kg) appeared effective against tapeworms in horses in field trials (Slocombe, 1979; Drudge et al., 1982), but this was probably because of its destrobilizing action, as critical trials showed only 15% activity (Slocombe, 1979). A double dose rate (13.2 mg pyrantel base/kg) has high efficiency (Slocombe, 1979; Drudge et al., 1982) and is an inexpensive and convenient treatment. While higher dose rates of morantel do not appear to have been tested, a mixture of the standard dose rate (6 mg/kg) and trichlorphon 30 mg/kg removed only 25% of A. perfoliata from one horse (Drudge et al., 1984). A double dose would probably give results similar to those achieved with pyrantel.

5. TAPEWORMS OF BIRDS

5.1. Introduction

Commercial poultry are hosts to many species of tapeworm, but modern husbandry methods prevent access to the various intermediate stages, thus preventing infection. However, free-ranging birds and cage birds in aviaries, particularly in those with earthen floors, can suffer severely from tapeworm infections. In moderate infections the birds may be depressed and lose weight, while heavier infections can cause an enteritis resulting in diarrhea, emaciation, and death. None of the modern compounds has been adequately tested in birds, and further work to define their efficacy and optimal dose rate is required.

5.2. Niclosamide

This compound appears to be safe and efficient in poultry and ducklings. Doses of 50 mg/kg in feed or as tablets have been satisfactory (Boisvenue and Hendrix, 1965), but Abrams (1976) required two doses of 50 mg/kg 2–3 weeks apart, followed by a further dose of 100 mg/kg to eliminate heavy infections of *Choanotaenia infundibulum* in poultry. In ducklings Bankov and Juperliev (1965) obtained 100% efficiency against *Hymenolepis* spp. and *Dicranotaenia* spp. using 50–80 mg/kg. Niclosamide has been widely used in cage birds, but no standard dose rate or method of administration can be recommended.

5.3. Praziquantel

Praziquantel has been tested in chickens, ducks, and geese at dose rates of 10 and 20 mg/kg, and high activity has been demonstrated against a range of cestodes (Vassilev *et al.*, 1977). However, the compound is too expensive for routine commercial use.

REFERENCES

Abrams, L., 1976, Cestodosis in battery and housed laying hens, *J. S. Afr. Vet. Assoc.* 47:171–173.

Allen, R. W., Enzie, F. D., and Samson, K. S., 1967, Trials with Yomesan and other selected chemicals against *Thysanosoma actinioides*, the fringed tapeworm of sheep, *Proc. Helminthol. Soc. Wash.* 34:195–199,

Anderson, F. L., Conder, G. A., and Marsland, W. P., 1979, Efficacy of injectable and tablet formulations of praziquantel against immature *Echinococcus granulosus*, *Am. J. Vet. Res.* 40:700–701.

Baeder, C., Bahr, H., Christ, O., Duwel, D., Kellner, H. M., Kirsch, R., Loewe, H., Schultes, E., Schultz, E., and Westen, H., 1974, Fenbendazole: A new, highly effective anthelmintic, *Experientia* 30:753–754.

Baldock, F. C., and Hopkins, T. J., 1977, Praziquantel: A new cestocide, *Proc.* 54th *Ann. Conf. Aust. Vet. Assoc.* pp. 127–128.

Baldock, F. C., Flucke, W. J., and Hopkins, T. J., 1977, Efficiency of praziquantel, a new cestocide, against *Taenia hydatigena* in the dog, *Res. Vet. Sci.* 23:237–238.

Bankov, D., 1976, Diagnosis and treatment of *Stilesia* infection in sheep, *Vet. Med. Nauk.* 13:28–36; 1977, *Vet. Bull.* 47:5050 (abst.).

Bankov, D. E., 1977, Comparative assessment of anthelmintics against *Echinococcus granulosus* in dogs, *Vet. Med. Rev.* 2:145–148.

Bankov, D., and Gradinarski, I., 1982, Cysticercosis (*Cysticercus tenuicollis*) in sheep and its treatment with Droncit, *Vet. Med. Rev.* 1:104–106.

Bankov, D., and Juperliev, W., 1965, Comparative studies of drugs for treatment of cestodes and trematodes of ducklings, *Vet. Sb.* 3:13; 1966, *Vet. Med. Rev.* 2:144–145 (abst.).

Barclay, W. P., Phillips, J. N., and Foerner, J. J., 1982, Intussusseption associated with *Anoplocephala perfoliata* infection in 5 horses, *J. Am. Vet. Med. Assoc.* 180:752–753.

Beck, A., Rassier, D., Chaplin, E., Picavea, J. P. C., and Almeida, A. F., 1980, The efficacy of Droncit in the control of *Echinococcus granulosus* in experimentally infected dogs, *Vet. Med. Rev.* 2:135–139.

Becker, W., 1975, Die Anwendung von Panacur bei trachtigen Tieren, in: *Proceedings of the Second European Multicolloquy on Parasitology, Trogir, Yugoslavia.*

Boisvenue, R. J., and Hendrix, J. C., 1965, Prophylactic treatment of experimental *Raillietina cesticillus* infections in chickens with Yomesan, *J. Parasitol.* 51:519–522.

Boray, J. C., Strong, M. B., Allison, J. R., von Orelli, M., Sarasin, G., and Gfeller, W., 1979, Nitroscanate, a new broad spectrum anthelmintic against nematodes and cestodes of dogs and cats, *Aust. Vet. J.* 55:45–53.

Borland, R., Sinclair, A. J., Allison, J. F., Embury, D., and James, R. E., 1978, Toxicity in cattle following exposure to combinations of fenbendazole and bromsalans-type anthelmintics, *Proc.* 55th *Ann. Conf. Aust. Vet. Assoc.* pp. 17–19.

Burrows, R. B., and Lillis, W. G., 1966, Treatment of canine and feline tapeworm infections with bunamidine hydrochloride, *Am. J. Vet. Res.* 27:1381–1384.

Campbell, W. C., 1961, Effects of thiabendazole upon infections of *Trichinella spiralis* in mice, and upon certain other helminthiasis, *J. Parasitol.* 47(2):37.

Ciordia, H., McCampbell, H. C., and Stuedemann, J. A., 1978, Cestocidal activity of albendazole in calves, *Am. J. Vet. Res.* 39:517–518.

Ciordia, H., Stuedemann, J. A., and McCampbell, H. C., 1983, Efficacy of fenbendazole against tapeworms in calves, *Am. J. Vet. Res.* 44:1091–1092.

Cobbold, T. S., 1872, *Worms*, J. & A. Churchill, London.

Craig, T. M., and Shepherd, E., 1980, Efficacy of albendazole and levamisole in sheep against *Thysanosoma actinioides* and *Haemonchus contortus* from the Edwards Plateau, Texas, *Am. J. Vet. Res.* 41:425–526.

Czipri, D. A., Nunns, V. J., and Shearer, G. L., 1968, Bunamidine hydroxynaphthoate: Activity against *Moniezia expansa* in sheep, *Vet. Rec.* 82:505–507.

Delatour, P., Lorgue, G., and Courtot, D., 1975, Embryotoxicity of some benzimidazolic anthelmintics, in: *Proceedings of the Twentieth World Veterinary Congress, Thessalonika.*

Drudge, J. H., Lyons, E. T., Tolliver, S. C., and Kubis, J. E., 1982, Pyrantel in horses: Clinical trials with emphasis on a paste formulation and activity on benzimidazole-resistant small strongyles, *Vet. Med. Small Anim. Clin.* 77:957–967.

Drudge, J. H., Lyons, E. T., and Tolliver, S. C., 1984, Critical tests of morantel-trichlorphon paste formulation against internal parasites of the horse, *Vet. Parasitol.* 14:55–64.

Duwel, D., 1978, Die Behandlung des Helminthen-Befaels bei Hunden mit Fenbendazole, *K. Prax.* 23:237–242.

Duwel, D., and Strasser, H., 1978, Versuche zur Geburt helminthenfrier Hundewelpen durch Fenbendazole-Behandlung, *Dtsch. Tierarztl. Wochenschr. (Berl.)* 85:239–241.

Fastier, F. N., Menrath, R. L. E., Sharard, A., and Ng, J., 1973, Toxicity of bunamidine. 1. Cardiovascular effects, *N.Z. Vet. J.* 21:201–204.

Forbes, L. S., and Whitten, L. K., 1961, Arecoline hydrobromide as a purgative in dogs: The effect of method of administration on its speed of action, *N.Z. Vet. J.* 9:101–104.

Gemmell, M. A., and Shearer, G. C., 1968, Bunamidine hydrochloride: Its efficiency against *Echinococcus granulosus*, *Vet. Rec.* 82:252–256.

Gemmell, M. A., Johnstone, P. D., and Oudemans, G., 1975, The effect of mebendazole on *Echinococcus granulosus* and *Taenia hydatigena* infection in dogs, *Res. Vet. Sci.* 19:229–230.

Gemmell, M. A., Johnstone, P. D., and Oudemans, G., 1977a, The effect of niclosamide on *Echinococcus granulosus, Taenia hydatigena* and *Taenia ovis* infection in dogs, *Res. Vet. Sci.* 22:389–391.

Gemmell, M. A., Johnstone, P. D., and Oudemans, G., 1977b, The lethal effect of some benzamidazoles on *Taenia hydatigena* in dogs, *Res. Vet. Sci.* 23:115–116.

Gemmell, M. A., Johnstone, P. D., and Oudemans, G., 1977c, The effect of micronised nitroscanate on *Echinococcus granulosus* and *Taenia hydatigena* infection in dogs, *Res. Vet. Sci.* 22:391–392.

Gemmell, M. A., Johnstone, P. D., and Oudemans, G., 1977d, The effect of praziquantel on *Echinococcus granulosus, Taenia hydatigena* and *Taenia ovis* infection in dogs, *Res. Vet. Sci.* 23:121–123.

Gemmell, M. A., Johnstone, P. D., and Oudemans, G., 1980, The effect of route of administration on the efficacy of praziquantel against *Echinococcus granulosus* infections in dogs, *Res. Vet. Sci.* 29:131–132.

Gibson, T. E., 1975, *Veterinary Anthelmintic Medication*, 3rd ed., technical Communication No. 33, Commonwealth Institute of Helminthology, St. Albans, U. K.

Gregor, W. W., 1963, A clinical assessment of 5-chloro-N-(2-chloro-4-nitrophenyl) salicylamide as a taeniacide for dogs and cats, *Vet. Rec.* 75:1421–1422.

Hall, C. A., 1966, Mansonil, a new cestocide for sheep, *Vet. Med. Rev.* 1:59–66.

Hatton, C. J., 1965, A new taeniacide, bunamidine hydrochloride: Its efficiency against *Taenia pisiformis* and *Dipylidium caninum* in the dog and *Hydatigera taeniaeformis* in the cat, *Vet. Rec.* 77:408–411.

Heath, D. D., and Lawrence, S. B., 1978, The effect of mebendazole and praziquantel on the cysts of *Echinococcus granulosus, Taenia hydatigena* and *T. ovis* in sheep, *N.Z. Vet. J.* 26:11–15.

Heath, D. D., Christie, M. J., and Chevis, R. A. F., 1975, The lethal effect of mebendazole on secondary *Echinococcus granulosus*, cysticerci of *Taenia pisiformis* and tetrathyridia of *Mesocestoides corti, Parasitology* 70:273–285.

Hromatka, von L., Kutzar, E., and Stettner, W., 1966, Versucher mit dem Bandwurmmittel Scolaban beim Hund, *Wien. Tierarztl. Mschr.* 53:616–617.

Johns, D. J., and Philip, J. R., 1977, Albendazole: Safety in sheep, in: *Proceedings of the Eighth International Conference of the World Association for Advancement of Veterinary Parasitology, Sydney,* No. 58.

Lloyd, S., Soulsby, E. J. L., and Theodorides, V. J., 1978, Effect of albendazole on the metacestodes of *Taenia saginata* in calves, *Experientia* 34:723–724.

Malan, F. S., 1980, Anthelmintic efficacy of fenbendazole against cestodes in sheep and cattle, *J. S. Afr. Vet. Assoc.* 57:25–26.

Michael, S. A., El-Rafaii, A. H., Mansour, W. H., Selim, M. K., and Higgins, A. J., 1979, Efficacy of oxfendazole against natural infestations of nematodes and cestodes in sheep in Egypt, *Vet. Rec.* 104:338–340.

Muermann, P., Eberstein, M. von and Frohberg, H., 1976, Notes on the tolerance of Droncit, *Vet. Med. Rev.* 2:142–153.

Pawlowski, Z., Kozakiewicz, B., and Wroblewski, H., 1978, The efficiency of mebendazole and praziquantel against *Taenia saginata* cysticercosis in cattle, *Vet. Sci. Comm.* 2:137–139.

Piercy, D. W. T., Reynolds, J., and Brown, P. R. M., 1979, Reproductive safety of oxfendazole in sheep and cattle, *Br. Vet. J.* 135:405–410.

Poole, P. B., Dooley, K. L., and Rollins, L. D., 1971, Efficacy of niclosamide for the removal of tapeworms (*Dipylidium caninum* and *Taenia pisiformis*) from dogs, *J. Am. Vet. Med. Assoc.* 159:78–80.

Prichard, R. K., 1978, Anthelmintics, in: *The Therapeutic Jungle, Postgraduate Committee on Veterinary Science, Sydney,* pp. 421–463.

Richards, R. J., and Somerville, J. M., 1980, Field trials with nitroscanate against cestodes and nematodes in dogs, *Vet. Rec.* 106:322–335.

Rickard, M. D., and Arundel, J. H., 1985, The chemotherapy of tapeworm infections; veterinary medicine, in: *Chemotherapy of Intestinal Helminths, Handbook of Experimental Pharmacology* 77:557–611.

Roberson, E. L., 1976, Comparative effects of uredofos, niclosamide and bunamidine hydrochloride against tapeworm infection in dogs, *Am. J. Vet. Res.* 37:1483–1484.

Roberson, E. L., 1977, Anticestodal and antitrematodal drugs, in: *Veterinary Pharmacology and Therapeutics* (L. M. Jones, N. H. Booth, and L. E. McDonald, eds.), 4th ed., The Iowa State University Press, Ames, Iowa.

Roberson, E. L., and Burke, T. M., 1980, Evaluation of granulated fenbendazole (22.2%) against induced and naturally occurring helminth infection in cats, *Am. J. Vet. Res.* 41:1499–1502.

Rommel, M., Grelck, H., and Horchner, F., 1976, The efficacy of praziquantel against tapeworms in experimentally infected dogs and cats, *Berl. Munch. Tierarztl. Wochenschr.* 89:255–257.

Safaev, Ya. S., 1972, Efficacy of phenasal against anoplocephalids in horses, *Veterinariya*, Moscow 49:68–69.

Sakamoto, T., 1977*a*, The anthelmintic effect of Droncit on adult tapeworms of *Hydatigera taeniaeformis, Mesocestoides corti, Echinococcus multilocularis, Diphyllobothrium erinacei* and *D. latum, Vet. Med. Rev.* 1:64–74.

Sakamoto, T., 1977*b*, The cestocidal effect of praziquantel on the larval stages of *Hydatigera taeniaeformis, Mesocestoides corti* and *Echinococcus multilocularis* in laboratory animals, *Vet. Med. Rev.* 2:153–162.

Schalkwyk, P. C. van, Geyser, T. L., Recio, M., and Erasmus, F. P. G., 1979, The anthelmintic efficiency of albendazole against gastrointestinal roundworms, tapeworms, lungworms and liver fluke in sheep, *J. S. Afr. Vet. Ass.* 50:31–35.

Schalkwyk, P. C. van, Geyser, T. L., Davies, P. V. A., and Recio, M., 1981, The efficacy of anthelmintics against *Thysaniezia giardi* in South Africa, *J. S. Afr. Vet. Assoc.* 52:207–209.

Schmidl, J. A., Cox, D. D., McCurdy, H. D., and Kohlenberg, M. L., 1981, Summary of safety evaluations for praziquantel in dogs, *Vet. Med. Small Anim. Clin.* 76:692–697.

Slocombe, J. O. D., 1979, Prevalence and treatment of tapeworms in horses, *Can. Vet. J.* 20:136–140.

Stampa, S., and Terblanche, H. J. J., 1961, Trials with Bayer 2353 and other drugs as cestocides for ruminants, *J. S. Afr. Vet. Assoc.* 32:367–371.

Standen, O. D., 1963, Chemotherapy of helminthic infections, in: *Experimental Chemotherapy* (R. F. Schnitzer and F. Hawkins, eds.), Vol. 1, p. 716, Academic Press, New York.

Strufe, R., and Gonnert, R., 1967, Über die Beeinflussung des Bandwurmstoffwechsels durch Arzneimittel, Z. Tropenmed. Parasitol. 18:193–202.

Thakur, A. S., Prezioso, U., and Marchevsky, N., 1979, Echinococcus granulosus: Ovicidal activity of praziquantel and bunamidine hydrochloride, Exp. Parasitol. 47:131–133.

Thomas, H., and Gonnert, L., 1978a, The efficacy of praziquantel against cestodes in cats, dogs and sheep, Res. Vet. Sci. 24:20–25.

Thomas, H., and Gonnert, R., 1978b, The efficacy of praziquantel against experimental cysticercosis and hydatidosis, Z. Parasitenkd. 55:165–179.

Todd, K. S., Jr., Howland, T. P., and Woerpel, R. W., 1978, The activity of uredofos, niclosamide, bunamidine hydrochloride and arecoline hydrobromide against Mesocestoides corti in experimentally infected dogs, Am. J. Vet. Res. 39:315–316.

Vassilev, I., Denev, J., and Kostov, R., 1977, Trials regarding the anticestodal activity of Droncit in poultry, Vet. Med. Rev. 2:149–152.

Verster, A., and Marincowitz, G., 1980, Treatment of Stilesia hepatica infection, J. S. Afr. Vet. Assoc. 51:249–250.

Walther, M., and Koske, J. K., 1979, The efficacy of praziquantel against Taenia saginata cysticercosis in naturally affected calves, Tropenmed. Parasitol. 30:401–403.

Westcott, R. B., 1967, Efficacy of niclosamide in the treatment of Taenia taeniaeformis infection in cats, Am. J. Vet. Res. 28:1475–1477.

Williams, J. F., and Keahey, K. K., 1976, Sudden death associated with treatment of three dogs with bunamidine hydrochloride, J. Am. Vet. Med. Assoc. 168:689–691.

25

Mode of Action of Anticestodal Agents

HUGO VANDEN BOSSCHE

1. INTRODUCTION

Mode of action of anticestodal agents is a pretentious title for a chapter that can only list the effects of anthelmintics on membranes, organelles, enzymes, and neuromuscular systems. In fact, essential information about the molecular mechanism of action of most anthelmintics is still lacking.

It is surprising that only few scientists are working on the mode of action of anthelmintic drugs, on the biochemical and molecular aspects of helminths, and on the mechanisms regulating host–parasite relationships, considering the myriad of interesting models available. To list just a few examples, many enzymes involved in nucleic acid and protein metabolism and in energy generation still await investigation at the molecular level. A better knowledge of the active sites of these enzymes, of their localization, orientation, and interaction with other cellular components, would be of great help in the study of the underlying mechanisms for the anticestodal activity of the chemical compounds discussed in this chapter. Investigation of the physicochemical properties of membranes, of the transport systems available, and of the neurotransmitters and their receptors will lead to a better understanding of the interaction of many of the anticestodal agents and will contribute to the development of chemicals that might act more selectively against the invader.

This review includes a limited number of publications that deal with the biochemical and biophysical aspects of anticestodal drugs. More details can be found in several comprehensive reviews that have summarized the interactions of common anthelmintics with biochemical and physiological processes in parasitic worms (Mansour, 1979; Rew, 1978; Sharma and Abuzar, 1983; Sharma et al., 1980; Vanden Bossche, 1976, 1978, 1980a,b, 1985; Vanden Bossche et al., 1982).

HUGO VANDEN BOSSCHE • Laboratory of Comparative Biochemistry, Department of Life Sciences, Janssen Pharmaceutica Research Laboratories, B-2340 Beerse, Belgium.

2. BENZIMIDAZOLES

Mebendazole, or methyl (5-(benzoyl)1H-benzimidazol-2-yl]carbamate has been proved active against a broad spectrum of gastrointestinal (GI) nematodes and cestodes in human and veterinary medicine. After it had been described as larvicidal against *Taenia taeniaeformis* larvae (Thienpont *et al.*, 1974), Heath and Chevis (1974) and Krotov *et al.* (1974, 1976) were the first to report the efficacy of mebendazole against secondary hydatid cysts in mice. The effects of this benzimidazole carbamate on *Echinococcus granulosus* and *E. multilocularis* have been reported in different experimental animals and in man (Schantz *et al.*, 1982; Bekhti *et al.*, 1977, 1980; Wilson and Rausch, 1980; Witassek *et al.*, 1981; Müller *et al.*, 1982; French, 1984).

The fluorine analogue of mebendazole, flubendazole (Schantz *et al.*, 1982) and of other benzimidazole derivatives, such as albendazole (Saimot *et al.*, 1983), also showed various degrees of larvicidal activity. Mebendazole and related benzimidazole carbamates interact with tubulin and prevent its polymerization. At high concentrations, the benzimidazole derivative, thiabendazole, also affects polymerization of tubulin (Ireland *et al.*, 1979).

The time-related micromorphological changes induced by mebendazole or flubendazole in *T. taeniaeformis* larvae or adult *Hymenolepis nana* have been reported by Borgers *et al.* (1975), Verheyen *et al.* (1976), and Laclette *et al.* (1981). The cytoplasmic microtubules of tegumental cells have almost completely disappeared from the tegument of *H. nana* collected from mice medicated for 6 hr with 500 ppm mebendazole in the food. After the disappearance of the microtubules, vesicles accumulate in the Golgi area, and the absorptive surface of the tegument degenerates. Examination of the hydatid cysts of mice treated with mebendazole revealed the same time-related deteriorative effect of the benzimidazole carbamate as described for other cestode species (Verheyen, 1982). Prolonged treatment with mebendazole of patients with hydatid disease often results in complete necrosis of the germinal layer of *E. granulosus* cysts. These cysts showed only remnants of degenerated germinal layer, including heterogeneous vesicular membranes, electron-dense amorphous structures, myeloid bodies, lipid globules, crystal-like precipitates, and remnants derived from muscular tissue (Verheyen, 1982). The hydatid germinal membrane tissue collected from sheep, treated daily with one or two courses of mebendazole (daily dose 6 g), each lasting 3 weeks, also showed complete degeneration of the tegumental and subtegumental structures (Al-Dabagh *et al.*, 1981).

Although a significant number of interesting studies have been reported, we have yet to learn whether the selective toxicity of mebendazole is attributable to differences between the parasite and host tubulin, to differences in their pharmacokinetic behavior (Köhler and Bachmann, 1980), or to differences in their metabolism.

Possible consequences of the block in transporting secretory substances following interruption of the microtubular system are impaired defense reactions, inadequate nourishment, and cellular autolysis. The inadequate nourishment induced by benzimidazole carbamates has been reported by several investigators. For example, mebendazole affects the glucose uptake by helminths both *in vitro* and *in vivo* (Vanden Bossche,

1976, 1980b, Vanden Bossche et al., 1982). This reduced glucose uptake is followed by an increased utilization or decreased synthesis of glycogen. It is interesting to note that mebendazole and cambendazole also diminished in vitro and in vivo ATP synthesis and/or turnover of adenine nucleotides. For example, in Moniezia expansa the effects on energy metabolism became apparent within a 30-min exposure to mebendazole or cambendazole in vitro (Rahman and Bryant, 1977). At the moment it is almost impossible to say which particular effect—interference with the microtubular system and/or energy-generating systems—is responsible for the eradication by benzimidazole derivatives of nematodes and cestodes. Rahman and Bryant (1977) conclude that "benzimidazoles are capable of exerting a number of effects which together account for their efficacy against parasites."

3. BITHIONOL

Bithionol sulfoxide has been used successfully in the treatment of human tapeworm infections (Gemmell and Johnstone, 1981). As could be expected from the presence of two hydroxyl groups, this 2,2'-thiobis[4,6-dichlorophenol] is an uncoupler of oxidative phosphorylation (Hamajima, 1973). According to Hamajima (1973), the phenolic OH groups of bithionol interfere in Paragonimus westermani with glycolysis, the tricarboxylic acid (TCA), or Krebs, cycle and the oxidation–reduction system transporting hydrogen to the succinate oxidation. So far no studies on the interaction of bithionol with the energy synthesis in cestodes have been found.

4. BUNAMIDINE

Ultrastructural studies revealed that bunamidine, or N,N-dibutyl-4-hexyloxy-1-naphthamidine, causes disruption of the outer layers of the integument of H. nana. Such an effect could be predicted from biochemical studies. In fact, a decrease in the rate of glucose uptake, an increase in the rate of glucose efflux, and the release of surface phosphatase activity into the incubation medium observed at 3×10^{-5} M bunamidine are suggestive of an interaction of bunamidine with the absorptive surface of H. nana (Hart et al., 1977). Bunamidine also inhibits the ATP-generating fumarate reductase system in a mitochondrial fraction of Hymenolepis diminuta (Chatfield and Yeary, 1979). The effects on the tegument and on the ATP-generating system might be unrelated.

5. NICLOSAMIDE

Niclosamide belongs, together with rafoxanide and closantel, to the salicylanilides. They disturb in vivo and/or in vitro the mitochondrial phosphorylation (Vanden Bossche et al., 1979; Vanden Bossche, 1980a; Vanden Bossche and Verhoeven, 1982). For example, Scheibel et al. (1968) found that niclosamide inhibits the anaerobic incorporation of ^{32}Pi into ATP and the ^{32}Pi–ATP exchange reaction in the mitochondria of *H. diminuta*. This salicylanilide also affects the mitochondrial ATP synthesis in *Ascaris* muscle mitochondria (Vanden Bossche, 1972). The failure to affect intact *Ascaris* may be the result of a permeability barrier (Saz, 1972). The fact that niclosamide is almost not absorbed in the GI tract of the host certainly protects the host against the uncoupling properties of niclosamide. In fact, this anthelmintic drug, like other salicylanilides, is a hydrogen-ionophore, tranlocating protons through the inner mitochondrial membrane. This results in uncoupling of oxidative phosphorylation from electron transport and inhibition of ATP synthesis in all isolated mitochondria investigated so far.

It should be noted that albumin prevents or at least abolishes *in vitro* the effects of salicylanilides on mitochondrial phosphorylation. Albumin was found not to counteract the effect of closantel on mitochondrial activity in intact *Fasciola hepatica*, as it had no effect on the uptake of closantel by the liver fluke. We presume that the formation of an albumin–closantel complex may be at the origin of the inability of closantel to interfere with host mitochondria *in vivo*, whereas the toxicity of closantel for *Fasciola* may originate from the ability of *Fasciola* to break down the complex (Vanden Bossche and Verhoeven, 1983). A similar mechanism might be involved in the selective toxicity of other salicylanilides.

6. NITROSCANATE

4-Isothiocyano-4′-nitrophenylether, nitroscanate, inhibits ATP synthesis in *Fasciola hepatica* (Cornish and Bryant, 1976). As far as I am aware, no data on the mode of action in cestodes have appeared in the literature.

7. PAROMOMYCIN

Paromomycin is an antibiotic related to streptomycin. Its mode of action is unknown. It has been suggested that the action against *Taenia saginata* may be affecting the ultrastructure of the tegumental membrane (Garin *et al.*, 1970). This effect should make the parasite susceptible to the host's digestive system.

8. PRAZIQUANTEL

The anthelmintic activity of the pyrazinoisoquinoline derivative, praziquantel, was discovered by Bayer A. G., Leverkusen and E. Merck, Darmstadt, in 1972, and was reported in 1975 (Andrews *et al.*, 1983; Groll, 1984).

8.1. Vacuolization of the Tegument

In vitro praziquantel is rapidly taken up by *Schistosoma mansoni*, *Fasciola hepatica*, *H. nana*, and isolated strobilocerci of *T. taeniaeformis*. For example, the concentration of the drug inside *H. nana* equaled that in the medium within less than 8 min (Andrews *et al.*, 1983). Uptake by *Cysticercus fasciolaris* (the larvae of *T. taeniaeformis*) in the cyst was markedly slower than that by the isolated larvae and adults. After 1 hr of incubation, the concentration of praziquantel in the larvae within the cyst was only 42% that of the medium (Thomas *et al.*, 1982). The cyst wall seems to be a barrier for praziquantel. Interesting is also the fact that the cuticle of the nematode, *Heterakis spumosa*, is impermeable to this drug. This may be one of the reasons why praziquantel lacks nematocidal properties.

Of course, uptake of a drug is no guarantee for therapeutic activity. An excellent example is *F. hepatica*. Although the liver fluke takes up praziquantel as rapidly as *S. mansoni* and *H. nana*, it is unaffected by the drug (Andrews *et al.*, 1980). The tegument of *F. hepatica* has been found to be refractory to the action of praziquantel that results in a rapid vacuolization of the tegumental layer in the growth zone of the neck region of adult *H. diminuta*, *H. microstoma*, *H. nana*, *E. multilocularis*, and *T. taeniaeformis* (Becker *et al.*, 1981). In the trematodes *S. mansoni* and *Dicrocoelium dendriticum*, the praziquantel-induced vacuolization of the tegument was confined to small areas scattered all over the surface of the parasites. This vacuolization led to the disruption of the apical tegumental layer. As already mentioned (Becker *et al.*, 1980), no changes were found in the tegument of *F. hepatica* after treatment with praziquantel. This result corresponds to those of Gönnert and Andrews (1977), who found no activity of this anthelmintic against mature *F. hepatica* in sheep and rats. The refractoriness of the tegument of *F. hepatica* to changes induced by praziquantel supports the hypothesis that one of the primary effects eventually leading to the death of the parasite is the disruption of the tegument in those parasites that are susceptible to praziquantel, e.g., the adult cestodes and *S. mansoni* (Becker *et al.*, 1980).

The molecular mechanism underlying tegumental alterations in both cestodes and susceptible trematodes is not well understood. In all species investigated, praziquantel at concentrations of 3.2×10^{-7} M to 3.2×10^{-4} M produced vacuolization at the base of the syncytial layer. The vacuoles increased in size, began to protrude above the surface becoming visible as blebs, and finally burst. In *H. diminuta* bursting of the blebs results in leakage of glucose, lactate, and amino acids into the bathing medium (Andrews *et al.*, 1983). The extensive damage also observed following treatment of adult *E. granulosus* with praziquantel for 1 hr suggests that massive losses of cellular constituents occur and contribute to the death of the tapeworm (Conder *et al.*, 1981). It should be noted that, in contrast with the findings of Conder *et al.* (1981); Becker *et al.* (1981) using praziquantel, in a drug concentration range from 0.1–100 μg ml, never observed rupture of the tegument of mature proglottides. Naturally, this is of great importance, since it reduces the possibility that parasite ova are released in the intestine of the host.

Scanning and transmission electron microscopic studies have shown that praziquantel causes a destruction of the tegument along the pseudostrobila and scolex of *C. fasciolaris*. This tegumental damage resembles that produced in adult tapeworms but, as could be expected from the slower uptake, the process takes much more time in the larvae than in the adults (Thomas *et al.*, 1982).

As pointed out by Andrews *et al.* (1983), vacuolization itself is not lethal to schistosomes. Death of parasites occurs as soon as tegumental damage is severe enough, so that phagocytic cells can invade the parasite. According to these investigators, it is plausible that tegumental erosion may render the schistosome helpless to the attack by the host's defense mechanism.

8.2. Contraction of the Parasite Musculature

At low concentrations (1 ng/ml), praziquantel stimulates movement of H. diminuta, H. microstoma, H. nana, and preadult E. multilocularis (collected 27 days after infection of dogs). At higher concentrations, the worms contract very rapidly. At concentrations of 1–10 μg/ml, they are immobilized and contracted within 10–30 sec (Andrews and Thomas, 1979). Terada et al. (1982) found praziquantel to induce spastic and/or paralytic actions against parasitic cestodes, trematodes, nematodes, and isolated host tissue preparations. Motility was paralyzed spastically at 10^{-8} M in Taenia pisiformis and at 10^{-7} M in Dipylidium caninum. On the other hand, the motility of nematodes such as Trichuris vulpis, Dirofilaria immitis, and Ascaris suum was less susceptible to praziquantel. Nematodes were paralyzed at $2-3 \times 10^{-4}$ M only.

The rapid contraction of, say, S. mansoni has been explained by a reduced influx of potassium and enhanced influx of sodium and calcium (Pax et al., 1978). Removal of Ca^{2+} or addition of Mg^{2+} to the incubation medium blocked the action of praziquantel on S. mansoni. It is suggested that this anthelmintic acts by permitting Ca^{2+} influx into the schistosomal muscle cells, causing them to contract (Coles, 1979). Since praziquantel does not combine with Ca^{2+} or Na^+ and carry them into a nonpolar organic phase, it does not act as an ionophore (Pax et al., 1978).

Depletion of external Ca^{2+} or the addition of Mg^{2+} does not abolish contraction in cestodes (Andrews et al., 1983). The perturbations in Ca^{2+} transport in H. diminuta are opposite to those induced by praziquantel in S. mansoni (Prichard et al., 1982). The praziquantel-induced contraction of H. diminuta musculature is accompanied by a strong inhibition of ^{45}Ca incorporation. Calcium efflux experiments showed that this drug stimulates the release of Ca^{2+} from the tapeworms preloaded with ^{45}Ca. The effluxed Ca^{2+} seems to be derived from a small fast pool and a larger slow pool. Both the stimulation of the efflux and the induced muscle contraction seem to be independent of external calcium. Praziquantel does not alter the activities of the ATPase-Ca^{2+} pump or of other ATPases found in H. diminuta (Prichard et al., 1982). The latter workers suggest that the sustained release of endogenous calcium produces the threshold concentration in the myoplasm, i.e., the contractile part of the muscle, needed for muscle contraction. In schistosomes this threshold concentration might be reached by the rapid uptake of external Ca^{2+}. Prichard et al. (1982) also propose that an increase in cytosol Ca^{2+} concentration could account for the vacuolization of the teguments of cestodes and schistosomes.

Although the molecular mechanism underlying both the tegumental alterations and muscle contraction remains to be studied, the work with praziquantel has already taught us that contraction of H. diminuta muscle depends on endogenous Ca^{2+} and thus resembles that of vertebrate skeletal muscle (Prichard et al., 1982). By contrast, muscle contraction in schistosomes is dependent on the uptake of external Ca^{2+} as in vertebrate smooth muscle (Pax et al., 1978).

REFERENCES

Al-Dabagh, M. A., Al-Moslih, M. I., Verheyen, A., Shafik, M. A., Al-Janabi, T. A., Al-Rawas, A. Y., Ismail, M. A., Fawzi, A. H., Al-Ani, M. S., and Rassam, S., 1981, The effect of mebendazole on sheep hydatid cysts as demonstrated by electromicroscopy, J. Parasitol. 67:709–712.

Andrews, P., and Thomas, H., 1979, The effect of praziquantel on Hymenolepis diminuta in vitro, Tropenmed. Parasitol. 30:391–400.

Andrews, P., Thomas, H., and Weber, H., 1980, The in vitro uptake of ^{14}C-praziquantel by cestodes, trematodes, and a nematode, J. Parasitol. 66:920–925.

Andrews, P., Thomas, H., Pohlke, R., and Seubert, J., 1983, Praziquantel, Med. Res. Rev. 3:147–200.

Becker, B., Mehlhorn, H., Andrews, P., and Eckert, J., 1980, Light and electron microscopic studies on the effect of praziquantel on Schistosoma mansoni, Dicrocoelium dendriticum, and Fasciola hepatica (trematoda) in vitro, Z. Parasitenkd. 63:111–128.

Becker, B., Mehlhorn, H., Andrews, P., and Thomas, H., 1981, Ultrastructural investigations on the effect of praziquantel on the tegument of five species of cestodes, Z. Parasitenkd. 64:257–269.

Bekhti, A., Schaaps, J. P., Capron, M., Dessaint, J.-P., Santore, F., and Capron, A., 1977, Treatment of hydatid disease with mebendazole: Preliminary results in four cases, Br. Med. J. (2):1047–1051.

Bekhti, A., Nizet, M., Capron, M., Dessaint, J.-P., Santoro, F., and Capron, A., 1980, Chemotherapy of human hydatid disease with mebendazole. Follow-up of 16 cases, Acta Gastroenterol. Belg. 43:48–65.

Borgers, M., De Nollin, S., Verheyen, A., Vanparijs, O., and Thienpont, D., 1975, Morphological changes in cysticerci of Taenia taeniaeformis after mebendazole treatment, J. Parasitol. 61:830–843.

Chatfield, R. C., and Yeary, R. A., 1979, The effects of bunamidine HCl on Hymenolepis diminuta in vitro, Vet. Parasitol. 5:177–193.

Coles, G. C., 1979, The effect of praziquantel on Schistosoma mansoni, J. Helminthol. 53:31–33.

Conder, G. A., Marchiondo, A. A., and Andersen, F. L., 1981, Effect of praziquantel on adult Echinococcus granulosus in vitro: Scanning electron microscopy, Z. Parasitenkd. 66:191–199.

Cornish, R. A., and Bryant, C., 1976, Changes in energy metabolism due to anthelmintics in Fasciola hepatica maintained in vitro, Int. J. Parasitol. 6:393–398.

French, C. M., 1984, Mebendazole and surgery for human hydatid disease in Turkana, East Afr. Med. J. 61:113–119.

Garin, J. P., Kalb, J. C., Despeignes, J., and Vincent, G., 1970, Action des antibiotiques oligo-saccharides sur Taenia saginata, J. Parasitol. 56:112 (abst.).

Gemmell, M. A., and Johnstone, P. D., 1981, Cestodes, Antibiot. Chemother. 30:54–114.

Gönnert, R., and Andrews, P., 1977, Praziquantel, a new broad-spectrum antischistosomal agent, Z. Parasitenkd. 52:129–150.

Groll, E., 1984, Praziquantel, Adv. Pharmacol. Chemother. 20:219–238.

Hamajima, F., 1973, Studies on metabolism of lung fluke genus Paragonimus. VII. Action of bithionol on glycolytic and oxidative metabolism of adult worms, Exp. Parasitol. 34:1–11.

Hart, R. J., Turner, R., and Wilson, R. G., 1977, A biochemical and ultrastructural study of the mode of action of bunamidine against Hymenolepis nana, Int. J. Parasitol. 7:129–134.

Heath, D. D., and Chevis, R. A., 1974, Mebendazole and hydatid cysts, Lancet 2:218–219.

Ireland, M., Gull, K., Gutteridge, W. E., and Pogson, C. I., 1979, The interaction of benzimidazole carbamates with mammalian microtubule protein, Biochem. Pharmacol. 28:2680–2682.

Köhler, P., and Bachmann, R., 1980, The possible mode of action of mebendazole in Ascaris suum, in: The Host Invader Interplay (H. Vanden Bossche, ed.), pp. 727–730, Elsevier, Amsterdam.

Krotov, A. I., Chernyaeva, A. I., Kovalenko, F. P., Bayandina, D. G., Budanova, I. S., Kuznetsova, O. E., and Voskoboinik, L. V., 1974, Experimental therapy of alveococcosis. II. Effectiveness of some antinematode agents against alveococcosis of laboratory animals *Med. Prazitol. Parazit. Bol.* 43:314–319 (in Russian).

Krotov, A. I., Chernyaeva, A. I., and Budanova, I. S., 1976, Experimental therapy of Echinococcus multilocularis hydatidosis. III. Effect of thiabendazole, sarcolysine acridine, levamisole and mebendazole on the development of *E. multilocularis* cysts in albino mice (In Russian), *Med. Parazitol. Parazitarnye Bol.* 45:164–168.

Laclette, J. P., Merchant, M. T., Willms, K., and Cañedo, L., 1981, Paracrystalline bundles of large tubules, induced *in vitro* by mebendazole in *Cysticercus cellulosae, Parasitology* 83:513–518.

Mansour, T. E., 1979, Chemotherapy of parasitic worms: New biochemical strategies, *Science* 205:462–469.

Müller, E., Akovbiantz, A., Ammann, R. W., Bircher, J., Eckert, J., Wissler, K., Witassek, F., and Wüthrich, B., 1982, Treatment of human echinococcosis with mebendazole. Preliminary observations in 28 patients, *Hepatogastroenterology* 29:236–239.

Pax, R., Bennett, J. L., and Fetterer, R., 1978, A benzodiazepine derivative and praziquantel: Effects on musculature of *Schistosoma mansoni* and *Schistosoma japonicum, Naunyn Schmiedebergs Arch. Pharmacol.* 304:309–315.

Prichard, R. K., Bachmann, R., Hutchinson, G. W., and Köhler, P., 1982, The effect of praziquantel on calcium in *Hymenolepis diminuta, Mol. Biochem. Parasitol.* 5:297–308.

Rahman, M. S., and Bryant, C., 1977, Studies of regulatory metabolism in *Moniezia expansa:* Effects of cambendazole and mebendazole, *Int. J. Parasitol.* 7:403–409.

Rew, R. S., 1978, Mode of action of common anthelmintics, *J. Vet. Pharmacol. Ther.* 1:183–197.

Saimot, A. G., Cremieux, A. C., Hay, J. M., Meulemans, A., Giovanangeli, M. D., Delaitre, B., and Coulaud, J. P., 1983, Albendazole as a potential treatment for human hydatidosis, *Lancet* 2:652–656.

Saz, H. J., 1972, Effects of anthelmintics on ^{32}P-esterification in helminth metabolism, in: *Comparative Biochemistry of Parasites* (H. Vanden Bossche, ed.), pp. 445–454, Academic Press, New York.

Schantz, P. M., Vanden Bossche, H., and Eckert, J., 1982, Chemotherapy for larval echinococcosis in animals and humans: Report of a workshop, *Z. Parasitenkd.* 67:5–26.

Scheibel, L. W., Saz, H. J., and Bueding, E., 1968, The anaerobic incorporation of ^{32}P into adenosine triphosphate by *Hymenolepis diminuta, J. Biol. Chem.* 243:2229–2235.

Sharma, S., and Abuzar, S., 1983, The benzimidazole anthelmintics—Chemistry and biological activity, in: *Progress in Drug Research* (E. Jucker, ed.), Vol. 27, pp. 85–161, Birkhäuser Verlag, Basel.

Sharma, S., Dubey, S. K., and Iyer, R. N., 1980, Chemotherapy of cestode infections, in: *Progress in Drug Research* (E. Jucker, ed.), Vol. 24, pp. 217–266, Birkhäuser Verlag, Basel.

Terada, M., Ishii, A. I., Kino, H., Fujiu, Y., and Sano, M., 1982, Studies on chemotherapy of parasitic helminths (IX). Effects of praziquantel on the motility of various parasitic helminths and isolated host tissues, *Experientia* 38:549–553.

Thienpont, D., Vanparijs, O., and Hermans, L., 1974, Anthelmintic activity against *Cysticercus fasciolaris, J. Parasitol.* 60:1052–1053.

Thomas, H., Andrews, P., and Mehlhorn, H., 1982, New results on the effect of praziquantel in experimental cysticercosis, *Am. J. Trop. Med. Hyg.* 31:803–810.

Vanden Bossche, H., 1972, Studies on the phosphorylation in *Ascaris* mitochondria, in: *Comparative Biochemistry of Parasites* (H. Vanden Bossche, ed.), pp. 455–468, Academic Press, New York.

Vanden Bossche, H., 1976, The molecular basis of anthelmintic action, in: *Biochemistry of Parasites and Host-Parasite Relationships* (H. Vanden Bossche, ed.), pp. 553–572, North-Holland Publishing Co., Amsterdam.

Vanden Bossche, H., 1978, Chemotherapy of parasitic infections, *Nature (Lond.)* 273:626–630.

Vanden Bossche, H., 1980*a*, Chemotherapy of *Hymenolepiasis*, in: *Biology of the Tapeworm Hymenolepis diminuta* (H. P. Arai, ed.), pp. 639–693, Academic Press, New York.

Vanden Bossche, H., 1980*b*, Peculiar targets in anthelmintic chemotherapy, *Biochem. Pharmacol.* 29:1981–1990.

Vanden Bossche, H., 1985, Pharmacology of anthelmintics, in: *Handbook of Experimental Pharmacology, Volume 77, Chemotherapy of Gastrointestinal Helminths,* (H. Vanden Bossche, P. G. Janssens, and D. Thienpont, eds.), pp. 125–181, Springer-Verlag, Heidelberg.

Vanden Bossche, H., and Verhoeven, H., 1982, Biochemical effects of the antiparasitic drug closantel, *Parasitology* 84:Li.

Vanden Bossche, H., and Verhoeven, H., 1983, Effects of albumin on the closantel-induced alterations of mitochondrial processes, in: *Fifteenth FEBS Meeting, Brussels, July 24–29*, abstract No. S-15-We-173, p. 305.

Vanden Bossche, H., Verhoeven, H., Vanparijs, O., Lauwers, H., and Thienpont, D., 1979, Closantel, a new antiparasitic hydrogen ionophore, *Arch. Int. Physiol. Biochim.* 87:851–852.

Vanden Bossche, H., Rochette, F., and Hörig, Ch., 1982, Mebendazole and related anthelmintics, *Adv. Pharmacol. Chemother.* 19:67–127.

Verheyen, A., 1982, *Echinococcus granulosus:* The influence of mebendazole therapy on the ultrastructural morphology of the germinal layer of hydatid cysts in humans and mice, *Z. Parasitenkd.* 67:55–65.

Verheyen, A., Borgers, M., Vanparijs, O., and Thienpont, D., 1976, The effects of mebendazole on the ultrastructure of cestodes, in: *Biochemistry of Parasites and Host-Parasite Relationships* (H. Vanden Bossche, ed.), pp. 605–618, North-Holland Publishing Co., Amsterdam.

Wilson, J. F., and Rausch, R. L., 1980, Alveolar hydatid disease. A review of clinical features of 33 indigenous cases of *Echinococcus multilocularis* infection in Alaskan Eskimos, *Am. J. Trop. Med. Hyg.* 29:1340–1355.

Witassek, F., Burkhardt, B., Eckert, J., and Bircher, J., 1981, Chemotherapy of alveolar echinococcosis, *Eur. J. Clin. Pharmacol.* 20:427–433.

VI

Arthropods

26

Chemistry of Drugs Used against Arthropod Parasites

G. WAYNE IVIE and LOYD D. ROWE

1. INTRODUCTION

The purpose of this chapter is to summarize the chemical data on control agents currently used against arthropod parasites of man and animal. Given the large number of different chemical structures that are active and useful in one or more host—parasite relationships—and given space limitations—this treatment is of necessity somewhat cursory. Our scope is limited to compounds that are intentionally and directly applied to man or animal for parasite control; thus, materials used in such applications as mosquito abatement, household pest control, and space sprays in livestock barns are not considered within the scope of this review. Also not presented in this section are generally widely known compounds or mixtures (e.g., xylene, chloroform, essential oils, petroleum fractions) that are often included in pesticidal formulations and that in fact may contribute to pesticidal activity. We have, perhaps paradoxically, opted to include the rather limited number of arthropod repellents used directly on man or domestic animals.

2. GENERAL CONSIDERATIONS

Pre-1940 pesticidal agents used against arthropod parasites included herbals (tincture of larkspur, California buhach, balsam of Peru), solvents (chloroform, benzene, carbon disulfide), inorganics (sulfur, lime-sulfur, arsenicals), aromatics (phenol, naphthalenes), petroleum derivatives (crude oils, creolin, coal tar, cresols, kerosene), and botanical insecticides [pyrethrum, tobacco (nicotine), derris (rotenone)] (Herms,

G. WAYNE IVIE and LOYD D. ROWE • Veterinary Toxicology and Entomology Research Laboratory, Agricultural Research Service, U.S. Department of Agriculture, College Station, Texas 77841.

1915; Hall, 1936; Culbertson, 1942). Sulfur and lime-sulfur preparations were quite effective in some antiparasite applications, and arsenical dips for tick control proved very successful in the containment and control of some important livestock diseases (e.g., cattle fever), but most of the pre-1940 control agents have passed by the wayside. Notable exceptions include pyrethrum, and to a much lesser extent, sulfur, lime-sulfur, and rotenone, which continue to have useful applications today. One of the most durable arthropod antiparasiticals is carbon disulfide, whose great utility in combatting horse bots was discovered as early as 1905 and which continues to be successfully used in that application even today.

Some of the early chlorinated hydrocarbon insecticides, whose low cost and great efficacy propelled them to rapid and widespread acceptance in many pest-control situations, still have major antiparasitical uses today. The fact that most members of the chlorinated hydrocarbon group were subsequently found to be "hard" pesticides with respect to their biological and environmental stability has led to dramatic restrictions or outright bans on usage in more developed, environmentally conscious nations. Yet in many parts of the world where such concerns are of necessity a lower priority, chemicals such as DDT and chlordane continue to have significant uses as antiparasiticals and in crop and public health protection.

Perhaps because of the rather limited scope of serious arthropod parasitism problems in man and the availability of long-standing therapeutics, there has apparently been little activity over the past few decades in developing new antiparasiticals for direct use on man. Such, however, has not been the case with animal insecticides and acaricides, for which the number of host–parasite combinations is large, economic considerations are paramount, and market competition is vigorous. In addition, acquired pest resistance—either real or anticipated—is a strong stimulus for continued efforts aimed at developing compounds of increased efficacy or pest selective modes of action. In the neighborhood of 100 pesticidal chemicals presently have utility against arthropod parasites of domestic animals, and certainly far more brand or trade name preparations of these various chemicals are currently available for use by the public or by veterinary practitioners.

Relative to other agricultural pesticide uses, the market and profit potential for specific domestic animal arthropod antiparasitical applications is usually "minor"; thus, the commercialization of arthropod antiparasiticals has generally been the offshoot of synthesis and screening efforts aimed primarily at compound development for major agricultural uses (e.g., field crops). For these reasons, many animal antiparasiticals are identical to compounds previously developed and established in major crop uses. Also, slight structural modifications of proven crop pesticides have commonly resulted in new compounds having efficacy, toxicological, and residual properties to make them highly satisfactorily animal antiparasiticals.

Because of the generally strict regulatory environments that have evolved in most developed countries during the past decade or so, rigid requirements must usually be met to gain approval of insecticides and acarcides proposed for use on or in domestic animals. Efficacious compounds must in almost all cases show a wide margin of animal safety under the proposed use patterns and, with food-producing animals, acceptable compounds must exhibit minimal tendency for retention of residues of the parent pesticide or its metabolites in edible tissues or their secretion into milk or eggs.

The development in the 1950s of the organic phosphate and carbamate pesticides, which act as anticholinesterase (AChE) agents, made available viable and generally preferred alternatives to many of the chlorinated hydrocarbons in most, including antiparasitical, pest-control applications. These compounds are, by and large, much less persistent in the environment, are highly biodegradable, and exhibit much more desirable properties than most chlorinated hydrocarbons with respect to residue potential in human foodstuffs obtained from treated animals. Although many organic phosphate and carbamate pesticides used in agriculture are potent mammalian poisons, a number of structural types (particularly among the organic phosphates) have been developed that have fully acceptable margins of safety, especially in dermal applications, such that they have been widely and successfully used as antiparasiticals for many years.

Within the past decade, tremendous advances in the development of highly pest-selective and economically competitive synthetic pyrethroids have resulted in the availability of compounds that currently have major agricultural uses, including some as animal antiparasiticals. Even more recently, much has been accomplished in efforts aimed at developing new classes of pesticidal chemicals that either have totally pest specific or highly pest selective modes of action. One insect juvenile hormone analogue (methoprene) has current applications as an animal feed through for manure breeding flies, and acceptance has now been obtained for multipest antiparasitical applications of the microbial fermentation product ivermectin, which acts by disrupting the normal function of γ-aminobutyric acid (GABA), an important neurotransmitter in the peripheral nervous system of invertebrates. Substantial progress has also been made at commercializing the benzoylphenyl ureas, a group of highly selective pesticides that act by inhibiting chitin synthesis. Although there are at present no animal antiparasitical applications for any of benzoylphenyl ureas, developmental work is now under way to gain approval for use of at least one of these compounds as an animal feed through for biting fly control.

3. ARTHROPOD ANTIPARASITICALS OF CURRENT UTILITY

A compilation of chemical and toxicological data on compounds of current utility against arthropod pests of man and domestic animals is given in Table I. These chemicals are grouped (by what we hope are reasonable criteria) as inorganic, chlorinated hydrocarbon, organic phosphate, carbamate, pyrethroid and pyrethroid-like, the inevitable "miscellaneous" and, finally, repellents. A total of 76 different active ingredients are indicated in Table I. Certain useful chemicals may have been omitted because of our unawareness of them and, a more likely problem, others may be included that are currently of marginal value as arthropod antiparasiticals. For the latter circumstance, we can only offer the justification that estimates of actual market volumes for most pesticide uses are difficult to obtain. Still other chemicals are included in Table I (most

Table I. Chemicals of Utility as Arthropod Antiparasiticals for Use in Man and/or Domestic Animals[a,b]

Name	Chemical name [CAS registry no.] [Empirical formula] [Molecular weight]	Structure	Solubility	Acute oral LD$_{50}$ in rat (mg/kg BW)
		Inorganics		
Arsenic trioxide	Arsenic oxide [1327-53-3] [As$_2$O$_3$] [197.8]	As$_2$O$_3$	Water (17 g/liter), ethanol (p. insol.), ether (p. insol.)	20
Lime-sulfur	Calcium sulfide [1344-81-6] [CaS$_x$] [variable]	CaS$_x$	Water (sol.)	Relatively nontoxic
Sodium arsenite	Arsenenous acid, sodium salt [7784-46-5] [NaAsO$_2$] [129.9]	NaAsO$_2$	Water (v. sol.), ethanol (sl. sol.)	41
Sulfur	Sulfur [7704-34-9] [S] [32.1]	S	Water (p. insol.)	Relatively nontoxic

Chlorinated hydrocarbons

Bromocyclen — 5-(Bromomethyl)-1,2,3,4,7,7-hexachlorobi-cyclo[2.2.1]hept-2-ene
[1715-40-8]
[C$_8$H$_5$BrCl$_6$]
[393.8]

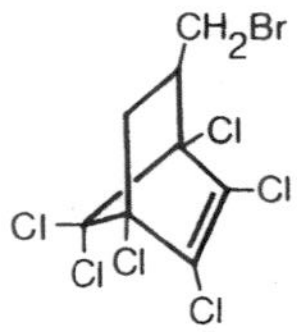

12,500

Chlordane — 1,2,4,5,6,7,8,8-Octachloro-2,3,3a,4,7,7a-hexahydro-4,7-methano-1H-indene
[52002-35-4]
[C$_{10}$H$_6$Cl$_8$]
[409.8]
(Technical chlordane contains 60–75% of chlordane isomers)

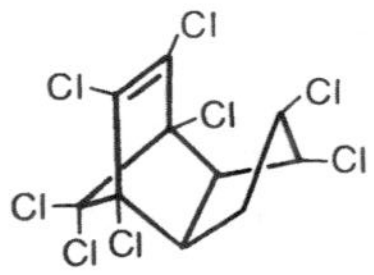

Water (0.1 mg/li-ter), EtOH (sol.), kerosene (sol.)

457–590

DDT — 1,1'-(2,2,2-Trichloroethylidene)bis[4-chloro-benzene]
[50-29-3]
[C$_{14}$H$_9$Cl$_5$]
[354.5]

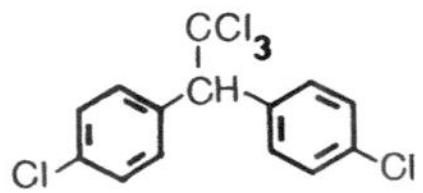

Water (p. insol.), most org. solv. (sol.)

113–118

Endosulfan — C,C'-(1,4,5,6,7,7-Hexachloro-8,9,10-trinor-born-5-en-2,3-ylene) (dimethyl sul-fite)-6,7,8,9,10,10-hexachlo-ro-1,5,5a,6,9,9a-hexahydro-6,9-meth-ano-2,4,3-benzodioxathiepin 3-oxide
[115-29-7]
[C$_9$H$_6$Cl$_6$O$_3$S]
[406.9]

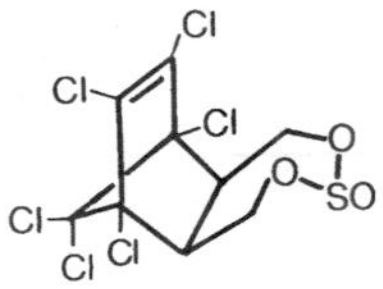

Water (0.33 mg/li-ter), EtOH (65 g/liter), hexane (24 g/liter)

80–110 (tech)

(continued)

Table 1 (Continued)

Name	Chemical name [CAS registry no.] [Empirical formula] [Molecular weight]	Structure	Solubility	Acute oral LD$_{50}$ in rat (mg/kg BW)
Lindane	$1\alpha,2\alpha,3\beta,4\alpha,5\alpha,6\beta$-Hexachlorocyclohexane [58-89-9] [C$_6$H$_6$Cl$_6$] [290.8]	(chlorocyclohexane structure with Cl substituents)	Water (7 mg/liter), EtOH (>50 g/liter), ether (>50 g/liter)	88–270
Methoxychlor	1,1'-(2,2,2-Trichloroethylidene)bis [4-methoxybenzene] [72-43-5] [C$_{16}$H$_{15}$Cl$_3$O$_2$] [345.7]	CH$_3$O—C$_6$H$_4$—CH(CCl$_3$)—C$_6$H$_4$—OCH$_3$	Water (0.1 mg/liter), MeOH (50 g/kg), CHCl$_3$ (440 g/kg)	6000 (tech)
Toxaphene	Toxaphene (a mixture of polychloro bicyclic terpenes with chlorinated camphene predominating) [8001-35-2] [C$_{10}$H$_{10}$Cl$_8$ approx] [432 approx]	Cl$_x$ (chlorinated camphene structure with CH$_3$, CH$_3$, CH$_2$)	Water (3 mg/liter), most org. solv. (sol.)	80–90
Bromophos	Organic phosphates 0-(4-Bromo-2,5-dichlorophenyl) 0,0-dimethyl phosphorothioate [2104-96-3] [C$_8$H$_8$BrCl$_2$O$_3$PS] [366.0]	(S)P(OCH$_3$)(OCH$_3$)—O—C$_6$H$_2$(Cl)(Cl)(Br)	Water (0.7 mg/liter), MeOH (100 g/liter), CH$_2$Cl$_2$, (sol.)	3750–8000

Name	Structure	Solubility	
Bromophos-ethyl	O-(4-Bromo-2,5-dichlorophenyl-O,O-diethyl-phosphorothioate [4824-78-6] [$C_{10}H_{12}BrCl_2O_3PS$] [394.0]	Water (0.14 mg/liter), most org. solv. (sol.)	48
Carbophenothion	S-[[(4-Chlorophenyl)thio]methyl] O,O-diethyl phosphorodithioate [786-19-6] [$C_{11}H_{16}ClO_2PS_3$] [342.9]	Water (<1 mg/liter), EtOH (sol.), kerosene (sol.)	20–79
Chlorfenvinphos	2-Chloro-1-(2,4-dichlorophenyl)ethenyldiethylphosphate [470-90-6] [$C_{12}H_{14}Cl_3O_4P$] [359.6]	Water (145 mg/liter), EtOH (sol.), xylene (sol.)	10–39
Chlorpyrifos	O,O-Diethyl O-(3,5,6-trichloro-2-pyridinyl) phosphorothioate [2921-88-2] [$C_9H_{11}Cl_3NO_3PS$] [350.6]	Water (2 mg/liter), MeOH (450 g/kg), benzene (sol.)	135–163
Coumaphos	O-(3-Chloro-4-methyl-2-oxo-2H-ben-zopyran-7-yl)O,O-diethylphosphorothioate [56-72-4] [$C_{14}H_{16}ClO_5PS$] [362.8]	Water (p. insol.), acetone (sl. sol.), CHCl₃ (sl. sol.)	56–230 (tech)

(continued)

Table I (Continued)

Name	Chemical name [CAS registry no.] [Empirical formula] [Molecular weight]	Structure	Solubility	Acute oral LD_{50} in rat (mg/kg BW)
Crotoxyphos	1-phenylethyl(E)-3-[(dimethoxyphosphinyl)oxy]-2-butenoate [7700-17-6] [$C_{14}H_{19}O_6P$] [314.3]		Water (1 g/liter), ErOH (sol.), xylene (sol.)	53
Cythioate	0,0-Dimethyl-0-(4-aminosulfonylphenyl)phosphorothioate [115-93-5] [$C_8H_{12}NO_5PS_2$] [297.3]		Water (insol.), EtOH (sol.), ether (sol.)	160 (tech)
Diazinon	0,0-Diethyl-0-[6-methyl-2-(1-methylethyl)-4-pyrimidinyl]phosphorothioate [333-41-5] [$C_{12}H_{21}N_2O_3PS$] [304.3]		Water (40 mg/liter), EtOH (sol.), ether (sol)	300–400 (tech)
Dichlofenthion	0-2,4-Dichlorophenyl-0,0-diethylphosphorothioate [97-17-6] [$C_{10}H_{13}Cl_2O_3PS$] [315.2]		Water (0.2 mg/liter), most org. solv. (sol.)	270
Dichlorvos	2,2-Dichloroethenyl dimethylphosphate [62-73-7] [$C_4H_7Cl_2O_4P$] [221.0]		Water (10 g/liter), most org. solv. (sol.), kerosene (2–3 g/kg)	56–108

Name	Compound	Structure	Solubility	
Dimethoate	O,O-Dimethyl-S-[2-(methylamino)-2-oxo-ethyl]phosphorodithioate [60-51-5] [C₅H₁₂NO₃PS₂] [229.2]	$CH_3NH-\overset{O}{\overset{\|}{C}}-CH_2-S-\overset{S}{\overset{\|}{P}}-OCH_3$, OCH_3	Water (25 g/liter), EtOH (>300 g/kg), CCl₄ (>50 g/kg)	180–325 (tech)
Dioxathion	S,S'-(1,4-Dioxane-2,3-diyl)-O,O,O',O'-tetraethyl di(phosphorodithioate) [78-34-2] [C₁₂H₂₆O₆P₂S₄] [456.5]	(1,4-dioxane-2,3-diyl) bis $S-\overset{S}{\overset{\|}{P}}-OC_2H_5$, OC_2H_5	Water (insol.), most org. solv. (sol.), hexane (10 g/kg)	23–43
Ethion	O,O,O',O'-Tetraethyl-S,S'-methylene di(phosphorodithioate) [563-12-2] [C₉H₂₂O₄P₂S₄] [384.5]	$C_2H_5O-\overset{S}{\overset{\|}{P}}-SCH_2S-\overset{S}{\overset{\|}{P}}-OC_2H_5$, C_2H_5O , OC_2H_5	Water (sl. sol.), most org. solv. (sol.), kerosene (sol.)	208
Famphur	O-{4-[(Dimethylamino)sulfonyl]phenyl}-O,O-dimethyl phosphorothioate [52-85-7] [C₁₀H₁₆NO₅PS₂] [325.3]	$(CH_3)_2N-\overset{O}{\underset{O}{\overset{\|}{\underset{\|}{S}}}}-\text{C}_6\text{H}_4-O-\overset{S}{\overset{\|}{P}}-OCH_3$, OCH_3	Water (sl. sol.), acetone (sol.), hexane (sl. sol.)	48 (tech)
Fenitrothion	O,O-Dimethyl-O-(3-methyl-4-nitrophenyl) phosphorothioate [122-14-5] [C₉H₁₂NO₅PS] [277.2]	$NO_2-\text{C}_6\text{H}_3(CH_3)-O-\overset{S}{\overset{\|}{P}}-OCH_3$, OCH_3	Water (14 mg/liter), MeOH (sol.), hexane (42 g/kg)	800
Fenthion	O,O-Dimethyl O-[3-methyl-4-(methylthio)phenyl]phosphorothioate [55-38-9] [C₁₀H₁₅O₃PS₂] [278.3]	$CH_3S-\text{C}_6\text{H}_3(CH_3)-O-\overset{S}{\overset{\|}{P}}-OCH_3$, OCH_3	Water (2 mg/kg), CH₂Cl₂ (sol.)	190–615

(continued)

Table 1 (Continued)

Name	Chemical name [CAS registry no.] [Empirical formula] [Molecular weight]	Structure	Solubility	Acute oral LD_{50} in rat (mg/kg BW)
Fospirate	Dimethyl-3,4,5-trichloro-2-pyridinyl phosphate [5598-52-7] $[C_7H_7Cl_3NO_4P]$ [306.5]			869
Iodofenphos	O-(2,5-Dichloro-4-iodophenyl)-O,O-dimethyl-phosphorothioate [18181-70-9] $[C_8H_8Cl_2IO_3PS]$ [413.0]		Water (<2 mg/liter), MeOH (30 g/liter), CH_2Cl_2 (sol)	2100 (tech)
Malathion	Diethyl(dimethoxyphosphinothioyl)thiobu-tanedioate [121-75-5] $[C_{10}H_{19}O_6PS_2]$ [330.3]		Water (145 mg/liter), most org. solv. (sol.)	2800
Naled	1,2-Dibromo-2,2-dichloroethyldimethylphosphate [300-76-5] $[C_4H_7Br_2Cl_2O_4P]$ [380.8]		Water (p. insol.), arom. solv. (sol.), hexane (sl. sol.)	430

Phosalone	S-[(6-Chloro-2-oxo-3(2H)-benzox-azolyl)methyl]-O,O-diethylphos-phorodithioate [2310-17-0] [C₁₂H₁₅ClNO₄PS₂] [367.8]		Water (10 mg/liter), EtOH (sol.), hexane (sl. sol.)	120–170
Phosmet	S-[1,3-Dihydro-1,3-dioxo-2H-isoindol-2-yl)methyl] O,O-dimethylphosphoro-dithioate [732-11-6] [C₁₁H₁₂NO₄PS₂] [317.3]		Water (22 mg/li-ter), acetone (650 g/liter), kerosene (5 g/liter)	113
Phoxim	α-[[(Diethoxyphosphinothioyl)oxy]imino]ben-zeneacetonitrile [14816-18-3] [C₁₂H₁₅N₂O₃PS] [298.3]		Water (7 mg/liter), CH₂Cl₂ (sol.)	1976–2170
Propetamphos	(E)-1-Methylethyl 3[[(ethylamino)methoxy-phosphinothioyl]oxy]-2-butenoate [31218-83-4] [C₁₀H₂₀NO₄PS] [281.3]		Water (110 mg/li-ter), EtOH (sol.), hexane (sol.)	119
Ronnel	O,O-Dimethyl-O-(2,4,5-trichlorophenyl)phos-phorothioate [299-84-3] [C₈H₈Cl₃O₃PS] [321.5]		Water (40 mg/li-ter), most org. solv. (sol.)	1740

(continued)

Table 1 (Continued)

Name	Chemical name [CAS registry no.] [Empirical formula] [Molecular weight]	Structure	Solubility	Acute oral LD$_{50}$ in rat (mg/kg BW)
Stirofos	(Z)-2-Chloro-1-(2,4,5-trichloro-phenyl)ethenyldimethylphosphate [22248-79-9] [C$_{10}$H$_9$Cl$_4$O$_4$P] [366.0]		Water (11 mg/liter), acetone (sol.), CH$_2$Cl$_2$ (sol.)	4000–5000
Trichlorfon	Dimethyl(2,2,2-trichloro-1-hydroxy-ethyl)phosphonate [52-68-6] [C$_4$H$_8$Cl$_3$O$_4$P] [257.4]		Water (154 g/liter), EtOH (sol.), eth-er (sl. sol.)	560–630
		Carbamates		
Carbaryl	1-Naphthalenylmethylcarbamate [63-25-2] [C$_{12}$H$_{11}$NO$_2$] [201.2]		Water (120 mg/li-ter), DMSO (400 g/kg)	850
Promacyl	3-Methyl-5-(1-methylethyl)phenylmethyl(1-oxobutyl)carbamate [34264-24-9] [C$_{16}$H$_{23}$NO$_3$] [277.4]		Water (sl. sol.), EtOH (sol.), hex-ane (sol.)	1220 (tech)

Propoxur	2-(1-Methylethoxyphenyl)methylcarbamate [114-26-1] $[C_{11}H_{15}NO_3]$ [209.2]		Water (2 g/liter), most org. solv. (sol.)	90–128

Pyrethroid and pyrethroid-like pesticides

Allethrin	2-Methyl-4-oxo-3-(2-propenyl)-2-cyclopenten-1-yl 2,2-dimethyl-3-(2-methyl-1-propenyl)cyclopropanecarboxylate [584-79-2] $[C_{19}H_{26}O_3]$ [302.4]		Water (p. insol.), MeOH (sol.), hexane (sol.)	425–875
Cyhalothrin	Cyano(3-phenoxyphenyl)methyl-3-(2-chloro-3,3,3-trifluoro-1-propenyl)-2,2-dimethylcyclopropanecarboxylate [68085-85-8] $[C_{23}H_{19}ClF_3NO_3]$ [449.9]		Water (<1 mg/liter), alcohols (sol.), ether (sol.)	144–243
Cypermethrin	(RS)-Cyano(3-phenoxyphenyl)methyl (1RS)-cis-trans-3-(2,2-dichloroethenyl)-2,2-dimethylcyclopropanecarboxylate [52315-07-8] $[C_{22}H_{19}Cl_2NO_3]$ [416.3]		Water (0.2 mg/liter), EtOH (>450 g/liter), hexane (103 g/liter)	251–4133
Deltamethrin	(1R)-[1α(S*),3α]-Cyano(3-phenoxyphenyl)methyl-3-(2,2-dibromoethenyl)-2,2-dimethylcyclopropanecarboxylate [52918-63-5] $[C_{22}H_{19}Br_2NO_3]$ [505.2]		Water (<2 µg/liter), EtOH (15 g/liter xylene (250 g/liter). acetone (500 g/liter)	135->5000

(continued)

Table 1 (Continued)

Name	Chemical name [CAS registry no.] [Empirical formula] [Molecular weight]	Structure	Solubility	Acute oral LD$_{50}$ in rat (mg/kg BW)
Fenvalerate	Cyano(3-phenoxyphenyl)methyl4-chloro-α-(1-methylethyl)benzeneacetate [51630-58-1] [C$_{25}$H$_{22}$ClNO$_3$] [419.9]		Water (<1 mg/liter), EtOH (sol.), hexane (155 g/kg)	451
Flucythrinate	(RS)Cyano(3-phenoxyphenyl)methyl(S)-4-(difluoromethoxy)-α-(1-methylethyl)benzeneacetate [70124-77-5] [C$_{26}$H$_{23}$F$_2$NO$_4$] [451.4]		Water (0.5 mg/liter), acetone (sol.), hexane (90 g/liter)	67–81 (tech)
Permethrin	(3-Phenoxyphenyl)methyl-3-(2,2-dichloroethenyl)-2,2-dimethylcyclopropanecarboxylate [52645-53-1] [C$_{21}$H$_{20}$Cl$_2$O$_3$] [391.3]		Water (0.2 mg/liter), MeOH (258 g/kg), hexane (sol.)	430–4000
Phenothrin	(3-Phenoxyphenyl)methyl-2,2-dimethyl-3-(2-methyl)-1-propenyl)cyclopropanecarboxylate [26002-80-2] [C$_{23}$H$_{26}$O$_3$] [350.5]		Water (2 mg/liter), MeOH (sol.), hexane (sol.)	>10,000

Pyrethrins	Mixture of active constituents: pyrethrins I and II; cinerins I and II; jasmolins I and II. [8003-34-7] (mixture)	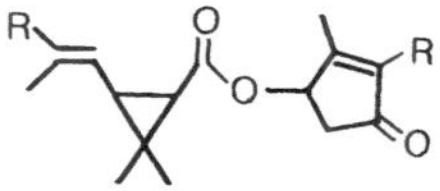	Water (p. insol.), most org. solv. (sol.)	584–900
Resmethrin	[5-(Phenylmethyl)-3-furanyl]methyl 2,2-dimethyl-3-(2-methyl-1-propenyl)cyclopropanecarboxylate [10453-86-8] [$C_{22}H_{26}O_3$] [338.4]	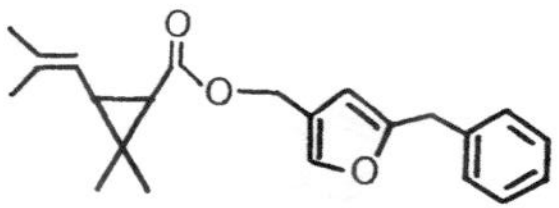	Water (<1 mg/liter), MeOH (81 g/kg), hexane (220 g/kg)	>2500

Miscellaneous compounds

Amitraz	N'-(2,4-Dimethylphenyl)-N-[[(2,4-dimethylphenyl)amino]methyl]-N-methylmethanimidamide [33089-61-1] [$C_{19}H_{23}N_3$] [293.4]	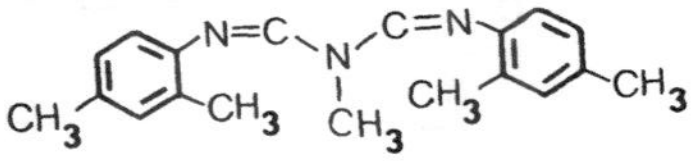	Water (1 mg/liter), acetone (>300 g/liter)	800
Benzyl benzoate	Phenylmethyl benzoate [120-51-4] [$C_{14}H_{12}O_2$] [212.2]	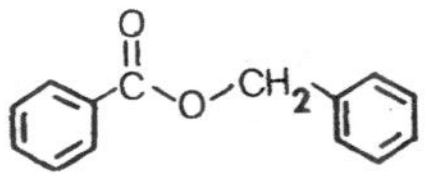	Water (insol.), $CHCl_3$ (sol.), ether (sol.)	500–5000
Carbon disulfide	Carbon disulfide [75-15-0] [CS_2] [76.1]	CS_2	Water (2.2 g/liter), EtOH (sol.), ether (sol.)	300 (sc) rabbit

(continued)

Table 1 (Continued)

Name	Chemical name [CAS registry no.] [Empirical formula] [Molecular weight]	Structure	Solubility	Acute oral LD$_{50}$ in rat (mg/kg BW)
Closantel	N-(5-Chloro-4-((4-chlorophenyl)cyanomethyl)-2-m-ethylphenyl)-2-hydroxy-3,5-diiodobenzamide [57808-65-8] [C$_{22}$H$_{14}$Cl$_2$I$_2$N$_2$O$_2$] [663.1]			
Crotamiton	N-Ethyl-N-(2-methylphenyl)-2-butenamide [483-63-6] [C$_{13}$H$_{17}$NO] [203.3]		EtOH (sol.), MeOH (sol.)	1500
Diflubenzuron	N-[[(4-Chlorophenyl)amino]carbonyl]-2,6-difluorobenzamide [35367-38-5] [C$_{14}$H$_9$ClF$_2$N$_2$O$_2$] [310.7]		Water (0.1 mg/liter), acetone (6.5 g/liter), hexane (p. insol.)	>4640
Diphenylamine	N-Phenyl-benzenamine [122-39-4] [C$_{12}$H$_{11}$N] [169.2]		Water (sol.), EtOH (sol.), MeOH (sol.)	>3,000
Disulfiram	Bis(diethylthiocarbamoyl)disulfide [97-77-8] [C$_{10}$H$_{20}$N$_2$S$_4$] [296.5]		Water (0.2 g/liter), EtOH (38 g/liter), ether (71 g/liter)	8.6

Name	Structure / description	Solubility	Value
Isobornyl thiocyanato acetate	*exo*-1,7,7-Trimethylbicyclo[2.2.1]hept-2-yl thiocyanatoacetate [115-31-1] [C₁₃H₁₉NO₂S] [253.4]		
Ivermectin	Complex macrocyclic lactone [70288-86-7] [C₄₈H₇₄O₁₄] [875.1]	Water (p. insol.), most org. solv. (sol.)	42–53
Methoprene	1-Methylethyl(E,E)-11-methoxy-3,7,11-trimethyl-2,4-dodecadienoate [40596-69-8] [C₁₉H₃₄O₃] [310.5]	Water (1.4 mg/liter), most org. solv. (sol.)	>34,600
Monosulfiram	Bis(diethylthiocarbamoyl)sulfide [95-05-6] [C₁₀H₂₀N₂S₃] [264.4]		
Phenothiazine	10H-Phenothiazine [92-84-2] [C₁₂H₉NS] [199.3]	Water (p. insol.), hexane (p. insol.), ether (sol.), EtOH (sl. sol.)	5,000

(Structural formulas shown for each compound)

(continued)

Table 1 (Continued)

Name	Chemical name [CAS registry no.] [Empirical formula] [Molecular weight]	Structure	Solubility	Acute oral LD$_{50}$ in rat (mg/kg BW)
Piperonylbutoxide	5-[2-(2-Butoxyethoxy)ethoxymethyl]-6-propyl-1,3-benzodioxole [51-03-6] [C$_{19}$H$_{30}$O$_5$] [338.4]		MeOH (sol.), EtOH (sol.)	~7500
Rotenone	(R)-1,2-Dihydro-8,9-dimethoxy-2-⟨1-methylethenyl⟩[1]benzopyrano[3,4-b]furo[2,3-b][1]benzopyran-6,12-dione [83-79-4] [C$_{23}$H$_{22}$O$_6$] [394.4]		Water (p. insol.), EtOH (sol.), acetone (sol.), CCl$_4$ (sl. sol.)	132–1500
Thiabendazole	2-(4-Thiazolyl)-1H-benzimidazole [148-79-8] [C$_{10}$H$_7$N$_3$S] [201.2]		Water (<50 mg/liter), EtOH (22 g/liter), hexane (5 g/liter)	3300
Triphenyltin acetate	(Acetyloxy)triphenylstannane [900-95-8] [C$_{20}$H$_{18}$O$_2$Sn] [409.0]		Water (9 mg/liter), EtOH (22 g/liter), hexane (5 g/liter)	140–298
Triphenyltin hydroxide	Hydroxytriphenylstannane [76-87-9] [C$_{18}$H$_{16}$OSn] [367.0]		Water (1 mg/liter), EtOH (10 g/liter), CH$_2$Cl$_2$ (171 g/liter)	110–171

Repellents

Deet	N,N-Diethyl-3-methylbenzamide [134-62-3] [C$_{12}$N$_{17}$NO] [191.3]		Water (p. insol.), EtOH (sol.)	2000

Deet	N,N-Diethyl-3-methylbenzamide [134-62-3] [C$_{12}$N$_{17}$NO] [191.3]		Water (p. insol.), EtOH (sol.)	2000
Dimethyl phthalate	Dimethyl-1,2-benzenedicarboxylate [131-11-3] [C$_{10}$H$_{10}$O$_4$] [194.2]		Water (4.3 g/kg), EtOH (sol.), ether (sol.)	8200
MGK-11	1,5a,6,9,9a,9b-Hexahydro-4a(4H)-dibenzo-furancarboxaldehyde [126-15-8] [C$_{13}$H$_{16}$O$_2$] [204.3]		Water (p. insol.), ethanol (sol.), xylene (sol.)	2500
MGK-264	2-(2-Ethylhexyl)-3a,4,7,7a-tetrahydro-4,7-methano-1H-isoindole-1,3(2H)-dione [113-48-4] [C$_{17}$H$_{25}$NO$_2$] [275.4]		Water (p. insol.), most org. solv. (sol.)	3640
MGK-326	Dipropyl-2,5-pyridinedicarboxylate [136-45-8] [C$_{13}$H$_{17}$NO$_4$] [251.3]		Water (p. insol.), EtOH (sol.), kerosene (sol.)	5230–7230
MGK-874	2-(Octylthio)ethanol [3547-33-9] [C$_{10}$H$_{22}$OS] [190.3]		Water (sl. sol.), most org. solv. (sol.), kerosene (sol.)	8530

[a]Data from Anonymous (1984a,b); Berg (1982); Blood et al. (1979); Drumond (1979, 1985); Gilman et al. (1980); Martin and Worthing (1977); Parish et al. (1983); Shotwell (1984); Sittig (1980, 1981); Spector (1956); Stecher (1968); and Worthing and Walker (1983).

[b]Abbreviations: sol., soluble; sl. sol., slightly soluble; p. sol., partly soluble; v. sol., very soluble.

notably under the pyrethroids) that have demonstrated considerable potential as arthropod antiparasiticals, but for which developmental efforts leading to regulatory approval for use have not yet culminated in most developed countries.

3.1. Inorganics

Only a very few inorganics remain of any significant use as arthropod antiparasiticals. It is probably safe to say that arsenical dips or sprays retain appreciable utility only in circumstances in which more efficacious organic pesticides are unavailable or their costs are prohibitive. Sulfur and lime-sulfur combinations remain safe, low-cost, and almost universally available remedies for ectoparasite control on humans and animals, but again the application of these long-standing remedies is likely to occur primarily in situations in which more efficacious remedies are, for whatever reasons, unavailable.

3.2. Chlorinated Hydrocarbons

Although the chlorinated hydrocarbons initiated a major revolution in arthropod pest control some four decades ago, many of these chemicals have been phased out of use in most developed countries in deference to pesticides of lesser environmental persistence and adverse impact. Nevertheless, some chlorinated hydrocarbons retain significant uses in modern animal husbandry and human medicine. Methoxychlor, a DDT analogue in which the aromatic chlorines of DDT are replaced by methoxy groups, retains high insecticidal activity, has much enhanced biodegradability and thus less tendency toward tissue retention of residues or their secretion into milk, and major uses worldwide against biting flies and lice of meat and milk-producing animals. Toxaphene, a complex mixture resulting from the chlorination of camphene, has for many years had major uses as a livestock antiparastic agent. The hexachlorocyclohexane isomer, lindane, continues to have significant animal and human antiparasitic uses. Other highly persistent chlorinated hydrocarbons whose livestock uses have been essentially eliminated in most developed countries (including chlordane, dieldrin, and particularly DDT) are still used as effective livestock and perhaps as human antiparasiticals in some parts of the world.

Major factors leading to the decline in use of many chlorinated hydrocarbons are their metabolic stability and lipophilicity, factors that lead to appreciable residue retention in lipid-rich tissues of exposed animals as well as to residue secretion into milk and eggs. The reader is referred to the comprehensive works of Brooks (1974, 1975) for details on the chemistry, structure–activity relationships, mode of action, and toxicological aspects of the chlorinated hydrocarbon pesticides.

3.3. Organic Phosphates

Since the 1950s, the organic phosphates have, as a class, achieved dominance in arthropod antiparasitical applications. As potent anticholinesterases, many of the early phosphates exhibited toxicities to warm-blooded animals (by both oral and dermal exposure routes) that were much too high to permit their direct use on man or domestic animals. Subsequent developmental efforts have, however, resulted in the availability of numerous compounds and associated use patterns in which adequate margins of safety are readily achieved. At least one organic phosphate, malathion, is used as a pediculocide in humans, as well as in numerous applications on domestic animals. The great selectivity and safety margins exhibited by malathion are attributable to the well-known fact that the compound is rapidly detoxified by carboxyesterases in most higher animals, a reaction that proceeds much slower in susceptible arthropods. The utility of some organic phosphates is greatly extended because they have sufficient metabolic stability and low toxicity in mammals that they are active systemically following oral or dermal administration (e.g., ronnel). Formulation of some organic phosphates in pest-control collars or in ear tags has also greatly extended the utility of this class of pest-control chemicals.

Although many organic phosphates have a moderate degree of lipid solubility, significant residue problems are usually not encountered under the use patterns employed. This is primarily attributable to the fact that organic phosphates are almost without exception highly biodegradable and are in most cases rapidly detoxified by exposed animals. Although some metabolic transformations (e.g., oxidative desulfuration of phosphorothionates, sulfur oxidation to sulfoxide and sulfone) are not detoxifications, essentially any esteratic cleavage around the phosphate moiety results in total loss of anticholinesterase activity, rendering the compounds essentially harmless and readily subject to excretory mechanisms. A recent treatment of the chemistry and biochemistry of organic phosphates (Fest and Schmidt, 1982) is recommended to those interested in an appreciation of the mode of action, toxicology, and structure–activity relationships of these chemicals.

3.4. Carbamates

Only a few carbamates have gained any significant application as animal antiparasiticals. The N-methylcarbamate carbaryl, however, possesses such desirable efficacy and toxicological characteristics that it has for many years been successfully used in a large number of animal ectoparasite control situations. Carbaryl is, in fact, quite probably the most widely used animal antiparasitical at this time. As with the organic phosphates, carbamates are anticholinesterases that are highly biodegradable in most higher animal species. Detoxification in exposed animals is usually rapid and the result of hydrolysis of the carbamic ester linkage—residues in food products from treated animals are generally very low and of no major toxicological consequences. Kuhr and Dorough (1976) reported a comprehensive analysis of the chemistry and biochemistry of this important class of pest-control chemicals.

3.5. Pyrethroid and Pyrethroidlike Pesticides

The natural pyrethrins, as crude preparations or in purified form from pyrethrum flowers, have been used effectively as control agents against human and animal ectoparasites dating back at least to the nineteenth century. The natural pyrethrins are still widely used today, generally in combination with synergists such as piperonyl butoxide to retard metabolic detoxification and thereby enhance efficacy. During the past decade, major advances have been made (and continue to be made at a rapid pace today) in the development of synthetic pyrethroids of greatly enhanced efficacy and selectivity. In addition to synthetic pyrethroids *per se,* pyrethroid analogues (lacking the cyclopropane ring) that retain a pyrethroid-like mode of action are similarly being developed as efficacious pest-control agents. Two of these pyrethroid analogues, fenvalerate and flucythrinate, are compounds that have considerable potential utility as animal anti-parasiticals. Although the synthetic pyrethroids are, for the most part, not in general use as animal antiparasiticals, there seems little doubt that several of the compounds shown in the table—and perhaps others as well—will shortly find major livestock uses.

Natural pyrethrins, synthetic pyrethroids, and pyrethroid-like pesticides are esters; the chemical complexity of both acid and alcohol moieties is such that most pyrethroids are susceptible to metabolic attack at a number of sites. However, the major factor related to the high degree of biodegradability of these compounds, once absorbed into the animal, is the susceptibility of the ester linkage to hydrolysis, which results in metabolites of little toxicological consequence and that are rapidly excreted. Many pyrethroids are quite lipid soluble, but metabolic considerations discussed above are such that residue appearance in foodstuffs from treated animals is not generally a significant problem. Volumes by Casida (1973) and Elliott (1977) are recommended to those interested in the historical aspects of pyrethrins and synthetic pyrethroids, their chemistry, mode of action, structure–activity relationships, and toxicological and environmental effects.

3.6. Miscellaneous

The chemicals shown in Table I under the miscellaneous category have little in common other than the fact that they do not lend themselves to categorization within any of the groups discussed above. Some of the more recent and significant efforts in developing arthropod antiparasiticals for domestic animal use have resulted in useful or potentially useful compounds that are not related to the major pesticidal classes; e.g., amitraz, the insect juvenile hormone analogue methoprene, the fermentation product ivermectin and the chitin synthesis inhibitor diflubenzuron.

3.7. Repellents

Although arthropod repellents cannot be considered drugs or pesticides in the usual sense, these compounds are widely used to minimize the annoying effects of some arthropod pests—a compilation of repellents having current utility is given in Table I.

REFERENCES

Anonymous, 1984a, *Animal Health Institute: Feed Additive Compendium,* Miller, Minneapolis.
Anonymous, 1984b, *Physicians' Desk Reference,* 38th ed., Medical Economics, Oradell, New Jersey.

Berg, G. L. (ed.), 1982, *Farm Chemicals Handbook*, Meister, Willoughby, OH.

Blood, D. C., Henderson, J. A., and Radostits, O. M., 1979, *Veterinary Medicine*, 5th ed., Lea & Febiger, Philadelphia.

Brooks, G. T., 1974, *Chlorinated Insecticides*, Vol. 1, CRC Press, Cleveland, Ohio.

Brooks, G. T., 1975, *Chlorinated Insecticides*, Vol. 2, CRC Press, Cleveland, Ohio.

Casida, J. E. (ed.), 1973, *Pyrethrum, The Natural Insecticide*, Academic Press, New York.

Culbertson, J. T., 1942, *Medical Parasitology*, Columbia University Press, New York.

Drummond, R. O., 1979, Livestock pests, in: *Guidelines for Control of Insect and Mite Pests of Foods, Fibers, Feeds, Ornamentals, Livestock, Forests and Forest Products* (J. W. Neal, ed.), USDA Agriculture Handbook 554, Washington, D.C.

Drummond, R. O., 1985, Acarine infestations of domestic animals, in: *Chemotherapy of Parasitic Diseases* (W. C. Campbell, and R. S. Rew, eds.), pp. 567–583, Plenum, New York.

Elliott, M. (ed.), 1977, *Synthetic Pyrethroids*, ACS Symposium Series 42, American Chemical Society, Washington, D.C.

Fest, C., and Schmidt, K.-J., 1982, *The Chemistry of Organophosphorus Pesticides*, Springer-Verlag, New York.

Gilman, A. G., Goodman, L. S., and Gilman, A. (eds.), 1980, *The Pharmaceutical Basis of Therapeutics*, 6th ed., Macmillan, New York.

Hall, M. C., 1936, *Control of Animal Parasites*, The North American Veterinarian, Evanston, Illinois.

Herms, W, B., 1915, *Medical and Veterinary Entomology*, Macmillan, New York.

Kuhr, R. J., and Dorough, H. W., 1976, *Carbamate Insecticides: Chemistry, Biochemistry and Toxicology*, CRC Press, Cleveland, Ohio.

Martin, H., and Worthing, C. R. (eds.), 1977, *Pesticide Manual*, 5th ed., British Crop Protection Council, Worchestershire, England.

Parish, L. C., Nutting, W. B., and Schwartzman, R. M., 1983, *Cutaneous Infestations of Man and Animal*, Praeger, New York.

Shotwell, T. K. (ed.), 1984, *Handbook of Approved New Animal Drug Applications in the United States*, Shotwell and Carr, Dallas, Texas.

Sittig, M., 1980, *Pesticide Manufacturing and Toxic Materials Control Encyclopedia*, Noyes Data Corp., Park Ridge, New Jersey.

Sittig, M., 1981, *Veterinary Drug Manufacturing Encyclopedia*, Noyes, Park Ridge, New Jersey.

Spector, W. S. (ed.), 1956, *Handbook of Toxicology*, Vol. 1, W. B. Saunders, Philadelphia.

Stecher, P. G. (ed.), 1968, *The Merck Index*, 8th ed., Merck & Co., Rahway, New Jersey.

Worthing, C. R., and Walker, S. B. (eds.), 1983, *Pesticide Manual*, 7th ed., Lavenham Press, Lavenham, Suffolk, England.

27

Insect Infestations of Man

WILLIAM C. CAMPBELL

1. INTRODUCTION

The field of medical entomology properly includes many insects that attack man directly but that are not parasitic in the conventional sense. Some inject poisons; others, coming closer to a parasitic way of life, feed on man with various degrees of exclusivity but do not dwell for extended periods in or on his body. Prime examples of the latter are mosquitoes, bedbugs, and fleas. Reactions to such stinging or biting insects and the diseases they transmit may require treatment, and the premises they inhabit may require treatment, but infection of the human body is not involved. They are controlled by environmental measures rather than by chemotherapy, and so generate a need for pesticides and exterminators rather than drugs and physicians; they are not considered herein. By contrast, certain fly larvae are truly parasitic, causing infections that may require treatment; they are considered briefly, even though treatment is usually not chemical. The lice, although not so deeply embedded in host tissue, have a prolonged and intimate contact with man; measures for the clinical management of these insects, and a few others, are also considered. While this review is thus limited to insect–man associations that might reasonably be described as infection, the term infestation is generally used in deference to convention.

2. GENERAL PRINCIPLES AND METHODS

The principles of treatment differ for the various groups of insect parasites of man and are therefore considered under the appropriate subheading. Perhaps the most important point they have in common is that the agents used for treatment are in the nature of pesticides rather than drugs in the conventional sense, and are intended to be applied to the exterior surfaces of man and his exterior surroundings. This is despite the

---

WILLIAM C. CAMPBELL • Merck Institute for Therapeutic Research, Rahway, New Jersey 07065.

selection for this chapter of insects that are in intimate contact with their host. The use of drugs for systemic efficacy against insect parasites is now widely practiced in the control of such parasites in domestic animals, but not yet in man. This is hardly surprising. In cattle, for example, the economic impact of larval *Hypoderma* infection calls for strenuous control efforts, whereas myiasis in man is neither an economic nor a public health problem of great magnitude.

A second point is that the lack of known or useful systemic efficacy does not presuppose lack of systemic absorption. Drugs that are applied to the skin may be absorbed to a greater or lesser extent from the skin; therefore, safety considerations must not be limited to a concern for skin damage.

Third, insect parasites, regardless of the permanency or the intimacy of their liaison with man, may provoke cutaneous reactions, especially those of an allergic nature. These may require lay or professional treatment. Such treatment is symptomatic in nature, frequently consisting of the topical application of antipruritic or anti-inflammatory agents, hence is not further discussed in this chapter. Methods for investigating the activity of compounds against parasitic insects have been developed mainly with a view toward their use in pets and livestock; extensive information on this subject may be found in Chapter 28.

The treatment and control of lice infestation have recently been reviewed by Orkin and Maibach (1985), Gratz (1985), Busvine (1985) and Juranek (1985).

3. LICE

3.1. *Pediculus humanus capitis, the Head Louse*

Head lice remain more or less constantly attached to the hairs of the head (cf. body lice), although they can survive for a few days off the body and readily forsake one host for another. Thus, the clinical management of pediculosis capitis usually requires application of insecticides to the scalp as well as the disinfecting of clothing and bed linens. The most widely used compounds for individual treatment are lindane (γ-benzene hexachloride), pyrethrins or synthetic pyrethroids (with or without the synergist piperonyl butoxide), and malathion. Destruction of all the louse eggs (the nits attached to the hairs) cannot be assured with most treatments, but it is no longer assumed that a second application should be given 5–10 days after the first. Repeat treatment should be contingent on the finding of live lice or on the finding of nits located on hair shafts not more than 6 mm (¼ inch) from the scalp. Nits further out on the shaft would be more than 1 week old and would have hatched (unless infertile) (D. D. Juranek, unpublished observations). Combs have been specially designed to remove nits from hair (e.g., LiceComb, Innomed, Inc.).

Bikowski (1983) provided a schema of recommendations for dealing with head louse infestation in institutional settings, including hospitals, mental institutions, nursing homes, correctional institutions, schools, camps, orphanages, day-care centers, and student dormitories. The recommendations include the treatment of (1) all individuals in whom the diagnosis is positively confirmed; (2) all individuals, whether symptomatic or not, who have had close personal contact with any proven case; (3) the immediate families of all members of the institution who are proven to have pediculosis; (4) the immediate families of all staff personnel of the institution who are proven to have pediculosis; (5) all employees who are symptomatic, even though a louse or nit is not isolated, but not their immediate families; and (6) all asymptomatic employees who request prophylactic treatment, but not the members of their families. Juranek (1985) presented a comprehensive and detailed set of recommendations for the control of head lice in schools.

There have been scattered reports of louse resistance to lindane and malathion as well as a more widely recognized resistance to DDT. The problem of regional drug resistance may therefore have to be taken into account in selecting a pediculocide for a given clinical situation.

3.1.1. Lindane (γ-Benzene Hexachloride)

Lindane has been the most popular pediculocide since its introduction in the 1950s, following the development of DDT resistance in lice (Taplin *et al.*, 1982). It is available, on prescription, in the United States as a 1.0% concentration in cream, lotion, or shampoo form (Kwell, Reed and Carnrick). It is sold over the counter at various concentrations in other countries (for other trade names, see under scabies in Chapter 28). Generally the most convenient formulation is the shampoo, and the following account of its application is based on reports by Orkin and Maibach (1984) and Witowski and Parish (1983) and on the manufacturer's instructions. The shampoo is applied in sufficient quantity (1 tablespoon or less) to thoroughly wet the hair and scalp. Small amounts of warm water are added to form a good lather, which should be worked into the hair for 4 min and then thoroughly rinsed out. When the hair has been dried with a towel, any remaining nits or nit shells may be removed with a fine comb. Dead nits remaining attached on the hair do not indicate continued infestation or reinfestation. If live lice can be found after 7 days, treatment should be repeated; persistent pruritis does not in itself justify repeated lindane treatment. Treatment must be followed by suitable hygienic measures (e.g., laundering of clothes, dry cleaning of hats).

The use of the 1% lindane cream or lotion is similar to the use of the shampoo, except that the product should be rubbed into the hair and scalp and left for 8–12 hr before being thoroughly washed out. Resistance of head lice to lindane has been reported in European studies (Maunder, 1978 la; Blommers *et al.*, 1978).

Lindane has long been regarded as a safe topical treatment, and indeed very few adverse reactions have been reported among the vast multitudes of treated people. In recent years, however, there has been much controversy over its safety, especially in children. Skin irritation may result from its application and some individuals may be highly sensitive—but that is not the point of concern. Lindane is absorbed to a degree through human skin, reaching peak plasma levels 6 hr after exposure and being slowly excreted in the urine (Ginsburg *et al.*, 1977; Solomon *et al.*, 1977). Repeated application may cause accumulation of drug, and studies in laboratory animals indicate that the drug has toxic effects on the CNS. Reports of such laboratory studies, together with circumstancial evidence of convulsions in man and conflicting evidence of carcinogenicity at high dosage in laboratory animals, have caused much disquiet and have led governmental regulatory authorities to investigate the potential hazard. The situation has been thoroughly reviewed by Rasmussen (1981) and Shacter (1981). It would seem that 1% lindane is very safe when used as directed and that adverse reactions are generally a consequence of overuse. Other available agents may be of lesser acute toxicity but are not known with certainty to have greater overall safety. At the same time, there is clearly a case to be made for minimizing the degree of exposure to lindane. It has therefore been recommended that physicians prescribe only the amount of drug needed, that they not allow the refilling of prescriptions, and that they give explicit warnings to patients (Orkin *et al.*, 1976; Rasmussen, 1981).

3.1.2. *Malathion*

This organophosphate has been used successfully against head lice, including lindane-resistant lice (Maunder, 1971a,b; Taplin *et al.*, 1982; Blommers *et al.*, 1978; Maguire and McNally, 1972). It is sold in the United States (by prescription) and elsewhere as a lotion containing 0.5% malathion in a vehicle consisting mostly of isopropyl alcohol (Prioderm, Purdue Frederick). The manufacturer of the lotion recommends that it be sprinkled onto the dry hair and gently rubbed in until the hair and scalp are thoroughly moistened. The hair should be allowed to dry without the use of heat or hair dryer and should be left uncovered. After at least 8 hr, the hair should be shampooed and rinsed; dead lice or eggs should be removed by combing. The lotion can conveniently be left on the skin overnight and, since the treatment is highly ovicidal, the need for repeat treatment is not likely to arise (D. D. Juranek, unpublished observations). However, if live lice are found after 7–9 days, treatment should be repeated. In a double-blind study, treatment with this lotion gave an ovicidal activity of 86% after 14 days, part of which could be attributed to the effect of the vehicle. At 7 days post-treatment, three of 65 treated subjects had live lice, while 26 of 47 vehicle-treated subjects had live lice (Taplin *et al.*, 1982). In another study, the malathion lotion was found to be highly active against head lice and to have (like the lindane shampoo used in the same trial) high but incomplete ovicidal efficacy (Mathias *et al.*, 1984). Resistance to malathion has been reported (Silverton, 1972).

Malathion is a relatively weak inhibitor of acetylcholinesterase (AChE) and is rapidly metabolized by the human liver. Its topical use in man appears to be well tolerated. The drug can be absorbed through human skin in some solvents. Its absorption from commercial pediculocide formulations does not seem to have been studied; appropriate caution should therefore be exercised, especially with respect to the treatment of nursing mothers. Regardless of absorption, direct contact may result in skin irritation. Concern has been expressed about the possible formation of isomalathion, a highly toxic isomer, in stored malathion products (WHO, 1979).

3.1.3. Pyrethrins

Pyrethrins, synergized by the addition of piperonyl butoxide, are widely used for louse infestations, although doubt has been expressed as to their ovidical efficacy (Taplin *et al.*, 1982). In the United States, the combination is sold without prescription under various trade names. One product (A-200 Pyrinate, Norcliff Thayer, Inc.) is available as a liquid containing 0.17% pyrethrins and 2% piperonyl butoxide or as a gel containing 0.33% pyrethrins and 4% synergist. The manufacturer recommends that either formulation be applied in an amount sufficient to wet the hair and scalp. After a maximum period of 10 min, the material is washed off and the hair rinsed with copious warm water. If necessary, the treatment may be repeated, but no more than two treatments should be given within a period of 24 hr. Another product (Rid, Pfipharmecs) contains 3.0% pyrethrins and 3.0% synergist.

3.1.4. Other Compounds

3.1.4a. DDT (Chlorophenothene). This compound has been used in the form of 2–5% emulsion or 10% powder but is no longer in common use. It has been reported to lack activity against nits, and drug-resistant louse strains have emerged. The chlorinated hydrocarbons have in general fallen into disfavor.

3.1.4b. MBIN. This designation refers to an emulsion consisting of 6% DDT, 68% benzylbenzoate, 12% benzocaine, and 14% polysorbate 80. Before use, it is to be diluted with water in a ration of 1 part emulsion to 5 parts water. Both DDT and benzylbenzoate are active against lice and, although neither compound is widely used alone, the combination is relatively inexpensive and therefore likely to be widely used in some areas. Its use has been recommended by the World Health Organization (Shacter, 1981).

3.1.4c. Temephos. This organophosphate compound has low acute mammalian toxicity and is available in some countries as a 2% dust (Shacter, 1981). An international panel of experts concluded that no significant hazard would be presented by the treatment of pediculosis capitis with 2% temephos "in a solvent commonly used for the oral administration of drugs" (WHO, 1979).

3.1.4d. Carbaryl. The carbamate insecticide carbaryl (Sevin) was very effective when applied as a lotion or shampoo containing 0.5% active ingredient, and in an amount equivalent to 50 mg per head. Treatment, especially in lotion form, was found to be highly ovicidal (Maunder, 1981). The drug was active against malathion-resistant lice and is widely used in the United Kingdom.

3.1.4e. Systemic Compounds. Although systemic treatment is used for the control of sucking lice on cattle, there has been no comparable use in man. The oral administration of cotrimoxazole (80 mg trimethoprim plus 400 mg sulfamethoxazole bid for 3 days) was reported effective in women with pediculosis capitis, while either drug alone was found ineffective (Shashindran *et al.*, 1978). Ivermectin, which is effective in cattle, might work in man but has not been tried in human pediculosis. As long as effective, safe topical remedies are available the use of systemic treatment would hardly be justified.

3.2. *Pediculus humanus humanus, the Body Louse*

Body lice are the most peripatetic of the human sucking lice, leaving the body between blood meals to dwell in the surrounding clothes, and laying most of their eggs in the seams of clothing. Control of pediculosis corporis in the individual patient is thus less dependent on the application of chemicals to the skin and can be accomplished to a large extent by the use of hot baths and changes or clothing. If substantial numbers of nits are found attached to body hairs (in heavy infestations, for example) lindane or pyrethrins can be applied as for the treatment of head louse infection (with minor modifications as appropriate). The synthetic pyrethroid known as permethrin has been tested against body lice as a single application in the form of a dust containing 1% drug. Efficacy was high and persisted for more than 1 month, and the treatment was considered safe (WHO, 1979). Inflammatory skin reactions, if any, should be treated symptomatically. Clothes and linens can be disinfected by heat, washing, or the application of insecticides (e.g., pyrethrins, pyrethroids, lindane). Spray formulations of synthetic pyrethroids are sold for application to mattresses and other household objects that cannot be laundered or dry cleaned (e.g., Li-Ban, Pfipharmecs; R. & C. Spray, Reed and Carnrick). Bikowski (1983) has formulated a set of recommendations for dealing with body louse infestation in institutions. They are similar to those for head louse infestations, but with less emphasis on the treatment of contact persons (unless they have symptoms of infestation).

3.3. *Phthirus pubis, the Crab Louse*

The crab louse is similar to the head louse in that it generally remains on the host's skin and its eggs are cemented to host hairs. The treatment of phthirias (pediculosis pubis) is therefore very similar to that for head louse infestation. *Phthirus pubis*, however, shuns areas of dense hair growth and dwells instead in areas where the hairs are about 2 mm apart, mainly but not exclusively in the pubic area (Witkowski and Parish, 1983); topical treatment is thus applied to such areas.

A common treatment is the topical application of 1% lindane. Treatment is often preceded by a warm soapy bath, but this may not be advisable in the case of pediculosis because it may lead to increased cutaneous absorption of drug. If a bath is taken, treatment should not be applied until the skin is dry and cool. A thin layer of lotion or cream is then applied to the hair and skin of the pubic and perianal regions. In hairy individuals treatment must be also applied to the thighs, trunk, and axillae (Orkin and Maibach, 1985). After 8–12 hr, the lotion or cream is thoroughly washed off. If the shampoo formulation of lindane is used, it should be allowed to remain in place for only

4 min. Hygienic measures (e.g., clean clothes, linens) should follow. Treatment should be repeated only if necessary. Treatment should be given simultaneously to sexual contacts, but it is not necessary to treat uninfested family members. Pyrethrin preparations may also be used (see Section 3.1, head lice), and their efficacy appears equal to that of the lindane preparations (Smith and Walsh, 1980; Newsom et al., 1979). In the Newsom study a 10-min application of a synergized pyrethrin lotion was as effective as a 12-hr application of a lindane lotion. Bitowski (1983) formulated recommendations for dealing with crab louse infestation in institutional environments. He recommends the treatment of sexual contacts even if asymptomatic, but not other contact persons; he does not recommend the application of pesticides to toilets or furniture or the shaving of scalp or body hair.

The case of P. pubis infestation of the eyebrows or eyelashes (pediculosis ciliaris) is clearly a special problem, since care must be taken in the use of insecticides in the region of the eye. The clinical management of pediculosis ciliaris has been described by Orkin et al. (1976) and Raber (1983). Lice and nits may be removed with forceps, but insecticidal treatment is usually indicated. The eyelashes may be smeared with petroleum jelly (petrolatum) with or without the inclusion of pyrethrin ointment, and treatment should be applied twice daily for 8–10 days. Ointments containing 1–2% yellow oxide of mercury were formerly used. Ophthalmic ointments containing 0.25–1.0% physostigmine are effective but are associated with undesirable side effects. Preparations of 1.0% lindane are also effective but are irritating to the eyes. Freezing (cryotherapy) was used to kill the lice and nits attached to the eyelashes of a young girl, with care taken to avoid damaging the eyelid skin (Awan, 1977). Secondary bacterial infections are often a problem and require appropriate adjunctive measures (topical or even systemic antibiotics, warm compresses, removal of encrustations).

4. PARASITIC FLY LARVAE (MAGGOTS)

Human myiasis, the infection of man by parasitic fly larvae, takes many forms, depending on the species of fly involved and the anatomical site of infection. Treatment, however, is similar in principle throughout the group of diseases, and chemotherapy plays essentially no role in it. In essence, treatment consists of the manual removal of the individual parasites. This will frequently involve debridement and surgical exploration of the wound and removal of parasites, with appropriate measures to enhance healing and prevent secondary infection. In principle, the parasites should not be damaged in the process of removal, since release of parasite fluids may provoke allergic reactions. In cutaneous myiasis, topical application of animal fat, petroleum jelly, or mineral oil can be used to stimulate the larvae to emerge. For example, in furuncular myiasis caused by Dermatobia hominis, the posterior end of the larva may be smeared with petroleum jelly to block the respiratory spiracles and stimulate emergence. Alternatively, chloroform may be applied to immobilize the larva before it is removed by needle or forceps. In the case of cutaneous invasion by Gastrophilus sp., mineral oil can be rubbed into the skin in front of the migration track in order to make the larva visible and susceptible to surgical removal.

When larvae have invaded tissues deeper or less accessible than the skin, their removal may have to be aided by measures appropriate to the particular site of infection. The following measures have been proposed: for nasal infection, 15% chloroform in vegetable oil used as a nasal douche and followed by saline rinses; for oral myiasis, saline rinses; for aural myiasis, minimal ether application to promote egress of maggots; for external ocular myiasis, immobilization by cocaine; for internal ocular myiasis, surgical removal if larvae are in the anterior chamber but photocoagulation if in the posterior; and for enteric, vaginal, or vesical myiasis, no special measures other than larval removal, where possible (Feinsod, 1984).

Systemic treatment of myiasis in man has not been practiced and would generally not be warranted. There might be instances, however, in which such chemotherapeutic measures would be indicated; the extraordinary potency of ivermectin against parasitic fly larvae and mites of domestic livestock raises the possibility that the drug might also be effective against myiasis (and scabies) in man. It is currently being tested in other human parasitic infections.

5. FLEAS

5.1. *Pulex irritans, the Common Flea*

This species is one of those "ectoparasites" that is a periodic feeder, and the use of a specific drug to rid the human host of the parasite is not warranted (see Section 1, Introduction).

5.2. *Tunga penetrans; the Chigoe or Jigger Flea*

The adult female of this species becomes embedded in the human skin, causing a painful lesion, usually on the soles of the feet. Clinical intervention may therefore be indicated, but this does not take the form of specific chemotherapy. Rather, each flea should be removed with a needle or scalpel, and the wound should be treated to prevent secondary infection. The use of footware is an effective form of control.

6. *LINGUATULA* AND *ARMILLIFER:* TONGUE WORMS

The tongue worms *Linguatula serrata* and *Armillifer armillatus* are occasional parasites of man. They are included here because the Pentostomida, to which they belong, are generally considered an atypical group of the Arthropoda. They are of minor medical significance, and essentially nothing is known of the efficacy of drugs against them.

ACKNOWLEDGMENT. The author is indebted to Dr. Dennis D. Juranek for helpful discussion.

REFERENCES

Awan, K. J., 1977, Cryotherapy in phthiriasis palpebrarum, *Am. J. Ophthalmol.* 83:906–907.

Bikowski, J. B., 1983, Institutional instructions for treatment of pediculosis, in: *Cutaneous Infestations of Man and Animal* (L. C. Parish, W. B. Nutting, and R. M. Schwartzman, eds.), pp. 169–175, Praeger, New York.

Blommers, L., van Lennep, M., and ven der Kaay, H. J., 1978, Gammexane and malathion in the treatment of pediculosis capitis, *Ned. Tijdschr. Geneeskd.* 122:664–668.

Busvine, J. R., 1985, Pediculosis: treatments on the horizon, in: Cutaneous Infestations and Insect Bites (O. M. Orkin, and H. I. Maibach, eds.), pp. 231–237, Marcel Dekker, New York.

Feinsod, F. M., 1984, Arthropods directly causing human injury, in: *Tropical and Geographical Medicine* (K. S. Warren and A. A. F. Mahmoud, eds.), pp. 499–516, McGraw-Hill, New York.

Ginsburg, C. M., Lowry, W., and Reisch, J. S., 1977, Absorption of lindane (gamma benzene hexachloride) in infants and children, *J. Pediatr.* 91:998–1000.

Gratz, N. G., 1985, Treatment resistance in louse control, *in: Cutaneous Infestations and Insect Bites* (O. M. Orkin and H. I. Maibach, eds.), pp. 219–230, Marcel Dekker, New York.

Juranek, D. D., 1985, *Pediculus capitis* in school children: Epidemiologic trends, risk factors, and recommendations for control, in: *Cutaneous Infestations and Insect Bites* (M. Orkin, and H. I. Maibach, eds.), pp. 199–211, Marcel Dekker, New York.

Maguire, J., and McNally, A. J., 1972, Head infestation in school children: Extent of the problem and treatment, *Community Med.* 128:374–375.

Mathias, R. G., Huggins, D. R., Leroux, S. J., and Proctor, E. M., 1984, Comparative trial of treatment with Prioderm lotion and Kwellada shampoo in children with head lice, *Can. Med. Assoc. J.* 130: 407–409.

Maunder, J. W., 1971a, Resistance to organochlorine insecticides in head lice and trials using alternative compounds, *Med. Off.* 125:27–29.

Maunder, J. W., 1971b, Use of malathion in the treatment of lousy children, *Community Med.* 126:145–147.

Maunder, J. W., 1981, Clinical and laboratory trials employing carbaryl against the human head-louse, *Pediculus humanus capitis* (de Geer), *Clin. Exp. Dermatol.* 6:605–612.

Newsom, J. H., Fiore, J. L., and Hackett, E., 1979, Treatment of infestation with *Phthirus pubis:* Comparative efficacies of synergized pyrethrins and gamma-benzene hexachloride, *Sex. Transm. Dis.* 6: 203–205.

Orkin, M., and Maibach, H. I., 1985, Treatment of today's pediculosis, in: *Cutaneous Infestations and Insect Bites,* (O. Orkin and H. I. Maibach, eds.), pp. 213–217. Marcel Dekker, New York.

Orkin, M., Epstein, E., and Maibach, H. I., 1976, Treatment of today's scabies and pediculosis, *J.A.M.A.* 236:1136–1139.

Raber, I. M., 1983, Pediculosis ciliaris, in: *Cutaneous Infestations of Man and Animal* (L. C. Parish, W. B. Nutting, and R. M. Schartzman, eds.), pp. 138–143, Praeger, New York.

Rasmussen, J. E., 1981, The problem of lindane, *J. Am. Acad. Dermatol.* 5:507–516.

Shacter, B., 1981, Treatment of scabies and pediculosis with lindane preparations: An evaluation, *J. Am. Acad. Dermatol.* 5:517–527.

Shashindran, C. H., Gandhi, I. S., Krishnasamy, S., and Ghosh, M. N., 1978, Oral therapy of pediculosis capitis with cotrimoxazole, *Br. J. Dermatol.* 98:699–700.

Silverton, N., 1972, Malathion-resistant pediculosis capitis, *Br. Med. J.* 3:646–647.

Smith, D. E., and Walsh, J., 1980, Treatment of pubic lice infestation: A comparison of two agents, *Cutis* 26:618–619.

Solomon, L. M., Fahrner, L., and West, D. P., 1977, Gamma benzene hexachloride toxicity, *Arch. Dermatol.* 113:353–357.

Taplin, D., Castillero, P. M., Spiegel, J., Mercer, S., Rivera, A., and Schachner, L., 1982, Malathion for treatment of *Pediculus humanus* var. *capitis* infestation, *J.A.M.A.* 247:3103–3105.

Witkowski, J. A., and Parish, L. S., 1983, The usual and not so usual forms of pediculosis, in: *Cutaneous Infestations of Man and Animal* (L. C. Parish, W. B. Nutting, and R. M. Schwartzman, eds.), pp. 125–137, Praeger, New York.

WHO, 1979, *Safe Use of Pesticides*, Technical Report Series 634, pp. 24–25, World Health Organization, Geneva.

28

Acarine Infestations of Man

JOHN E. GEORGE

1. INTRODUCTION

A variety of acarine species will bite or feed on humans to the extent that they may cause discomfort or a more serious health problem. These mites and ticks may be categorized as continuous or permanent parasites, temporary parasites, or those that do not colonize on their host, incidental or accidental parasites, and nonparastic mites that under certain circumstances attack humans. The approach to chemotherapy or control varies considerably, depending on the species causing a problem.

The human scabies mite (*Sarcoptes scabiei*) and the human follicle mites (*Demodex folliculorum* and *D. brevis*) are continuous or permanent parasites of humans. Chemotherapy is required to eliminate the disease caused by these mites, especially scabies. Chiggers and ticks cause health problems because of hypersensitivity to allergens introduced during feeding, the toxicity of the saliva of some ticks, and disease transmission. Because they do not colonize on their hosts, chemotherapy is not required to eliminate infestations. Preventive medicine is the best course to follow to protect people against health problems associated with chiggers and ticks. To some extent, chemical agents in the form of repellents or pesticides applied to the skin or clothing can provide protection against these organisms.

Mites, such as the chicken mite (*Dermanyssus gallinae*), the northern fowl mite (*Ornithonyssus sylviarum*), the tropical rat mite (*O. bacoti*), the cat fur mite (*Cheyletiella blakei*), and the dog fur mite (*C. yasguri*), are not parasites of humans, but people come into contact with them incidentally and are bitten or used as a facultative host. Other mites, such as the hay itch mite (*Pyemotes tritici*) or various saprophagous mites found in association with stored food (e.g., *Acarus siro, Tyrophagus putrescentiae*, and *Glycyphagus domesticus*), will often bite humans who handle or contact contaminated materials. In many cases, the lesions from the bites of these mites may be associated with consider-

JOHN E. GEORGE • U.S. Department of Agriculture, Agricultural Research Service, Southern Plains Area, U.S. Livestock Insects Laboratory, Kerrville, Texas 78029.

able irritation or discomfort caused by reactions to toxic salivary secretions or hypersensitivity to nontoxic mite saliva (Krinsky, 1983). Medical attention to such cases of dermatitis requires that the lesions be recognized as the first step in the determination of the etiologic agent. The patient's history can then be helpful in pinpointing the kind of mite causing the problem and the situation in which the mite–patient contact is occurring. None of these mites colonizes on humans, and in most cases these mites will not be found on the person or in his/her clothing. Treatment in such cases does not require application of an acaricide to the patient, but rather requires the detection and elimination of the source of the mites. The control of these incidental parasites is not covered in this book. For information on methods used to study the chemotherapy of acarine infections, see Chapter 29.

2. SCABIES

2.1. Overview

Throughout the world, the prevalence of scabies steadily increased through the mid-1960s, and by 1978 the number of patients with the disease was large enough to classify the outbreak as a pandemic (Orkin et al., 1977). γ-Benzene hexachloride (lindane), a highly effective scabicide, is the most frequently used chemotherapeutic agent in scabies treatment, although controversy about the safety of lindane has prompted reexamination of available scabicides to determine the safest and most effective materials.

2.2. Individual Agents

2.2.1. Lindane

2.2.1a. Formulations of Lindane. The γ-isomer of hexachlorocyclohexane is often referred to by the generic names of γ-benzene hexachloride (GBHC) or lindane. It has been marketed as a scabicide around the world in several formulations and under a variety of proprietary names, including Kwell, Hexicid, Jacutin, Gammene, Quellada, Lorexane, and Scabisan. The concentration of lindane in the various formulations varies from 0.3 to 2% (Orkin et al., 1977; Hurwitz, 1977; Taylor, 1979; Lange et al., 1981; Shacter, 1981).

2.2.1b Toxicity of Lindane. Lindane has a long history of use against human infestations of S. scabiei (Cannon and McCrae, 1948; Halpern et al., 1950; Kornblee and Combes, 1950), but questions have been raised about the safety of this compound. Information on its toxicity includes reports on the relationship among exposure, blood dyscrasias and hematopoietic depression, CNS toxicity, and damage to the liver and kidneys (Solomon et al., 1977). However, these toxic reactions were all related to agricultural or industrial contact, usually involving chronic exposure or misuse of the chemical. There is no concrete evidence of a relationship between lindane and adverse drug reactions (ADRs) in humans treated for scabies with topical applications of 1% lindane. However, knowledge of the overall toxicity, industrial and agricultural accidents, and some clinical incidents prompted recommendations (Orkin *et al.*, 1977; Hurwitz, 1977; Solomon *et al.*, 1977; Pramanik and Hansen, 1979) for the exercise of considerable caution in the use of lindane as a scabicide, particularly in the treatment of pregnant women, infants, and small children.

More recent reviews (Schacter, 1981; Rasmussen, 1981) and a systematic analysis of case histories of patients suspected of experiencing lindane toxicity (Kramer *et al.*, 1980) have also pointed out the need to exercise prudence in the use of 1% lindane formulations for treating scabies but concluded that abuse of the drug is more of a problem than is the toxicity of lindane. There have been an estimated 24,000,000 applications over the past 17 years of the formulation of lindane marketed under the proprietary name of Kwell. But, in all the published reviews and case reports found in the English language medical literature and in the files of the U.S. Food and Drug Administration (FDA), there are only 26 reported cases of alleged toxicity to 1% lindane applied for scabies treatment. Seven of these cases clearly represented inappropriate use of the drug (Kramer *et al.*, 1980).

2.2.1c. Clinical Considerations. In spite of extensive use of lindane for the treatment of *S. scabiei* infestations of humans and the limited documentation of incidents of ADRs associated with the drug, all parameters related to possible toxic effects are not well defined, and caution should be exercised, particularly when lindane is to be used on infants and small children. The minimum effective concentration of lindane needed to cure scabies has not been established. A 1% concentration is the standard formulation used in most parts of the world (Rasmussen, 1981), but a 0.3% lindane emulsion is available in Europe (Zesch *et al.*, 1982). In contrast to efforts to decrease the concentration of lindane in standard lotion or cream formulations, Taylor (1979) recommends using 2% lindane in a liquid paraffin formulation. He obtained effective coverage of an adult body with only 7–10 ml (140–200 mg lindane) of the preparation and needed 3–5 ml (60–100 mg lindane) for children. Percutaneous absorption is enhanced by the organic solvent (chloroform) in the formulation but, because of the small quantities required for whole-body coverage, appreciably less lindane is actually applied than the recommended (Orkin *et al.*, 1977) 30-g dose of a 1% lotion needed to cover the average adult. Recommended procedure for using lindane 1% creams or lotions for scabies treatment is as follows:

1. Do not apply lindane after a hot, soapy bath (Solomon *et al.*, 1977; Kramer *et al.*, 1980; Rasmussen, 1981), as bathing will enhance percutaneous absorption and will not significantly improve efficacy.
2. Apply 1% lindane only one time unless there is evidence of failure. A concentration of less than 1% may be equally effective, particularly for use on a person with badly excoriated skin (Solomon *et al.*, 1977).
3. The application of lindane should be left on for 12 hr to maximize mite

mortality without altering the probability of adverse toxic effects and then thoroughly washed off in a warm, soapy bath (Shacter, 1981). An infant or young child should be fully clothed or under the direct supervision of an adult to ensure that none of the medication is licked or mouthed during or after application (Kramer *et al.*, 1980). Some physicians (Orkin *et al.*, 1977; Solomon *et al.*, 1977) prefer not to use lindane, or recommend extreme caution when treating infants, young children, pregnant women, and patients with massively excoriated skin. Rasmussen (1981) concluded after review of studies of the effects of lindane on test animals and their fetuses that the compound does not appear to be teratogenic and that there is no justification for suggestions that lindane is mutagenic. He also warned that it is not appropriate on the basis of any clinical evidence to assume that lindane is safe (or unsafe) to use topically during pregnancy. Unfortunately, clinical experience with alternative drugs such as sulfur, crotamiton, or benzyl benzoate is limited, and virtually nothing is known about their possible toxicities (Kramer *et al.*, 1980).

4. A routine second application of lindane is unnecessary unless a 0.3% formulation is used. Retreatment with 1% lindane should not occur before 8 days, and then only if the presence of live mites is demonstrated (Kramer *et al.*, 1980). The recommended course of treatment with 0.3% lindane is once every 24 hr for 3 days (Lange *et al.*, 1981).

2.2.2. Crotamiton

Crotamiton (crotonyl-*N*-ethyl-*O*-toluidine) is a colorless, odorless, oily liquid. The standard formulation for treatment of scabies is either a cream or lotion containing 10% crotamiton (Cubela and Yawalkar, 1978; Konstantinov *et al.*, 1979; Shacter, 1981).

The results of the first clinical trial with crotamiton on patients with scabies were reported by Burckhardt and Rymarowicz in 1946. The recent controversy over the safety of lindane preparations prompted recommendations that alternative drugs, such as crotamiton, should be used when the patient is an infant, a young child, or a pregnant woman (Orkin *et al.*, 1977; Hurwitz, 1977; Solomon, 1977). The 10% crotamiton formulation had to be applied daily for 5 days to cure the scabies infestations of 69% of the infants and small children treated as outpatients (Cubela and Yawalkar, 1978). A 100% scabies cure rate was obatined when 50 hospitalized infants or young children were treated daily for 5 days with 10% crotamiton cream or lotion (Konstantinov *et al.*, 1979). A nonspecific antipruritic effect of crotamiton was observed in both studies, as was an antibacterial effect against the secondary bacterial skin infections commonly associated with scabies in children. No adverse reactions following crotamiton applications were noted.

The recommended treatment regimen is to bathe with soap and warm water and to dry the skin before 10% crotamiton cream or lotion is applied from the neck downward to the whole body. The application is repeated daily for a total of five applications. Once treatment has begun, the patient should not bathe until the sixth day (Cubela and Yawalkar, 1978; Konstantinov *et al.*, 1979).

2.2.3. Benzyl Benzoate

Benzyl benzoate is a clear, oily, colorless liquid that has been used since 1937 for the treatment of scabies. It is formulated as an emulsion in concentrations from 20 to 35% (Mellanby, 1972; Gulati and Singh, 1978; Shacter, 1981). Although it is an effective scabicide, benzyl benzoate is less convenient to use than lindane because it is applied nightly, or every other night, for three applications (Shacter, 1981). Benzyl benzoate does not have a disagreeable odor nor does it stain clothing or bedding. Objections include frequent complaints of burning on contact and many instances of irritation or sensitivity (Cannon and McCrae, 1948).

2.2.4. Benzyl Benzoate in Combination with Other Drugs

Since 1947 the proprietary preparation Tenutex (an aqueous emulsion containing 0.5% DDT, 2% disulfiram, and 22% benzyl benzoate) has been used in Sweden as a scabicide, with few reported treatment failures. Concern about possible adverse effects from the percutaneous absorption of DDT (Kolmodin-Hedman et al., 1979) prompted testing of a DDT-free emulsion of disulfiram and benzyl benzoate. Efficacy of the emulsion containing 2% disulfiram and 22.5% benzyl benzoate was not reduced in comparison with the Tenutex formulation (Landeren et al., 1979).

Benzyl benzoate is also a component of a formulation recommended by the World Health Organization as a scabicide. The preparation is an emulsion concentrate, designated NBIN, that contains 68% benzyl benzoate, 6% DDT, 12% benzocaine, and 14% polysorbate 80 and diluted with 5 vol of water before application. The preparation is reportedly advantageous for use in underdeveloped countries because it can be compounded from relatively inexpensive and readily obtainable materials (Shacter, 1981).

2.2.5. Sulfur

Sulfur has a long history of use as a scabicide and, although once considered outmoded, it is recommended as an alternative to such compounds as lindane or crotamiton for use on infants, children, or pregnant women because it is presumed to be more safe (Orkin et al., 1977; Solomon, 1977; Jen, 1978; Shacter, 1981). Typically, sulfur is prescribed as precipitated sulfur at a concentration of 5–10% in petrolatum. The recommended course of treatment involves nightly application for 3 nights with a bath immediately before the first application and a bath 24 hr after the third application. Sulfur ointment is messy, stains, and has an unpleasant odor but, in spite of these drawbacks, most patients treated with sulfur do not complain about it (Orkin et al., 1977).

2.2.6. Other Chemicals

A 0.5% liquid formulation of malathion, an organophosphate insecticide, was evaluated for use in the treatment of scabies. Twenty-nine adult patients received a single application to all the skin below the neck with a hot bath immediately before the malathion was applied and a second bath 24 hr later. The cure rate was 83% (Hanna *et al.*, 1978).

Permethrin, a synthetic pyrethroid insecticide in a 1% liquid paraffin formulation, was tested on 38 patients as a scabicide (Taylor, 1979). The preparation was supplied to patients for self-application with instructions that all of the contents be used at one time (7 ml for adults and 3 ml for children). Sixty-one percent of 38 patients were completely cured. This compares favorably with a cure rate of 69% for a separate group of patients in the same study who were treated with 2% lindane in liquid paraffin. Most unsuccessful treatments were traced to a failure to apply all of the scabicide at one time or to contact with an untreated, infested person.

Thiabendazole, [2-(4-thiazolyl)benzimidazole], has been administered orally and applied topically for the treatment of scabies. The daily oral dose rate is 25 mg/kg body weight for 10 days. Although this course of treatment of scabies is relatively effective, side effects such as nausea, diarrhea, and dizziness limit its usefulness by oral administration (Hernández-Perez, 1976; Mendoza-Buiza *et al.*, 1976). A 5% thiabendazole cream applied topically one to three times daily for 5 days cured scabies in 73–83% of cases, but some cases required additional treatment (Villalobos and Neuman, 1975; Mendoza-Buiza *et al.*, 1976; Hernández-Perez, 1976). A few patients experienced a mild transient dermatitis, but no other side effects were observed (Villalobos and Neuman, 1975).

3. DEMODICIDOSIS

3.1. Overview

Demodex folliculorum and *D. brevis* are both found in different parts of the pilosebaceous complex of human skin, and both may occur simultaneously on the same individual. Both mites are low-grade pathogens, and there is evidence that in some circumstances *D. folliculorum* is more than mildly pathogenic, but definitive evidence of the precise relationship between these mites and specific skin disorders is lacking (Desch and Nutting, 1972). Mites identified as *D. folliculorum* have been associated with certain cutaneous disorders including dermatitis of the scalp, dermatitis of the face (especially the forehead and nose), rosacea, blepharitis, *pityriasis folliculorum,* and pigmentation (Gear, 1972). Several drugs have been used to treat skin conditions related to demodicidosis.

3.2. Individual Agents

3.2.1. Metronidazole

Metronidazole, (2-methyl-5-nitroimidazole-1-ethanol), is a widely used antiprotozoal agent (Martin, 1982) that has been successfully employed in the treatment of rosacea-like demodicidosis (Pye and Burton, 1976). In a double-blind trial, patients administered oral doses of 200 mg metronidazole daily for 6 weeks responded favorably to treatment, as compared with individuals given a lactose placebo on the same schedule. The mode of action of metronidazole is unknown. Mazabrey and Bonafe (1982), who used metronidazole successfully to treat seven patients with severe rosacea or seborrheic dermatitis associated with the presence of *D. folliculorum*, inferred that the disappearance of the mite and the concomitant cure resulted from a modification of the composition of the sebum under the action of metronidazole. *Demodex folliculorum* survivied *in vitro* exposure to concentrations of metronidazole of as much as 1 mg/ml; therefore, it seems unlikely that this compound acts directly on these mites (Persi and Rebora, 1981).

3.2.2. Sulfur

Skin conditions attributable to *D. folliculorum* respond to treatment with sulfur ointments. Gear (1972) recommended treatment with 10% sulfur ointment every night for at least 3 nights per week, with the face and other affected areas thoroughly washed with soap and water each morning after application of the ointment. Successful treatment may require several months of applications. Ayres and Mihan (1967) used a compound sulfur ointment (Danish ointment) that contained potassium polysulfide, potassium thiosulfate, and sulfur. Patients are instructed to wash their face at night with soap and water, to apply the Danish ointment to the entire face, except the eyelids, and to wash the face again in the morning. The routine is followed for 3 consecutive nights for 1 week and then twice the next week.

3.2.3. Lindane

Topical applications of a lotion containing the combination of 0.25% lindane and 0.25% phenylmethyl benzoate (Rufli *et al.*, 1981) or 1% lindane lotion (Phadke *et al.*, 1977) nightly for 2–7 weeks were considered effective treatments for patients suffering from demodicidosis.

4. TICKS AND CHIGGERS

The transmission of disease agents, irritation, and toxic reactions caused by the attachment and feeding of ticks and chiggers make it desirable to protect people against these arthropods. Personal protection against all hemophagous arthropods and chiggers has primarily been dependent on the application of repellents. Among the hundreds of compounds screened for repellent effect, deet (*N,N*-diethyl-*meta*-toluamide) is the most widely used product; it is favored because of the longer duration of its repellency to a variety of insects, acarines, and leeches (Kochhar *et al.*, 1974). However, deet is not equally effective against all tick species and their life stages. It appears that the more active species and older instars within a species have higher thresholds of sensitivity to repellents than do less active species and younger instars. Dimethylphthalate (DMP) is another popular repellent, but it also is not equally effective against all tick species (Obenchain, 1979). Research to find more effective repellents is a continuing process that to date has not led to the identification and marketing of any repellent products superior to those already available. In laboratory screens, certain ethylene glycol acetamides (Skinner et al., 1982) and N-substituted azacyclopentanones and azacyclopentenones (Skinner et al., 1983) have been effective as repellents of *Rhipicephalus sanguineus*, the brown dog tick; however, the safety and efficacy of these chemicals for use on humans has not been established.

Permethrin, at a concentration of 0.125 mg/cm^2, has been successfully tested as a clothing impregnant for human protection against the lone star tick (*Amblyomma americanum*) (Schreck et al., 1978, 1982). The effect of the permethrin against the ticks is apparently caused by rapid intoxication and not by repellency. Treated clothing was nonirritating and nonodorous, unlike clothing treated with deet (Breeden et al., 1982). Permethrin-impregnated clothing provides useful protection to personnel whose work exposes them for days at a time to ticks. Those who desire a high level of protection without impregnated clothing can apply pressurized sprays of 0.5% permethrin directly to outer clothing. A 1-min application of permethrin to the exterior surface of pants and shirt provided 100% protection against both the American dog tick, *Dermacentor variabilis*, and the lone star tick (Mount and Snoddy, 1983). It has also been an effective spray application to clothing against *D. occidentalis* and *Ornithodoros coriaceus* (Lane and Anderson, 1984).

Clothing treated with permethrin (0.125 mg/cm^2) provided 74.2% better protection for 3 consecutive days of exposure to natural infestations of chiggers (*Trombicula* spp.) than was found with untreated clothing and use of the repellent deet (Breeden et al., 1982). *In vitro* assays of a variety of repellents and acaricides against another chigger species, *Leptotrombidium* (L.) *fletcheri*, provided evidence that permethrin as a repellent is less effective than either deet or DMP (Buescher et al., 1984). As was the case with ticks, a repellent or toxicant that is effective against one chigger species will not necessarily prove effective against other species.

REFERENCES

Ayres, S., Jr., and Mihan, R., 1967, Rosacea-like demodicidosis involving the eye lids, *Arch. Dermatol.* 95:63–66.

Breeden, G. C., Schreck, C. E., and Sorensen, A. L., 1982, Permethrin as a clothing treatment for personal protection against chigger mites (Acarina: Trombiculidae), *Am. J. Trop. Med. Hyg.* 31(3):589–592.

Buescher, M. D., Rutledge, L. C., Wirtz, R. A., Nelson, J. H., and Inase, J. L., 1984, Repellent tests against *Leptotrombidium (Leptotrombidium) fletcheri* (Acari: Trombiculidae), *J. Med. Entomol.* 21(3):278–282.

Burckhardt, W., and Rymarowicz, R., 1946, Erfahrungen mit dem neuen Antiscabiosum "Eurax," *Schwiez. Med. Wochenschr.* 47:1213.

Cannon, A. B., and McCrae, M. E., 1948, Treatment of scabies, *J.A.M.A.* 138(8):557–560.

Cubela, V., and Yawalkar, S. J., 1978, Clinical experience with crotamiton cream and lotion in treatment of infants with scabies, *Br. J. Clin. Pract.* 32:229–231.

Desch, C., and Nutting, W. B., 1972, *Demodex folliculorum* (Simon) and *D. brevis* Akbulatova of man: Redescription and reevaluation, *J. Parasitol.* 58(1):169–177.

Gear, J. H. S., 1972, The pathogenicity of *Demodex folliculorum*, in: *Essays on Tropical Dermatology* (J. Marshall, ed.), Vol. 2, pp. 209–215, Excerpta Medica, Amsterdam.

Gulati, P. V., and Singh, K. P., 1978, A family based study on the treatment of scabies with benzyl benzoate and sulphur ointment, *Indian J. Dermatol.* 44(5):269–273.

Halpern, L. K., Wooldridge, W. E., and Weiss, R. S., 1950, Appraisal of the toxicity of the gamma isomer of hexachlorocyclohexane in clinical usage, *Arch. Dermatol.* 62:648–650.

Hanna, N. F., Clay, J. C., and Harris, J. R. W., 1978, *Sarcoptes scabiei* infestation treated with malathion liquid, *Br. J. Vener. Dis.* 54(5):354.

Hernandez-Perez, E., 1976, Topically applied thiabendazole in the treatment of scabies, *Arch. Dermatol.* 112(10):1400–1401.

Hurwitz, S., 1977, Scabies in infants and children, in: *Scabies and Pediculosis* (M. Orkin, H. I. Maibach, L. C. Parish, and M. B. Schwartzman, eds.), pp. 31–38, J. B. Lippincott, Philadelphia.

Jen, I., 1978, Scabies in babies, *Can. Fam. Physician* 24:250–251.

Kochhar, R. K., Dixit, R. S., and Somaya, C. I., 1974, A critical analysis of "deet" as a repellent against arthropods of public health importance and water leeches, *Indian J. Med. Res.* 62(1):.125–133.

Kolmodin-Hedman, B., Borglund, E., and Werner, Y., 1979, Percutaneous absorption of DDT from a parasiticide used for treatment of scabies, *Acta Derm. Venereol. (Stockh.)* 59(3):276–278.

Konstantinov, D., Stanoeva, L., and Yawalkar, S. J., 1979, Crotamiton cream and lotion in the treatment of infants and young children with scabies, *J. Int. Med. Res.* 7(5):443–448.

Kornblee, L. V., and Combes, F. C., 1950, Gammexane in treatment of scabies, *Arch. Dermatol.* 61:407–412.

Kramer, M. S., Hutchinson, T. A., Rudwick, S. A., Leventhal, J. M., and Feinstein, A. R., 1980, Operational criteria for adverse drug reactions in evaluating suspected toxicity of a popular scabicide, *Clin. Pharmacol. Ther.* 27(2):149–155.

Krinsky, W. L., 1983, Dermatoses associated with the bites of mites and ticks (Arthropoda: Acari), *Int. Soc. Trop. Dermatol.* 22:75–91.

Landegren, J., Borglund, E., and Storgards, K., 1979, Treatment of scabies with disulfiram and benzyl benzoate emulsion: A controlled study, *Acta Derm. Venereol. (Stockh.)* 59(3):274–276.

Lane, R. S., and Anderson, J. R., 1984, Efficacy of permethrin as a repellent and toxicant for personal protection against the Pacific Coast tick and the Pajaroello tick Acari: Ixodidae and Argasidae, *J. Med. Entomol.* 21(6):692–702.

Lange, M., Nitzsche, K., and Zesch, A., 1981, Percutaneous absorption of lindane in healthy volunteers and scabies patients, *Arch. Dermatol. Res.* 271(4):387–399.

Martin, A. R., 1982, Anti-infective agents, in: *Wilson and Gisvold's Textbook of Organic Medicinal and Pharmaceutical Chemistry*, 8th edition (R. F. Doerge, ed.), pp. 129–188, J. B. Lippincott–Harper & Row, Philadephia.

Mazabrey, D., and Bonafe, J. L., 1982, Acné rosacée, dermatite seborrhéique, *Demodex folliculorum* et metronidazole, *Rev. Med. Toulouse* 18(7):349–350.

Mellanby, K., 1972, *Scabies*, E. W. Classey, London.

Mendoza-Buiza, E., Cabrera, U., G., Posadas, A., B., Daoud, S., G., and Contaris, A., 1976, Tratamiento de la escabiosis con tiabendazol, *Arch. Venez. Pueric. Pediatr.* 39(3):103–108.

Mount, G. A., and Snoddy, E. L., 1983, Pressurized sprays of permethrin and deet on clothing for personal protection against the lone star tick and the American dog tick (Acari: Ixodidae), *J. Econ. Entomol.* 76(3):529–531.

Obenchain, F. D., 1979, Non-acaricidal chemicals for the management of acari of medical and veterinary importance, in: *Recent Advances in Acarology* (J. G. Rodriguez, ed.), Vol. II, pp. 35–43, Academic Press, New York.

Orkin, M., Epstein, E., Sr., and Maibach, H. I., 1977, Treatment of today's scabies, in: *Scabies and Pediculosis* (M. Orkin, H. I. Maibach, L. C. Parish, and M. B. Schwartzman, eds.), pp. 108–116, J. B. Lippincott, Philadelphia.

Persi, A., and Rebora, A., 1981, Metronidazole and Demodex folliculorum, Acta Derm. Venereol. (Stockh.) 61(2):182–183.

Phadke, S. N., Gupta, D. K., and Gupta, J. C., 1977, Demodectic disease in human beings, Indian J. Dermatol. Venereol. Leprol. 43(2):114–115.

Pramanik, J. R., and Hansen, R. C., 1979, Transcutaneous gamma benzene hexacholoride absorption and toxicity in infants and children, Arch. Dermatol. 115:1224–1225.

Pye, R. J., and Burton, J. L., 1976, Treatment of rosacea by metroniazole, Lancet 1:1211–1213.

Rasmussen, J. E., 1981, The problem of lindane, J. Am. Acad. Dermatol. 5:507–516.

Rufli, T., Mumcuoglu, Y., Cajocab, A., and Buchner, S., 1981, Demodex folliculorum: Zur Atiopathogenese und Therapie der Rosazea und der perioralen Dermatitis, Dermatologica 162(1):12–26.

Schreck, C. E., Posey, K., and Smith, D., 1978, Durability of permethrin as a potential clothing treatment to protect against blood-feeding arthropods, J. Econ. Entomol. 71:397–400.

Schreck, C. E., Mount, G. A., and Carlson, D. A., 1982, Wear and wash persistence of permethrin used as a clothing treatment for personal protection against the lone star tick (Acari: Ixodidae), J. Med. Entomol. 19(2):143–146.

Shacter, B., 1981, Treatment of scabies and pediculosis with lindane preparations: An evaluation, J. Am. Acad. Dermatol. 5:517–527.

Skinner, W. A., Rosentreter, U., and Elward, T., 1982, Tick repellents. I: Ethylene glycol acetamides, J. Pharm. Sci. 71:837–839.

Skinner, W. A., Rosentreter, U., and Elward, T., 1983, Tick repellents. II: N-substituted azacyclopentanones and azacyclopentenones, J. Pharm. Sci. 72:1354–1356.

Solomon, L. M., Fahrner, L., and West, D. P., 1977, Gamma benzene hexachloride toxicity: A review, Arch. Dermatol. 113:353–357.

Taylor, P., 1979, Scabies in Zimbabwe Rhodesia: Distribution on the human body and the efficacy of lindane and permethrin as scabicides, Cent. Afr. J. Med. 25(8):165–168.

Villalobos, D., and Neuman, V., 1975, Estudio de la acción antisárnica del thiabendazol al 5% en uso topica, Bol. Chil. Parasitol. 30(1/2):2–5.

Zesch, A., Nitzsche, K., and Lange, M., 1982, Demonstration of the percutaneous resorption of lipophilic pesticide and its possible storage in the human body, Arch. Dermatol. Res. 273(1–2):43–49.

29

Insect Infestations of Domestic Animals

WILLIAM N. BEESLEY

1. INTRODUCTION AND GENERAL PRINCIPLES

Insects that attack animals may do so quite temporarily (biting flies and most fleas); they may attack or invade for weeks or even months (cattle grubs and sticktight fleas), or they may be fully dependent on the host (lice). The parasitic stage that invades the host is always the larva (screwworms, fleeceworms, cattle grubs, bots) or adult (fleas, lice). Feeding patterns vary considerably, and as extreme examples some larval fleas feed on the hemorrhagic droppings of their blood-sucking parents, while certain adult flies are unable to feed at all, relying for their activity on the energy stored away in the juvenile stages, as in the cattle grub.

Because of the many and varied lifestyles of the parasites considered here, chemical control methods have had to become correspondingly diverse, from simple conventional dusting, spraying, dipping, or aerosol treatments to the use of medicated ear tags and collars and pour-on, spot-on, and injection treatments with systemically active organophosphorus insecticides. Drugs used for the control of insect infestations of domestic animals are listed in Tables I–III. [a]

[a] Data from Tables I–III are taken from lists published by the Departments of Agriculture in various countries. Not all formulations of a given insecticide may be available in a particular country. Individual label instructions should always be followed very carefully, especially with regard to dilution of concentrate, method of application, minimum age of animal on which the insecticide can be used, use of protective clothing, and other considerations. These detailed requirements have been omitted from the tables, which are intended only to give an overall view of the preparations available.

WILLIAM N. BEESELY • Department of Veterinary Parasitology, Liverpool School of Tropical Medicine, Liverpool L3 5QA, England.

1.1. Myiases

Myiasis-producing insects, all of them *Diptera*, have larval stages that actively invade the living tissue of animals or birds. As they usually do not require the prior damage of the host before they penetrate, the myiasis is normally primary.

1.1.1. Fleeceworms, Screwworms

The temperate zone fleeceworms or blowflies (e.g., *Lucilia sericata, L. cuprina*) and the tropical or semitropical screwworms (*Cochliomyia hominivorax* in the New World, *Chrysomya bezziana* in the Old World) cause considerable damage to animals, leaving the way open for further myiasis attack and secondary bacterial infections. Screwworm infestation may also follow skin damage caused by ticks, shearing wounds, dehorning, and so forth.

1.1.2. Oestrids: Cattle Grub, Horse Bot, Sheep Nasal Bot

The larvae of oestrids grow inside the host from a newly hatched 1 mm to around 20–25 mm when they vacate the animal and pupate. Different species invade the wall of the upper or lower gut, nasal passages, connective tissue, or the fatty tissue associated with nerves. Their often deep penetration of the tissue makes them ideal targets for the systemically active OP insecticides and ivermectin.

1.2. Lice

Sucking lice ingest blood and so can be killed externally or by systemics, whereas chewing (biting) lice are much more mobile and feed superficially. As all lice, like sheep ticks, spend their entire lifetime on the host, they form a "captive audience" for insecticidal control.

1.3. Fleas

Adult fleas are susceptible to treatment while on the host, but fleas in the immature stages must be sought in dust, household debris, and other environmental surroundings.

2. EXPERIMENTAL METHODS

2.1. Myiases

A laboratory LD_{50} test with adult houseflies (*Musca domestica*) is a common primary insecticide screen, but it has to be borne in mind that the larvae, not the adults, of myiasis flies are the ultimate target. Also, insecticide resistance levels among fleeceworms, for example, may differ considerably between the adults and the larvae recovered from actual field infestations. Again, the appropriate adult flies may (*Lucilia, Callitroga*) or may not (*Hypoderma*) be easily accessible for, or relevant to, work on myiasis larvae.

2.1.1. Fleeceworms, Screwworms

Discovery by a pharmaceutical firm of a potentially marketable insecticide will be followed by tests against many different potential targets, from mealworms to mosquitoes but, as far as myiasis larvae are concerned, attention will be paid particularly to the easily cultured fleeceworms (blowflies) or screwworms. These are not obligatory myiasis parasites and so can be kept easily and indefinitely on liver or meat. Adult *Lucilia sericata*, for example, lay most eggs on days 3–20, placing these on liver, especially in slits cut into the tissue; *Phormia* females lay maximum numbers of eggs on days 5–7. The eggs with their substrate can be removed from their cages each day in paper cups or petri dish halves to a separate series of cages or screened jars. The egg masses are left in their dishes, on a 5–15-cm depth of sawdust or vermiculite. The eggs hatch within 12–24 hr and the larvae pass through the three stages in only 4–5 days at 27°C and 60–70% relative humidity. The larvae can easily penetrate coarse gauze, so that several layers provide better security for the culture jars. The prepupae leave the meat containers and burrow into the sawdust, so that the tissue remnant can then be shaken out and removed. Pupation lasts 5–6 days at 25–27°C. The flies can be allowed to mass-emerge in communal cages or the container of pupae in their sawdust can be moved from cage to cage each day in order to produce flies of given ages. It is convenient to keep 200–800 flies in each cage. Because of the unpleasant smell of the decomposing meat used in blowfly cultures, artificial cultures can be used incorporating such materials as agar, yeast, casein and salt (Lennox, 1939). A good extractor fan is usually essential.

Crude larvicidal tests can be done by placing batches of 100–250 first-stage larvae on a liver mince incorporating insecticides at ppm levels and examining the eventual development of the pupae and adults. At the end of the test, a careful count is made of the surviving pupae and adults, including any semiemergent, deformed, or nonfertile adults. Eggs then laid by flies that develop from dosed larvae may be fertile or infertile; all these parameters are useful in the assessment of possible sublethal effects of insecticides (Beesley, 1960). A small practical point is that the poisoned liver substrate must not be allowed to dry out or skin over; otherwise the larvae, already weak from the effects of the insecticide, may become trapped and die. To prevent this problem, the liver can be gently mixed each day and a small amount of water added.

For the more precise tube test, small pieces (say 0.2 g) of cellulose, cotton wool, or dental plugs are saturated with serial dilutions of the candidate insecticide, in acetone, in triplicate. An automatic dispenser is useful if large numbers of tests are carried out (Shaw and Blackman, 1971). The impregnated cotton can be dried and stored for later use, but it is best used immediately. The plug is placed at the bottom of a 7.5 × 2.5-cm glass vial and 1–3 ml serum added, followed by a counted 25–30 fleeceworm larvae. The tubes are then plugged with cotton; some insecticides repel the larvae, which try to migrate upward, but a strip light situated a few centimeters above the tube will prevent this. After 24–72 hr, the contents of each tube are teased out in a dish of water and examined under a dissecting microscope. Results can be expressed as dead/alive larvae or as dead/moribund/alive larvae.

The implant test (*in vivo*) is used to observe the persistence of candidate insecticides in the fleece/skin of treated sheep. Approximately 100–500 newly hatched fleeceworm larvae from a standard strain are placed on intact or lightly scarified skin and covered with a small pad of damp cotton wool, held in place by tying the wool over it, stapling, or using an elastic band. Larvae are implanted each week until some remain alive after 24–48 hr, indicating breakdown of that particular test. At this point the surviving larvae are removed in order to prevent injury and further fly attack. In a "patch" modification of the implant test, small areas of wool are treated, allowed to dry off, and then implanted with larvae as before (James *et al.*, 1980).

Field tests may have to be organized to investigate the breakdown of known insecticides on dipped, sprayed, or jetted sheep under natural fleeceworm or screwworm attack (Roxburgh and Shanahan, 1973). For this work, simple fly attractants can be added as an additional stress on the insecticide, e.g., ammonium sulfide, mercaptans, or fleece extracts seeded with bacteria such as *Proteus mirabilis* (Emmens and Murray, 1983).

Unfortunately, the period of insecticide persistence provided against blowfly strike under field conditions may be only one-half that anticipated from laboratory *in vitro* tests, because of the attraction of wild flies to skin and wool soiled by mycotic dermatitis, bacterial or worm infections, and so forth. Consequently, it is necessary to mimic field conditions as closely as possible in laboratory tests. One way of doing this is by deliberately adding to a clean laboratory sheep dip wash a mix of skin material, wool or hair, urine, mud, and feces ("shumf"). Insecticidal activity will then have had to overcome the competition from stripping (exhaustion) effects, as well as the attraction of the wash for egg-laying flies.

Rearing methods for the larvae of the screwworm, *Cochliomyia hominivorax*, are basically the same as for the fleeceworms. However, because 200 million screwworm flies were needed each week in the U.S. eradication program, culture methods had to be thoroughly researched (Goodenough *et al.*, 1983). Maggots were reared in large vats and fed dried whole blood, dried whole egg, nonfat dried milk, formalin, and water. Larvae for field studies of insecticide susceptibility are collected from tethered bait sheep or goats, as was also done in the final stages of the U.S. eradication program.

Larval tests can be supplemented by work with adult fleeceworms and screwworms to investigate reports of possible resistance to insecticides. Direct application of 0.2–1.0 μl of an acetone solution of insecticide to the dorsal surface of the thorax is accomplished with an Agla micrometer syringe, using a foot pedal or hand-operated trigger delivery system. As insecticide susceptibility can vary several fold depending on sex, the sex of flies is determined under CO_2 anesthesia; each subject is then held in fine forceps or by finger and thumb while acetone or oil solution of insecticide is deposited on the fly. Because acetone is extremely volatile, handling should be done as quickly as possible, or the insecticide may solidify at the tip of the needle. The 24-hr survival of the flies at each concentration is noted and the LD_{50} and slope of the probit line compared with standard data from a known susceptible strain. Exposure of flies to deposits of insecticide on filter paper may also be used to assess resistance.

The speed at which a systemic insecticide reaches the blood after oral or dermal (pour-on, spot-on) application may be followed by taking venous blood samples $\frac{1}{2}$–24 hr after treatment. The serum can then be used in tube tests with *Lucilia* larvae to show that, for example, orally applied trichlorphon, or at least its insecticidal moiety, reaches the peripheral blood circulation in 20–30 min, while dermally applied fenthion (Tiguvon) takes up to 4 hr (Beesley, unpublished observations). The HPLC technique will detect the presence of insecticide and its metabolites, regardless of their insecticidal activity, so that both the tube test and HPLC complement one another in overall assessment of the fate of the insecticide.

2.1.2. Oestrids

Adult oestrid flies are not used in insecticidal tests, as the primary effort of practical control is directly against the larvae. It is difficult to mass-culture these larvae for any reasonable length of time (Chamberlain, 1964), but first-instar *Hypoderma* larvae have been exposed to organophosphorus insecticides in Earle's or similar media (Barrett and Wells, 1948; Beesley, 1962). The first-stage larvae of *H. lineatum* are remarkably tolerant of OP insecticides, taking about 1 week to die, even in concentrations of 32 ppm of fenchlorphos, for example.

The logical method of implanting larvae into natural or laboratory hosts has been used for *Hypoderma* (Bishopp et al., 1926; Beesley, 1962), but this technique is tedious and expensive. In rabbits and guinea pigs, implanted cattle grub larvae will reach and penetrate the skin of the back, but then immediately escape to the outside, without moulting and resting, as in natural bovine infections. Nevertheless, some useful basic data has been collected in this way.

A simpler technique is to use one of the rodent bot flies (*Cuterebra jellisoni, C. fontinella*) in laboratory rats or mice, which are infected intraorbitally (Ostlind et al., 1979). Test systemic insecticides are then dosed, and any surviving larvae appear in the inguinal region within 4 days of the infestation. (Drummond, 1979).

A three-parasite guinea pig test devised by Drummond (1958) assesses a wide range of systemic insecticidal activity. On the first day, 10 nymphal *Amblyomma americanum* ticks are allowed to attack; 24 hr later, screwworm larvae are placed on the host, and after a further 24 hr the insecticide is dosed at a standard rate of 100 mg/kg; 4 and 24 hr later, adults of *Stromoxys calcitrans* are allowed to feed. Promising compounds are then taken into the field for similar tests on sheep or goats.

2.2. Lice

In vitro culture of animal lice has rarely been successful, but Hopkins and Chamberlain (1972) set up a long-running colony of the cattle-biting lice, *Damalinia*

(Bovicola) bovis. These workers collected 200 adults and nymphs by clipping hair from an infested Hereford steer, placing the hair on a screen and collecting the lice that dropped through. The lice were then incubated at 37°C and 80% relative humidity (RH) in a beaker containing cowskin scrapings. These environmental conditions were chosen as being similar to those previously used in work on the colonization of goat and sheep lice. The flakey outer portion of a fresh-frozen cow skin was scraped off, dried, and ground to provide the "bovine" constituent of the culture. The lice survived well at 80% RH, but after 1 week they were moved to 70% RH to lessen the possibility of growth of molds.

Sucking lice can be fed artificially on heparinized or defibrinated blood through a chicken skin or crop membrane; this technique has been used for culturing the pig louse, *Haematopinus suis,* and dog louse, *Linognathus setosus* (Nelson, 1955).

Preliminary insecticide tests on lice can be carried out using impregnated paper and then extended to include natural infestations on laboratory animals, e.g., *Polyplax serrata* on rats or *Gliricola porcelli* in guinea pigs. Screening work is usually taken into the field soon afterward. In the case of the sheep-biting louse, *Damalina (Bovicola) ovis,* a standard method of examination used by Hall (1978) involves the counting of live lice seen when the fleece is parted five times at sites over the shoulders, the ribs, and the loins. The numbers of lice are determined on 2 days the week after treatment.

After the first week, a 14-day cycle is introduced. Two lousy sheep from the challenge group are introduced into each pen of three treated sheep and kept in close contact for 8 days. The challenge sheep are removed on the 8th day, and during the next 6 days the treated sheep are inspected on two separate occasions for the presence of live or dead lice. This cycle is repeated until live lice are recorded on the treated sheep for two consecutive contact periods. Discovery of living lice on the sheep is accepted as indicating a failure of protection. At the same time, counts are also made on the untreated challenge sheep to ensure that their louse population has not decreased.

Insecticides may (chlorpyrifos, famphur) or may not (fenchlorphos) show ovicidal effects (Loomis, 1976), the condition of the eggs being graded as viable (tan color and firm, with embryonic structures often visible) or nonviable (semitransparent and deflated, with few or no embryonic structures visible). Flat and transparent hatched eggs lacking their opercula were not counted.

The timings of laboratory tests must include adequate cover for the speed of activity of the insecticide. For example, insecticide-tolerant human lice (*Pediculus humanus*) are killed by exposure for 1 day to paper impregnated with 4.0% DDT or 0.1% dieldrin, yet die only 5 hr after exposure to 1.0% fenitrothion and only 2.5 hr after exposure to 1.0% trichlorfon (Neguvon) (WHO, 1980).

2.3. Fleas

Insecticides are tested as dusts, sprays, or aerosols against flea colonies *in vitro* or against natural infections on dogs, cats, or laboratory animals. The rodent flea (*Xenopsylla cheopis*) and cat flea (*Ctenocephalides felis*) are in frequent use, the latter being the commonest flea on both cats and dogs.

For laboratory tests, 9-cm-diameter filter papers (Whatman no. 9) are treated with the test insecticide and allowed to dry off for 24 hr. They are then folded and placed in 75 × 25-mm glass tubes; 10–12 fleas are placed in each tube and mortality observed after 24 hr. One test showed an LC_{50} of 50ppm for carbamate bendiocarb, 150 ppm for propoxur, 330 ppm for malathion, and 400 for bromocyclen (Goose, 1980).

As with lice, fleas differ in their susceptibility to various insecticides. For example, deaths of the rat flea are best assessed after 24-hr exposure to 1.0% DDT paper, while only $2\frac{1}{2}$-hr exposure to 1.0% fenitrothion and $1\frac{1}{4}$-hr exposure to 1.0% trichlorfon paper are necessary for meaningful results (WHO, 1980).

Tests on cats and dogs should involve 50–100 fleas for each test. The fleas should be placed on the host 20–30 min before treatment is given (Goose, 1980). If the compound is effective, the fleas begin to drop off the host $\frac{1}{2}$–2 hr after treatment; flea challenges can be made each week after treatment.

Systemically active insecticides can be tested by dosing guinea pigs or rats at the rate of, say, 2.5–400 mg/kg and exposing them for 10–15 min to 20 fleas 1–5 hr later (Clark and Cole, 1965). In a test with *X. cheopis*, 100 mg/kg of trichlorfon killed all the fleas that fed 1 hr after dosing and 85% of those that fed after 4 hr, while with fenthion a dose of only 50 mg/kg killed all the fleas that fed up to 4 hr after dosing. An alternative technique is to give medicated feed to rats (Clark and Cole, 1968); kills of fleas can reach 100% after steady exposure for up to 2 days to rats on feed treated with diazinon, or to 2 weeks of dimethoate.

Flea repellents can be screened in animal tests or by using the human arm exposed in cages containing up to 1000 hungry fleas (Lindquist *et al.*, 1944) but individual people and animals vary in their attractiveness to fleas. Repellents may not necessarily prevent fleas from jumping onto the skin, but feeding will be inhibited; thus, the degree of repellency may be judged by the proportion of fleas that leave wheals after feeding.

3. THE DRUGS AND THEIR USES

Because of their persistent residues in tissues, organochlorine insecticides lost favor during the mid-1960s, and many have since been replaced by organophosphorus compounds, carbamates, photostable pyrethroids, ivermectin, and other agents. Dieldrin, for example, was voluntarily withdrawn from use as a sheep dip in Britain in 1965. Unfortunately, there is an extremely narrow gap between the ideal of maximum efficacy and persistence on the skin on the one hand and unduly long tissue persistence of the insecticide and its metabolites on the other; the optimum combination to suit all views is virtually unobtainable, at least on public health grounds.

Much progress has been made in the control of myiasis larvae, fleas, and lice, but actual eradication is rare. The 1958 U.S. Screwworm Eradication Program is an example of what can be achieved with massive planning and minimum insecticide usage, while several European countries have reduced cattle grub infestation to very low levels.

3.1. Myiases

3.1.1. Fleeceworms, Screwworms

As noted already, *Cochliomyia* (= *Callitroga*) *hominivorax* was the subject of a huge and very successful sterile male eradication scheme, now extended to include a wide no-go zone along the U.S./Mexican border. Screwworm remains a severe problem in many of the warmer countries of the world, and preventive measures have included the smear preparations "62" (benzene and diphenylamine) and EQ 335 (3% hexachlorocyclo-hexane (HCH) in a gel base).

Current formulations in use against screwworms include dips, sprays, (wettable powder, WP, and emulsifiable concentrate, EC,) spray foams, dusts, and aerosols containing the OPs coumaphos or ronnel (cattle, swine), with HCH for use on sheep and nonlactating goats. Fleeceworms are controlled with a similar range of insecticides, plus diazinon, dioxathion, propetamphos, dichlorvos, and toxophene, for example. These OP and OC insecticides should be used not more frequently than once every 2 weeks. Ivermectin also shows excellent activity against calliphorine myiasis larvae and is effective against acarines and gut roundworms of livestock as well. There is great potential for these wide-spectrum pesticides, such as trichlorfon (helminths, insects, acarines) and rafoxanide (trematodes and sheep nasal bot).

Sublethal effects of insecticides have been studied for many years (Beesley, 1960; Moriarty, 1969). Hall (1982) exposed *Lucilia cuprina* females *in vitro* to wool treated with cypermethrin, deltamethrin, (decamethrin), and cyhalothrin. No eggs were laid for 6 months with many of the exposed flies dying with their ovipositors extruded.

3.1.2. Oestrids

The cattle grubs are the most economically important of the oestrid parasites, doing great damage to the skin of the host. Horse bots and sheep nasal bots are generally of much less importance.

Younger animals tend to be the most severely affected, but the whole herd should be treated prophylactically with systemic OPs at the end of the adult fly season. Treatments should be given not later than 8–12 weeks before the anticipated first appearance of the larvae in the back, because larvae of *H. bovis* and *H. lineatum* can cause severe reactions if killed in the epideral fat or esophagus, respectively. Cytotoxic material escaping from dying *H. bovis* larvae in the spinal canal can produce severe paraplegia, which may necessitate euthanasia; there may also be anaphylactic reactions.

Pour-on and spot-on OPs have replaced the original oral applications of the first systemics; currently used insecticides include fenthion, famphur, coumaphos, phosmet, and trichlorfon, at concentrations of 6–20%; coumaphos and phosmet can also be used as 0.25–0.5% sprays Table I. Ivermectin gives excellent control of cattle grub, at a dose rate of only 0.2 mg/kg, and also kills roundworms. Great Britain, Eire, and Switzerland have made very good progress with their national grub-eradication programs, although the prospects of eradication are much more limited in areas that are not geographically isolated.

Table 1. Insecticides Suitable for the Control of Myiases on Farm Livestock, Dogs, and Cats

Host	Insect pest	Insecticide	Recommended dosage (%)	Remarks
Cattle	Cattle grub (warble)			
	BL[a]	Derris	5	Scrub-on
	BNL[b]	Coumaphos	0.375–0.5	Pressure spray
			0.25	Spray, dip
			4	Pour-on
		Famphur	12.5, 13.2	Pour-on
		Fenthion	2–3	Pour-on
			20	Spot-on
		Phosmet	0.2	Dip
			0.25	Spray
			4, 13.3, 20	Pour-on
		Trichlorfon	8	Pour-on
		Ivermectin	1	sc injection
	Screwworm			
	BL[a]	Coumaphos	5	Dust
			3	Spray foam
		Ronnel	2.5	Aerosol
	BNL[b]	Coumaphos	0.25	Spray
		Ronnel	0.5	Spray
Sheep/goats	Screwworm	Bromocyclen	—	Aerosol
		Coumaphos	5	Dust
			3	Spray foam
			0.25	Spray, dip
		HCH	3	Aerosol
		Ronnel	2.5	Aerosol
			0.5	Spray
		Chlorfenvinphos	0.05–0.1	Dip, spray
	Fleeceworm	Coumaphos	0.125	Dip
		Dioxathion	0.15	Dip, spray
		Dioxathion + dichlorvos	0.15 + 0.005	Dip or spray
		HCH	3	Aerosol
		Ronnel	0.5	Spray
		Carbophenothion	0.04	Dip
		Diazinon	0.025	Dip
		Chlorpyrifos	0.05	Dip, jet
			0.2	Spray
		Chlorfenvinphos	0.05	Dip
	Nasal bot	Trichlorfon	40	In feed or water; not in young or pregnant animals
		Ivermectin	0.08	Oral drench
	Horse bot	Dichlorvos	17.5	Pellets in feed
		Trichlorfon	40	Paste

(*continued*)

Table 1 (Continued)

Host	Insect pest	Insecticide	Recommended dosage (%)	Remarks
Horses	Screwworm	HCH	3	Aerosol
		Ronnel	2.5	Aerosol
		Coumaphos	0.25	Wash
			3.0	Spray foam
			5.0	Dust
Swine	Screwworm	Coumaphos	5	Dust
			3	Spray foam
			0.25	Spray
		Ronnel	2.5	Aerosol
Dogs/cats	Screwworm	Diazinon	—	Wash
		Ronnel		

*a*BL, beef and lactating dairy cattle.
*b*BNL, beef and nonlactating dairy cattle.

Where costs are particularly important, the older insecticide rotenone (derris) can be used. Rotenone is very effective as a contact insecticide, but it has little persistence, necessitating that treatments be given at 4–6-week intervals, while the larvae are arriving in the skin of the back. Unfortunately the skin has already been damaged when the insecticide is applied. The tropical warble fly, *Dermatobia hominis* (berne, nuche, forcel), which affects livestock in Central and South America, causes very severe damage to the skin, but it is controllable by trichlorfon and other OP insecticides.

Suitable insecticides for the control of *Gasterophilus* include the OP trichlorfon, given dry in the food, dissolved in water, or as a 40% paste applied by syringe to the back of the tongue. The chemically similar insecticide dichlorvos can be given as 17.5% pellets in the feed. Combinations of thiabendazole and trichlorfon are useful against both intestinal strongyles and *Gasterophilus*.

Instillation of 1–4% HCH in oil into the nostrils while the sheep is lying on its back has given excellent results in South Africa. Various systemic OP insecticides, such as trichlorfon, coumaphos, and crufomate, have also proved effective. Rafoxanide, given orally at 7.5 mg/kg, is also satisfactory and has the added advantage of being a suitable drug against the liver fluke *Fasciola hepatica*.

3.2. Lice

Pediculosis is an important economic problem of many species of livestock and poultry; consequently, a large number of insecticides are available to control the condition Table II. These include the OPs (chlorpyrifos, coumaphos, crotoxyphos, dichlorvos, diazinon, dioxathion, famphur, fenitrothion, fenthion, malathion, phosmet, propoxur, stirophos, and ronnel), the OCs (HCH, which is not recommended for use on animals less than 3 months old, methoxychlor, bromocyclen, and toxaphene), the older synergized pyrethrins, and the photostable pyrethroids (cypermethrin, the carbamate

Table II. Insecticides Suitable for the Control of Lice on Farm Livestock, Birds, Dogs, and Cats

Host	Insecticide	Concentration (%)	Remarks
Cattle BL[a]	Coumaphos	1	Dust or dust bags
		0.03	Spray
	Crotoxyphos	0.15–0.3	Spray
	Crotoxyphos + dichlorvos	0.25–0.3 + 0.06–0.02	Spray
		1 + 0.25	Mist spray
	Pyrethrins + piperonyl butoxide	(oily) 0.06/+ 0.48	Mist spray
	Stirofos (= tetrachlorvinphos)	3	Dust or dust bags
BNL[b] (BL range also)	Chlorpyrifos	43	Spot-on
	Dioxathion	0.15	Spray, dip
		1.5 (oily)	Backrubber
	Dioxathion + dichlorvos	0.15 + 0.005	Spray, dip
		1.5 + 0.05 (oily)	Backrubber
	HCH	0.03–0.06	Dip, spray
		0.625	Dust
		0.25	Spray
		0.2	Dip
	Phosmet	4, 20	Pour-on
		1	Dust or dust bags
	Ivermectin	1	sc injection
	Coumaphos	0.06–0.125	Dip, spray
	Bromocyclen	0.2–0.5	Wash
		0.82	Aerosol spray
		4.25	Dust
	Famphur	13.2	Pour-on
	Fenthion	20	Spot-on
		1 or 3	Pour-on
	Malathion	0.5	Spray
		2 (oily)	Backrubber
		4 or 5	Dust or dust bag
	Methoxychlor	3	Dust bag
		3–5	Dust
		0.5	Spray, dip
		5 (oily)	Backrubber
	Methoxychlor + malathion	5 + 4	Dust
	Methoxychlor + toxophene	5 + 5	Dust
	Ronnel	0.25	Spray
		1 (oily)	Backrubber
	Stirofos	0.35	Spray
	Stirofos + dichlorvos	0.35 + 0.1	Spray
	Toxaphene	0.4–0.5	Spray, dip
		2–5 (oily)	Backrubber
	Toxaphene + dichlorvos	0.35 + 0.015	Spray
	Toxaphene + HCH	5 + 1	Dust
		0.3 + 0.003–0.02	Spray or dip
		4.5 + 0.5 (oily)	Backrubber

(continued)

Table II (Continued)

Host	Insecticide	Concentration (%)	Remarks
BNL[b] (BL range also) (*cont.*)	Toxaphene + malathion	0.5 + 0.02–0.5	Spray or dip
		2.5 + 0.25–0.5 (oily)	Backrubber
	Toxaphene + methoxychlor	0.25 + 0.25	Spray or dip
	Trichlorfon	8	Pour-on
	Diazinon	0.013	Spray or wash
Sheep/goats	Cypermethrin	2.5	Pour-on
	Carbophenothion	0.021	Dip
	Coumaphos	0.025	Dip
	HCH	0.6	Dust
	Chlorfenvinphos	0.01	Dip
	Chlorfenvinphos	0.05	Spray
	Diazinon, with or without	0.025	Dip
	chlorfenvinphos, chlor-	0.045	Dip
	pyrifos	0.05	Dip, jet
		0.2	Spray
Horses	Bromocyclen	0.2–0.5	Wash
		0.82	Aerosol
		4.2	Dust
	HCH	0.6	Dust
	Diazinon	0.013	Spray or wash
Swine	Bromocyclen	4.25	Dust
		0.82	Aerosol
		0.07–0.2	Wash
	Diazinon	0.013–0.02	Spray or wash
	Coumaphos	1.0	Dust
	HCH	0.016	Spray
	Crotoxyphos	0.15–0.3	Spray
	Phosmet	20	Pour-on
Dogs/cats	Bromocyclen	0.07	Wash (care needed with cats)
		0.82	Aerosol
		4.25	Dust
	Dichlorvos + fenitrothion	0.2 + 0.8	Aerosol
	Derris	2–5	Dust
	Carbaryl	0.5	Wash
	Chlorfenvinphos	0.1	Wash
Poultry	DDT[c]	5	Dust
	HCH[c]	0.1–1.0	Dust
	Derris	10	Dip
	Pyrethrins	10	Dip
	Malathion	4	Dust
	Coumaphos	0.5	Dust
Cage birds	As for poultry, also bro-mocyclen		

[a]BL, beef and lactating cattle.
[b]BNL, beef and nonlactating cattle.
[c]Can taint eggs and flesh.

carbaryl, and ivermectin). Methods of application range from sprays, dips, dusts, and self-treat dust bags to the newer pour-ons, e.g., fenthion, chlorpyrifos, cypermethrin. (Henderson and McPhee, 1983), spot-ons, e.g., fenthion, and slow-release insecticidal plastic ear tags, e.g., cypermethrin. *Solenopotes capillatus* often feeds around the eyes of cattle, and cypermethrin sprays can give much better results at this site than do ear tags, which are otherwise excellent (Titchener, 1982). Cypermethrin killed *Damalina (Bovicola) ovis* on Australian sheep at dip concentrations as low as 1 ppm, and at 5 and 19 ppm prevented reinfestation from contact challenge on sheep for 7 and 19 weeks, respectively (Hall, 1978). Resistance by *D. ovis* to 0.06% HCH was detected in England in 1965 but was overcome by the use of 0.021% carbophenothion. An interesting spinoff from the cattle grub eradication program in Eire was that farmers who used skin dressings containing crufomate reported excellent control of sucking lice; this dual activity helped the campaign immensely: the immediate killing of the lice compensated for the "nothing-to-see" prophylactic effect against grub holes the next spring. Single injections of ivermectin are effective against sucking and biting lice of cattle (Lloyd *et al.*, 1981).

Swine are often infested with sucking lice, *Haematopinus suis*, and most of the insecticides already listed can be used, generally as sprays. Ivermectin was very effective against pig lice by subcutaneous injection at 0.2 mg/kg (Barth and Brokken, 1980). A pour-on formulation of 20% phosmet has also been found doubly useful against lice and *Sarcoptes* on swine. As with the use of OPs on other livestock, care should be taken not to treat too frequently. For example, coumaphos, famphur, toxaphene, and trichlorfon can be harmful to animals of many species under 3 months of age, while HCH and toxaphene may be harmful for dogs and cats.

Horses commonly have lice; as horses are normally not used for human consumption, a wide range of insecticides are available with virtually no restrictions, from HCH and toxaphene to malathion, usually applied as sprays or dusts. Dog lice may be controlled with such agents as coumaphos, ronnel, chlordane, malathion, and carbaryl, but insecticides must be used with care on cats because of their self-grooming habits. Safer insecticides for these animals include pyrethrum and bromocyclen.

Poultry lice were formerly controlled by painting the perches with a strong extract of tobacco or nicotine, or by treating the birds with rotenone or the rather toxic sodium fluoride. Carbaryl, bromocyclen, coumaphos, malathion, stirofos, and dichlorvos are among the insecticides now in common use, generally as sprays or dusts, including dust baths. Kunz and Hogan (1970) used dichlorvos-impregnated resin strands attached to laying hens or to the bottom of their cages, obtaining good louse control for 4–6 months.

3.3. Fleas

Fleas are mainly a problem on dogs, cats and poultry; pets can be treated with dusts, sprays or aerosols containing pyrethrins, bromocyclen, HCH (not cats), iodofenphos, malathion, ronnel, coumaphos, or carbaryl, for example Table III. A combination of 0.2% dichlorvos and 0.8% fenitrothion, in an aerosol, is also very popular, and a quietening valve can be incorporated for use on pets which may be

Table III. *Insecticides Suitable for the Control of Fleas on Dogs, Cats, and Poultry*

Host	Formulation	Insecticide	Concentration (%)	Remarks
Dog/cat	Dusts	Bromocyclen	4.25	
		Pyrethrins +	0.25	
		piperonyl bu-toxide	2.5	
		Permethrin	1.0	Useful for treatment of host and its bedding
		HCH	0.5–0.6	Care with cats
		Derris	2.0–5.0	
		Bendiocarb	0.1	
		Coumaphos	0.5	Not cats
	Aerosol sprays	Bromocyclen	0.82	Aerosol sprays may cause
		Dichlorvos + fenitrothion	0.2 + 0.8	fright, especially with cats—
		Permethrin	1.0	can spray onto cotton wool, then used to wipe the ani-
		Propoxur	0.25	mal
	Baths	Bromocyclen	0.7	Dogs; not desirable to bathe cats: may leave residue in coat especially in long-haired breeds: self-grooming
		Carbaryl	0.5	Dog/cat; not for use on ani-mals under 4 weeks old
		Ronnel	0.25	Dogs/cats
		HCH	0.01	Dogs/cats
		Iodofenphos	0.5	Dogs
		Derris	2	Dogs
		Permethrin	1.0	Dogs
		Chlorfenvinphos	0.1	Dogs
	Collars	Diazinon	15	Cats/dogs
		Dichlorvos	9.3	Dogs
			4.65	Cats
			18.6	Dogs (medallions)
	Oral	Ronnel	Tablet (0.25, 0.5, 1.0 g a.i.)	Dog/cat
		Cythioate	Tablet (0.03 g a.i.)	Dog/cat
Poultry	Chicken flea	Bromocyclen	4.25	Dust for pigeons (residue prob-lem on poultry)
		HCH	0.1–0.2	Dust
		Malathion	4.0	Dust, dust box
		HCH	0.06	Spray
		Coumaphos	0.5	Dust box
	Sticktight flea	Carbaryl	10.0	Dust head
			5.0	Dust, dust box
		Carbaryl + sulfur	5% + 10%	Dust head region, Dust box
		Malathion	0.45	Treat head region
			4–5	Dust box
			3.5	Mist spray
			0.45	Spray

alarmed by the noise of the aerosol (8 sec for dogs, 5 sec for cats over 3 kg, with one-half the dose for smaller animals, repeated at 2-week intervals).

Flea collars consist of plastic impregnated with dichlorvos (9.3% for dogs, 4.65% for cats; 18.6% for flea medallions for dogs). The dog may also be placed in a bag containing an insecticidal collar, with just his head protruding. As dichlorvos (and other OPs) are cholinesterase inhibitors, animals wearing flea collars should not be exposed to or treated with other anticholinesterases. Dog flea collars should not be used on cats. Also, some breeds of dogs, such as greyhounds, can show mild toxic effects from flea collars.

The poultry sticktight flea, *Echidnophaga gallinacea*, and the European hen flea, *Ceratophyllus gallinae*, can be controlled with sprays or dusts at 7−10-day intervals of HCH, bromocyclen, malathion, or carbaryl. Dipping in 0.1−1.0% DDT may be necessary against *E. gallinacea*, as the adults of this species spend most of their time attached to the comb and wattle of the host. A 3 : 1 mixture of lard : kerosene will cause the fleas to fall off the host but, of course, there are no insecticidal or residual effects. As with the control of fleas on pets, care must be taken to treat the environment thoroughly, as at any one time many more fleas may be hiding within a few feet of the host than we actually know of.

REFERENCES

Barrett, W. L., and Wells, R. W., 1948, Transplantation of *Hypoderma* larvae and testing chemicals for control of larvae in experimental hosts, *J. Econ. Entomol.* 41:779−782.

Barth, D., and Brokken, E. S., 1980, The activity of 22, 23-dihydroavermectin B$_1$ against the pig louse, *Haematopinus suis*, *Vet. Rec.* 106:388.

Beesley, W. N., 1960, Persistence of insecticide in fleece, *Vet. Rec.* 72:638−640.

Beesley, W. N., 1962, Experimental techniques for evaluation of systemic insecticide against ox warble fly larvae, *Exp. Parasitol.* 12:102−108.

Bishopp, F. C., Laake, E. W., Brundrett, H. M., and Wells, R. M., 1926, The cattle grub or ox warbles, their biologies and suggestions for control, U.S. Dept. Agric. Bull. no. 1369, Washington, D. C.

Chamberlain, W. F., 1964, Survival of first-instar common cattle grub under anaerobic conditions in vitro, *J. Econ. Ent.* 57:799−800.

Clark, P. H., and Cole, M. M., 1965, Laboratory evaluation of promising systemic insecticides in guinea pigs against oriental rat fleas, *J. Econ. Entomol.* 58:83−86.

Clark, P. H., and Cole, M. M., 1968, Systemic insecticides for control of oriental rat fleas, *J. Econ. Entomol.* 61:505−508.

Drummond, R. O., 1958, Laboratory screening tests of animal systemic insecticides, *J. Econ. Entomol.* 51:425−427.

Drummond, R. O., 1979, Mouse-*Cuterebra* systemic test, *Proc. Entomol. Soc. Am.* 5:230−231.

Emmens, R. L., and Murray, M. D., 1983, Bacterial odours as oviposition stimulants for *Lucilia cuprina*, *Bull. Entomol. Res.* 73:411−415.

Goodenough, J. L., Brown, H. E., Wendel, L. E., and Tannahill, F. H., 1983, Screwworm eradication program: A review of recent mass-rearing technology, *Southwest. Entomol.* 8:16−30.

Goose, J., 1980, The use of bendiocarb to control fleas, in: *Fleas* (R. Traub and H. Starcke, ed.), pp. 315−320, A. A. Balkema, Rotterdam.

Hall, C. A., 1978, The efficiency of cypermethrin (NRDC 149) for the treatment and eradication of the sheep louse *Damalinia ovis*, *Aust. Vet. J.* 54:471−472.

Hall, C. A., 1982, Ovipositional deterrents for the control of blowfly strike on sheep, in: *Ectoparasites of Veterinary and Medical Importance in Temperate Areas, London, November 1982*, pp. 64–66.

Henderson, D., and McPhee, I., 1983, Cypermethrin pour-on for control of the sheep body louse (*Damalinia ovis*), *Vet. Rec.* 113:258–259.

Hopkins, D. E., and Chamberlain, W. F., 1972, *In vitro* colonization of the cattle biting louse, *Bovicola bovis*, *J. Econ. Entomol.* 65:771–772.

James, P. S., Picton, J., and Riek, R. F., 1980, Insecticidal activity of the avermectins, *Vet. Rec.* 106:59.

Kunz, S. E., and Hogan, B. F., 1970, Dichlorvos impregnated strands for control of chicken lice on laying hens, *J. Econ. Entomol.* 63:263–266.

Lennox, F. G., 1939, *Studies of the Physiology and Toxicology of Blowflies*, Council for Scientific Industrial Research, Australia, Pamphlet no. 90, 24 pp.

Lindquist, A. W., Madden, A. H., and Watts, C. N., 1944. The use of repellents against fleas, *J. Econ. Entomol.* 37:485–486.

Lloyd, J. E., Kumar, R., and Jones, C. J., 1981, Cattle lice control, *Proc. Entomol. Soc. Am.* 6:190–191.

Loomis, E. C., 1976, Trials with chlorpyrifos (Dursban) as a systemic insecticide against the cattle louse, *Vet. Rec.* 98:168–170.

Moriarty, F., 1969, The sublethal effects of synthetic insecticides on insects, *Biol. Rev.* 44:321–357.

Nelson, W. A., 1955, Artifical feeding of certain ectoparasites through membranes, *J. Parasitol.* 41:635–636.

Ostlind, D. A., Cifelli, S., and Lang, R., 1979, Insecticidal activity of the anti-parasitic avermectins, *Vet. Rec.* 105:168.

Roxburgh, N. A., and Shanahan, G. J., 1973, A method for the detection and measurement of insecticide resistance in larvae of *Lucilia cuprina*, *Bull. Entomol. Res.* 63:99–102.

Shaw, R. D., and Blackman, G. G., 1971, A method of measuring the susceptibility to insecticides of larvae of the sheep blowfly *Lucilia* spp., *Aust. Vet. J.* 47:268–271.

Titchener, R. N., 1982, The prevalence and control of cattle lice, in: *Ectoparasites of Veterinary and Medical Importance in Temperate Areas, London, November 1982*, pp. 64–66.

WHO, 1980, Resistance of vectors of disease to parasites, WHO *Tech. Rep. Ser.* 655.

30

Acarine Infestation of Domestic Animals

ROGER O. DRUMMOND

1. INTRODUCTION

Acarine pests, ticks, and mites, found on all domestic and wild animals and pets, often represent a serious threat to the health, productiveness, and well-being of animals because they inflict direct physical damage to their hosts and transmit a variety of disease organisms (Drummond *et al.*, 1978). The use of chemotherapeutic agents for the control of acarine pests in some instances is essential to prevent death of animals. This chapter presents a review of experimental techniques used to evaluate chemotherapeutic agents (commonly called acaricides) and lists important acarine pests and acaricidal treatments for their control on cattle, horses, sheep, goats, swine, poultry, dogs, and cats.

2. TESTING OF ACARICIDES

2.1. Laboratory Trials

In vitro laboratory testing of acaricides should allow for the rapid, repeatable, and precise evaluation of small amounts of chemicals (Matthewson 1977; Drummond *et al.*, 1974). Much of the *in vitro* screening work has been conducted with single-host ticks (Drummond, 1979). There are several commonly used techniques: (1) the packet larvae test (Stone and Haydock, 1962; FAO, 1971), a test used principally for resistance testing; (2) the sandwich larvae test (Shaw, 1966; Matthewson and Hughes, 1976); (3) the engorged female immersion test (Drummond *et al.*, 1971); (4) the disposable pipette test (Foulk and Matthysse, 1964); (5) the teabag test (Fiedler, 1968; Gladney *et al.*, 1972; Kigaye and Matthysse, 1974); and (6) the filter paper residue test (Mount *et*

ROGER O. DRUMMOND • U.S. Livestock Insects Laboratory, U.S. Department of Agriculture, Agricultural Research Service, Kerrville, Texas 78028.

al., 1968). Different tests use different solvents; some allow for direct treatment of ticks, while others expose ticks to residues of acaricides. Barnard *et al.* (1981) compared all the tests except no. 3 and concluded that test no. 4 "provided the best combination of precision and ease of use." Stendel (1980) compared methods 1, 2, and 3 with a minidip *in vivo* technique (Downing *et al.*, 1977), and concluded that the best test (albeit the most expensive and time consuming) in terms of accuracy of use concentration and of ability to provide data on acaricides with different modes of action was the *in vivo* test and that each *in vitro* test had shortcomings. Stendel (1977*a*) presented a unique test that monitered the movement of treated ticks.

In vitro tests have also been used to evaluate acaricides against other acarines. Matthysse *et al.* (1975) used the disposable pipette technique to evaluate residues of acaricides for the control of *Chorioptes bovis* and *Ornithonyssus sylviarum*. Stendel (1977*b*) described a technique in which *Psoroptes cuniculi* were treated while being held in blister packaging; further testing involved treating pieces of sheep skin infested with *P. ovis*. Wright and Riner (1979) used the teabag technique to confine either *P. ovis* or *P. cuniculi* and dipped bags in acaricides. Matthewson *et al.* (1981) described an *in vitro* technique to screen repellents against tick larvae.

Acaricides may be tested against ticks *in vivo* by the minidip procedure or by treating infested cattle. Cattle are confined in stanchions or in isolated stalls, and numbers of female ticks that engorge and reproduce are recorded (Roulston and Wilson, 1965). Baker *et al.* (1977) reviewed *in vivo* testing of acaricides. Detection of systemic acaricides for control of ticks has been accomplished by *in vivo* tests with laboratory animals (Drummond, 1976; Hunt and Gilbert, 1979) and with cattle (Teel *et al.*, 1977; Drummond *et al.*, 1981).

In vivo testing of acaricides for the control of *P. ovis* on sheep has been accomplished by use of a cell technique (Page *et al.*, 1968). Ears of rabbits were washed with acaricides to determine effects on populations of *P. cuniculi* (Fisher *et al.*, 1979). Hadani *et al.* (1977) described an *in vivo* test for evaluating repellents against ticks by applying materials to gerbils, *Meriones trestrami*.

2.2. Field Trials

Drummond *et al.* (1977) presented the details for a variety of techniques used to evaluate the efficacy of insecticides applied to cattle, horses, sheep, goats, swine, and poultry.

2.2.1. Cattle

Numbers of ticks on specific body areas of treated cattle are compared with numbers on untreated cattle (Drummond and Gladney, 1978; Bernard and Jones, 1981). Also, counting numbers of *Boophilus microplus* females >4.5 mm was used by Wharton *et al.* (1970) to measure efficacy of acaricides. Other techniques are necessary to evaluate acaricides applied to ears or other specific sites (Gladney *et al.*, 1977). Techniques for field evaluation of contact and systemic acaricides for control of *P. ovis* have been presented by Guillot *et al.* (1983) and Meleney (1982), respectively.

2.2.2. Horses

Little has been published on the evaluation of acaricides for control of ticks and mites on horses. Drummond and Graham (1964) described techniques for evaluating contact and systemic treatments for the control of *Anocentor nitens* in ears and nasal diverticulae and on horses' bodies. Drummond and Medley (1965) devised techniques for evaluating sprays for control of *Ixodes scapularis* and Boersema (1978) for *Chorioptes bovis*.

2.2.3. Sheep and Goats

Techniques for evaluation of acaricides for control of psoroptic and other mange mites on sheep have been presented by Alcaino *et al.* (1982), Kirkwood and Quick (1982), Meleney and Roberts (1979), and Ram *et al.* (1980). Evaluation of acaricides for control of other acarines has been presented by Diplock and Hyne (1975) for *Chorioptes* and by Euzeby *et al.* (1976) and Thomson and MacKenzie (1982) for *Demodex*.

2.2.4. Swine

Evaluation of acaricides for the control of *S. scabiei* on swine consists of monitoring the number of mites and extent of skin lesions before and after treatment (Griffiths, 1975; Hewett and Heard, 1982). Effectiveness of a systemic acaricide against *S. scabiei* on swine has been determined by Courtney *et al.* (1983).

2.2.5. Poultry

Techniques to evaluate acaricides for the control of *O. sylviarum* on poultry were presented by Arthur and Axtell (1982), Collison *et al.* (1981), DeVaney *et al.* (1982), Hall *et al.* (1978, 1983), and Loomis and Dunning (1980).

2.2.6. Dogs and Cats

Techniques to evaluate acaricides for acarines on dogs have been reported for *Demodex* by Folz *et al.* (1978), Scott (1979), and Vollset (1980), for *Sarcoptes* by Berge and Joerstad (1981), and for *Otodectes cynotis* by Pott and Riley (1979) and Rose (1976). A technique to evaluate acaricides as dips for control of ticks on dogs was presented by Koch *et al.* (1985). Techniques to evaluate acaricides for control of mites on cats were presented by Fox and de Leon (1982).

3. MAJOR ACARINE PESTS OF ANIMALS AND THEIR CONTROL

3.1. Cattle

3.1.1. Acarine Pests

Cattle are infested with four major species of mange, itch, or scab mites. Mites can be identified by recognition of the type and location of lesions and by microscopic examination of organisms from scrapings of infested skin. Chorioptic mange, caused by *Chorioptes bovis*, is generally located on the tail and legs and may spread to all parts of the body, but pathogenicity of this species is not as severe as that of *Psoroptes ovis*. Psoroptic mange, caused by *P. ovis*, usually appears on the neck, shoulders, and back; infestations cause severe irritation and itching, and infested areas are thickened, crusty, heavily wrinkled, and scabby. Infested cattle lose weight, are unthrifty, and may die unless treated. Cattle are also infested with *Sarcoptes scabiei*, the cause of sarcoptic mange or barn itch. Symptoms include irritation, scratching, serous exudate, scabs, thickened and folded skin, and loss of hair. Heavily infested cattle are unthrifty and poor producers. Often, the disease disappears or diminishes in severity during summer months. Finally, cattle are infested with *Demodex bovis*, the agent of demodectic mange. These minute mites live in hair follicles and glands in the skin. Infestations cause small lesions on the head, neck, and shoulders that may increase in size and appear over the entire body of older animals. Infestations may cause blemishes in hides.

The large variety of ticks that attack cattle often need to be controlled (Bram, 1975). Attached ticks cause irritation, unrest, and loss of blood and weight—a variety of symptoms called "tick worry." Tick attachment sites may provide loci for infection of animals with pathogens or other arthropods and may also cause permanent blemishes in cattle skins that lower the value and utility of the hides. Several species of ticks inject toxins that cause paralysis, sweating sickness, or tick toxicosis in cattle. Symptoms are usually reversed once ticks are removed or killed.

The major tick vectors and diseases of cattle that they vector are *Boophilus* spp.—*Babesia* spp. and *Anaplasma* spp.; *Hyalomma* spp.—*Theileria annulata*; *Amblyomma* spp.—*Cowdria ruminantium*; *Rhipicephalus* spp.—*Theileria* spp. and *Babesia* spp. Losses in worldwide cattle production as a result of ticks and tickborne diseases were estimated by McCosker (1979) to be >$7 billion per year resulting from decreased vigor, lowered milk and meat production, inefficient reproduction, poor feed conversion, and death of cattle. The control of tick parasites of cattle in certain areas is essential before cattle production can be undertaken or improved.

Important hard ticks of the family Ixodidae that attack cattle are found in the genera *Amblyomma, Boophilus, Dermacentor, Haemaphysalis, Hyalomma, Ixodes,* and *Rhipicephalus*. Important soft ticks of the family Argasidae that attack cattle are found in the genera *Otobius* and *Ornithodoros*. Ticks have a variety of life cycles, portions of which are spent off and on hosts. It is necessary to identify ticks accurately in order to know the life cycle, seasonal appearance, and other facets of their biology.

3.1.2. Treatment

Most acaricides are applied dermally to cattle (and other animals) as emulsions, suspensions, or solutions. Dipping vats permit complete immersion of animals in a large volume (often >10,000 liters) of acaricide. Properly executed dippings provide complete and thorough application of acaricides to animals. Acaricides in vats, if properly recharged, replenished, and monitored, can be reused for long periods without loss of acaricidal activity. However, vats have disadvantages in that they are generally not portable (although small portable vats are available), the cost of initial acaricide charge can be high, and used vat fluids must be disposed of properly to prevent a hazard to the environment.

Spray dips or spray races are mechanical devices that utilize many nozzles to apply a large volume of spray at low pressure. Runoff from the animals is collected, filtered, and recirculated through the spraying system. Spray races are generally stationary, whereas spray dips are portable. These machines use smaller volumes than do dipping vats, but the pumps and nozzles are difficult to maintain in proper working order unless cared for constantly.

Animals may be sprayed with acaricides applied with hand- or motor-powered sprayers. Spray applications are as thorough as the attention of the spray operator. Spray equipment is portable, and it is necessary only to mix enough spray to treat available animals; however, mechanical aspects of sprayers need attention to make sure that the equipment functions satisfactorily.

Methods for control of acarines with acaricides depend on the biology of the species. Whole-body treatments control acarines attached to the surfaces of cattle— especially necks, flanks, and backs. Specific body areas such as ears, axillae, and tails may be treated by hand with acaricides in water, oil, or as aerosols, dusts, and other forms in order to kill acarines found there. Animals need to be restrained so that the areas can be treated thoroughly. The application of a limited volume of acaricide along the back line of animals (the pour-on technique) has been used to control some ecto-parasites but has not been widely used to control acarines. Acaricide-impregnated ear tags attached to the ears of cattle control ticks in or on the ears. Certain acarines on cattle can be controlled through the oral or parenteral administration of animal systemic insecticides.

It may be possible to treat small pastures, pens, and so forth with acaricides to kill off-the-host stages of certain ticks. Acaricides used on cattle are listed in Table I.

3.2. Horses

3.2.1. Acarine Pests

Horses are often infested with the same mites that infest cattle. Mange mites, such as *Chorioptes bovis*, *Psoroptes equi*, and *Sarcoptes scabiei*, cause itching, irritation, and severe dermatitis and the skin may become thickened and scabby. Horses are also infested with many of the ticks found on cattle. Of special note is *Anocentor nitens*, found in tropical areas of the new world. All parasitic stages of this single-host species may be found in ears, nasal diverticulae, and other body areas of horses. This species, along with other species in the genera *Dermacentor*, *Hyalomma*, and *Rhipicephalus*, are vectors of equine piroplasmosis. Ticks may also cause paralysis of horses.

3.2.2. Treatment

Acarines on horses can be controlled by applying acaricides by hand-pumped or power-driven sprayers. Because of the excitable nature of many horses, it may be safer

Table 1. Acaricides for Control of Mites and Ticks on Cattle

Acaricide (formulation)	Treatment	Remarks and safety restrictions
Psoroptic Mange and Ticks		
Amitraz EC	0.018–0.025% dip/spray	Dip should be stabilized with lime; replenish dip at 1.5 times original charge rate.
Coumaphos EC, WP	EC 0.016–0.15%; WP 0.05–0.15% dip/spray	Replenish EC at two times original charge; replenish WP at original charge rate; use highest concentrations for psoroptic mites.
Diazinon EC	0.025% spray/wash	Treat again every 10 days.
Dioxathion + chlorfenvinphos EC	0.025% + 0.023% dip/spray	Replenish at 1.7 times original charge.
Flumethrin EC	0.003–0.005% dip/spray	Replenish at original rate; use higher levels for multihost ticks.
Ivermectin (10 mg/ml injectable)	Subcutaneous injection, 1 ml/50 kg (200 μg/kg)	Inject in neck area; eradicates *Psoroptes* and *Sarcoptes*; controls single-host ticks 20 days and three-host ticks 5 days.
Lindane EC	0.025–0.06% dip/spray	Replenish at 1.6 times original charge.
Phosmet EC	0.25 dip/spray	Do not repeat treatment within 7–10 days.
Phoxim EC	0.025% spray/wash	For mites, two or three treatments are necessary.
Toxaphene EC	0.25–0.5% dip/spray	Use highest concentration for mites; replenish dip at 1.3 times original charge.
Toxaphene + dioxathion EC	0.25% + 0.04% dip/spray	Replenish 1.2 times original charge.
Toxaphene + malathion EC	0.4–0.5% + 0.04–0.05% dip/spray	Treat again in 10 days if needed.
Toxaphene + methoxychlor EC	0.25% + 0.25% dip/spray	Do not treat calves <6 months old.
Ticks and Other Mange Mites		
Closantel 30% solution	Oral treatment 1 ml/13.3 kg (22.5 mg/kg)	
Crotoxyphos EC	0.15–0.3% spray	Do not spray more often than every 7 days.
Crotoxyphos + dichlorvos EC	0.25% + 0.06% spray	
Deltamethrin EC	0.0025–0.003% dip/spray	Replenish at 1.2–1.5 times original charge.
Deltamethrin + ethion EC	0.005% + 0.025% dip/spray	Replenish at 1.2 times original charge.
Dioxathion EC	0.03–0.15% dip/spray	Replenish at 1.4 times original charge.
Ethion EC	0.05–0.075% dip/spray	Replenish at 1.3 times original charge.
Fenvalerate WDL	0.05% whole-body spray or 0.25% wash	Not more frequently than once every 2 weeks; 20 ml of wash/animal.
Permethrin EC	0.014% whole-body spray; 0.057% spray	Whole-body spray; 1–2 liters/animal

Table 1 (Continued)

Acaricide (formulation)	Treatment	Remarks and safety restrictions
Quintiofos EC	0.02% dip/spray	Replenish at 1.5 times original charge.
	0.06% hand application	Brush or rub in well to areas where ticks are attached.

Ticks Only

Arsenic EC	0.16–0.32% dip	
Chlormethiuron EC	0.2% spray	
Chlorpyrifos EC	0.02% spray	
Coumaphos dust	5% dust, treat ears	Effective against *Otobius megnini*.
spray foam	3% aerosol, treat ears	Effective against *Otobius megnini*.
Cyhalothrin	0.007% dip/spray	
Dioxathion + dichlorvos EC	0.15% + 0.005% dip/spray	Do not retreat within 2 weeks.
Malathion EC, WP dust	0.5–1% spray, 4 or 5% dust	Dust thoroughly.
Propetamphos EC	0.0175% spray	
Propoxur	0.1% EC spray	
EC, WP	0.2% WP spray	
Dust	1% dust	
Tetrachlorovinfos, WP, EC	0.5% spray	
Tetrachlorovinfos + dichlorvos EC	0.5% + 0.1% spray	
Trichlorfon SP	1% dip/spray	

Ear Tags[a]

Chlorpyrifos	10% in ear tag	Apply 1 tag to each ear.
Fenvalerate	8% in ear tag	Apply 1 tag to each ear.
Flucythrinate	7.5% in ear tag	Apply 1 tag to each ear.
Permethrin	10% in ear tag	Apply 1 tag to each ear.
Tetrachlorovinfos	10% in ear tag	Apply 1 tag to each ear.

[a]Effective against ticks in or near ears.

and easier to brush, wash, or sponge acaricides onto horses by hand. Horses may be treated in a dipping vat with great care so that horses do not injure themselves or their handlers. Ticks in ears, e.g., *Otobius megnini*, *R. appendiculatus*, or *A. nitens*, may be controlled by applying acaricides in oil or as dusts into the ears. *Anocentor nitens* in nasal diverticulae can be treated with acaricides in oils applied lightly with the fingers to the surface of the diverticulae. Ticks in paddocks, stalls, and pens can be controlled by treating the areas or structures with an appropriate acaricide spray or dust.

Because of the reactive, sensitive, and tender nature of the skin of horses, it is important that persons treating horses use acaricide formulations specifically approved and recommended for horses. Solvents and other chemicals tolerated by cattle and other

Table II. Acaricides for the Control of Mites and Ticks on Horses

Acaricide formulation	Treatment	Remarks and safety restrictions
Coumaphos EC, WP	0.05–0.15% spray/wash	Repeat after 8–10 days.
Crotoxyphos + dichlorvos EC	0.3% + 0.02% spray	Do not treat more often than once weekly.
Dioxathion EC	0.15% dip/spray	
Dioxathion + dichlorvos EC	0.15% + 0.005% dip/spray	
Ethion EC	0.056–0.075% dip/spray	Replenish vat at 1.3 times original charge.
Flumethrin EC	0.004% spray/wash	
Lindane EC	0.025–0.05% dip/spray	Repeat at 10–14-day intervals.
Malathion EC, WP, dust	0.5–1% spray; 4–5% dust	Do not treat foals under 1 month of age.
Permethrin Sol., EC	1% wipe-on, 0.0125–0.025% spray 0.156% wash	Apply directly to ticks; treat thoroughly— never more than once every 2 weeks; treat ears thoroughly for ear ticks.
Phoxim EC	0.025–0.05% spray/wash	Treat again weekly 2–3 times.
Quintiofos EC	0.02–0.04% spray/wash	
Toxaphene EC	0.25–0.5% dip/spray	Do not treat animals <3 months of age.
Toxaphene + malathion EC	0.2–0.5% + 0.02–0.05% dip/spray	

livestock may cause severe reactions of the skin of horses. Acaricides used on horses are listed in Table II.

3.3. Sheep and Goats

3.3.1. Acarine Pests

Sheep are infested with several species of mange or scab mites. Sheep scab, caused by *Psoroptes ovis,* is of considerable economic importance. Losses in wool production from excessive rubbing of sheep, the hardened, thickened, and scabby skin, anemia, and even death of infested sheep have caused a number of countries (United States, Argentina, Australia, United Kingdom) to undertake massive progams to eradicate *P. ovis.* Sheep are also infested with *Sarcoptes scabiei,* found chiefly around the face. The tunneling of this species causes severe irritation and loss of wool. *Chorioptes ovis* causes foot mange; damage is generally limited to lower extremities, including the scrotum of males. Sheep are rarely infested with *Demodex ovis,* the cause of reddened skin around eyelids and genital organs. Other mites that have been reported to cause mange in sheep are *Psorergates ovis,* which can be of economic importance, and *Caloglyphus berlesei.*

Sheep may be infested with a variety of ticks in the genera *Amblyomma, Boophilus, Dermacentor, Haemaphysalis, Hyalomma, Ixodes,* and *Rhipicephalus* that cause toxicosis, anemia, and paralysis and are vectors of sheep babesiosis, Nairobi sheep disease, heartwater, louping ill, and sweating sickness. Ears of sheep may be infested with *Otobius megnini.*

Goats are infested with many of the same acarines that infest sheep. Ears of Angora goats may be infested with *Psoroptes cuniculi*, which may spread to the body. Goats may also be heavily infested with *Demodex caprae* that forms large nodules on the skin that damage the hides. In South Africa, Angora goats are especially susceptible to Karoo paralysis caused by *Ixodes rubicundus*.

3.3.2. Treatment

Acarine pests can be controlled by treating sheep and goats dermally with acaricides. Sarcoptic and psoroptic mange are difficult to control and require special dip treatments (Kirkwood *et al.*, 1978). Other mites and ticks can generally be controlled with a variety of acaricides applied as dips, sprays, pour-ons, and dusts. Mites in ears of goats may be treated with ointments of concentrated insecticides. Acaricides used on sheep and goats are listed in Table III.

Table III. Acaricides for the Control of Mites and Ticks on Sheep and Goats[a]

Acaricide	Treatment	Remarks and safety restrictions
	Sheep and Goats	
Amitraz EC	0.05% dip/spray	Treat 2 or 3 times at 7–10-day intervals.
Bromophos + lindane EC	0.05% + 0.016% dip/spray	
Carbophenothion + lindane EC	0.021% + 0.016% spray	14-day slaughter intervals.
Chlorpyrifos + lindane EC	0.05% + 0.016% dip/spray	
Closantel 30% Sol	Oral treatment, 1 ml/60 kg (5 mg/kg)	For control of mites.
Coumaphos WP	0.1–0.25% dip/spray	
Cypermethrin EC	0.005% dip/spray	
Cythioate	Oral treatment (3 mg/kg)	Two times per week
Deltamethrin EC	0.00375–0.005% dip/spray	Treat twice at 8–10-day intervals.
Diazinon EC	0.02% dip/spray	
Flumethrin EC	0.003% dip/spray	
Lindane EC	0.0125–0.06% dip/spray	
Phoxim EC	0.05% dip/spray	Replenish dip at 0.1%.
Propetamphos EC	0.032% dip/spray	
Quintiofos EC	0.02% dip/spray	Replenish at 0.03%.
Toxaphene EC	0.5% dip/spray	
Trichlorfon SP	1.0% spray or pouron	
	Goats: Demodectic mange	
Rotenone	In surgical spirit	Treat daily.
Trichlorfon SP	1% spray	

[a]Only certain acaricides and application techniques may be approved for official use in programs to eradicate *P. ovis* of sheep.

3.4. Swine

3.4.1. Acarine Pests

The most important acarine pest of swine is *Sarcoptes scabiei,* the cause of sarcoptic mange. These mites live in the epidermis and their burrowing causes severe itching and loss of vitality and productiveness. The skin becomes thickened, rough, and heavily folded. Lesions are found on the head and forward areas of the body. Swine may also be infested with *Demodex phylloides.*

Swine can be parasitized by soft ticks of the genus *Ornithodoros,* reservoirs and vectors of African Swine Fever, a highly contagious viral disease, which has been recently eradicated by isolation and slaughter of swine in Brazil, Cuba, and Hispaniola.

3.4.2. Treatment

Sarcoptic mange mites of swine can be controlled by treating swine thoroughly by dipping, spraying, or washing. Multiple treatments may be necessary with certain acaricides. Light spraying or dusting, which may control lice, is often not thorough enough to control mange mites. A pour-on treatment is also effective against sarcoptic mange. A single subcutaneous injection of a systemic acaricide eradicates sarcoptic scabies in swine. Some of the treatments that control sarcoptic mange may aid in the control of demodectic mange. Acaricides used on swine are listed in Table IV.

Table IV. Acaricides for the Control of Sarcoptic Mites on Swine

Acaricide (formulation)	Treatment	Remarks and safety restrictions
Amitraz EC	0.05% spray	Two treatments at 14-day intervals.
Coumaphos EC, WP	0.1–0.125% spray/wash	Repeat three times at weekly intervals.
Crotoxyphos + dichlorvos EC	0.3% + 0.02% spray/wash	
Diazinon EC	0.025% spray/wash	Repeat every 10 days.
Dioxathion EC	0.15% dip/spray	Do not treat sows within 2 weeks of farrowing or while nursing.
Ivermectin, 10 mg/ml injectable	Subcutaneous injection, 1 ml/50 kg (200 µg/kg)	
Lindane EC, WP	0.02–0.06% dip/spray	Repeat every 12 days.
Malathion EC, WP	0.25–0.5% spray/wash	
Permethrin EC	0.0125% spray/wash	Treat again in 14 days.
Phosmet pour-on	Pour-on, 1 ml/10 kg (20 mg/kg)	Pour along backline.
Phoxim EC	0.05% spray/wash	Repeat every 14 days.
Toxaphene EC	0.2–0.5% spray/wash or dip	Do not treat swine <6 months of age.

3.5. Poultry

3.5.1. Acarine Pests

A very important mite pest of poultry is *Ornithonyssus sylviarum*. This blood-sucking mite spends its life cycle on the host and can build up very large populations, especially in the vent areas of birds, in very short periods. Heavy infestations may lead to loss of vitality, decreased weight gains and egg production, and even death. A less common, closely related mite species is *Ornithonyssus bursa*. Another important mite pest of poultry is *Dermanyssus gallinae* that lives in cracks and crevices of poultry houses and roosts and feeds on resting poultry. Populations of this species generally are not as large as those of *O. sylviarum*, but it transmits spirochetosis and fowl pox and can cause anemia in poultry. Poultry may also be infested occasionally with *Knemidokoptes mutans* and *K. laevis* or *gallinae*. These minute mites burrow under leg scales or into skin, damage legs of poultry, and can cause loss of feathers. A mite of considerable economic importance to turkey raisers in certain parts of the southern United States is *Neoschongastia americana*. The larval stage, called chigger, attaches in clusters to turkeys; the resultant feeding lesions decrease the value of processed turkeys.

The most important tick pest of poultry is *Argas persicus*, principally an Old World species; closely related New World species are *A. radiatus*, *A. sanchesi*, and *A. miniatus*. Generally, the biology of all these species is similar. Fowl ticks live for long periods in poultry structures and feed for very short periods on resting poultry. Fowl ticks can cause emaciation, weakness, decreased egg production, and death of heavily infested birds; they are vectors of spirochetosis and fowl piroplasmosis and may cause paralysis of poultry.

3.5.2. Treatment

Control of mites that live on poultry is accomplished by direct application of low-volume, low-pressure sprays or dusts, especially toward the vent area where mites and eggs are found. Poultry may be allowed access to dust boxes that contain acaricides. Also, poultry may be dipped, vent-tail area only, in acaricides. Plastic strips, impregnated with insecticides, attached to cages that contain laying hens provide adequate control of mites on the hens. The scaley-legged mite or the depluming mite can be eliminated by removing the infested poultry from the flock or treating infested body areas with acaricides. To control mites and ticks off of the host, it is necessary to treat poultry buildings, roosts, and other structures and the ground with acaricides. Acaricides used on poultry are listed in Table V.

3.6. Dogs and Cats

3.6.1. Acarine Pests

The most important mite pest of dogs is *Demodex canis*, found in hair follicles and adjacent glands. These very tiny mites are found on many healthy dogs without causing

Table V. Acaricides for the Control of Mites and Ticks on Poultry[a]

Acaricide (formulation)	Treatment	Remarks and safety restrictions
Amitraz EC	0.05–0.1% spray	
Carbaryl	3.5% mist spray	5–6 liters/1000 birds.
S, WP	0.45% spray	4 liters/100 birds.
Dust	5–10% dust	0.25–0.5 kg/100 birds or in dust boxes.
Coumaphos WP	0.006% spray	4 liters/100–125 birds.
Fenvalerate WDL	0.025% spray	4 liter/100 birds.
Malathion	0.4–0.5% spray	4 liters/100–150 birds.
EC, WP	0.2% tail dip	140 ml/bird.
Dust	4–5% dust	Treat birds individually or in dust boxes.
Permethrin	0.05% spray	40 ml/bird.
EC, WP	0.1% mist spray	20 ml/bird.
Dust	0.25% dust	4.5 g/bird.
Tetrachlorovinfos	0.05% spray	4 liters/100 birds.
EC, WP	50% WP use as dust	Place in dust boxes.
Dust	3% dust	Treat birds or 0.5 kg/9.3 m^2 on litter.
Trichlorfon SP	2% spray	

[a]For direct application to poultry: Other acaricides can be applied to poultry environs for control of mites and ticks.

symptoms. Large populations produce clinical manifestations called demodicosis. A mild form, localized or squamous demodicosis, is limited to areas of the face and/or foreleg. A serious form, generalized or pustular demodicosis, is characterized by large areas of alopecia, seborrhea, and edema and can cause anorexia, debilitation, and pruritis. Often, dogs with localized demodicosis self-cure, but it is usually necessary to treat dogs with an acaricide to cure generalized demodicosis.

Dogs may also be infested with *Sarcoptes scabiei*, which lives in the skin. Their burrowing activity causes intense itching, and the skin becomes dry, thickened, and wrinkled. Scabies lesions are usually first found on the head and then spread to other areas of the body. Another mite, *Cheyletiella yasguri*, found on the skin and hair of dogs, can cause a dermal pruritis. Dogs may be infested with *Otodectes cynotis*, which lives on the inner surface of the ear; feeding causes irritation, inflammation, and crusting of the ear, a condition called otitis externa parasitica. Also, *Pneumonyssus caninum* has been found in the nasal sinuses of dogs.

The most important mite pest of dogs is *Demodex canis*, found in hair follicles and adjacent glands. These very tiny mites are found on many healthy dogs without causing symptoms. Large populations produce clinical manifestations called demodicosis. A mild form, localized or squamous demodicosis, is limited to areas of the face and/or foreleg. A serious form, generalized or pustular demodicosis, is characterized by large areas of alopecia, seborrhea, and edema and can cause anorexia, debilitation, and pruritis. Often, dogs with localized demodicosis self-cure, but it is usually necessary to treat dogs with an acaricide to cure generalized demodicosis.

Demodectic mange caused by *Demodex cati* is occasionally found in cats, but it is of general lesser clinical consequence than *Demodex* in dogs. Cats may also be infested with

Table VI. Acaricides for the Control of Mites and Ticks on Dogs and Cats

Acaricide (formulation)	Treatment	Remarks and safety restrictions
Amitraz EC	0.025–0.05% dip/wash	Retreat at 14-day intervals (do not use on cats).
Benzyl benzoate	15% solution in alcohol	For otitis externa.
Bromocyclen WP	0.2% wash	Three applications.
Dust	3% dust	
Carbaryl EC	0.1% wash	
Dust	5% dust	
Chlorfenvinphos EC	0.1% wash	
Chlorpyrifos EC	0.07% wash	
Coumaphos WP, EC	0.05–0.1% spray/wash	Treat again after 8–10 days (do not use on cats).
Cythioate	Oral treatment, 1.5 mg/0.5 kg in feed (3 mg/kg)	Treat every third day.
Diazinon EC	0.025% wash, 15% in collar[a]	Treat again; 4–6 treatments every 7 days (not for use on cats).
Dichlorvos EC	0.05% bath, 5% in collar[a]	
Dioxathion EC	0.075% wash	
Disulfiram Sol	5% drops in ears	For otitis externa.
Fenchlorphos EC	0.5% wash	Treat every 3–4 days.
Fenitrothion EC	0.125% wash/swab	
Dust	1% dust	
Flumethrin EC	0.003–0.005% spray/wash	
Fospirate	15% in collar[a]	
Lindane EC	0.025% bath/wash	
Lime sulfur Sol	0.06% wash	
Malathion EC	0.3% wash	
Naled	10% in collar[a]	
Permethrin EC	0.05–0.1% wash	
Dust	1% dust	
Phoxim EC	0.1% bath/wash	Not completely effective against *Demodex*.
Phosmet EC	0.09% bath/wash	
Piperonyl butoxide EC	5% dressing	
Propoxur EC	0.12% wash	
Dust	1% dust	
	9.4% in collar[a]	
Pyrethrum + piperonyl butoxide EC	0.01% + 0.1% bath/wash	
Quintiofos EC	0.06% spray/wash	
Rotenone EC	1% wash in surgical alcohol	Retreat every 2–3 days.
Tetrachlorovinphos	9.5% in collar[a]	
Trichlorfon SP	0.2% bath	

[a]Collars provide tick control.

Notoedres cati, Sarcoptes scabiei, and *Cheyletiella blakei,* with clinical conditions similar to those seen in dogs. Ears of cats are also infested with *Otodectes cynotis.* In addition, cats are infested with a fur mite, *Lynxacarus radovskyi,* and a chigger mite, *Walchia americana.* Generally, cats are rarely infested with ticks. A number of the mites on dogs and cats can also be transmitted to humans, in whom they can cause severe dermatitis.

3.6.2. Treatment

Treatment of dogs for the control of sarcoptic mites is accomplished by applying acaricides as whole-body sprays, washes, shampoos, or dips. Demodectic mange, which is difficult to cure, can be treated with acaricides applied as thorough whole-body treatments, applied topically to infested areas, or with systemic acaricides given orally. Often, treatments have to be repeated before complete cure can be achieved. Otoacariasis can be treated with acaricides applied directly to the ears. Ticks may also be controlled by treating dogs with dips, sprays, washes, or shampoos. Acaricidal dusts and insecticide-impregnated plastic collars may provide some control of ticks. Where brown dog ticks have invaded dwellings, it is necessary to treat the structures with dusts or sprays in order to control ticks not on the hosts.

Care must be exercised in using acaricides on cats. Cats may be washed with acaricides, although dusts are effective if thoroughly applied and rubbed on the skin. Ears may be treated with acaricides applied as washes, drops, or ointments. Insecticide-impregnated collars may be used on cats to control ticks, but caution must be used in the selection of collars because of susceptibility of cats to poisoning. Acaricides used on dogs and cats are listed in Table VI.

REFERENCES

Alcaino, H. A., Gorman, T. R., and Sabureau, J., 1982, Acaricidal effect of three dilutions of a synthetic pyrethrum (cypermethrin) in sheep, *Arch. Med. Vet. Chile* 14:121–125.

Arthur, F. H., and Axtell, R. C., 1982, Comparisons of permethrin formulations and application methods for northern fowl mite control on caged laying hens, *Poult. Sci.* 61:879–884.

Baker, J. A. F., Stanford, R. J., and Taylor, R. J., 1977, Techniques involved in the *in vivo* screening of candidate ixodicidal compounds, in: *Crop Protection Agents* (N. R. McFarlane, ed.), pp. 583–593, Academic Press, London.

Barnard, D. R., and Jones, B. G., 1981, Field efficacy of acaricides for control of the lone star tick on cattle in Southeastern Oklahoma, *J. Econ. Entomol.* 74:558–560.

Barnard, D. R., Jones, B. G., Rogers, G. D., and Mount, G. A., 1981, Acaricide susceptibility in the lone star tick: Assay techniques and baseline data, *J. Econ. Entomol.* 74:766–769.

Berge, G., and Joerstad, A., 1981, Mange in dogs—Treatment, *Norsk. Vet.* 93:361–362.

Boersema, J. H., 1978, Effectiveness of coumaphos against *Chorioptes bovis* in a horse with foot-mange, *Tijdschr. Diergeneesk.* 103:377–380.

Bram, R. A., 1975, Tick-borne livestock diseases and their vectors. 1. The global problem, *Wld. Anim. Rev.* 16:1–5.

Collison, C. H., Danka, R. G., and Kennell, D. R., 1981, An evaluation of permethrin, carbaryl and amitraz for the control of northern fowl mites *Ornithonyssus sylviarum* on caged chickens, *Poult. Sci.* 60:1812–1817.

Courtney, C. H., Ingalls, W. L., and Stitzlein, S. L., 1983, Ivermectin for the control of swine scabies: Relative values of prefarrowing treatment of sows and weaning treatment of pigs, *Am. J. Vet. Res.* 44:1220–1223.

DeVaney, J. A., Beerwinkle, K. R., and Ivie, G. W., 1982, Residual activity of selected pesticides on laying hens treated for Northern fowl mite control by dipping, *Poult. Sci.* 61:1630–1637.

Diplock, P. T., and Hyne, R. H. J., 1975, Chorioptic mange in cattle associated with a severe fall in milk production, *N.S.W. Vet. Proc.* 11:31–33.

Downing, F. S., Stubbs, V. K., and Bowyer, S., 1977, A technique for localizing infestations of the cattle tick *Boophilus microplus* (Can.) on small areas of the host and subjecting each area to dip treatments, in: *Crop Protection Agents* (N. R. McFarlane, ed.), pp. 609–622, Academic Press, London.

Drummond, R. O., 1976, *Materials Screened as Animal Systemic Insecticides at Kerrville, Texas, 1967–1973*, USDA ARS-S-101, 57 pp.

Drummond, R. O., 1979, *Chemicals Tested as Acaricides to Control One-Host Ticks at U.S. Livestock Insects Laboratory 1962–1977*, USDA-SEA ARM-S-3, 60 pp.

Drummond, R. O., and Gladney, W. J., 1978, Acaricides applied to cattle for control of the lone star tick, *Southwest. Entomol.* 3:96–105.

Drummond, R. O., and Graham, O. H., 1964, Insecticide tests against the tropical horse tick, *Dermacentor nitens*, on horses, *J. Econ. Entomol.* 57:549–553.

Drummond, R. O., and Medley, J. G., 1965, Field tests with insecticides for the control of ticks on livestock, *J. Econ. Entomol.* 58:1131–1136.

Drummond, R. O., Gladney, W. J., Whetsone, T. M., and Ernst, S. E., 1971, Laboratory testing of insecticides for control of the winter tick, *J. Econ. Entomol.* 64:686–688.

Drummond, R. O., Gladney, W. J., and Graham, O. H., 1974, Recent advances in the use of ixodicides to control ticks affecting livestock, *Bull. Off. Int. Epiz.* 81:47–63.

Drummond, R. O., Lancaster, J. L., and Ludwig, P. D., 1977, *Analysis of Specialized Pesticide Problems: Invertebrate Control Agents—Efficacy Test Methods, Livestock, Poultry, Fur & Wool Bearing Animals*, Vol. IV, EPA 540/10-77-002, 68 pp.

Drummond, R. O., Bram, R. A., and Konnerup, N., 1978, Animal pests and world food production, in: *World Food, Pest Losses and the Environment* (D. Pimentel, ed.), pp. 63–93, Westview Press, Boulder, Colorado.

Drummond, R. O., Whetstone, T. M., and Miller, J. A., 1981, Control of ticks systemically with Merck MK-933, an Avermectin, *J. Econ. Entomol.* 74:432–436.

Euzeby, J., Chermette, R., and Gevrey, J., 1976, Demodectic mange in goats in France, *Bull. Acad. Vet. Fr.* 49:423–430.

FAO, 1971, Recommended methods for the detection and measurement of resistance of agricultural pests to pesticides. Tentative method for larvae of cattle ticks, *Boophilus* spp.—FAO Method No. 7, *FAO Plant Prot. Bull.* 19:15–18.

Fiedler, O. G. H., 1968, A new biological method for evaluating the efficacy of acaricides against ticks, *J. S. Afr. Vet. Med. Assoc.* 39:84–87.

Fisher, W. F., Robbins, W. E., Wilson, G. I., Thompson, M. J., Kochansky, J. P., and Page, S. N., 1979, Control of the rabbit ear mite, *Psoroptes cuniculi* (Delafond), with experimental alkyl amines, *Southwest. Entomol.* 4:249–253.

Folz, S. D., Geng, S., Nowakowski, L. H., and Conklin, R. D., Jr., 1978, Evaluation of a new treatment for canine scabies and demodicosis, *J. Vet. Pharmacol. Ther.* 1:199–204.

Foulk, J. D., and Matthysse, J. G., 1964, A new toxicological test method for haematophagous mites, *J. Econ. Entomol.* 57:602–604.

Fox, I., and de Leon, D., 1982, Evaluation of insecticides in collars and powders against the cat fur mite *Felistrophorus radofskyi* (Tenorio) on Persian cats, *J. Agric. Univ. Puerto Rico* 66:139–144.

Gladney, W. J., Dawkins, C. C., and Drummond, R. O., 1972, Insecticides tested for control of nymphal brown dog ticks by the "tea-bag" technique, *J. Econ. Entomol.* 65:174–176.

Gladney, W. J., Price, M. A., and Graham, O. H., 1977, Field tests of insecticides for control of the Gulf Coast tick on cattle, *J. Med. Entomol.* 13:579–586.

Griffiths, A. J., 1975, Amitraz—For the control of animal ectoparasites with particular reference to sheep tick (*Ixodes ricinus*) and pig mange (*Sarcoptes scabiei*), in: *Proceedings of the Eighth British Insecticide and Fungicide Conference*, pp. 557–563.

Guillot, F. S., Wright, F. C., and Meleney, W. P., 1983, Efficacy of four acaricides applied as dips for control of the sheep scabies mite, *Psoroptes ovis*, on cattle, *Prev. Vet. Med.* 1:179–186.

Hadani, A., Ziv, M., and Rechav, Y., 1977, A laboratory study of tick repellents, *Entomol. Exp. Appl.* 22:53–59.

Hall, R. D., Townsend, L. H., Jr., and Turner, E. C., Jr., 1978, Laboratory and field tests to compare the effectiveness of organophosphorous, carbamate, and synthetic pyrethroid acaricides against Northern fowl mites, *J. Econ. Entomol.* 71:315–318.

Hall, R. D,, Vandepopuliere, J. M., Fischer, F. J., Lyons, J. J., and Doisy, K. E., 1983, Comparative efficacy of plastic strips impregnated with permethrin and permethrin dust for Northern fowl mite control on caged laying hens, *Poult. Sci.* 62:612–615.

Hewett, G. R., and Heard, R. T. W., 1982, Phosmet for the systemic control of pig mange, *Vet. Rec.* 111:558.

Hunt, L. M., and Gilbert, B. N., 1979, An improved method of evaluating acaricides and other candidate chemicals for systemic activity against ticks, *Southwest. Entomol.* 4:269–272.

Kigaye, M. K., and Matthysse, J. G., 1974, Testing acaricide susceptibility of the brown dog tick *Rhipicephalus sanguineus* (Latreille 1806). II. Teabag method, *Bull. Epiz. Dis. Afr.* 22:279–285.

Kirkwood, A. C., and Quick, M. P., 1982, Propetamphos for the control of sheep scab, *Vet. Rec.* 111:367.

Kirkwood, A. C., Quick, M. P., and Page, K. W., 1978, The efficacy of showers for control of ectoparasites of sheep, *Vet. Rec.* 102:50–54.

Koch, H. G., Burkwhat, H. E., and Tuck, M. D., 1985, Field method for evaluating the effectiveness of acaricides against lone star ticks (Acari: Ixodidae) on domestic dogs, *J. Econ. Entomol,* 78:287–289.

Loomis, E. C., and Dunning, L. L., 1980, Synthetic pyrethroids effective against fowl mite, *Calif. Agric.* 34:10–11.

Matthewson, M. D., 1977, Techniques involved in the *in vitro* screening of ixodicidal compounds, in: *Crop Protection Agents* (N. R. McFarlane, ed.), pp. 571–581, Academic Press, London.

Matthewson, M. D., and Hughes, G., 1976, The establishment of cultures of two and three-host ticks in the laboratory and their use in the screening of candidate ixodicides, in: *Tick-borne Diseases and Their Vectors, Proceedings of the International Conference, Edinburgh, Sept. 27–Oct. 1, 1976* (J. K. H. Wilde, ed.), pp. 231–240, Lewis Reprints Ltd., Tonbridge, Great Britain.

Matthewson, M. D., Hughes, G., Macpherson, I. S., and Bernard, C. P., 1981, Screening techniques for the evaluation of chemicals with activity as tick repellents, *Pesticide Sci.* 12:455–462.

Matthysse, J. G., van Vreden, G., Purnasiri, A., Jones, C. J., Netherton, H. R., and McClain, D. S., 1975, Comparative susceptibility of the chorioptic mange mite, northern fowl mite, and brown dog tick to acaricides, *Search Agric. Entomol.* 14:31.

McCosker, P. J., 1979, Global aspects of the management and control of ticks of veterinary importance, in: *Recent Advances in Acarology* (J. G. Rodriquez, ed.), Vol. II, pp. 45–53, Academic Press, New York.

Meleney, W. P., 1982, Control of psoroptic scabies on calves with ivermectin, *Am. J. Vet. Res.* 43:329–331.

Meleney, W. P., and Roberts, I. H., 1979, Trials with eight acaricides against *Psoroptes ovis* the sheep scabies mite, in: *Recent Advances in Acarology* (J. G. Rodriguez, ed.), Vol. II, pp. 95–101, Academic Press, New York.

Mount, G. A., Hirst, J. M., McWilliams, J. G., Lofgren, C. S., and White, S. A., 1968, Insecticides for control of the lone star tick tested in the laboratory and as high- and ultra-low-volume sprays in wooded areas, *J. Econ. Entomol.* 61:1005–1007.

Page, K. W., Ault, C. M., and Nunez, J. L., 1968, Psoroptic mange in sheep: Cell test use and application in diagnostic and research work, *Rev. Med. Vet.* 49:3–7.

Pott, J. M., and Riley, C. J., 1979, The efficacy of a topical ear preparation against *Otodectes cynotis* infection in dogs and cats, *Vet. Rec.* 104:579.

Ram, S. M. T., Gupta, S. L., Chhabra, M. B., and Gautam, O. P., 1980, Psoroptic mange in sheep and evaluation of some acaricides, *Indian Vet. Med. J.* 4:71–75.

Rose, W. R., 1976, Otitis externa-5: Otoacariasis, *Vet. Med/SAC* 71:1280–1283.

Roulston, W. J., and Wilson, J. T., 1965, Chemical control of the cattle tick *Boophilus microplus* (Can.), *Bull. Entomol. Res.* 55:617–635.

Scott, D. W., 1979, Canine demodicosis, *Vet. Clin. North Am. Small Anim. Pract.* 9:79–92.

Shaw, R. D., 1966, Culture of an organophosphorus-resistant strain of *Boophilus microplus* (Can.) and an assessment of its resistance spectrum, *Bull. Entomol. Res.* 56:389–405.

Stendel, W., 1977a, A novel and simple device for characterization of compounds active against ticks, in: *Crop Protection Agents* (N. R. McFarlane, ed.), pp. 595–608, Academic Press, London.

Stendel, W., 1977b, Development and assessment of a test-method suitable to select substances effective against mange mites, in: *Crop Protection Agents* (N. R. McFarlane, ed.), pp. 547–555, Academic Press, London.

Stendel, W., 1980, The relevance of different test methods for the evaluation of tick controlling substances, *J. S. Afr. Vet. Assoc.* 51:147–152.

Stone, B. G., and Haydock, K. P., 1962, A method for measuring the acaricide-susceptibility of the cattle tick *Boophilus microplus* (Can.), *Bull. Entomol. Res.* 53:563–578.

Teel, P. D., Hair, J. A., and Randolph, T. C., 1977, Continuous administration of famphur for control of ticks and bed bugs feeding on ruminants, *J. Econ. Entomol.* 70:664–666.

Thomson, J. R., and MacKenzie, C. P., 1982, Demodectic mange in goats, *Vet. Rec.* 111:185.

Vollset, I., 1980, Demodicosis in the dog—Treatment, *Norsk. Vet.* 92:675–677.

Wharton, R. H., Roulson, W. J., Utech, K. B. W., and Kerr, J. D., 1970, Assessment of the efficiency of acaricides and their mode of application against the cattle tick, *Boophilus microplus, Aust. J. Agric. Res.* 21:985–1006.

Wright, F. C., and Riner, J. C., 1979, A method of evaluating acaricides for control of psoroptic mites, *Southwest. Entomol.* 4:40–45.

31

Mode of Action of Agents Used against Arthropod Parasites

RICHARD JOHN HART

1. INTRODUCTION

This chapter provides a brief guide to the mode of action of the antiparasitic compounds in current use. The emphasis reflects more the chemical usage than the extent of the literature. In particular, references to the action of DDT are condensed to a brief note in view of the virtual abolition of this compound as a treatment in parasite control. The desire for brevity has meant that inclusion of referenced work has to be particularly selective in some areas that have been extensively explored. All work carried out with parasite species has, as far as possible, been included. However, much of the work to elucidate the mode of action of chemical treatment is carried out in nontarget species. All the hypotheses presented in this chapter are derived from studies of either vertebrates or arthropods that have proved suitable for laboratory experimentation. Arthropods such as lobster, crayfish, American cockroach, and locust are large and easier to work with than are ticks, mites, and fleas. Insect and acarine parasites are all more or less specialized, and less is known of their physiology. It is therefore wise to exercise some caution in extrapolating general theories to this group.

Most antiparasitic compounds have an initial effect on the nervous system. A smaller group of compounds act primarily as tissue poisons with effects on energy production. Detailed symptoms vary from compound to compound, but in general the two groups can be distinguished by the initial symptoms of poisoning. Arthropods affected by compounds acting on the nervous system show a rapid onset of behavioral changes, with detachment from the host, cessation of feeding, rapid uncoordinated movements being typical. Paralysis develops, appendages may contract or remain flaccid, and a period of hyperactivity may precede the terminal paralysis, which may occur within minutes or hours of the onset of symptoms. The major difference in symptoms

RICHARD JOHN HART • Wellcome Research Laboratories, Berkhamsted Hill, Berkhamsted HP4 2DY, United Kingdom.

caused by treatment with tissue poisons is one of time: paralysis occurs more gradually and may take several days to develop fully (Brown, 1963).

Before dealing in detail with the mode of action of compounds, a note of caution must be introduced. Much of the work deals with the physiological effects often thought responsible for the initial symptoms of poisoning. It must be emphasized that this does not necessarily explain what kills the parasite. While long-lasting or gradual paralysis will prevent feeding and cause death by starvation or desiccation, it is likely that primary disruption, certainly in the case of nerve poisons, may initiate secondary modes of action. There are well-supported theories that such secondary effects may be much less compound specific. For example, organophosphates, chlorinated hydrocarbon compounds, and pyrethroids all affect the hormonal centers of insects (Singh, 1984; Singh and Orchard, 1982).

The chapter is organized in two main divisions describing compounds that affect the nervous system and those that affect bioenergetic pathways. A brief résumé of each area introduces the terminology used in the descriptions of mode of action. Section 2 describes compounds that affect the nervous system, including the pyrethroids, avermectins, formamidines, organophosphates, carbamates, and cyclodienes. The pyrethroids are well established and replace organophosphates and carbamates. Avermectin is just beginning to appear as an ectoparasiticide and will probably be used in special areas, as are the formamidines. Lindane and the cyclodienes are included, as they are still in use despite widespread restrictive legislation. Section 3 deals with just two long-lived compounds that affect bioenergetics: rotenone and arsenic. The latter is still being used for the control of mites on animals some 100 years after its introduction. Brief references to other compounds occasionally encountered or whose mode of action is unknown are collected in Table I.

2. COMPOUNDS AFFECTING THE NERVOUS SYSTEM

Arthropod parasites exhibit a wide range of physical adaptation to their hosts and environment. This affects the gross structural arrangement of the nervous system, but the underlying cellular arrangement is remarkably consistent. Sensory neurons linked to receptors in sensory structures transmit information to central ganglia. Information is integrated, and motor nerves carry efferent nerve signals to the effector organs. The neurons appear typical of the invertebrate type, but there may be some tendency to simplification of supporting structures. The nervous system of cattle ticks has been examined more extensively than that of most ectoparasites. It has been shown that changes in the glial cells, which surround the nerve cells, make the ganglia more accessible to diffusible ions in the hemolymph (Binnington and Lane, 1980; Hart et al., 1980).

Several aspects of nervous system function are affected by pesticides, but they can be divided simply into those compounds that affect electrically excitable membranes and those that affect chemically mediated synaptic events. The membranes of neurons and some muscle cells are electrically excitable. The membranes are sensitive to voltage

Table I. Compounds in Limited Current Use or for Which Mode of Action is Unknown

Compound	Site of action	Comment
Nicotinoids (eg. nor-nicotine)	Nervous system: synapse	Cholinergic agonists in the ganglia; compounds bind to the ACh receptor and depolarize the neuron, causing hyperexcitation followed by block.
Cartap	Nervous system: synapse	Binds to ACh receptor; kinetics may differ from nicotine, explaining more rapid onset of paralysis.
DDT	Nervous system: axon	Affects ion channels in nerve membrane, especially sodium current, permitting the time course of the action potential to lengthen; in turn causing generation of repetitive potentials; characteristic symptoms of tremors superimposed on spasms indicate that nerves to both tonic and phasic muscles are affected in arthropods.
Dinitrophenols (e.g., DNOC)	Nervous system: axon; respiration: uncoupler	Rapid onset of hyperactivity and convulsions correlates with initial effects on the nervous system, but terminal paralysis caused by impairment of oxidative phosphorylation.
Organic thiocyanates (e.g., Lethane)	Respiration: inhibitor	A gradual decrease in oxygen consumption parallels the progressive block of muscle contraction.
Organotin (e.g., triphenyl tin)	Respiration: inhibitor	A gradual decrease in oxygen consumption parallels the progressive block of muscle contraction.
Urea analogues (e.g., Dimilin)	Chitin synthesis	Inhibits the enzyme, chitin synthetase (assumed from accumulation of precursor: UDP-N-acetylglucosamine); prevents proper cuticle formation in developing instars.
Thiabenzole (TBZ)	Microtubules (anthelmintic, antifungal)	Used as an ectoparasiticide for scab mite control only, where mode of action is unknown.
Benzyl benzoate	—	Mode of action unknown.
Vetrazin	—	Mode of action unclear, but growth is severely retarded.
Sulfur	—	Mode of action unclear—sulfur dust causes tissue necrosis and paralysis.
Calcium polysulfide (lime sulfur)	—	Calcium polysulfide generates hydrogen sulfide, a nonspecific enzyme inhibitor.

change and respond by forming transitory channels in the membrane. The channels selectively allow ions to cross the membrane and alter its charge, locally biased either to hyperpolarize or to depolarize. Most information is carried by regenerative action potentials, referred to as spikes because they appear as brief, discrete voltage changes on analogue records of nerve activity. Some neurons convey much smaller depolarizing potentials and are distinguished as nonspiking. Signals are transmitted between neurons or between neuron and muscle cell by chemical messengers at the synapse. Nerve terminals are specialized to release chemical neurotransmitter across the synapse. Areas of receptor membrane generate electrical signals in response to the chemical message. Differentiation of nerve signals at synapses is controlled by the identity of neurotransmitter. Arthropods use acetylcholine (ACh) at excitatory synapses in the CNS, glutamic acid to excite muscle cells at the neuromuscular junction, and 4-aminobutyric acid (GABA) as a modifying inhibitory transmitter at both central and peripheral synapses. Biogenic amines also have a transmitter role, octopamine having been associated with nonspiking neurons.

The nervous system and the effect of chemicals can be studied by recording and analyzing the electrical signals in nerve and muscle cells using a variety of electrodes and techniques to study the small voltage and current changes which occur. More direct information on the chemical transmitters is obtained from biochemical studies. Enzyme inhibition kinetics and the binding of compounds to membrane receptors can be measured, and more recently, the uptake and release of neurotransmitters has been studied. An important technique enables nerve terminals to be isolated *in vitro* from insect central nervous tissue. The isolated terminals, called synaptosomes, will take up and release neurotransmitters, permitting the study of mechanistic factors (Breer, 1984).

Most compounds in use today act on the nervous system. They are rapid acting and of increasing safety to mammals. The differential toxicity is often attributable not to different target sites in parasite and host nervous systems, but to differential metabolism.

2.1. Pyrethroids

Pyrethroids cause hyperexcitation followed by convulsions and death in arthropods. Predominance of particular symptoms can be linked to specific classes of chemical structure (Elliott, 1977). A simple classification of compounds, based on two major divisions of symptoms and neurophysiological effects in laboratory use has been proposed by Gammon et al. (1981).

Compounds causing predominantly behavioral changes associated with a rapid onset of hyperactivity and repetitive action potentials in the nervous system are classed as type I. Those characterized by a lethal action at low doses with few behavioral effects are type II. Chemically, type II compounds are distinguished by the presence of a cyanophenoxybenzyl moiety in the structure.

Information on mode of action has been obtained from *in vitro* studies using electrodes to record electrical impulses in the nervous system or biochemically measuring the behavior of isolated nerve membrane systems. This is still an active field of research, but the available evidence suggests that the primary effect is an interaction with ion channels in the nerve membrane. The disturbance to the gating of ions across the membrane leads to the generation of repetitive trains of electrical signals or to blocking or nerve conduction.

The first observations of pyrethroid effects on arthropod nerves were made by

Lowenstein (1942), recording abnormal repetitive action potentials in cockroach nerve treated with pyrethrins. Similar symptoms were seen in crayfish (Welsh and Gordon, 1947) with conduction block following the bursts of repetitive action potentials (Camougis and Davis, 1977). Studies in insects were taken further by Burt and co-workers (Burt and Goodchild, 1971; Burt et al., 1971), who showed that axons and ganglia were not equally sensitive. Manipulation of electrodes into a living cockroach enabled Gammon (1978) to monitor signals from the nervous system and simultaneously observe behavioral changes during the poisoning process. Initial symptoms of hyperactivity seen as the insect was treated with type I pyrethroids correlated well with increased signal traffic in the peripheral nerve. Uncoordinated limb movements followed trains of impulses in the nerve. The trains continued until after the animal became prostrate, and eventual block of nerve conduction occurred after the insect was paralyzed (Gammon, 1978). Interpretation of these and other effects of pyrethroids is complicated by the effect of temperature. It was observed that the repetitive activity in the nervous system returned to normal if the insect was cooled from 32°C to 15°C. This finding suggests that the symptoms are unrelated to overall lethal effect of pyrethroids, which are generally more toxic at lower temperatures.

A preparation of tethered flies using either houseflies (Musca domestica) (Miller and Kennedy, 1972; Adams and Miller, 1980) or the more robust Lucilia sericata (Fig. 1) also allows nervous system records to be compared with behavioral symptoms. The motor output from the ganglion is responsible for initiating and sustaining flight. A wide range of pyrethroids has been tested, those compounds having a rapid effect in vivo cause an almost instantaneous disturbance of the ganglionic output. Increasing frequency of bursts of signals parallel the violent and uncoordinated wing movements. All pyrethroids appear to cause the breakup of the normal pattern of output and, although (as in Gammon's cockroach) signals continue, the distorted impulses cannot activate the muscles and tetany occurs.

Repetitive nerve activity has been described in a wide range of arthropods including cattle ticks (Nicholson et al., 1980; Binnington and Obenchain, 1982). The origin of disturbance appears to be at or near the cell body of the neuron in sensory nerves, demonstrated in the frog (Wouters and van den Berken, 1978), crayfish (Osborne, 1980), and insect (Clements and May, 1977). In insect motor nerves there is evidence that the disturbance occurs at the nerve terminal, with distorted signals passing back into the CNS as well as on to the muscle (Adams and Miller, 1980). Examination of the distorted signals suggests an association with modified ion currents flowing across the nerve membrane in both arthropods (Narahashi, 1971) and vertebrates (Wouters and van den Berken, 1978). These currents have been studied in detail using electrophysiological voltage-clamp techniques (Narahashi, 1976). Experiments with crustaceans and insects show that all type I pyrethroids increase sodium ion permeability. The ion gates are held open longer than normal, and the prolonged current causes distorted nerve impulses. Deltamethrin, representative of type II compounds, also holds the sodium gates open, but its action is more prolonged and cumulative. Gradually, as more and more gates are opened, the polarity of the membrane is reduced to a point where the axon is blocked for impulse transmission. Pyrethroids probably interact

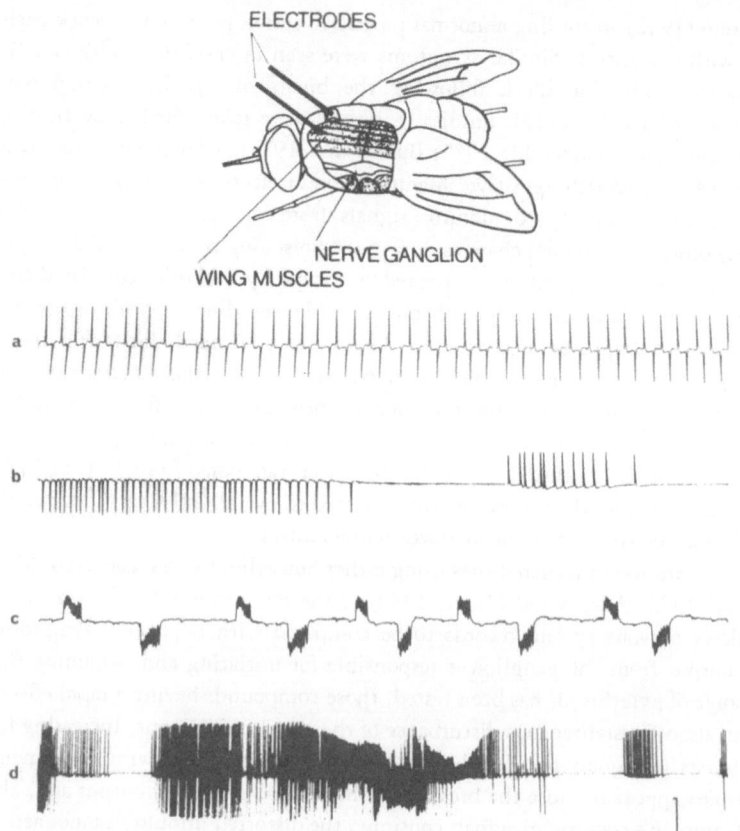

Figure 1. (*Top*) Preparation used to record electrical signals from the nervous system of a tethered flying insect, the sheep maggot fly (*Lucilia sericata*). Tungsten wire electrodes implanted in the large flight muscles detect signals and hold the fly away from the substrate without impeding normal flight activity. (*Bottom*) (a) Electrical recordings show action potentials during normal flight, as positive and negative spikes. These represent signals from the ganglion to the left and right wing muscles, respectively. (b) Uncoupled signals follow treatment with organophosphate (paraoxon 1 μg). The insecticide affects the control mechanism in the ganglion. (c) Action potentials become repetitive after application of DDT (1 μg). (d) A pyrethroid (permethrin 0.1 μg) causes uncoupling, repetitive activity, and amplitude changes. All these treatments cause tetany with no wing movement in response to the severely distorted signals in (b), (c), and (d). Calibration time bar: (a, b) 0.5 sec, (c) 0.1 sec, (d) 3 sec. Amplitude bar: 50 mV.

directly with the membrane components to alter ion channel properties but there may be some effect due to inhibition of the ion pumps responsible for actively maintaining the membrane potential. The ATPase group of enzymes involved in ion pumps and in producing energy to operate them are susceptible to inhibition by pyrethroids (Desaiah and Cutkomp, 1973), but the theory of how this would explain the symptoms has not been worked out in detail.

Some studies have revealed a direct depolarisation of the membrane in crayfish sensory nerve axon (Osborne, 1980) and in leech and locust neurons (Leake *et al.*, 1980). This effect of type I compounds occurred before changes in action potentials were observed. Depolarization of nerve terminals occurs at neuromuscular junctions in Dipteran insect larvae (Salgado *et al.*, 1983) with both type I and type II compounds. The depolarization causes release of excess neurotransmitter, which in turn generates enhanced miniature potentials in the muscle cell. Measurement of these potentials after treatment at different temperature showed increasing effects at lower temperatures with the more toxic type II compounds. This action is therefore different from the repetitive nerve activity, which is enhanced at higher temperature (Adams and Miller, 1980) and reflects the lethal effects of pyrethroids that increase as the temperature is reduced. Both the repetitive nerve activity and direct depolarization are likely to be mediated by increased sodium permeability. Further information on the mode of action of type II pyrethroids is now accumulating to suggest the involvement of chloride channels (Gammon *et al.*, 1982; Lawrence and Casida, 1983). Interaction with receptors for the neurotransmitter γ-aminobutyric acid (GABA) may possibly interfere with the chloride mediated inhibition of central synapses and neuromuscular junctions. This may account for the enhanced toxicity of deltamethrin and other type II pyrethroids, but further work is needed, particularly to correlate *in vitro* and *in vivo* effects related to temperature change.

2.2. Avermectins

Avermectin controls ectoparasites by a systemic action; the symptoms of toxicity develop more slowly than most other compounds active on the nervous system. Experiments with ticks show normal feeding is affected and the life cycle interrupted by failure to moult or to lay eggs (Wilkins *et al.*, 1981). *In vitro* studies indicate that avermectin has an action at particular neuromuscular junctions. Work with the lobster shows that avermectin blocks postsynaptic potentials in leg muscles by opening of chloride ion channels in the membrane (Fritz *et al.*, 1979). Similar results in locust muscle have been obtained by Duce and Scott (1983). The insect experiments suggest that at low concentrations (10^{-10} M) avermectin acts on chloride channels specifically associated with the action of GABA as a neurotransmitter at inhibitory nerve muscle junctions. In addition, at higher concentrations (10^{-6} M) there is an effect on non-specific chloride channels. The effect of opening chloride channels is to increase the electrical conductance of the membrane, induce hyperpolarization, and overall reduce the excitability of the muscle, so that normal muscle contraction is reduced or abolished.

Apart from a direct action as a type of GABA agonist, avermectin appears to cause the release of transmitter GABA (but not glutamate) from nerve terminals. These experiments were conducted on isolated synaptosomes from rat brain (Pong *et al.*, 1980) but reinforce the hypothesis that the mode of action is associated with inhibitory mechanisms in the nervous system.

The importance of inhibition and GABA systems as potential targets for pest control agents has been reviewed by Miller (1978) and Beeman (1983). Not only do inhibitory synapses modify muscle action, but they are also essential in the control of central neurons. Therefore, it seems likely that avermectin may well act on both central and peripheral systems in parasite control.

2.3. Formamidines

The use of formamidines for the control of ectoparasites depends quite largely on the marked behavioral changes induced, as well as the overall toxicity. For example, initial hyperactivity leads to detachment of blood sucking parasites (Stone and Knowles, 1974). Careful analysis of the symptoms from both insects and acarines suggests that several different effects may occur. These may be marked by similar overall expressions of toxicity as in repellency and antifeeding (Beeman and Matsumara, 1974) or clearly separated as in the association of hyperactivity and paralysis with different experimental compounds (Stendel, 1978). A wide range of biochemical and physiological effects have been described from in vitro studies of the compounds, but no clearly defined mode of action has emerged. No studies have made direct correlations between overt symptoms and the simultaneous measurement of physiological effects. Much of the in vitro work demonstrates the action of formamidines (particularly chlordimeform) on amine systems in the nervous system. This may help explain the behavioral effects, if not the overall toxicity.

The enzyme monamine oxidase (MAO) is inhibited by formamidines (Atkinson et al., 1974; Beeman and Matsumura, 1974, 1978). MAO metabolizes neurotransmitter amines in the nervous system and is found in high concentrations in ticks and mites (Atkinson et al., 1974). Treatment of feeding ticks with known inhibitors of the mammalian MAO does cause detachment but no lasting toxicity (Stone and Knowles, 1974). Insects probably have little MAO in the nervous system, amines being metabolized by n-acetyltransferase (Dewhurst et al., 1972). Perhaps significantly, chlordimeform does inhibit cockroach n-acetyltransferase (Beeman and Matsumura, 1978). Electrophysiological recordings have detected repetitive activity of nerve impulses in treated tobacco hornworm (Manduca sp.) (Lund et al., 1979) and contractions in the artery wall muscle of the rabbit (Robinson and Bittle, 1979). The muscle effect is consistent with that for an aminergic α-receptor agonist, and this supports work in insects suggesting an action as octopamine agonists. Desmethylchlordimeform, a putative metabolite of chlordimeform, stimulates the octopamine adenylate cyclase enzyme system in the firefly light organ (Murdock and Hollingworth, 1980; Hollingworth and Murdock, 1980). Both desmethylchlordimeform and chlordimeform activate octopamine receptors on locust leg muscle, the threshold dose being lower for the metabolite (Evans and Gee, 1980; Evans, 1981). The normal function of the octopamine receptors on muscle is thought to be in modifying tonic contraction. Interference with this control could be expected to cause some behavioral changes, but little is known of the distribution of octopamine receptors in the parasite nervous system; no conclusions can be drawn about their possible involvement in formamidine toxicity. Recent work (Osborne, 1984a) shows that neurosecretory nerve fibers from isolated neurohemal organs of the stick insect are activated by low (10^{-7} M) concentrations of chlordimeform, desmethylchlordimeform, and Amitraz. This effect was not mimicked by octopamine or affected, except at high concentrations, by aminergic antagonists; Osborne concludes that the formamidine compounds act directly on the voltage-sensitive ion channels in the nerve membrane. This would support the evidence of a direct action of chlorodimeform on crayfish axons (Hollingworth and Lund, 1983). The effect was analyzed in detail and found to result from an inhibition of sodium inactivation gates, causing a prolongation of the nerve spike—rather similar to the effect of DDT but caused by a different mechanism.

2.4. Organophosphates

Organophosphates are employed as effective killing agents in parasite control, although the toxic action may involve an initial behavioral effect of antifeeding or expellency caused by general hyperactivity. Most of the work on mode of action has involved biochemical studies of enzyme kinetics. The general conclusions show that organophosphates inhibit a number of esterase and other hydrolase enzymes, but it is the inhibition of acetylcholinesterase (AChE) in the nervous system which is critical (see O'Brien, 1973, for review). Nerve cells that communicate through ACh-mediated synapses depend on this enzyme. The release of ACh as a neurotransmitter from the nerve terminal triggers a response in a synapsing cell. The enzyme then hydrolyzes transmitter in the synapse to inactivate the system. Inhibition of AChE permits excess ACh to accumulate, causing abnormally high levels of activation and total block of nerve function. AChE occurs at synapses in the CNS of mammals and at nerve muscle junctions. In insect and acarine parasites, it appears to be restricted to the CNS. Toxicity to parasites is then limited to effects expressed through central control, whereas muscle twitch and tremors in mammals may be caused by a direct action on nerve muscle junctions.

Inhibition of AChE has been demonstrated in a range of insect and some acarine parasites. The involvement of the enzyme in the toxic action of organophosphates is supported by evidence of changes that occur in pesticide resistance. Insensitivity of some tick species to organophosphate treatment can be correlated with a parallel decrease in the sensitivity of the AChE to inhibition (Schunter et al., 1968; Hart and Batham, 1969).

Electrophysiological measurements of treated flies (Miller, 1976) indicate that paralysis and other symptoms involve disruption of the CNS, but it is difficult to demonstrate a precise link between enzyme inhibition and symptoms of toxicity. Several isoenzymes can exist in the insect nervous system, each showing up to a fivefold difference in sensitivity to inhibition (O'Brien, 1973). However, Burt et al. (1966) found that abnormal electrical activity and eventual block of ganglionic output in treated cockroaches did show some correlation with a decrease in enzyme activity when measured histochemically. (See Figures 2 and 3.)

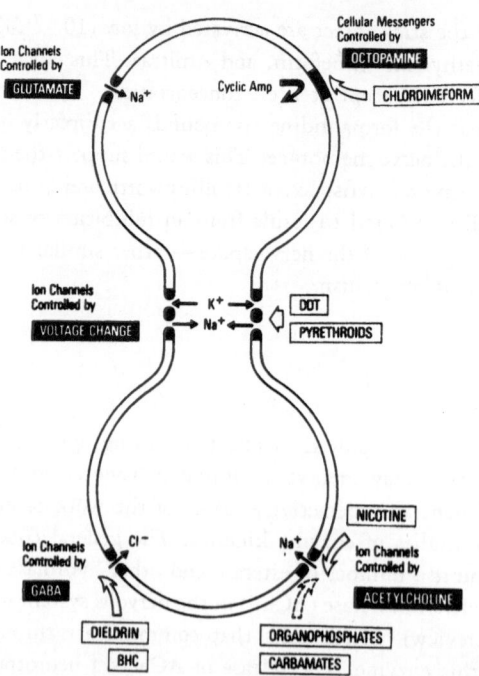

Figure 2. Summary of compounds affecting the nervous system. Diagram of a stylized excitable cell showing open ion channels through the membrane. Ion channels controlled by voltage change occur in the nerve axon and in some muscle cells. The chemically mediated channels operate at synapses between neurons or neurons and muscle cells. Solid lined arrows show the direct affect of compounds on receptors associated with channel operation. Dotted arrow indicates the indirect effect of compounds causing receptor block by inhibition of the enzyme controlling the amount of natural transmitter. (See also Fig. 3.)

2.5. Carbamates

The action of carbamates on the nervous system is believed to be similar to that of organophosphates. Both groups inhibit the enzyme AChE, but the kinetics of inhibition are different. The carbamylated enzyme is the less stable complex; it rapidly decarbamylates to release free enzyme when excess inhibitor is metabolized away.

The symptoms of carbamate and organophosphate poisoning can differ in detail. A survey of the effect of 37 compounds on houseflies, correlating behavioral and nervous system symptoms, showed that the two classes could be distinguished (Miller, 1976). Carbamates generally acted faster and caused more hyperactivity. Electrophysiology showed that flies treated with carbamates could recover after the ganglionic signals became disrupted but flies treated with organophosphates did not. The recovery factor can be related to the reversible nature of the carbamate inhibited enzyme in the CNS. The overall greater sensitivity of the nervous system in early stages of poisoning could reflect a difference in the initial rate of enzyme inhibition.

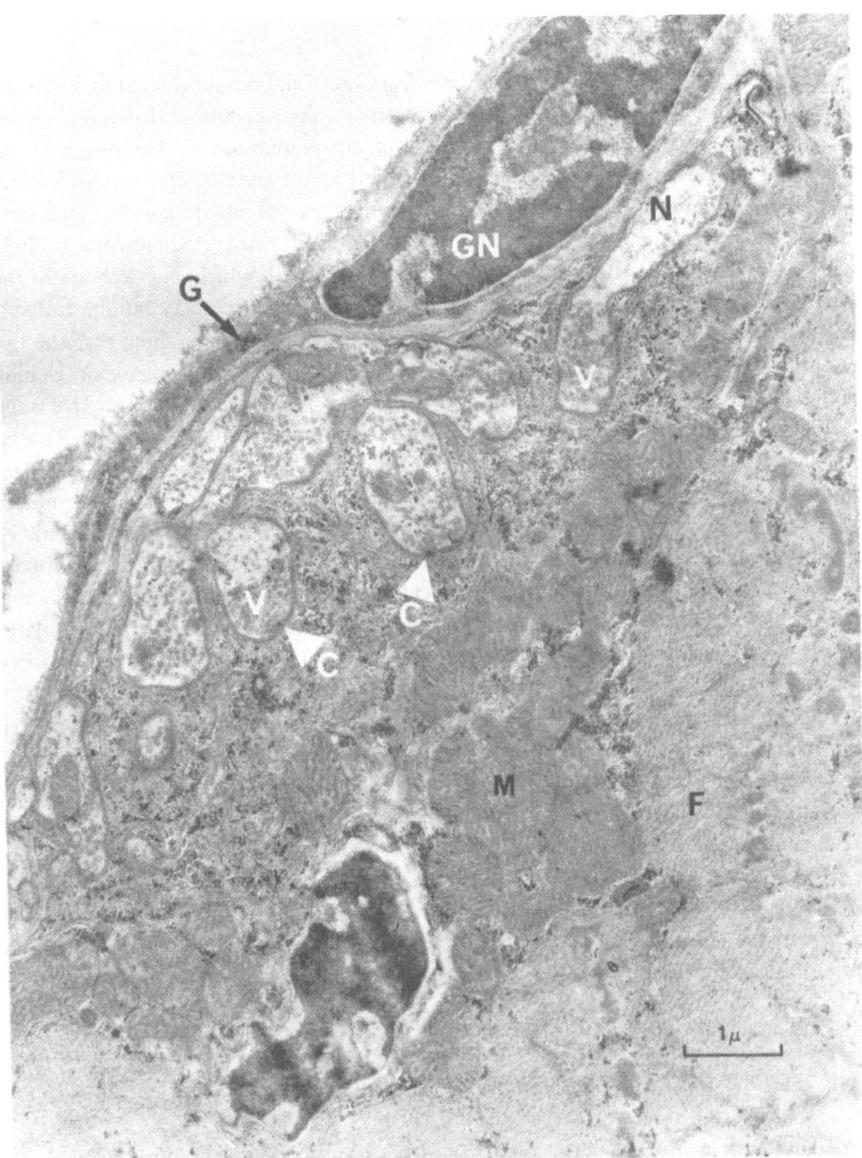

Figure 3. Electron micrograph of nerve and muscle from the cattle tick (*Boophilus microplus*) illustrating the types of cellular elements involved in the mode of action studies. A glial cell (G) with dark-stained cytoplasm and nucleus (GN) is close to a nerve ending (N). The nerve terminals are packed with vesicles (V) containing chemical neurotransmitter. Transmitter is released into the synaptic cleft (C). The postsynaptic cell shown is a somatic muscle fiber, but a similar arrangement of neuronal synapses and glial cells occurs in the CNS. The muscle cell section illustrates contractile myofibrils (F) and the large mitochondria (M) housing the respiratory mechanism. The small dots between the nerve terminals and mitochondria are reserves of glycogen.

2.6. Lindane (BHC/γ-HCH) and Cyclodienes

These compounds differ in their effects from DDT and its chlorinated hydrocarbon analogues. Symptoms of poisoning include tremors, convulsions, and paralysis in arthropods, qualitatively similar to the effects of organophosphates. The origin of the symptoms appears to be in the CNS. The severed leg of a cyclodiene-poisoned insect will stop twitching. A DDT-treated insect will continue its tremors. Biochemical investigations into the cause of the CNS disruption show that cyclodienes and γ-HCH affect nerve terminals. They cause excess ACh to be released, which may account for the symptomological similarity with organophosphates (see Brooks, 1974, for review). Electrophysiological recordings from the cockroach nervous system show that the hyperactivity induced by insecticide is suppressed by a cholinergic blocking agent (Uchida et al., 1978). The precise mechanism of this action is not clear. The hyperactive stage caused by γ-HCH is accompanied by distinct cytological changes in the glial cells, which are closely associated with the nerves (Osborne, 1984b). The biochemical mechanism proposed by Yamaguchi et al. (1980) is based on in vitro studies of transmitter release from nerve terminals prepared as synaptosomes. The common factor in a number of processes causing transmitter release is calcium. Calcium- (and magnesium-) linked ATPase enzyme activity and the binding of calcium ions were inhibited and uptake was enhanced. Current attention is focused on the development of a theory that correlates convincingly with a study of cyclodiene resistance in insects. Matsumura and coworkers (Ghiasuddin and Matsumura, 1982; Kardous et al., 1983) discovered that picrotoxinin is less toxic to the resistant cockroach, and binding of picrotoxinin to nerve terminals is reduced. This finding suggests an altered receptor–ionophore complex involving the neurotransmitter GABA, which is affected by picrotoxinin binding to an associated receptor. Further studies using cockroach muscle showed γ-HCH reduced GABA-dependent uptake of chloride. Like picrotoxinin, γ-HCH and cyclodienes may antagonize GABA action. GABA is an inhibitory neurotransmitter that modifies the excitatory synaptic activity. Suppression of this inhibition is thought to account for the neuroexcitant effects of picrotoxinin and thus may also be involved in the mode of action of cyclodienes.

3. COMPOUNDS AFFECTING BIOENERGETIC PATHWAYS

The mechanisms of energy production in parasitic arthropods do not appear to differ, as far as is known, from other insects. Differences do occur in the substrates used to fuel respiration and in their initial breakdown, but the final stage of releasing energy from food and storing it as high energy phosphate in adenosine-5'-triphosphate (ATP) is probably general. The flying insects are specialized for high aerobic activity. Calliphorine flies have oxygen consumption rates for flight of up to 5 ml/min per g, the highest recorded. The primary carbohydrate supply is glycogen but this is switched to trehalose to fuel the longer flights of these flies. (Tsetse differs from the other flies in using proline to fuel its long flights.)

The mobilization of fuels is controlled by hormones, e.g., hyperglycaemic hormone for carbohydrate, adipokinetic hormone for fats, and these may be sensitive, at least to secondary effects, of a wide range of chemicals. However, the compounds thought to act primarily on energy systems have their effect further along the chain of events in the respiratory pathway. The breakdown products of carbohydrate, fats, and proteins are oxidized to produce $NADH_2$ (reduced nicotinamide adenine dinucleotide). The $NADH_2$ is then oxidized in a controlled way, the released electrons being passed down a chain of electron carriers to combine with oxygen in a low-energy state. The energy of oxidation is used to produce ATP by the phosphorylation of ADP in stepwise reactions.

It is difficult to correlate symptoms of pesticide treatment *in vivo* with activity on respiration except by measurement of the reduced oxygen consumption. As this is affected by any change in behavior, the effects can be misleading. Symptoms of most respiratory poisons are characteristically gradual in their development (and most nerve poisons cause an initial increase in oxygen consumption). Action *in vitro* is monitored using isolated respiring mitochondria. Homogenized tissue is centrifuged under appropriate conditions to separate mitochondria from other cell components. Addition of substrates (e.g., succinate) increases oxygen consumption only slightly, addition of substrate together with ADP permits respiration coupled to oxidative phosphorylation to proceed with a high demand for oxygen, and addition of compounds inhibiting respiration slows oxygen uptake and compounds uncoupling phosphorylation permit oxygen to be consumed independently of the addition of ADP.

3.1. Arsenic (Trioxide)

Insect and acarine parasites treated with arsenic compounds show a gradual reduction in activity, followed by paralysis and death. Tremors are rare. Symptoms are those of a tissue poison, with degeneration of cells, vacuolation and disintegration occurring in gut epithelial cells before death occurs. The mode of action is thought to be the inhibition of respiration (Brown, 1963). Arsenical compounds used in ectoparasite control are mainly arsenic trioxide or mixtures that release arsenite ions in the tissue. The arsenite ion is thought to interfere with oxidative enzymes. *In vitro* experiments with insect mitochondria have shown inhibition of the enzyme α-ketoglutarate dehydrogenase (Hoskins *et al.*, 1956; Gonda *et al.*, 1957). Comparative work in vertebrates showed that pyruvate dehydrogenase is also affected (Webb, 1977) and that both enzymes are probably inhibited in arthropods as they are in mammals and birds. Inhibition of cellular respiration would account for the necrosis of tissues and slow death of the parasite.

3.2. Rotenone

Symptoms of rotenone poisoning (like those of arsenic) include inhibition of respiration with a gradual reduction in oxygen consumption. Some insects exhibit restlessness, but there is always a slow enfeebling that can be so prolonged as to allow appendages to decay before the heart stops beating (Brown, 1963). The nervous system of the cockroach has been shown to be affected by rotenone. A period of excitation is followed by conduction block with a progressive decrease in muscle contraction. These effects are not thought to be associated with the initial onset of symptoms but do follow the dose—response curve for toxicity (Fukami, 1976). Experiments with *in vitro* preparations of vertebrate mitochondria have shown a direct effect of rotenone on the respiratory pathway. Mitochondrial uptake of oxygen was inhibited by rotenone when the respiratory substrate was α-ketoglutarate, L-glutamate, malate, or fumarate. Rotenone had no effect on oxygen uptake with succinate as substrate. Oxidation of the former group of compounds requires the involvement of the coenzyme $NADH_2$, but oxidation of succinate does not. This suggests a site of action blocking the respiration between $NADH_2$ and the flavoprotein where succinate enters the chain of events. These studies were all carried out on mammalian mitochondria, but work by Mitsui, reviewed by Fukami (1976), to establish the mode of action of another natural insecticide (Piericidin extracted from *Streptomyces* sp.), obtained some confirmatory evidence in the insect. Piericidin has a similar mode of action and inhibits NADH oxidation at the same site in cockroach mitochondria; like rotenone, it kills by inhibition of respiration, thus preventing the formation of ATP.

REFERENCES

Adams, M. E., and Miller, T. A., 1980, Neural and behavioral correlates of pyrethroid and DDT-type posioning in the housefly: *Musca domestica* L., *Pestic. Biochem. Physiol.* 13:137–147.

Atkinson, P. W., Binnington, K. C., and Roulston, W. J., 1974, High monoamine oxidase activity in the tick, *Boophilus microplus* and inhibition by chlordimeform and related compounds, *J. Aust. Entomol. Soc.* 13:207–210.

Beeman, R. W., 1983, Recent advances in mode of action of insecticides, *Annu. Rev. Entomol.* 27:253–281.

Beeman, R. W., and Matsumura, F., 1974, Studies on the action of chlordimeform in cockroaches, *Pestic. Biochem. Physiol.* 4:325–336.

Beeman, R. W., and Matsumura, F., 1978, Formamidine pesticides—Actions in insects and acarines, in: *Pesticide and Venom Neurotoxicity* (D. L. Shankland, R. M. Hollingworth, and T. Smyth, Jr., eds.), pp. 179–188, Plenum Press, New York.

Binnington, K. C., and Lane, N. J., 1980, Perineural and glial cells of the tick nervous system: A tracer and freeze fracture study, *J. Neurocytol.* 9:343–362.

Binnington, K. C., and Obenchain, F. D., 1982, Structure and function of the circulatory, nervous and neuroendocrine systems of ticks, in: *Physiology of Ticks* (F. D. Obenchain and R. Galun, eds.), pp. 351–398, Pergamon Press, Oxford.

Breer, H., 1984, Neurochemical analysis of cholinergic elements in insect synaptosomes, in: *Insect Neurochemistry and Neurophysiology* (A. B. Borkovec and T. Kelly, eds.), pp. 329–331, Plenum Press, New York.

Brooks, G. T., 1974, *Chlorinated Insecticides*, Vol. II, Biological and Environmental Aspects, CRC Press, Cleveland.

Brown, A. W. A., 1963, Chemical injuries, in: *Insect Pathology: An Advanced Treatise* (E. A. Steinhaus, ed.), Vol. 1, pp. 67–131, Academic Press, New York.

Burt, P. E., and Goodchild, R. E., 1971, The site of action of pyrethrin I in the nervous system of the cockroach *Periplaneta americana*, *Entomol. Exp. Appl.* 14:179–189.

Burt, P. E., Gregory, G. E., and Molloy, F. M., 1966, A histochemical and electrophysiological study of the action of diazinon on cholinesterase activity and nerve conduction in ganglia of the cockroach *Periplaneta americana*, *Ann. Appl. Biol.* **58**:341–354.

Burt, P. E., Lord, K. A., Forrest, J. M., and Goodchild, R. E., 1971, The spread of topically-applied pyrethrin I from the cuticle to the central nervous system of the cockroach *Periplaneta americana*, *Entomol. Exp. Appl.* **14**:255–269.

Camougis, G., and Davis, W. M., 1971, A comparative study of the neuropharmacological basis of action of pyrethrins, *Pyrethrum Post.* **11**(1):7–14.

Clements, A. N., and May, T. E., 1977, The actions of pyrethroids upon the peripheral nervous system and associated organs in the locust, *Pestic. Sci.* **8**:661–680.

Desaiah, D., and Cutkomp, L. K., 1973, The effect of pyrethrins on ATP ases in cockroach and blue gillfish, *Pyrethrum Post.* **12**(2):70–75.

Dewhurst, S. A., Crocker, S. G., Ikeda, K., and McCaman, R. E., 1972, Metabolism of biogenic amines in *Drosophila* nervous tissue, *Comp. Biochem. Physiol.* **43B**:975–981.

Duce, I. R., and Scott, R. H., 1983, Reversible and irreversible action of dihydroavermectin B1a on GABA mediated responses in insect muscle, *Br. J. Pharmacol.* **80**:524.

Elliott, M., 1977, Synthetic Pyrethroids, in: *Synthetic Pyrethroids*, ACS Symposium Series 42 (M. Elliott, ed.), pp. 1–28, American Chemical Society, Washington, D. C.

Evans, P. D., 1981, Multiple receptor types for octopamine in the locust, *J. Physiol.* **318**:99–122.

Evans, P. D., and Gee, J. D., 1980, Action of formamidine pesticides on octopamine receptors, *Nature (Lond.)* **287**:60–62.

Firtz, L. C., Wang, C. C., and Gorio, A., 1979, Avermectin B1a irreversibly blocks postsynaptic potentials at the lobster neuromuscular junction by reducing muscle membrane resistance, *Proc. Natl. Acad. Sci. USA* **76**(4):2062–2066.

Fukami, J., 1976, Insecticides as inhibitors of respiration, in: *Insect Biochemistry and Physiology* (C. F. Wilkinson, ed.), pp. 353–396, Plenum Press, New York.

Gammon, D. W., 1978, Neural effects of allethrin on the free walking cockroach *Periplaneta americana:* An investigation using defined doses at 15° and 32°C, *Pestic. Sci.* **9**:79–91.

Gammon, D. W., Brown, M. A., and Casida, J. E., 1981, Two classes of pyrethroid action in the cockroach, *Pestic. Biochem. Physiol.* **15**:181–191.

Gammon, D. W., Lawrence, L. J., and Casida, J. E., 1982, Pyrethroid toxicology: Protective effects of diazepam and phenobarbital in the mouse and the cockroach, *Toxicol. Appl. Pharmacol.* **66**:290–296.

Ghiasuddin, S. M., and Matsumura, F., 1982, Inhibition of GABA induced chloride uptake by γ-BHC and heptachlor epoxide, *Comp. Biochem. Physiol.* **73C**:141–144.

Gonda, O., Traub, A., and Avi-Dor, Y., 1957, The oxidative activity of particulate fractions from mosquitoes, *Biochem. J.* **67**:487–493.

Hart, R. J., and Batham, P., 1969, A biochemical explanation for resistance to organophosphate ixodicides shown by a strain of blue tick (*Boophilus decoloratus*) from South Africa, *J. S. Afr. Vet. Med. Assoc.* **40**(3):284–289.

Hart, R. J., Beadle, D. J., and Botham, R. P., 1980, The penetration of ionic lanthanum into the central nervous system of the tick, *Amblyomma variegatum*, *Physiol. Entomol.* **5**:401–405.

Hollingworth, R. M., and Lund, A. E., 1983, Behavioral and lethal actions of amidines on invertebrates, in: *The Fifth International Conference of Pesticide Chemistry. Pesticide Chemistry, Human Welfare and the Environment* (J. Miyamoto and P. C. Kearney, eds.), Vol. 3, p. 15, Pergamon Press, Oxford.

Hollingworth, R. M., and Murdock, L. L., 1980, Formamidine pesticides: Octopamine-like actions in a firefly, *Science* **208**:74–76.

Hoskins, D. D., Cheldelin, V. H., and Newburgh, R. W., 1956, Oxidative enzyme systems of the honey bee *Apis mellifera* L., *J. Gen. Physiol.* **39**:705–713.

Kardous, A. A., Ghiasuddin, S. M., Matsumura, F., Scott, J. C., and Tanaka, K., 1983, Differences in the picrotoxin receptor between the cyclodiene resistant and susceptible strains of the German cockroach, *Pestic. Biochem. Physiol.* **19**:157–166.

Lawrence, L. J., and Casida, J. E., 1983, Stereospecific action of pyrethroid insecticides on the γ-aminobutyric acid receptor–ionophore complex, *Science* **221**:1399–1401.

Leake, L. D., Lauckner, S. M., and Ford, M. G., 1980, Relationship between neurophysiological effects of selected pyrethroids and toxicity to the leech *Haemopsis sanguisuga* and the locust *Schistocerca gregaria*, in: *Insect Neurobiology and Pesticide Action* (Neurotox '79), pp. 423–430, Society of Chemical Industry Publication, London.

Lowenstein, O., 1942, A method of physiological assay of pyrethrum extracts, *Nature (Lond.)* 150:760–762.

Lund, A. E., Hollingworth, R. M., and Shankland, D. L., 1979, Chlordimeform: Plantprotection by a sublethal, noncholinergic action on the central nervous system, *Pestic. Biochem. Physiol.* 11:117–128.

Miller, T., 1976, Distinguishing between carbamate and organophosphate insecticide poisoning in houseflies by symptomology, *Pestic. Biochem. Physiol.* 6:307–319.

Miller, T. A., 1978, The insect neuromuscular system as a site of insecticide action, in: *Pesticide and Venom Neurotoxicity* (D. L. Shankland, R. M. Hollingworth, and T. Smyth, Jr., eds.), pp. 95–111, Plenum Press, New York.

Miller, T. A., and Kennedy, J. M., 1972, Flight motor activity of houseflies as affected by temperature and insecticides, *Pestic. Biochem. Physiol.* 2:206–222.

Murdock, L. L., and Hollingworth, R. M., 1980, Octopamine-like actions of formamidines in the firefly light organ, in: *Insect Neurobiology and Pesticide Action* (Neurotox '79), pp. 415–422, Society of Chemical Industry Publication, London.

Narahashi, T., 1971, Mode of action of pyrethroids, *Bull. W.H.O.* 44:337–345.

Narahashi, T., 1976, Nerve membrane as a target of pyrethroids, *Pestic. Sci.* 7:267–272.

Nicholson, R. A., Chalmers, A. E., Hart, R. J., and Wilson, R. G., 1980, Pyrethroid action and degradation in the cattle tick (*Boophilus microplus*), in: *Insect Neurobiology and Pesticide Action* (Neurotox '79), pp. 289–295, Society of Chemical Industry Publication, London.

O'Brien, R. D., 1973, Acetylcholinesterase and its inhibition, in: *Insecticide Biochemistry and Physiology* (C. F. Wilkinson, ed.), pp. 271–296, Plenum Press, New York. .

Osborne, M. P., 1980, The insect synapse: Structural functional aspects in relation to insecticidal action, in: *Insect Neurobiology and Pesticide Action* (Neurotox '79), pp. 28–40, Society of Chemical Industry Publication, London.

Osborne, M. P., 1984a, Actions of formamidines, local anesthetics, octopamine and related compounds upon the electrical activity of neurohaemal organs of the stick insect (*Carausius morosus*) and sense organs of fly larvae (*Musca domestica*); (*Calliphora erythrocephala*), *Pestic. Biochem. Physiol.* 23:190–204.

Osborne, M. P., 1984b, DDT, γ-HCH and the cyclodienes, in: *Comprehensive Insect Physiology, Biochemistry and Pharmacology* (G. A. Kerkut, ed.), Pergamon Press, Oxford, in press.

Pong, S. S., Wang, C. C., and Fritz, L. D., 1980, Studies on the mechanism of action of avermectin B1a: Stimulation of release of γ-aminobutyric acid from brain synaptosomes, *J. Neurochem.* 34:351–358.

Robinson, C. P., and Bittle, I., 1979, Vascular effects of demethyl chlordimeform, a metabolite of chlordimeform, *Pestic. Biochem. Physiol.* 11:46–55.

Salgado, V. L., Irving, S. N., and Miller, T. A., 1983, The importance of nerve terminal depolarization in pyrethroid poisoning of insects, *Pestic. Biochem. Physiol.* 20:169–182.

Schunter, C. A., Roulston, W. J., and Snitzerling, H. J., 1968, A mechanism of resistance to organophosphorus acaricides in a strain of the cattle tick *Boophilus microplus*, *Aust. J. Biol. Sci.* 21:97–109.

Singh, G. J. P., 1984, Hormone release in *Locusta migratoria* in relation to insecticide poisoning syndrome, in: *Insect Neurochemistry and Neurophysiology* (A. B. Borkovec and T. J. Kelly, eds.), pp. 475–477. Plenum Press, New York.

Singh, G. J. P., and Orchard, I., 1982, Is insecticide induced release of insect neurohormones a secondary effect of hyperactivity of the central nervous system?, *Pestic. Biochem. Physiol.* 17:232–242.

Stendel, W., 1978, Cyclic amidines, compounds with a new mode of action against ticks, in: *Tickborne Diseases and Their Vectors* (J. K. H. Wilde, ed.), pp. 219–225, University of Edinburgh, Centre for Tropical Veterinary Medicine.

Stone, B. F., and Knowles, C. O., 1974, A laboratory method for evaluation of chemicals causing the detachment of the cattle tick *Boophilus microplus*, *J. Aust. Entomol. Soc.* 12:163–172.

Uchida, M., Fujita, T., Kurihara, N., and Nakajima, M., 1978, Toxicities of γ-BHC and related compounds, in: *Pesticide and Venom Neurotoxicity*, (D. L. Shankland, R. M. Hollingworth, and T. Smyth, Jr., eds.), pp. 133–151, Plenum Press, New York.

Webb, J. L., 1977, *Enzyme and metabolic inhibitors*, Vol. III, Academic Press, New York.

Welsh, J. H., and Gordon, H. T., 1947, The mode of action of certain insecticides on the arthropod nerve axon, *J. Cell. Comp. Physiol.* 30:147–171.

Wilkins, C. A., Conroy, J. B. A., Ho, P., O'Shanny, W. J., and Capizzi, T., 1981, The effect of Ivermectin on the live mass period of attachment and percent control of ticks, in: *Tick Biology and Control* (G. B. Whitehead and J. D. Gibson, eds.), pp. 137–142, Rhodes University, R.S.A.

Wouters, W., and van den Berken, J., 1978, Action of pyrethroids, *J. Gen. Pharmacol.* 9:387–398.

Yamaguchi, I., Matsumura, F., and Kardous, A. A., 1980, Heptachlor epoxide: effects on calcium mediated transmitter release from brain synaptosomes in rat, *Biochem. Pharmacol.* 29:1815–1823.

32

Drug Resistance in Arthropod Parasites

JAMES NOLAN and HERBERT J. SCHNITZERLING

1. INTRODUCTION

Despite considerable progress during the past 20 years in the development of non-chemical means of ectoparasite management, chemotherapy remains the basis, or an important adjunct, of many control programs designed to maximize production. There can be no argument that the greatest threat to stable chemical control and progress in the management of ectoparasites, and the diseases of which they are vectors, is the continued, and probably inevitable, emergence of pesticide resistance. The threat comes not only from the crises that are likely to arise in vector and disease outbreaks with the emergence of new resistant strains of parasites, but more importantly every new strain makes the task of finding replacement compounds more difficult. This difficulty arises partially because of ever-increasing costs associated with the development, and registration, of new materials. Of greater concern is the accumulation of resistance alleles in the population, which, with their associated biochemical and physiological defense mechanisms, constitute a formidable array of obstacles for any new chemical class to overcome. The latter problem can pose a difficult and expensive barrier to discovery and development, particularly as experience has shown that resistance mechanisms, selected by contemporary and previously used chemicals, often operate against structurally unrelated compounds. Thus, predictions on the expected life of even new chemical classes are difficult to make.

2. OCCURRENCE OF RESISTANCE

In an effort to present a concise picture of the current status of pesticide resistance in ectoparasites, reports of individual cases of resistance, already adequately docu-

JAMES NOLAN and HERBERT J. SCHNITZERLING • CSIRO, Division of Tropical Animal Science, Long Pocket Laboratories, Indooroopilly, Queensland 4068, Australia.

Table 1. *Geographical and Chronological Records of Resistance in Ectoparasite Species Not Previously Recorded by Brown and Pal (1971)*

Order/species	Chemical	Place of occurrence	Year reported
Siphonaptera			
Pulex irritans	DDT	Egypt	1968
	Dieldrin		
	DDT	Czechoslovakia	1972
	Dieldrin		
Ctenocephalides canis	DDT	Puerto Rico	1968
	Dieldrin		
	Malathion		
Xenopsylla cheopis	DDT	Ecuador	1969
	DDT	Egypt	1970
	Dieldrin		
	DDT	India	1971
	DDT	Libya	1971
	DDT	India	1972
	BHC		
	Malathion		
	DDT	Vietnam	1974
	Dieldrin		
	Malathion		
	DDT	India	1974
	Dieldrin		
	BHC		
	DDT	Burma	1978
	DDT	Java	1980
	DDT	U.S.S.R.	1981
Phthiraptera			
Pediculus humanus humanus	DDT	Egypt	1970
	BHC		
	DDT	Libya	1971
	BHC		
	Dieldrin		
	DDT	Burundi	1972
	BHC		
	Malathion		
Pediculus humanus capitis	BHC	Netherlands	1978
Linognathus africanus	Rotenone	South Africa	1969
	Dioxathion		
Hemiptera			
Cimex hemipterus	DDT	India	1973
	Malathion		
Cimex lectularis	DDT	USSR	1970
	Trichlorphon		
	DDT	Korea	1970
	Dieldrin		

Table I (Continued)

Order/species	Chemical	Place of occurrence	Year reported
	DDT Dieldrin BHC	Libya	1970
	DDT Dieldrin	Rumania	1971
Rhodnius prolixus	Dieldrin BHC	Venzuela	1969
Triatoma maculata	Dieldrin BHC	Venezuela	1976
Diptera			
Chrysomyia albiceps	Diazinon	South Africa	1975
Cochliomyia hominivorax	Coumaphos	U.S. El Salvador Mexico Jamaica	1983
Culicoides furens	DDT Dieldrin BHC	Puerto Rico	1968
Haematobia irritans exigua	DDT Fenvalerate	Australia	1982
Lucilia cuprina	Arsenic Diazinon	South Africa	1975
Lucilia sericata	Dieldrin	Ireland	1968
Phlebotomus papatasi	DDT	India	1979
Sarcophaga peregrina	BHC	Japan	1968
Acarina			
Psoroptes ovis	BHC Diazinon	Argentina	1970
Chorioptes bovis	Coumaphos	Netherlands	1978

mented by Brown and Pal (1971), will not be repeated in this chapter. In addition because of the extensive, up-to-date, and detailed listings of the chronology, distribution, and spectrum of resistance in ticks already presented by Wharton (1976), Drummond (1977), Baker (1978), Nolan and Roulston (1979), and Solomon (1983), another such listing is superfluous. The more recent developments in other ectoparasites of medical and veterinary importance, not covered by the Brown and Pal review in 1971, are given in Table I. The comparison of data presented in Table I and in the previous publications listed above reveals interesting points of difference between resistance development in ticks and other species, and even between single and multihost ticks.

In the one-host *Boophilus* tick, resistance has progressed (or degenerated) from arsenic, through the chlorinated hydrocarbons and a wide range of organophosphorus compounds to, more recently, the amidines. In contrast, the spectrum of compounds affected in species of bugs, fleas, flies, lice, and mites, which live as ectoparasites, is much narrower, and the geographical distribution of resistance to the compounds that have failed is limited. Although it is difficult, and probably dangerous, to generalize about such a wide range of pest species, one must suspect that the salient feature contributing to this contrast is the variation in treatment regimens adopted across the range. Heavy reliance has been placed on chemicals for control of *Boophilus* in the past, treatments have been frequent and often haphazard in timing and intensity, and control rather than eradication has usually been the aim. Treatment for mites and, to a slightly lesser extent, other ectoparasites infesting domestic animals, although spasmodic, is usually intensive when applied, with eradication the aim and resistance a relatively rare occurrence.

It is probably not surprising, in view of the smaller proportion of the total population of a multihost species, such as *Rhipicephalus appendiculatus*, treated at any one time, and the single generation per year for this species compared with the four or five for *Boophilus*, that acaricide resistance has not developed to the same extent in multihost species. What is puzzling is that in those areas, such as East Africa, in which intensive treatments are carried out to control multihost species, and where *Boophilus* is prevalent, the wide spectrum of resistance that exists in Australia for this species is not found. It can only be concluded that where intensive treatments are applied, a virtual saturation strategy for *Boophilus* ensues, with consequent suppression of the one-host tick population gene pool. This strategy is in contrast to that practiced in many instances in Australia where, for the first 70 years of tick control, treatments were applied at best at economic threshold levels of tick infestation, or at worst only when convenient.

3. TOXICOLOGY

3.1. Spectrum of Effect between Drugs

Ticks, and in particular the one-host cattle tick *Boophilus microplus*, have developed resistance to a wide array of chemicals used for their control (see Section 2). It is therefore logical that within the resistance mechanisms developed by this species are many examples of cross-resistance between and within chemical classes. Basically five types of resistance have emerged in ticks, and these can be categorized by the drug types to which resistance is expressed: arsenic, DDT-pyrethrum, organochlorine, organophosphorus-carbamate, and more recently amidine resistance. Although these represent distinctly different resistance categories, it does not mean that ticks in a field population cannot exhibit a spectrum of resistance encompassing several or all of the mechanisms. The lack of any successful attempts to eradicate newly emerged mechanisms has meant that in several areas a steady accumulation of unrelated resistance alleles has occurred in the population (Roulston *et al.*, 1981).

Du Toit *et al.* (1941) first described resistance in ticks to arsenic in the East London area of South Africa, and Whitehead (1961) demonstrated that resistance to sodium arsenite did not confer cross-resistance to any other pesticidal group. This was a simple case of a specific resistance mechanism and certainly of a relationship that did not hold for many other subsequent cases of tick resistance.

DDT resistance, first reported in one-host ticks in Australia in 1955 (Legg *et al.*, 1955) and subsequently in South Africa (Whitehead, 1956), also showed limited effect on other acaricides. However, the finding that DDT resistance also conferred resistance to pyrethrum (Whitehead, 1959), although possibly not of great significance at that time, was subsequently to have an important influence on the development and use of synthetic pyrethroids for tick control (Nolan *et al.*, 1979). DDT resistance in ticks was found to be independent of resistance to the organochlorines BHC, dieldrin, and toxaphene (Stone, 1957), although between the latter group cross-resistance occurred in single- and multihost ticks (Norris and Stone, 1956; Whitehead, 1965).

In the three types of resistance discussed so far for ticks, only single resistance mechanisms exist in each case. However, with the onset of organophosphorus (OP) and carbamate resistance, first reported by Shaw and Malcolm (1964) for *Boophilus microplus*, a more complex resistance pattern based on multiple mechanisms, each with specific limited effects within the one class of compounds, began to emerge. In Australia some nine forms of OP-carbamate resistance in *Boophilus microplus*, each having characteristic toxicological and biochemical features (Roulston and Nolan, 1975) and each affecting a discrete range of OP compounds (Fig. 1), have been documented. This pattern of specific resistance mechanisms, within a group, has important implications for decisions on the choice of alternative effective acaricides to replace those affected by resistance (see further discussion in Section 6).

The similar sequence and spectrum of arsenic, DDT, and organochlorine resistance that has occurred in both single- and multihost tick species in widely separated tick-infested countries poses the important question of whether identical patterns of cross-resistance, between and within chemical groups, for tick species will continue in all areas. Obviously, if this were so, the Australian experience with *Boophilus* could be used as a guide for the selection of alternative chemicals when problems occur in other areas or with other species, in cases where resistance is not as advanced. OP-carbamate resistance has been demonstrated in both single- and multihost ticks in several other countries besides Australia (Baker, 1978; Lourens and Lyaruu, 1979), although the range of compounds involved is not as extensive. A strain that was apparently toxicologically similar to the Ridgelands strain emerged in *Boophilus* in Africa (Shaw *et al.*, 1967), South America (Amaral *et al.*, 1974), and New Caledonia (Brun *et al.*, 1983), but subsequent cross-resistance patterns within the OP group, for single- and multihost ticks, have differed in different areas. Certainly the evidence accumulated so far does not provide a strong scientific basis to support the view that the spectrum of resistance within the OP group for *Boophilus* and multihost ticks will be identical in all areas infested by ticks. At least, where tick strains emerge that are shown to be toxicologically similar to those already established elsewhere, the choice of alternative effective compounds is simplified considerably. There is also still reason to expect that the lack of cross-resistance patterns between groups such as the OPs, amidines, and pyrethroids found for *Boophilus* in Australia will be maintained.

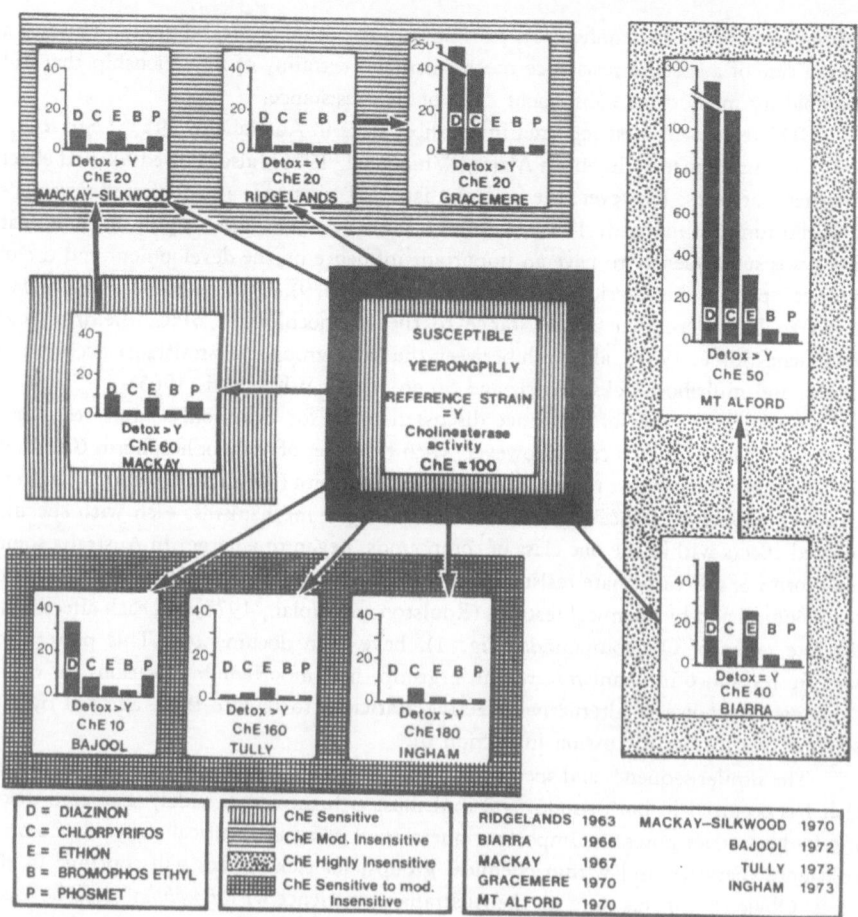

Figure 1. Biochemical and toxicological characteristics of nine strains of the cattle tick, *Boophilus microplus* resistant to organophosphorus compounds. Resistance factors shown on vertical axes. (After Nolan and Roulston, 1979.)

As would be expected, a similar sequence of different pesticide groups has been used for most ectoparasites, with unsatisfactory control due to emergence of resistant strains being the usual stimulus for change to a new group. Exceptions to this sequential usage pattern have occurred when it has been found that compounds may be unsuitable, or too toxic, for application to the host, often man, for ectoparasites such as bugs, fleas, and lice or when legislation has required that certain compounds, e.g., DDT, be replaced because of concern over residues and other problems in meat or dairy products.

Fortunately in no other ectoparasite has the complexity and spectrum of resistance of *Boophilus* been seen. The lack of cross-resistance between DDT and the organochlorine group has been a consistent feature and has been reported for fleas

(Shalaby, 1971), lice (Soliman and Soliman, 1966; Ardalan, 1977), and bugs (Bhatia and Deshpande, 1975). Only limited development of resistance within the OP-carbamate group has occurred in most nonacarine ectoparasite species, with the exception of the Australian and South African sheep blowfly, *Lucilia cuprina.*

Malathion has been the most commonly used OP compound to replace DDT and the organochlorine group for the control of nonacarine ectoparasites other than flies. Specific malathion resistance has occurred in fleas (Fox *et al.*, 1968) and bugs (Shetty *et al.*, 1975), although later work (Feroz, 1974) has shown nonspecific OP resistance in a different species of *Cimex*, and lice (Maunder, 1981). No information is available on the spectrum of compounds affected in other cases of OP resistance reported in Table I. The resistance picture for most of the nonacarine ectoparasites currently ends at the stage of limited OP resistance. However, the cross-resistance reported by Schnitzerling *et al.* (1982) between DDT-resistant *Haematobia* and the synthetic pyrethroids fenvalerate and cypermethrin provides a timely warning on the necessity for careful planning in the use of this effective new group of pesticides, especially in ectoparasites in which DDT resistance is well established.

The sheep blowfly, *Lucilia cuprina,* has a resistance picture that is beginning to emulate that of the cattle tick. No field reports of arsenic resistance in *Lucilia* spp. were documented in Australia, although Shanahan and Roxburgh (1974) pointed out that a laboratory-selected OP-carbamate-resistant strain did develop a low level of cross-resistance to arsenic, and Blackman and Baker (1975) reported arsenic resistance in *Lucilia* in South Africa. Resistance did not develop in the field to DDT, which was used for several years for control of this parasite. However, as mentioned by Shanahan, this exception in the ectoparasite resistance sequence probably occurred because DDT was an oviposition deterrent rather than a larvicide. The use of DDT for blowfly control in Australia also occurred during a period of persistent dry conditions with low incidence of body strike (M. D. Murray, personal communication). Combined with the rapid and complete replacement of DDT by organochlorines, this meant the potential for selection of DDT resistance in this species was limited. Resistance to the organochlorines and cross-resistance within the group, however, did occur in Australia (Busvine and Shanahan, 1961). Resistance to diazinon, the first OP compound used to control this species, appeared within 8 years of its introduction; the mechanism was nonspecific, affecting several other OPs used for blowfly control (Shanahan and Hart, 1966). The broad spectrum of this resistance was in contrast to the pattern found in ticks and in certain other coprophagous blowfly species, e.g. *Chrysomyia putoria* (Busvine *et al.*, 1963), and it ruled out the introduction of new OP compounds as effective diazinon substitutes. It is of interest, however, that a subsequent report demonstrated that diazinon resistance did not confer cross-resistance to carbophenothion (Treeby, 1974) and, in an evaluation of the resistance status of some 41 field samples of *Lucilia*, Hughes (1981) demonstrated that two diazinon-resistant samples were not cross-resistant to coumaphos. Butacarb was developed and released specifically for the control of OP-resistant *Lucilia* (Harrison, 1967). Initial tests failed to find any evidence of cross-resistance between diazinon-resistant *Lucilia* and this carbamate, again a variation from the picture established in the cattle tick (J. Wilson, unpublished observations). This finding provided grounds for optimism that this compound would be a suitable long-term diazinon replacement. Unfortunately, the optimism was not warranted, as butacarb resistance was widespread by 1969 (Shanahan and Roxburgh, 1974): So far no evidence of cross-resistance, or of emergence of specific resistance, to the triazine insect growth regulator cyromazine, which is currently being used for *Lucilia* control, has been found.

4. MECHANISMS

Of the number of possible resistance mechanisms given in Fig. 2, only those of behavior, penetration, detoxication, and insensitivity have been verified experimentally. Behavioral resistance has not yet arisen in any of the ectoparasites of interest, and therefore our discussion focuses on the other three mechanisms. While the numbers of species studied are small, they are wide ranging and include ticks, blowflies, lice, and bugs. Again, the cattle tick *Boophilus microplus* has been studied most comprehensively. This section emphasizes mechanisms, rather than species, as we believe this provides the more informative and concise approach. Of the total of 23 ectoparasites, not including separate tick species in which resistance has been documented, only in four has the mechanism been identified.

4.1. Penetration

This mechanism of resistance has been found only in *B. microplus*, and then only in a laboratory strain. It is present in the permethrin-selected Malchi, DDT- and pyrethroid-resistant strain (Schnitzerling *et al.*, 1983). Strangely, reduced penetration occurred only with cypermethrin isomers and not with the isomers of the selecting agent, permethrin.

4.2. Detoxication

Detoxication (see Fig. 3 for reactions) has been identified as a causative resistance mechanism in ticks, blowflies, and bed bugs. Of the nine strains of OP- and carbamate-resistant ticks investigated (Fig. 1), only in the Mackay strain (a transitory situation) has the resistance been accounted for entirely by detoxication (Roulston *et al.*, 1969). Later, in this strain, and in all others in which detoxication was of significance, it was found to be supplemented by insensitivity of acetylcholinesterase (AChE) in the expression of a dual OP resistance mechanism (Fig. 1). Feroz (1974) found that increased degradation of malathion acted as a resistance mechanism in *Cimex*, but this degradation was apparently not specific for the carboxyl-ester. OP resistance in the Q strain of the sheep blowfly was shown by Hughes and Devonshire (1982) to be mainly attributable to a microsomal phosphatase, hydrolyzing the phosphate moiety, with some evidence of additional detoxication of the parent phosphorothionate by a microsomal oxidase.

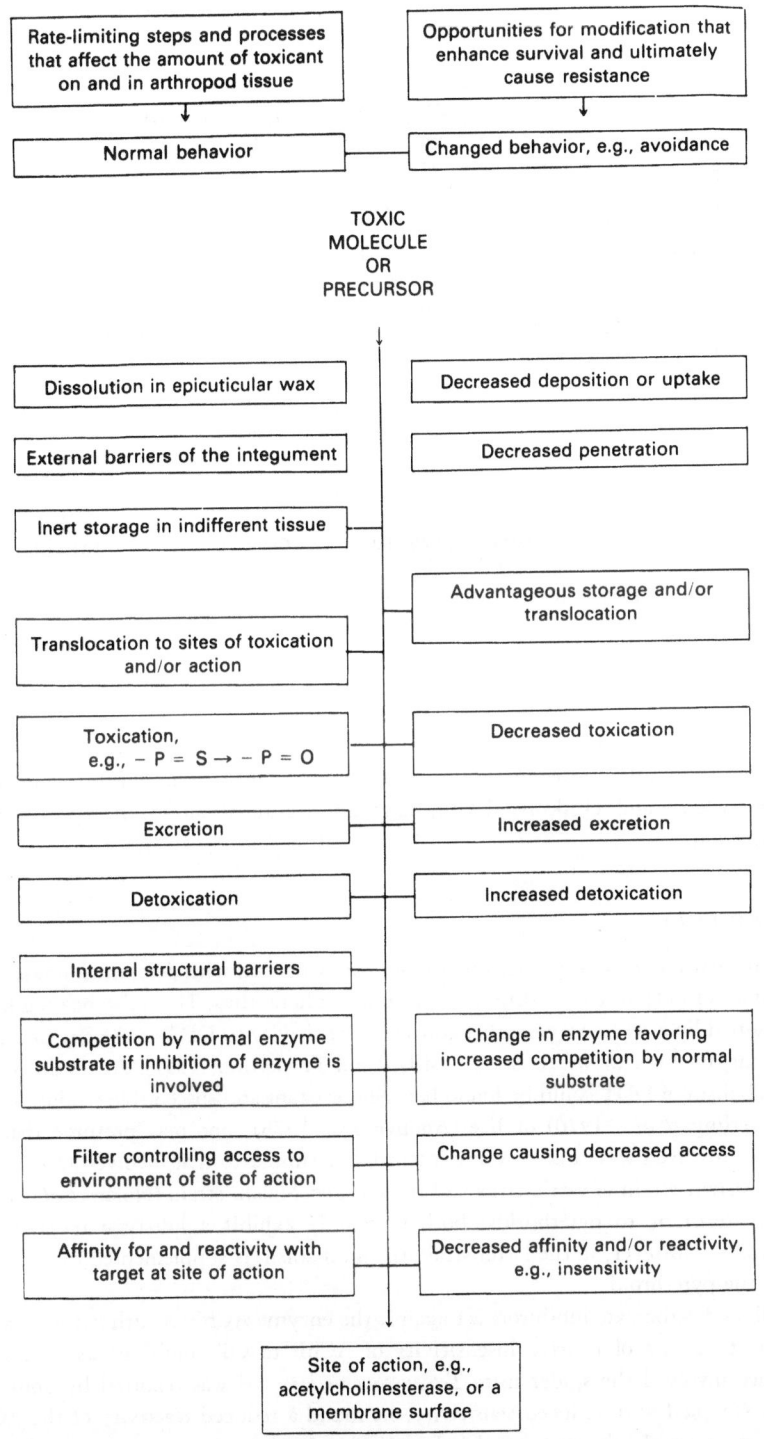

Figure 2. Factors influencing effectiveness of toxicants and opportunities for the development of resistance. (Adapted from Winteringham, 1969, and Brooks, 1976.)

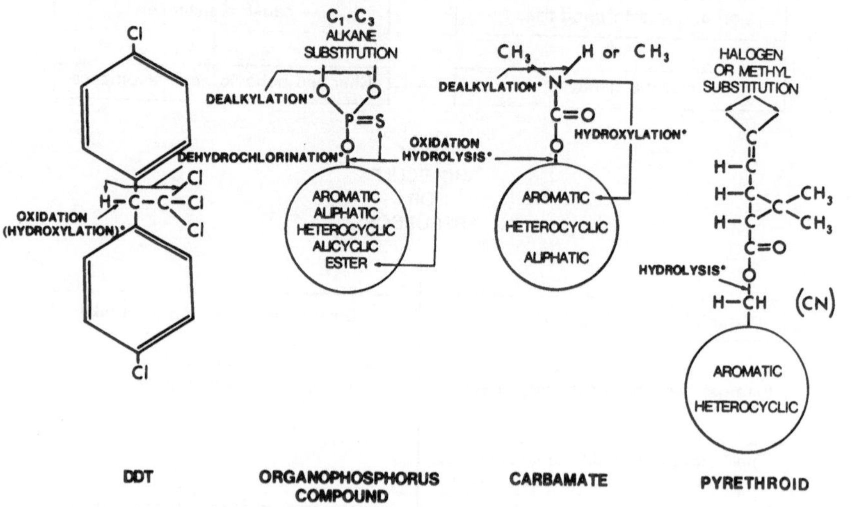

Figure 3. Important metabolic reactions (*) of some pesticide molecules, modification of which may lead to resistance.

The most well known of causative detoxication mechanisms, dehydrochlorination, associated with DDT resistance (Fig. 3) and first identified in the housefly *Musca domestica* (Perry and Hoskins, 1950), does not figure at all in the species under consideration.

4.3. Insensitivity

The first report of resistance other than that associated with detoxication was made by Busvine (1951) in relationship to DDT-resistant houseflies. The resistance was found to be caused by a recessive gene that conveys insensitivity to DDT at the site of action, called kdr, for knockdown resistance (Milani and Travaglino, 1957). As no differences in metabolism of DDT could be found between resistant and susceptible strains of ticks (Schnitzerling *et al.*, 1970) or lice (Anonymous, 1973), one may presume that the resistance involved was caused by site insensitivity similar to that involved in kdr. The DDT-resistant strain of cattle ticks and the selected Malchi strain (Nolan *et al.*, 1979) are cross-resistant to pyrethorids; both seemingly exhibit a kdr-type resistance to pyrethroids. However, in the latter strain the mechanism is supplemented by detoxication of the pyrethroid.

OP and carbamate inhibitors act against the enzyme AChE as outlined in Chapter 31. The first case of relative insensitivity of AChE to OP inhibitors as a cause of resistance involved the spider mite *Tetranychus urticae* and was reported by Smissaert (1964). Coupled with reduced sensitivity, he found a reduced reactivity of the AChE toward the normal substrate acetylcholine (ACh). In ticks these two aspects are intimately related, being controlled by the same altered active site on AChE (Roulston and

Nolan, 1975). AChE insensitivity was first recognized in M strain ticks later known as Ridgelands (see Fig. 1) by Lee and Batham (1966). This was followed by a stream of reports on the subject in Australia (summarized in Fig. 1) and later by a report from Argentina (Reich *et al.*, 1978). The AChE in ticks occurs in particulate form, seems irreversibly bound, and occurs as two components, only one of which becomes modified (Nolan *et al.*, 1972; Nolan and Schnitzerling, 1975). The genetic character of the strain concerned determines the degree of the ensuing insensitivity. The alteration of the site has occurred in such a way as to reduce affinity as well as the rate of deacylation (Schnitzerling *et al.*, 1982). For the normal substrate, the latter process is rate limiting, and thus the hydrolysis of normal substrate is directly proportional to the rate constant for this step. For OP inhibitors (reacting as substrates), the reduction in affinity determines the degree of insensitivity, as the rate of dephosphorylation is extremely small, and the enzyme cannot resume its hydrolytic activity, i.e., for practical purposes, the enzyme becomes irreversibly inhibited.

Where insensitivity is the cause, resistance levels may be low, but more importantly they can be very high (1000× and more). On the other hand, where detoxication is the cause, resistance levels are generally low (50× and less). It follows that in situations in which resistance levels exceeding 50× prevail, one will confidently be able to ascribe the cause to insensitivity. For instance, DDT resistance in the buffalo fly *Haematobia irritans exigua*, which is 1000× (Schnitzerling *et al.*, 1982), will be attributable to site insensitivity. Similarly, this mechanism will have been involved also in the dieldrin resistance of ticks reported by Stone and Meyers (1957) to be on the order of 2000×.

5. COUNTERMEASURES

Given the number, variety, and different classes of chemicals to which pests have developed resistance, we may now regard the development of resistance as an inevitable outcome of control by chemicals. From the point of view of prolonging the useful life of pesticides, we might be wise to consider the appropriateness of measures to combat resistance other than the obvious change to a new chemical class.

This section considers two approaches to the problem: first that of eradicating the resistant strain from the scene, and second that of adopting strategies to control resistance and so nullify or minimize its effects. Once again, this discussion leans heavily on the information available from research on cattle ticks. However, some of the conceptual notions discussed here have in some instances been scrutinized in the previous reviews by Brown and Pal (1971) and Nolan and Roulston (1979). Little new information has come to hand since 1979, and the reader is referred to the latter review if supplementary information is required on a particular point.

5.1. Eradication of Resistant Strains

If the resistant individuals can be removed from the immediate population, the continued efficacy of the chemical should be maintained. This proposition has been put to test successfully on two separate occasions. One reported by Nolan and Roulston (1979) involved a local eradication of the OP-resistant Ridgelands strain of *B. microplus* using dioxathion, to which the strain first had become resistant. It took 10 3-weekly treatments of normal-strength dioxathion (0.075%) to eradicate a resistant strain, as opposed to four 3-weekly treatments for a susceptible strain. The other instance involved a local eradication of a strain of *Boophilus decoloratus* in Rhodesia (Zimbabwe) (Matthewson *et al.*, 1971). This strain, which exhibited a 200× resistance to the OP compound oxinthiophos, was eradicated by the frequent use of a mixture of chlorfenvinphos/dioxathion, to which the ticks exhibited an 11× resistance. The overriding needs for success are that the resistance should be localized and characterized and that the area be defined to prevent movement of hosts out of the area before eradication has begun. The situation is further complicated by the imponderable question as to whether the strain would appear independently in new areas.

5.2 *Control of Resistant Strains*

5.2.1. *Manipulation of the Structure*

Some 80 OP compounds have found their way into accepted agricultural use since the 1950s. It is probably safe to say that the number synthesized with biological activity would be 100 times greater and almost without exception that they would have been synthesized on the basis of Schrader's structural model:

$$R^1 \diagdown \quad \diagup O(S) \\ P \\ R^2 \diagup \quad \diagdown Acyl$$

With the ready manipulability of these compounds in mind, we set about making homologous changes to an arbitrarily chosen model, the phosmet molecule (Schnitzerling *et al.*, 1982). This provided the basis for a study of the reactivity of these homologues with cattle tick AChE extracted from various resistant strains. The objective was to develop a rationale for an attack on the resistance mechanism. Because of the different types of insensitive AChE involved in OP resistance in ticks (Nolan *et al.*, 1972; Nolan and Schnitzerling, 1975), we were unable to arrive at an inhibitor configuration that would provide optimum reactivity with all AChEs. This particular experience gives little encouragement to the feasibility of custom synthesis as a strategy to defeat resistance mechanisms, although such a strategy is often advocated.

5.2.2. *Increased Concentration*

Where in a particular situation resistance is low enough and a reduced level of control may be tolerated, increasing the concentration of chemical will provide an effective and simple means of dealing with resistance. Of course, it is implied in this approach that the margin of safety remaining is sufficient to ensure that no significant hazard to man or the animal will result from the increased concentration of the chemical involved. When DDT was in use in Australia to control the cattle tick, it was used at a concentration of 0.5% p,p-isomer. Increasing the concentration to 1% p,p-isomer provided a satisfactory means of dealing with the $8\times$ resistance when it arose and prolonging the useful life of DDT. Similarly, increasing the concentration of chlorpyrifos from 0.025% to 0.05% also provided satisfactory control of the Biarra OP-resistant strain of ticks when it arose. However such a strategy is dependent on the nature and level of the resistance mechanism. Doubling the concentration of amitraz from 0.025% to 0.05% raised the control of the recently developed, highly amidine-resistant Ulam strain from 61% to only 66% (J. Nolan, unpublished observations).

5.2.3. Alteration of Formulation

It is well established in cattle tick control that the type of formulation used has profound effects on the deposition and toxicological performance of the chemical (Roulston et al., 1958; Roulston and Schnitzerling, 1965; Schnitzerling and Stone, 1968). Most acaricides are insoluble in water and, as a result, they need to be specially prepared to provide suspensions on addition to water, e.g., as in melts, emulsifiable concentrates (EC) wettable powders or flowable pastes. In general, the more chemical deposited the more effective is the formulation. Cattle ticks are usually controlled by dipping cattle in large immersion vats, which with use become heavily fouled with urine, feces, dirt, and hair. Such a medium will affect the performance of most formulations in suspension. Fortuitously with ECs, for example, deposition increases with fouling and ageing and to a degree this enhances effectiveness. Even in the absence of fouling, different types of formulation and changes made to a particular formulation will increase the amount deposited on the host (Roulston and Schnitzerling, 1965). Thus, without resorting to increasing the concentration of the chemical in suspension, it is possible to achieve the same effect by manipulating the formulation. An enhancement could also be achieved by a change in formulation that aided penetration of the toxicant through the arthropod integument.

5.2.4. Synergism and Additives

Synergists have potential application when the resistance mechanism is known to be detoxication. The type of synergist chosen will depend on the type of detoxication involved. Where oxidative mechanisms prevail, as in carbaryl metabolism, oxidase inhibitors such as piperonyl butoxide should be synergistic; where hydrolytic mechanisms prevail, as in pyrethroid metabolism, esterase inhibitors such as OP compounds should be synergistic. Experimental trials with tick-infested cattle have confirmed the potential of carbaryl synergized by piperonyl butoxide (Schuntner et al., 1974) and of pyrethroids synergized by the OP compounds chlorfenvinfos and ethion (Nolan and Bird, 1977). The latter combination is being used effectively for field control of ticks, particularly in relationship to DDT-resistant ticks that exhibit cross-resistance to pyrethroids. Unfortunately, compounds that are useful as synergists for certain classes of compounds may have the opposite effect with others. OP compounds that require activation before becoming toxic are antagonized by piperonyl butoxide; amidines are also antagonized by this compound (Knowles and Roulston, 1972). Other problems, such as the cost of the high concentration of synergist needed in the combination, the synergist : acaricide ratio often being as high as 10 : 1, instability, and formulation difficulties, have mitigated against the use and acceptance of synergized mixtures. Because synergists tend to be nonspecific in their action, there is also the added danger of increased toxicity to the host, which is itself often protected by the same types of detoxication mechanisms that operate in the pest.

Another method of prolonging the life of an acaricide is the addition of a compound that is additively toxic. For instance, chlordimeform added at 0.04% to a vat containing ethion restored control of the OP-resistant Biarra strain of ticks that hitherto could not be controlled by ethion alone (Roulston et al., 1971).

6. RATIONAL CHOICE OF ALTERNATIVE DRUGS

Although various strategies have been tried as countermeasures to control resistant strains of ectoparasites and prolong the useful life of particular drugs (see Section 5), the usual procedure adopted is to change to an alternative pesticide that is unaffected by the resistance mechanism. This practice provides the simple convenient answer, but always at the cost of preserving yet another resistance allele in the population. When several such effective alternatives are available, it is important to consider whether the experience gained so far in pesticide resistance management can be used to provide a rational basis for making the choice on other than economic grounds. To illustrate the problems that need to be considered, a few examples have been selected from experience in Australia with the much-researched cattle tick and sheep blowfly.

The common temptation, when faced with a resistance problem, is to change to an entirely new class of compounds in the belief that this represents the safest procedure to adopt. Experience has shown that new chemistry may not always provide the most reliable alternative. During the use of OP compounds as tickicides, between 1959 and 1975, when control failed, recourse was often made to a different type of anticholinesterase agent, as the spectrum of effect of each resistance mechanism in terms of control did not extend to other, closely related structures. Thus, ethion and coumaphos were used in place of dioxathion when Ridgelands resistance developed, chlorpyrifos was able to be used in place of coumaphos and ethion when Biarra resistance developed, promacyl (acylated promecarb-a carbamate) replaced chlorpyrifos when Mt. Alford resistance developed, and this latter compound remains effective. Table II illustrates the sequential introduction of these tickicides essentially all from the one class of compounds: a sequence that provided efficient tick control for many years after resistance was first reported for one member of the class in 1963.

A rather different picture has emerged for OP resistance in the sheep blowfly in

Table II. Percentage Control of Susceptible and the Four Major OP-Resistant Strains of the Cattle Tick (Boophilus microplus) in Stall Trials on Infested Animals with Chemicals Applied at Normal Recommended Concentrations

Chemical	Recommended field concentration (% w/v)	Susceptible reference strain	Ridgelands (1963)	Biarra (1966)	Mackay-Silkwood (1967)	Mt. Alford (1970)
Dioxathion (1958)[a]	0.075	99	76	—	68	—
Coumaphos (1959)	0.025	99	99	41	69	—
Ethion (1962)	0.075	99	99	74	90	34
Chlorpyrifos (1967)[b]	0.025	99	99	90[b]	99	46
Phosmet (1967)	0.075	99	99	97	—	98
Promacyl (1975)	0.15	99	—	—	96	99

[a]Figures in brackets show year of introduction of the chemical and, under strain names, year when resistance problems first developed.
[b]Until new acaricides became available, the concentration of chlorpyrifos was doubled for control of this strain.

Australia, where diazinon resistance was first reported by Shanahan and Hart in 1966. Butacarb was introduced as a replacement in 1967 (see Section 3), but the failure of this compound, which occurred in 2 years, prompted the return to diazinon, with its low level of resistance and shorter period of fly protection. This situation applied until 1980, when the effective alternative, cyromazine, was released.

Despite detailed knowledge of biochemical mechanisms of resistance and of the chemistry and mode of action of new compounds, it is difficult to predict the problems that candidate compounds will face from established resistant strains of ectoparasites, even when such candidates belong to entirely new chemical classes. This enigma was recently illustrated by the spectrum of drug susceptibility of the recently emerged Ulam amidine-resistant tick strain. The strain showed an unsatisfactory level of response to the widely used, and structurally related, tickicides amitraz, chloromethiuron, and cymiazole, yet remained susceptible to the cyclic amidine clenpyrin (J. Nolan, unpublished observations). To confuse the picture further, a completely unrelated and promising new tickicide with a triazine-thione structure, which had given satisfactory control of all known resistant strains up to that stage, provided only a 24% control of the Ulam strain. The lesson to be learned, from experience with these ectoparasites, is that the conservation of resources should be a guiding principle in dealing with pesticide resistance. There are often as many problems to be faced in leaping ahead to a new chemical class as there are in attempting to utilize what is available within a current group when a new resistance problem emerges.

REFERENCES

Anonymous, 1973, *Proceedings of the International Symposium on the Control of Body Lice and Louse-borne Diseases, Washington, D.C., December 4–6, 1972*, Pan American Health Organization Scientific Publication No. 263.

Amaral, N. K., Noumany, L. G. S., and Carvalho, L. A. D., 1974, Acaricide AC 84,633: First trials for control of *Boophilus microplus*, *J. Econ. Entomol.* 67:387–389.

Ardalan, A., 1977, Preliminary survey on susceptibility of *Pediculus humanus corporis* to insecticides in Teheran Iran, *Bull. Soc. Pathol. Exot.* 69:538–540.

Baker, J. A. F., 1978, Resistance to ixodicides by ticks in Africa south of the Equator with some thoughts on tick control in this area, in: *Tick-borne Diseases and Their Vectors* (J. K. H. Wilde, ed.), pp. 101–109. University of Edinburgh Centre for Tropical Veterinary Medicine, Edinburgh.

Blackman, G. G., and Baker, J. A. F., 1975, Resistance of the sheep blowfly *Lucilia cuprina* to insecticides in the Republic of South Africa, *J. S. Afr. Vet. Assoc.* 46:337–339.

Bhatia, S. C., and Deshpande, L. B., 1975, A note on malathion resistance in bed bug (*Cimex hemipterus*) in Jahwar area of Palghar Unit of Thana District, Mahasashtra State, India, *J. Commun. Dis.* 7:72–73.

Brooks, G. T., 1976, Penetration and distribution, in: *Insecticide Biochemistry and Physiology* (C. F. Wilkinson, ed.), pp. 3–58, Plenum Press, New York.

Brown, A. W. A., and Pal, R., 1971, *Insecticide Resistance in Arthropods*, WHO Mongraph Series No. 38, World Health Organization, Geneva.

Brun, L. O., Wilson, J. T., and Daynes, P., 1983, Ethion resistance in the cattle tick (*Boophilus microplus*) in New Caledonia, *Trop. Pest Mgmt.* 29(1):16–22.

Busvine, J. R., 1951, Mechanism of resistance to insecticide in houseflies, *Nature (Lond.)* 168:193–195.

Busvine, J. R., and Shanahan, G. J., 1961, The resistance spectrum of a dieldrin resistant strain of the sheep blow-fly (*Lucilia cuprina*) (Wied), *Entomol. Exp. Appl.* 4:1–6.

Busvine, J. R., Bell, J. D., and Guneidy, A. M., 1963, Toxicology and genetics of two types of insecticide resistance in *Chrysomyia putoria* (Wied.), *Bull. Entomol. Res.* 54:589–600.

Drummond, R. O., 1977, Resistance in ticks and insects of veterinary importance, in: *Pesticide Management and Insecticide Resistance* (D. L. Watson and A. W. A. Brown, eds.), pp. 303–319, Academic Press, New York.

DuToit, R., Graf, H., and Bekker, P. M., 1941, Resistance to arsenic as displayed by the single host blue tick *Boophilus microplus* (Koch) in a localised area of the Union of South Africa, *J. S. Afr. Vet. Med. Assoc.* 12:50–58.

Feroz, M., 1974, The effect of additives on the toxicity of malathion and fenchlorphos to a susceptible and an organophosphorus resistant strain of the bed bug *Cimex lectularius* L., *Biol. (Lahore)* 20:103–110.

Fox, I., Rivera, G. A., and Bayona, I. G., 1968, Toxicity of six insecticides to the cat flea, *J. Econ. Entomol.* 61:869–870.

Harrison, I. R., 1967, The development of organophosphorus insecticide resistance in Australian sheep blowfly *Lucilia cuprina* (Wied.), *Vet. Rec.* 80:205–206.

Hughes, P. B., 1981, Spectrum of cross resistance to insecticides in field samples of the primary sheep blow-fly *Lucilia cuprina*, *Int. J. Parasitol.* 11:475–479.

Hughes, P. B., and Devonshire, A. L., 1982, The biochemical basis of resistance to organophosphorus insecticides in the sheep blowfly, *Lucilia cuprina*, *Pest. Biochem. Physiol.* 18:289–297.

Knowles, C. O., and Roulston, W. J., 1972, Antagonism of chlorphenamidine toxicity to the cattle tick *Boophilus microplus* by piperonyl butoxide, *J. Aust. Entomol. Soc.* 11:349–350.

Lee, R. M., and Batham, P., 1966, The activity and organophosphate inhibition of cholinesterases from susceptible and resistant ticks (Acari), *Entomol. Exp. Appl.* 9:13–24.

Legg, J. Brooks, O. M., and Joyner, C. N., 1955, A note on the appearance of a DDT-resistant cattle tick *Boophilus microplus* (Canes.) in Queensland, *Aust. Vet. J.* 31:148.

Lourens, J. H. M., and Lyaruu, D. M., 1979, Susceptibility of some East African strains of *Rhipicephalus appendiculatus* to cholinesterase inhibiting acaricides, *Pest. Artic. News Summ.* 25:135–142.

Matthewson, M. D., Wilson, R. G., and Hammant, C. A., 1971, The development of resistance to certain organophosphorus and carbamate ixodicides by the blue tick, *Boophilus decoloratus* (Koch) (Acarina, Ixodidae), in Rhodesia, *Bull. Entomol. Res.* 66:553–560.

Maunder, J. W., 1981, Clinical and laboratory trials employing carbaryl against the human head-louse *Pediculus humanus capitis* (de Geer), *Clin. Exp. Dermatol.* 6:605–612.

Milani, R., and Travaglino, A., 1957, Ricerche genetiche sulla resistenza al DDT in *Musca domestica* concatenazione del gene kdr (knockdown-resistance) con due mutanti morfologigi, *Riv. Parassitol.* 18:199–202.

Nolan, J., and Bird, P. E., 1977, Co-toxicity of synthetic pyrethroids and organophosphorus compounds against the cattle tick (*Boophilus microplus*), *J. Aust. Entomol. Soc.* 16:252.

Nolan, J., and Roulston, W. J., 1979, Acaricide resistance as a factor in the management of acari of medical and veterinary importance, in: *Recent Advances in Acarology* (J. G. Rodriguez, ed.), Vol. 2, pp. 3–13, Academic Press, New York.

Nolan, J., and Schnitzerling, H. J., 1975, Characterization of acetylcholinesterases of acaricide-resistant and susceptible strains of the cattle tick *Boophilus microplus* (Can.). 1. Extraction of the critical component and comparison with enzyme from other sources, *Pest. Biochem. Physiol.* 5:178–188.

Nolan, J., Schnitzerling, H. J., and Schuntner, C. A., 1972, Multiple forms of acetylcholinesterase from resistant and susceptible strains of the cattle tick, *Boophilus microplus* (Can.), *Pest. Biochem. Physiol.* 2:85–94.

Nolan, J., Roulston, W. J., and Schnitzerling, H. J., 1979, The potential of some synthetic pyrethroids for control of the cattle tick (*Boophilus microplus*), *Aust. Vet. J.* 55:463–466.

Norris, K. R., and Stone, B. F., 1956, Toxaphene-resistant cattle ticks (*Boophilus microplus* (Canestrini)) occurring in Queensland, *Aust. J. Agric. Res.* 7:211–226.

Perry, A. S., and Hoskins, W. M., 1950, The detoxification of DDT by resistant house flies and inhibition of this process by piperonyl cyclonene, *Science* 111:600–601.

Reich, C. I., Grillo Torrado, J. M., Peréz Arrieta, A., and Zorzópulos, J., 1978, *Boophilus microplus:* Strain differences in the cholinesterase system, *Exp. Parasitol.* 44:50–55.

Roulston, W. J., and Nolan, J., 1975, Resistance in *Boophilus microplus* to cholinesterase inhibition and alteration in the site of action, *Environ. Qual. Saf. (Suppl.)* 3:416–420.

Roulston, W. J., and Schnitzerling, H. J., 1965, Relation of the formulation of cattle sprays to the deposition and loss of DDT, *J. Sci. Food Agric.* 16:179–185.

Roulston, W. J., Norris, K. R., Schnitzerling, H. J., and Meyers, R. A. J., 1958, Comparison of two formulations of DDT as dipping fluids for the control of the cattle tick, *Aust. J. Agric. Res.* 9:587–598.

Roulston, W. J., Schuntner, C. A., Schnitzerling, H. J., and Wilson, J. T., 1969, Detoxification as a mechanism of resistance in a strain of the cattle tick *Boophilus microplus* (Canestrini) resistant to organophosphorus and carbamate compounds, *Aust. J. Biol. Sci.* 22:1585–1589.

Roulston, W. J., Wharton, R.H., Schnitzerling, H. J., Sutherst, R. W., and Sullivan, N. D., 1971, Mixtures of chlorphenamidine with other acaricides for the control of organophosphorus-resistant strains of cattle tick *Boophilus microplus, Aust. Vet. J.* 47:521–528.

Roulston, W. J., Wharton, R. H., Nolan, J., Kerr, J. D., Wilson, J. T., Thompson, P. G., and Schotz, M., 1981, A survey for resistance in cattle ticks to acaricides, *Aust. Vet. J.* 57:362–371.

Schnitzerling, H. J., and Stone, B. F., 1968, Loss of toxicity to cattle ticks of a wettable powder formulation of coumaphos, *Aust. Vet. J.* 44:7–10.

Schnitzerling, H.J., Roulston, W. J., and Schuntner, C. A., 1970, The absorption and metabolism of [^{14}C] DDT in DDT-resistant and susceptible strains of the cattle tick *Boophilus microplus, Aust. J. Biol. Sci.* 23:219–230.

Schnitzerling, H. J., Nolan, J., and Davey, P. A., 1982, A comparative study of the reactivity of acetylcholinesterases of the cattle tick *Boophilus microplus* and cattle erythrocytes with organophosphorus and carbamate inhibitors, *Pest. Biochem. Physiol.* 18:216–225.

Schnitzerling, H. J., Noble, P. J., Macqueen, A., and Dunham, R. J., 1982, Resistance of the buffalo fly, *Haematobia irritans exigua* (De Meijere), to two synthetic pyrethroids and DDT, *J. Aust. Entomol. Soc.* 21:77–80.

Schnitzerling, H. J., Nolan, J., and Hughes, S., 1983, Toxicology and metabolism of some synthetic pyrethroids in larvae of susceptible and resistant strains of the cattle tick *Boophilus microplus* (Can.), *Pest. Sci.* 14:64–72.

Schuntner, C. A., Roulston, W. J., and Wharton, R. H., 1974, Toxicity of piperonyl butoxide to *Boophilus microplus, Nature (Lond)* 249:386.

Shalaby, A. M., 1971, Susceptibility status of the rat flea *Xenopsylla cheopis* Roths. (Pulicidae) to DDT, gamma BHC and dieldrin in Libya, *Z. Angew. Entomol.* 69:64–71.

Shanahan, G. J., and Hart, R. J., 1966, Change in response of *Lucilia cuprina* Wied. to organophosphorus insecticides in Australia, *Nature (Lond.)* 212:1466–1467.

Shanahan, G. J., and Roxburgh, N. A., 1974, The sequential development of insecticide resistance problems in *Lucilia cuprina* Wied in Australia, *Pest. Artic. News. Summ.* 20:190–202.

Shaw, R. D., and Malcolm, H. A., 1964, Resistance of *Boophilus microplus* to organophosphorus insecticides, *Vet. Rec.* 7:210–211.

Shaw, R. D., Thompson, G. E., and Baker, J. A. F., 1967, Resistance to cholinesterase inhibitors in the blue tick *Boophilus decoloratus* in South Africa, *Vet. Rec.* 81:548–549.

Shetty, K. M., Subbiah, K. V., Panickar, K. K., 1975, A comparative evaluation fenitrothion Dursban and malathion for the control of bed bugs, *Indian J. Publ. Health* 19:79–83.

Smissaert, H. R., 1964, Cholinesterase inhibition in spider mites susceptible and resistant to organophosphate, *Science* 143:129–131.

Soliman, S. A., and Soliamn, A. A., 1966, Susceptibility levels of the body louse *Pediculus humanus corporis* DeGeer, to DDT and BHC, *Bull. Soc. Entomol. Egypte* 1:43–46.

Solomon, K. R., 1983, Acaricide resistance in ticks, *Adv. Vet. Sci. Comp. Med.* 27:273–296.

Stone, B. F., 1957, Resistance to DDT in the cattle tick *Boophilus microplus* (Canestrini), *Aust. J. Agric. Res.* 8 424–431.

Stone, B. F., and Meyers, R. A. J., 1957, Dieldrin-resistant cattle ticks, *Boophilus microplus* (Canestrini), in Queensland, *Aust. J. Agric. Res.* 8:312–317.

Treeby, P., 1974, OP tolerant *cuprina*, *Vet. Rec.* 94:505.

Wharton, R. H., 1976, Tick-borne livestock diseases and their vectors. 5. Acaricide resistance and alternative methods of tick control, *World Anim. Rev.* 20:8–15.

Whitehead, G. B., 1956, DDT-resistance in the blue tick *Boophilus decoloratus*, Koch, *J. S. Afr. Vet. Med. Assoc.* 27:117–120.

Whitehead, G. B., 1959, Pyrethrum resistance conferred by resistance to DDT in the blue tick, *Nature (Lond.)* 184:378–379.

Whitehead, G. B., 1961, Investigation of the mechanism of resistance to sodium arsenite in the blue tick *Boophilus decoloratus* Koch., *J. Insect. Physiol.* 7:177–185.

Whitehead, G. B., 1965, Resistance in the Acarina: Ticks, *Adv. Acarol.* 2:53–70.

Winteringham, F. P. W., 1969, Mechanisms of selective insecticidal action, *Annu. Rev. Entomol.* 14:409–442.

Appendix

Generic (non-proprietary) and proprietary (trade) names of antiparasitic drugs. Where a drug is sold in numerous forms, especially in the case of over-the-counter products, no attempt has been made to list all of the trade names. Inclusion of a name does not imply endorsement or current availability of a product or legitimacy of the name. Omission of a name does not imply the converse. For the most part, spelling variants of a given name are not listed.

PART I: ANTIPROTOZOAL AGENTS

Generic names	Proprietary names
acedapsone	Hansolar, Rodilone
acranil	
acriflavine·HCl	Panflavin
aklomide	*In:* Aklomix, Novastat
amicarbalide, diisethionate	Diampron
amodiaquine HCl	Basoquin, Camoquin HCl, Flavoquine, Miaquin
amphotercin·B	Ampho-Moronal, Amphozone, Fungillin, Fungizone
amprolium	Amprol, Amprovine, Corid
	In: Amprol Plus, Amprol Hi-E, Amprolmix, Pancoxin, Supacox
amquinate	
antimony potassium tartrate	
antimony sodium gluconate	Myostibin, Pentostam, Stibanate, Stibanose, Stibatin, Stibinol, Solustibosan, Solyusurmin, Triostam, T.S.A.G.
arprinocid	Arpocox
arsanilic acid	Arsonic Powder, Pro-Gen
arsthinol	Balarsen, Mercaptoarsenol
azanidazole	Triclose
bamnidazole	
berythromycin	Erythromycin B
bialamicol·HCl	Camoform·HCl
buquinolate	*In:* Bonaid
butynorate	Davainex, Tinostat, Wormal Granules

(*continued*)

Generic names	Proprietary names
carbarsone	Amabevan, Ameban, Amebarsone, Amibiarson, Aminarsone, Arsambide, Carb-O-Gain, Carb-O-Sep, Fenarsone, Histocarb, Leucarsone
carnidazole	Spartrix
chlorguanide	Diguanyl, Drinupal, Guanatol, Paludrin, Palusil, Proguanil, Tirian
chloroquine	Aralen HCl, Arechin, Artrichin, Avloclor, Bemaphate, Bipiquin, Imagon, Malaquin, Nivaquine B, Resochin, Resoquine, Reumachlor, Sanoquin, Silbesan, Tresochin _In:_ Daraclor
chlorphenoxamide	Mebinol
chlorproguanil	Lapudrine
chlortetracycline	Acronize, Aureociclina, Aureocina, Aureomycin, Biomycin, Bitomitsin, Chryomykine, CTC Soluble, Isphamycin
clamoxyguin HCl	Clamoxyl
clindamycin	Cleocin, Dalacin C, Dalactine, Sobelin
clopidol	Coyden
clotrimazole	Canesten, Empecid, Gyne-Lotrimin, Mycelax, Mycosporin, Trimysten
cycloguanil pamoate	Camolar
cyproquinate	Coxytrol
dapsone	Avlosulfon, Avlosulphone, Croysulfone, Croysulphone, Diphenasone, Diphone, Disulone, Dumitone, Eporal, Novophone, Sulfona-Mae, Sulphadione, Udolac, _In:_ Maloprim
decoquinate	Deccox
dehydroemetine	Mebadin
diloxanide	Ame-Boots, Entamide, Furamide
dimetridazole	Dimetryl, Emtryl, Emtrylvet, Unizole
diminazene aceturate	Azidin, Babesin, Berenil, Ganasag
dinitolmide	Salcostat, Zoalene, Zoamix
dinsed	
doxycycline·HCl	Doxigalumicina, Doxitard, Doxy-II, Doxy-Tablinen, Ecodex, Hydramycin, Liomycin, Liviatin, Mesafin, Midoxin, Nivocilin, Novadox, Retens, Roximycin, Samecin, Tanamicin, Tecacin, Tetradox, Vibradox, Vibramycin, Vibra-Tabs, Vibravenos
emetine·HCl	Arsemtine, Canforemetina, Emetoplix
ethopabate	_In:_ Amprol Hi-E, Amprol Plus, Pancoxin, Supacox
ethyl stibamine	Astral, Neostibosan, Stibosamine
flubendazole	Flumoxal, Flumoxane
flunidazole	
fumagillin	Amebacilin, Fugillin, Fumadil B, Fumidil
furazolidone	Furox-100, Furoxane, Furoxone, Furovag, Giardil, Giarlam, Medarone, Neftin, Nicolen, Nifulidone, Ortazol, Roptazol, Tikofuran, Topazone, Unidone
gloxasone	Contrapar
glycobiarsol	Broxolin, Dysentulin, Milibis, Viasept, Wintodon
halofunginone·HBR	Stenorol
homidium	Babidium, Dromilac, Novidium·Cl
hydroxychloroquine·SO_4	Ercoquin, Plaquenil·SO_4, Quensyl

Generic names	Proprietary names
hydroxystilbamidine isethionate	
imidocarb dipropionate	Imizad Equine Injection
iodochlorohydroxyquin	Alchloquin, Amebil, Amoenol, Bactol, Barquinol, Budoform, Chinoform, Clioquinol, Eczecidin, Entero-quinol, Entero-Septol, Entero-Vioform, Enterozol, En-trokin, Hi-Enterol, Iodoenterol, Nioform, Quinambicide, Rometin, Vioform
iodoquinol	Dinoleine, Diodoquin, Diodoxylin, Di-Quinol, Direxiode, Disoquin, Dyodin, Embequin, Enterosept, Floraquin, Io-quin, Moebiquin, Quinadome, Rafamebin, Searlequin, Stanquinate, Yodoxin, Zoaquin
ipronidazole·HCl	Ipropran
isometamidium·HCl	Samorin, Trypamidium
lasalocid·Na	Avatec, Bovatec
levofuraltadone	Altabactina, Altafar, Furazolin, Ibifur, Medifuran, Nitral-done, Otifuril, Sepsinol, Ultrafur, Unifur, Valsyn
maduramicin	Cygro, Prinocin
mefloquine	Larian, Laricur
meglumine	*See* N-Methylglucamine antimonate
melarsoprol	Arsobal, Mel B
menoctone	Menocton
mepacrine	*See* quinacrine·HCl
N-methylglucamine antimonate	Glucantime, Protostib
metronidazole	Arilin, Clont, Cont, Danizol, Deflamon, Flagyl, Fossyol, Gineflavir, Klion, Orvagil, Sanatrichom, Trichazol, Tri-chocide, Tricho Cordes, Tricho-Gynaedron, Tricocet, Trivazol, Vagilen, Vagimid
miconazole	Albistat, Andergin, Brentan, Conofite, Daktar, Daktarin, Deralbine, Dermonistat, Epi-Monistat, Florid, Gyno-Daktarin, Gyno-Monistat, Micatin, Monistat, Vodol
mirincamycin·HCl	
misonidazole	Radelar, Riadelar, Riasch
monensin	Coban, Elancoban, Romensin, Rumensin
	In: Sweetlix with Rumensin
moxnidazole	
narasin	Monteban
nequinate	Statyl
nicarbazin	Nicarb, Nicoxin, Nicrazin
nifuratel	Inimur, Macmiror, Magmilor, Omnes, Polmiror, Tydantil
nifuroxime	Micofur
nifursemizone	Etafurazone
nifursol	Histomon, Salfuride
nifurtimox	Lampit
nimorazole	Acterol, Esclama, Naxofen, Naxogin, Nulogyl, Sirledi, Radanil, Rochagan
niridazole	Ambilhar
nitarsone	
nitrimidazine	
nitrofurazone	Aldomycin, Amifur, Chemofuran, Coxistat, Furacin, Furacinetten, Furacoccid, Furaplast, Furazol W, Furesol, Mammex, Nefco, Nifuzon, Nitrofural, Nitrozone, Vabrocid

(continued)

Generic names	Proprietary names
nitromide	*In:* Tristat, Unistat, Unistat-3
ormetoprim	*In:* Rofenaid-40
oxyquinoline	
oxytetracycline	Abbocin, Arcospectron, Aquacycline, Berkmycen, Bio-Mycin, Biostat, Clinimycin, Duphacycline, Geomycin, Gynamousse, Imperacin, Liquamycin, Macocyn, Macodyn, Occrycetin, Oxacycline, Oxatets, Oxlopar, Oxybiocycline, Oxybiotic, Oxycycline, Oxydon, Oxy-Dumocyclin, Oxyject, Oxymycin, Oxypan, Oxytetracid, Ryomcin, Stecsolin, Stevacin, Terraject, Terramycin, Tetramel, Tetran, Tetra-Tablinen, Toxinal, Vendarcin, Vendracin
pamaquine	Aminoquin, Beprochine, Gamefar, Plasmochin, Plasmoquine, Praequine, Quipenyl
paromomycin·SO_4	1600 Antibiotic, Farmiglucin, Farminosidin, Gabbromicina, Gabbromycin, Gabbroral, Humatin, Pargonyl, Paramicina, Paricina, Tricardil
partricin	Mepartricin, Tricandil
pentamidine isoethionate	Lomidine
phenamidine	
polymixin B	Aerosporin
	In: Thiosporin
primaquine·PO_4	
puromycin	Stylomycin
	Note: Pre-1953 was Achromycin, now Achromycin is assigned to Tetracycline·HCl.
pyrimethamine	Chloridin, Darapram, Daraprim, Malocide, Tindurin, Whitsan
	In: Fansidar, Daraclor, Maloprim, Supacox
pyrithidium·Br	Prothidium
quinacrine·HCl	Acrichine, Acriquine, Atabrine·diHCl, Atebrin·HCl, Chinacrin·HCl, Erion, Italchin, Metoquine, Palacrin
quinapyramine	Antrycide
quinfamide	
quinine	Aristochin, Aristoquin, Aristoquinine, Bi-Quinate, Coco-Quinine, Dentojel, Diquinine carbonate, Quinamin, Quinamm, Quinate, Quinbisan, Quine, Quinoform, Quinsan, Quiphile, Tasteless Quinine
quinuronium·SO_4	Acaprin, Akiron, Atral, Babesan, Baburan, Ludobal, Pirevan, Piroplasmin, Zothelone
rifampin	Rifa, Rifadin, Rifadine, Rifaldin, Rifaprodin, Rifobac, Riforal, Rifoldine, Rimactan
robenidine·HCl	Cycostat, Robenz
rolitetracycline	Bristacin, Reverin, Superciclin, Syntetrex, Syntetrin, Synotodecin, Tetraverin, Transcycline, Velacicline, Velacycline
ronidazole	Dugro, MCMN, Ridzol
roxarsone	Korum, Ren-O-Sal, Ristat, Ruco, Russell's Lift Tabs, Tunum, Zuco
	In: Unistat-3
salinomycin	Coxistac, Sacox

Generic names	Proprietary names
sinefungin	
spiramycin	Calactin vet, Foromacidin, Provamycin, Rovamicina, Rovamycin, Selectomycin, Sequamycin, Suanovil, Suanozil
stibamine glucoside	Neostam
stibophen	Corystibin, Fantorin, Fouadin, Fuadin, Heyden 611, Neo-antimosan, Pyrostib, Repodral, Sodium Antimosan, Trimon
stilbamidine isethionate	
sulfabenz	
sulfachloropyrazine·Na	Cosulfa, Cosulid, Nefrosul, Prinzone, Sorilyn, Vetisulid
sulfadiazine	Adiazine, Debenal, Diazyl, Eskaiazine, Flamazine, Flammazine, Pyrimal, Silvadene, Sterazine, Sulfolex, Ultradiazin
	In: Coptin, Triglobe
sulfadimethoxine	Agribon, Albon, Ancosul, Bactrovet, Diasulfa, Diasulfyl, Dimetazina, Dinosol, Madribon, Maxulvet, Memcozine, Metoxidon, Neostreptal, Radonia, Roscosulf, SDM, Sudine, Suldixine, Sulfasol, Sulxin, Symbio, Theracanzan
	In: Rofenaid 40
sulfadimidine	Unidim
sulfadoxine	Fanasil, Fanzil
	In: Fansidar
sulfaguanidine	Abiguanil, Aterian, Diacta, Ganidan, Guamide, Guanicil, Resulfon, Ruocid, Shigatox, Suganyl, Sulfaguine, Sulfoguenil
sulfalene	Farmitalia, Dalysep, Kelfizina, Longum, Polycidal
sulfamethazine	Azolmetazin, Diazil, Dimezathine, Dimidin-R, Mefenal, Neazina, Pirmazin, S-Dimidine, S-Mez, Sulfadine, Vesadin, Vertolan
sulfamethoxazole	*In:* Abacin, Apo-Sulfatrim, Bactramin, Bactrim, Bactromin, Baktar, Drylin, Eltrianyl, Eusaprim, Fectrim, Gantanol, Gantaprim, Gantrim, Kepinol, Linaris, Microtrim, Momentol, Nopil, Omsat, Septra, Septrim, Sigaprim, Sinomin, Sulfotrim, Sulfotrimin, Sulprim, Sumetrolim, Suprim, Tacumil, Teleprim, TMS 480, Trigonyl, Trimesulf, Trimforte, Uro-Septra
sulfamethoxypyridazine	Davosin, Depovernil, Durox, Kynex, Lederkyn, Lentac, Midicel, Midikel, Myasul, Mylo-Sulfdurazin, Sultirene, Vinces
sulfanitran	*In:* Novastat, Polystat, Unistat
sulfaquinoxaline	Aviochina, Embazin, Dr. Hess SQX, Quinatrol, Quinel, Solquin, Sol-Quinel, S.Q., Sulfa-Nox, Sulfa-Q, Sul-Q-Nox, Vineland Liquid Sulfaquinoxaline
	In: Pancoxin, Supacoxin
sulfisoxazole	Entusil, Entusil, Gantrisin, Gantrosan, Neazolin, Renosulfan, Sosol, Soxisol, Soxo, Soxomide, Suladrin, Sulfalar, Sulfazin, Sulfium, Sulfoxol, Sulsoxin, V-Sul
sulnidazole	
suramin	Antrypol, Germanin, Moranyl, Nagarol, Naganin, Naphuride·Na

(continued)

Generic names	Proprietary names
symetine·HCl	Symetinum
tebuquine	
teclozan	Falmanox
tetracycline	Abricycline, Achro, Achromysin, Agromicina, Ala Tet, Ambracyn, Ambramicina, Ambramycin, Artomycin, Bio-Tetra, Bristaciclina, Cefracycline, Criseociclina, Cyclomycin, Cyclopar, Democracin, Diacycline, Dumocyclin, Hostacyclin, Lauracycline, Mephacyclin, Omegamycin, Panmycin, Partrex, Polycycline, Purocyclina, Quadracycline, Quartex, Remicyclin, Ricycline, Ro-cycline, Sanclomycine, Steclin, Stilciclina, Subamycin, Sumycin, Supramycin, Sustamycin, Tefilin, Teline, Telotrex, Tetrabakat, Tetrabid, Tetrablet, Tetrachel, Tetracompren, Tetracyn, Tetra-D, Tetradecin, Tetrakap, Tetralution, Tetramavan, Tetramycin, Tetra-Wedel, Tetrex, Tetrosol, Topicycline, Totomycin, Triphacyclin, Unicin, Unimycin, Upcyclin, Vetquamycin-324
tiazuril	
tinidazole	Fasigin, Fasigyn, Pletil, Simplotan, Sorquetan, Tricolam
trimethoprim	Monotrim, Proloprim, Syraprim, Tiempe, Trimanyl, Trimopan, Trimpex, Wellcoprim
	In: Abacin, Apo-Sulfatrim, Bacatramin, Bactrim, Bactromin, Baktar, Co-Fram, Coptin, Drylin, Eltrianyl, Eusaprim, Fectrim, Gantaprim, Gantrim, Kepinol, Lidaprim, Linaris, Microtrim, Momentol, Nevin, Nopil, Omsat, Septra, Septrim, Sigaprim, Sulfotrim, Sulfotrimin, Sulprim, Sumetrolim, Suprim, Supristol, Tacumil, Teleprim, TMS-480, Triglobe, Trigonyl, Trimesulf, Trimforte, Uro-Septra
trypan blue	Benzamine Blue, Benzo Blue, Congo Blue, Diamine Blue, Dianil Blue, Naphthylamine Blue, Niagara Blue
tryparsamide	Glyphenarsine, Tryparsone, Tryponarsyl, Trypothane
urea stibamine	Carbantine, Carbostimamide, Carbostibamine, Stiburea

PART II: ANTHELMINTICS (AGENTS ACTIVE AGAINST NEMATODES, TREMATODES, CESTODES)

Generic names	Proprietary names
abamectin	Avomec
acetarsol	Spirillizine, Spirocid, Stovarsol
	In: Osarcide
acetarsone, *see* acetarsol	
albendazole	Albazine, Valbazen, Zentel
amphotalide	Schistomide
amphotericin B	Fungizone
antimony dimercaptosuccinate	Astiban, TWSb
arecoline derivatives	Anthelin, Areco-Caine, Cestarsol, Hydarex, Nemural, Nemurol, Neumural, Tenoban

Generic names	Proprietary names
arsenamide, *see* thiacetarsamide	
ascaridole, *see* chenopodium	
aspidin, *see* male fern	
aspidium, oleoresin (aspidin, de-saspidin, filicin, filmaron)	Distol, Filmaron, Rosapin
bephenium	Alcopar, Frantin
bithionol	Actamer, Bitin, Lorothidol
bithionol sulfoxide	Bitin-S, Disto-5
bitoscanate	Jonit
bromonaphtol	Disthelmin, Wormin
bromophenophos	Acedist
bromsalans	Diaphene, Fascol, Hilomid, Mitenyl, Trinoin
brotianide	Dirian
	In: Flukombin, Vermadax
bunamidine	Buban, Scolaban
butamisole	Styquin
butynorate, *see* dibutyl tin dilaurate	
cambendazole	Ascapilla, Bonlam, Camvet, Equiben, Equicam, Novazole, Noviben, Porcam
cantrodifene, *see* nitroscanate	
caparsolate, *see* thiacetarsamide	
carbon disulfide	*In:* Thiprazole
carbon tetrachloride	Avipar, Benzinoform, Didakol, Fasciol, Flukoids, Necatorina
	In: Distocain, Fasciolin
chenopodium oil	Ascaridol, Nematol
clioxanide	Tremerad
clorsulon	Curatrem
closantel	Flukiver, Seponver
coumaphos	Asuntol, Baymix, Co-Ral, Meldane, Muskatox
cyacetazide	Armazal, Benecid, Cyanazid, Dictycide, Dictyfuge
cyanacethydrazide, *see* cyacetazide	
diamfenetide	Coriban
dibutyl tin dilaurate	Davainex
dichlorophene	Antiphen, Dicestal, Didroxane, Diphenthane-70, Parabis, Teniathane, Teniatol
	In: Dichlosal, Difolin, Paracide, Teniazine, Vermiplex
dichlorvos	Atgard, Dichlorman, DDVP, Equigard, Equigel, Task, Tenac
diethylcarbamazine	Banocide, Caricide, Carbam, Caritol, Cypip, Decanine, Dicacid, Dicarocide, Difil, Digacid, Dirocide, Diro-form, Ethodryl, Filaribits, Filariosan, Franocide, Hetrazan, Loxwran, Luwucit, Nemacide, Neo Paulvermin, Notezine, Pet-Dec, Pulmocid, Supatonin, Unicarbazan
	In: Anthelworm L, Banmith D, Control Diet HRH, Styrid Caricide
dimethylstyrylquinolinium	Styguin
disophenol	Ancylol, DNP, Iodophene, Syngamix
dithiazanine	Abminthic, Delvex, Deselmine, Dilombrin, Dizan, Telmid
ditrazine, *see* diethylcarbamazine	
diuredosan, *see* uredofos	

(continued)

Generic names	Proprietary names
divezid, *see* diethylcarbamazine	
drocarbil, *see* arecoline	
dymanthine	Thelmesan
febantel	Amatron, Bayverm, Provet, Rintal
	In: Combotel
fenbendazole	Panacur, Safe-Guard
fenchlorphos	Dermaphos, Ectoral, Ronnel, Trolene
fenthion	Lysoff, Mercaptophos, Talodex, Tiguvon, Spotton, Pro-spot
flubendazole	Flubenol, Flumoxal, Fluvermal
gentian violet	Aksuris, Oxiuran, Viocid
glycobiarsol	Milibis, Viasept, Wintodon
haloxon	Eustidil, Halox, Loxon
	In: Haloxil
hetolin	Dicodren, Hetolin
hexachloroethane	Avlothane, Distomatol, Egitol
hexachloroparaxylene	Bitriben, Hetol
hexachlorophene	Bilevon, Coopaphene, Distocid, Distodin, Fasciophene, Fascol Super
	In: Bisophene, Hepadist, Hexaphen
hexylresorcinol	Ascaricid, Caprokol, Crystoids, Gelovermin
	In: Contrahelmin
hycanthone	Etrenol, Hycanthone
hygromycin	Hygramix, Phylascar
ivermectin	Cardomec, Eqvalan, Heartquard 30, Ivomec, Oramec, Zymectrin
kainic acid	Digenin, Helminal
	In: Camin, Seetonin
levamisole	Anthelpor, Aviverm, Bionem, Cevasol, Citarin-L, Cyverm, Dilarvon, Duphamisole, Ketrax, Levadin, Levipor, Levacide, Levasole, Narpenol 5, Nemacide, Nilvern, Ripercol L, Solaskil
	In: Ambex, Nilvax, Nilzan, Spectril
lucanthone	Miracil, Nilodin, Tixanthone
mebendazole	Equivurm, Fugacar, Mebenvet, Mebutar, Multispec, Nemasole, Ovitelmin, Pantelmin, Parmeben, Rumatel, Sirben, Telmin, Telmintic, Vermirax, Vermox
	In: Trivexan, Telmin B
melarsonyl potassium	Mel W, Trimelarsen
methylbenzene, *see* toluene	
methyridine	Dekelmin, Mintic, Promintic
metrifonate, *see* trichlorphon	
morantel	Banminth II, Ibantic, Paratec, Rumatel
	In: Banminth D, Equiban
naphthalophos	Amdax, Maretin
niclofolan	Bilevon, Dertil, Distolon, Menichlopholan
niclosamide	Cestocid, Devermin, Fenasal, Lintex, Mansonil, Radeverm, Sagimid, Tredemine, Vermitin, Yomesan
	In: Ambex
niridazole	Ambilhar, Bulgarstan
nitroclofene, *see* nitroclofenum	

Generic names	Proprietary names
nitroclofenum	Distoject
nitrodan	Nidanthel
nitroscanate	Canverm, Lopatol
nitroxynil	Fasciolid, Dovenix, Trodax
oxamniquin	Mansil, Vansil
oxantel pamoate	*In:* Quantrel
oxfendazole	Benzelmin, Synanthic, Systamex
oxibendazole	Anthelcide, Anthelworm, Equipar, Equitac, Loditac, Verzine, Widespec
	In: Anthelworm L, Nemtrem, New Duospec
oxyclozanide	Diplin, Metiljin, Zanil
	In: Duospec, Haloxil, Nemtrem, Nilzan, Spectril
parathion	Thiophos
parbendazole	Helmatac, Topclip, Triban, Verminum, Worm Guard
paromomycin	Humatin
phenasal, *see* niclosamide	
phenothiazine	Contraverm, Coopazine, Fenopur, Helmetina, Neoavilep, Phenovis, Phenoxur, Radiol
	In: Bisophene, Coopex, Dyrex T.F., Helmox, Hexaphen, Parvex Plus
phenzidole	Gainex
phthalofyne	Whipcide
picadex, *see* piperazine	
piperazine adipate	Antivermin, Ascatrix, Askarat, Coopane, Entacyl, Equinol, Helmirazin, Mapiprin, Nematocton, Pipadox, Piperaskat, Piperfesa, Pipero-vet, Piperwin, Pipradin
	In: Helmifen, Tenarids
piperazine carbodithioic acid	Choisine, Parvex, Polyver, Safersan
	In: Parvex Plus
piperazine citrate	Antelmin, Antiren, Antoban, Bioscaridina, Byrel, Moncasan, Multifuge, Parazine, Pipcide, Piperasol, Pipizan, Piprelix, Pipricide, Radiol, Safersol, Verocid
	In: Paulvermin Plus
piperazine, various	Antepar, Bexin, Candizine, Digenin, Eraverm, Helmezine, Nematorazine, Noveril, Novivermol, Ovilon, Oxyzin, Paravermin, Piavetrin, Pilanin, Pipa-Tabs, Piperaverm, Piperazate, Pip-pop, Pripsen, Tasnon, Upixon, Verban, Vermicompren, Wiperazine
	In: Alvetuna, Ancaris, Avisan, Camin, Certuna, Dyrex T.F., Eludon, Equizole, Nebusin, Swiverm, Thenatol, Vanpar, Vericid
praziquantel	Biltricide, Cesol, Droncit
pyrantel pamoate	Antiminth, Cobantril, Combantrin, Felex, Helmex, Imathal, Nemex, Piranver, Pyraminth, Strongid T
	In: Trivexan
pyrantel tartrate	Banminth, Exhelm, Nemex, Pyreguan, Strongid
pyrvinium pamoate	Alnoxin, Molevac, Neo-Oxypaat, Pamovin, Parvanol, Poquil, Povan, Povanyl, Pyr-Con, Pyr-Pam, Vanguil, Vanguin, Vermigal, Vermitiber
	In: Ciamin, Quantrel, Tricocefal, Vanpar

(continued)

Generic names	Proprietary names
rafoxanide	Flukanide, Ranide
	In: New Duospec, Ranizole
resorantel	Resorcylam, Terenol
santonin	Santosol, Semenen
stibophen	Corystibin, Fantorin, Fuadin, Pyrostib, Repodral
stilbazium iodide	Monopar
styrylpyridinium	Styrid
	In: Control Diet HRH, Styrid Caricide
suramin	Antrypol, Germanin, Moranyl, Naganol
tetrachlorethylene	Didakene, Miranon, Nema, Terit, Tetracap
	In: Askis-E, Neobedermin
tetrachlorodifluoroethane	Freon 112, Troyfon
tetramisole	Anthelvet, Ascaridil, Citarin, Nemicide, Ripercol, Spartakon
thenium	Bancaris, Canopar
	In: Ancaris, Thenatol
thiabendazole	Bovizole, Coglazol, Equizole, Helmintazole, Hyozole, Mintezole, Nemapan, Omnizole, Polival, Soldrin, TBZ, Thibenzole
	In: Equizole A, Equizole B, Ranizole, Suiverm, Thiprazole, Tresaderm, Tricocefal
thiacetarsamide	Arsphenamide, Caparside, Caparsolate, Filaramide, Filicide
thiophanate	Helminate, Nemafax
	In: Flukembin, Vermadax
tin compounds	Cestodin
	In: Laparin, Stannotaen
toluene	Methacide
	In: Anaplex, Difolin, Paracide, Teniazine, Vermiplex
trichlorphon	Anthon, Bilarcil, Combot, Dipterex, Difrifon, Dylox, Dyrex, Mastotem, Neguvon, Tugon
	In: Bubulin, Combotel, Dyrex T.F., Equizole, Neguvon A, Telmin B
triclabendazole	Fasinex
uredofos	Sansalid

PART III: AGENTS ACTIVE AGAINST ARTHROPOD PARASITES

Generic names	Proprietary names
allethrin	Felethrin, Pynamin, Pyresyn
	In: Alleviate, Aparasit koncentrat, Matas sproejtemiddel, mod lopper, Lop-A′ utoejsspray, Mycodex, Spectro-CF and -F
amitraz	Azadiene, BAAM, Mitaban, Mitac, Mitex, Taktic
arsenic trioxide	
benzyl benzoate	Ascabin, Ascabiol, Benylate, Demodek, NBIN, Scabana, Temedex, Tenutex, Vanzoate, Venzonate
bromocyclen	Alugan Concentre
bromophos	Bromex, Nexagan, Nexion, formerly Brophene

Generic names	Proprietary names
carbaryl, + pyrethrins, rotenone, synergists	Arylam, Carbamine, Carylderm, Cekubaryl, Denapon, Derasect, Devicarb, Dicarbam, Diryl, E-Z Dip, F-L-T Bomb or Powder, Hexavin, Karbaspray, Mycodex, Nac, Norsect, Para, Paradip, Para-Go, Para S-1, Pet Spray, Ravyon, Sect-A-Spray, Seffein, Septene, Sevin, Spectro-Spray, Tercyl, Tricarnam, Vet Kem
carbon disulfide	*In:* Parvex, Parvex Plus
carbophenothion	Dagadip, Garrathion, Trithion (Endyl and Lethox, discontinued)
chlorfenvinphos (clofenvinfos)	Apachlor, CVP, Dermaton, Marmaduke Spray or Dip, Sapecron, Secta-A-Chlor, Steladone, Supona, Vinylphate (Unitax, discontinued)
chlorophenothane	*see* DDT
chlorpyrifos	Brodan, Dursban, Eradex, Liqui-Ban, Lorsban, Pyrinex, Sect-A-Chlor
	In: Siphotrol Plus II
closantel	*See* Anthelmintics
coumaphos (coumafos)	Diolice, Resitox, Umbethion (*see* Anthelmintics)
	In: Negasunt
crotamiton	Crotamitex, Euraxil, Veteusan
	In: Eurax
crotoxyphos (crotoxyfos)	Ciodrin, Cio-Rid, Cypona E.C., Decrotox, Duo-Kill, Duravos, Rycovet
	In: Ciovap
crufomate	Montrel, Ruelene, Rulex
cyhalothrin	Grenade
cypermethrin	Amino, Avicade, Barricade, Flectron, Imperator, Parasol, Ripcord, Rycopel, Rycovet Ovipur, Siperin, Stockade, Topclip
cypothrin	
cythioate	Cyflee, Proban
DDT	Agritan, Anofex, Arkotine, Dedelo, Didimac, Digmar, Genitox, Gesapan, Gyron, Hildit, Ixodex, Kopsol, Neocid, Pentachlorin, Rukseam, Zerdane, *see* chlorophenothane
	In: Tenufex, MBIN
deltamethrin	Butoflin, Butox, Decis, K-Orthrin (previously decamethrin), Sput-Op, Sputop-S
diazinon	Absolut D, Demodin, Escort Plus, Fly-Toxol, Knox out, Neocidal, Parasitox, Penngar, Turboblan
dichlofenthion	Bromex, Nemacide
dichlorovos	Apavap, Astrobot, Canogard, Cekusan, Cypona, Devikol, Divipan, Duo-Kill, Duravos, Estrosol, Fly-Die, Fly Fighter, Herkol, Mafu, Marvex, No-Pest, Nuvan, Oko, Phosvit, Tetravos, Vapona, Vaponite, Vapora II, Verdican, Verdipor, Verdisol (*see* Anthelmintics)
	In: Ciovap, Vet-Fog, Zeprox
N,N-diethyl-*m*-toluamide	Autan, DEET, Detamide, Dieltamid, Flypel, M-Det, m-DETA, Metadelphene, Off, Repel
diflubenzuron	Astonex, Dimilin

(continued)

Generic names	Proprietary names
dimethoate	Cekuthoate, Cygon, Daphene, De-Fend, Demos-L40, Devigon, Dimate, Dimethogen, Fostion MM, Perfekthion, Rebelate, Rogodial, Trimetion
dimethyl phthalate	Avolin, DMP, Fermine, Mipax, Palatinol M, Ritamide
dioxathion	Co-Nav, Delnav, Deltic, Diveley, Hercules 528, Kemtox, Lohr, Speck
diphenylamine	Big Dipper, DPA, Scaldip
disulfiram	*In:* Tenutex
endosulfan	
ethion	
famphur (famophos)	Bo-Ana, Dovip, Famfos, Grub-Kil, Warbex
fenitrothion	AA-spray, Nuvanol, Nuvan Top, Sumithion
	In: Stallfly Permanent
fenthion	Baycid, Baytex, Entex, Grub-Louse, Lebaycid, Lysoff, Mercaptophos, Queletox, Spotton, Talodex, Tiguvon
fenvalerate	Ectrin, Sanmarton, Sumifly, Sumipower, Tirade
flucythrinate	Guardian
flumethrin	
fospirate	Torelle
iodofenphos	Alfacron, Nuvanol N
isobornylthiocyanato acetate	
ivermectin	(*see* Anthelmintics)
lime sulfurated	Vleminckx's solution
D-limonene	Organic Formula Flea and Tick
lindane in combination (γ-benzene hexachloride)	Agrox 3-Way, Aparsin, Aphtiria, Benzyl Benzoate with Lindane, γ-BHC, Carnick, Cooper's Lice and Mange Liquid, Cooper's Louse Powder, Cooper's Skin Dressing, Demsardex, Duo-Tox, Exagama, Fenatox, Forlin, Framomycin, Galogama, Gamaphex, Gamatin, Gamene, Gamiso, Gamma-col, Gammalin, Gammexane, Gammex, Gammophele, Gexane, Granol, Hexicid, Hog Mange Powder, Inexit, Isotox, Jacutin, Kil-A-Mite, Kwell, Lacco Hi Lin, Lindafor, Lindagam, Lindagrain, Lindagranox, Lindalo, Lindamul, Lindapoudre, Lindatox, Linspray, Lindaterra, Lintox, Lorexane, Louse and Insect Powder, Mycodex Shampoo with Lindane, Myzin, Novigam, Parasitic, Quelada, Reed, Rigo Lindane Concentrate, Rycovet Louse, Scabisan, Sectilin Shampoo, Silvanol, Skin-Dressing No. 2, Streunex, SW-T Bomb, Temedex, Theradex with Lindane, Thionium Shampoo with Lindane, Tri-6, Viton
malathion	Calmathion, Celthion, Cython, Detmol MA 96%, Emmatos, Emmatos Extra, Flea Off, For-Mal, Fyfanon, Hilthion, Karbofos, Kop-Thion, Kypfos, Malaspray, Malamar, Malaphele, Malathion ULV Concentrate, Malatol, Malmed, Maltox, MLT, Priorderm, Sumitox, Vegfru Malatox, Zithiol
	In: Kemal, Kill-A-Mite, Lindox M, Para Bomb-M-1, Pet Pest Spray, Vet-Kem Dairy and Livestock Dust

Generic names	Proprietary names
methomyl	Lannate, Nu-Bait II, Nudrin
methoprene	Altosid, Aparasit pre-lop spray, Precor, Siphotrol 10
	In: Siphotrol Plus with Precor or Plus II
methoxychlor	Atex, Blitz-Stop, Lintox, Marlate, Reina-Vloeibar, Sixanol, Veecide
	In: Para S-1 Aerosol, Alfa-tox, Double-M
monosulfiram	Parasitex
naled	Bromex, Dibex, Dibrom, Ortho-Dibrom
nicotine	
nifluridide	
N-octyl bicycloheptene dicarboximide	*In:* Pyrocide, Pestrin
permethrin	Atroban, Ectiban, Expar, Indothrin, Kafil, Outflank, Permasect, Perthrine, Pulvex, Stomoxin, Talcord, Wellcare
	In: Aparasit koncentrat, Matas sproejtemiddel mod lopper, Lop-A'utoejsspray, Siphotrol Plus with Precor
phenothiazine	AFI-Tiazin, Antiverm, Biverm, Fenoverm, Fentiazin, Lethelmin, Nemazine, Orimon, Padaphene, Phenegic, Phenoverm, Reconox, Souframine (*see* Anthelmintics)
	In: Parvex Plus
phenothrin	Shelltox, Sumithrin
phosalone	
phosmet	Appa, Cooper Warble Fly Liquid, Dermol, Escort, Imidan, O-bisect, Kemolate, Nupov, Paramite, Porect, Profacte, Prolate, Rycovet
phoxim	Baythion, Sebacil
piperazine	*See* Anthelmintics
	In: Parvex, Parvex Plus
piperonyl butoxide	Butacide, Prentox Piperonyl Butoxide Tech.
	In: Alleviate, Many pyrethrum and rotenone combinations
promacyl	
propetamphos	Blotic, Safrotin
	In: Prodip
propoxur	Baygon, Bifex, Blattanex, Bolfo, Breakaway, Invisi-Gard, Pestisol-R, Pro Dip 50, Propyon, Sendran, Sprecto, Suncide, Tugon Fliegenkugel, Unden, Zodiac Tick Collar
	In: Negasunt, Pestisol-R, Prentox Carbamate Concentrate
pyrethrins or pyrethrins +	Aurimite, Buzzoff, Caniderm, Cerumite, Controller Flea-Kill, D-Flea, Diryl, Feliderm, Flair, Fleatol, F.L.T. Powder, Fleaban, Flick, Hava-cide, Heathcliff's Flea and Tick Spray for Cats, K.F.L. Shampoo, L-Ban, Liqua-sect, Liquidate, Mycodex, Novalcide, Paladin, Para Bomb-M, Para-Go, Para S-1, Pestisol-R, Pet Pest Spray, Pro-Kill, Pyrenone, Pyresept Shampoo, Pyrinate, Rid, Sebbatix, Sectrol, Sect-A-Spray, Spectro, Theradex, Thera-Groom, Tick Kill, Trisect, Vet-Kem Pet Spray, Zero-Mite
rafoxanide	*See* Anthelmintics
	In: New Duospec
repellents	MGK Repellent II, MGK Repellent 874, MGK Repellent 326, MGK Repellent 264

(*continued*)

Generic names	Proprietary names
resmethrin	Benzofuroline, Chryson, Durakyl, Premgard, Pyretherm, Synthrin *In:* Tetralate, Pynosect
ronnel (fenchlorphos)	Catron, Ectoral, Etrolene, Nankor, Rid-Ezy, Ron-245, Trolene, Viozene *In:* Golden Decoy
rotenone + synergists	Benzylhex, Canex, Canolene, Derris, Derrisic, Goodwinol, Mitone, Motax, Nicouline, Parago, Pro-Kill, Prentox, Tubatoxin, Skin Dressing No. 1
sodium arsenite	Chem Pels C, Chem-Sen 56, Kill-All, Penite, Prodalumnol Double
sodium fluoride	Chemifluor, Florocid, Flura-Drops, Karidium, Lemoflur, Luride-SF, Ossalin, Ossin, Villiaumite, Zymafluor
squalene and piperonyl butoxide	Cerumite
stirofos (tetrachlorvinphos)	Appex, CVMP, Debantic, Dietreen, Dust M, Gardcide, Gardona, Rabon, Rabond, ROL, Unipet *In:* Ravap, Tetravos
sulfur (lime)	Orthorix, Sebbafon, Sebtar, Skin Dressing No. 3, Sultex
temefos (temephos)	Abate, Abathion, Biothin, Difenthos, Ecopro, Nimitox
tetraethyl thiuram monosulphide	Tetmosol
thiabendazole	*See* Anthelmintics
toxaphene	Allotox, Cooper-Tox, Geniphene, Motox, Phenacide, Phenatox, Penphene, Strobane-T, Toxakil, Toxon, Vertac Toxaphene
trichlorfon (metrifonate)	Bovinox, Briten, Casect, Cekufon, Ciclosom, Combot Equine, Crinex, Danex, Equino-Aid, Grub and Louse Pour-on, Leivasom, Proxol, Trinex (*see* Anthelmintics)
(2)-9-tricosene	Muscalure
triphenyl tin	Batasan, Brestan, Dunter, Phentinoacetate, Suzu, Tinestan, TPTA

Index

This Index includes all generic drug names listed in the Appendix or mentioned in the main text. Trade names are included only if mentioned in the text.